Hemato-Oncology with Case Studies

Hemato-Oncology with Case Studies

Editor: Elliot King

AMERICAN
MEDICAL PUBLISHERS
www.americanmedicalpublishers.com

AMERICAN
MEDICAL PUBLISHERS
www.americanmedicalpublishers.com

Cataloging-in-Publication Data

Hemato-oncology with case studies / edited by Elliot King.
p. cm.
Includes bibliographical references and index.
ISBN 979-8-88740-643-5
1. Hematological oncology. 2. Lymphoproliferative disorders. 3. Blood--Cancer.
4. Oncology. I. King, Elliot.
RC280.H47 H46 2023
616.994 18--dc21

American Medical Publishers,
41 Flatbush Avenue,
1st Floor, New York,
NY 11217, USA

ISBN 979-8-88740-643-5 (Hardback)

Contents

Preface

The purpose of the book is to provide a glimpse into the dynamics and to present opinions and studies of some of the scientists engaged in the development of new ideas in the field from very different standpoints. This book will prove useful to students and researchers owing to its high content quality.

Hemato-oncology, also known as hematologic oncology, is a medical specialty that focuses on the diagnosis, treatment, and management of cancers affecting the blood, bone marrow, and lymphatic system. It is an interdisciplinary field that combines aspects of hematology (the study of blood disorders) and oncology (the study of cancer). Hemato-oncology deals with hematologic malignancies, which include various types of leukemia, lymphoma and myeloma. Some of the major aspects of hemato-oncology are diagnosis, chemotherapy and stem cell transplantation. There are numerous procedures which are used for the diagnosis of blood related cancers such as bone marrow biopsies, blood tests, genetic testing, imaging studies, and lymph node biopsies. They can be treated through chemotherapy, radiation therapy, targeted therapy, immunotherapy, bone marrow transplantation, or a combination of these approaches. This book includes some of the vital pieces of works being conducted across the world, on various topics related to hemato-oncology. It will also provide interesting topics for research which interested readers can take up. The book will serve as a valuable source of reference for graduate and postgraduate students.

At the end, I would like to appreciate all the efforts made by the authors in completing their chapters professionally. I express my deepest gratitude to all of them for contributing to this book by sharing their valuable works. A special thanks to my family and friends for their constant support in this journey.

Editor

1

Alectinib Monotherapy in Isolated Central Nervous System Relapse of ALK-Positive Anaplastic Large Cell Lymphoma

Julian Verran and Vidya Mathavan

Department of Haematology, Waikato Hospital, 183 Pembroke Street, Hamilton 3204, New Zealand

Correspondence should be addressed to Vidya Mathavan; vidya.mathavan@waikatodhb.health.nz

Academic Editor: Kostas Konstantopoulos

Anaplastic lymphoma kinase-positive anaplastic large cell lymphoma (ALK-positive ALCL) is an aggressive form of peripheral T cell lymphoma (PTCL), harbouring an underlying pathogenic ALK fusion gene that produces a constitutively activated tyrosine kinase. The ALK tyrosine kinase provides a targeted treatment option in the form of ALK inhibitors. ALK-positive ALCL may rarely involve the central nervous system (CNS), either at presentation or on relapse of disease. The outcomes of CNS relapse in PTCL are historically extremely poor. We present a case of a 20-year-old man diagnosed with stage IVB ALK-positive ALCL. He responded favourably to six cycles of cyclophosphamide, doxorubicin, vincristine, etoposide, and prednisone (CHOEP). He unfortunately relapsed with isolated CNS involvement only 3 weeks after completing his sixth cycle of CHOEP chemotherapy. The CNS-penetrating ALK inhibitor alectinib was identified as a targeted treatment option, as he was not a candidate for CNS-penetrating chemotherapy due to significant iatrogenic renal impairment. After commencing alectinib monotherapy, he rapidly achieved a clinical and radiological response. He has now remained in a durable remission for more than two years on alectinib monotherapy.

1. Introduction

ALCL is an aggressive form of PTCL. It is characterised morphologically by the presence of large anaplastic cells that express CD30. ALCL can be categorised into two distinct entities based on the presence or absence of a rearrangement in the ALK gene. The majority of cases of ALCL (up to 80%) harbour a rearrangement in the ALK gene located on chromosome 2p23 [1] that leads to the formation of a pathogenic fusion gene that produces a constitutively activated tyrosine kinase, promoting cell growth and inhibiting apoptosis [1, 2]. The most common ALK translocation partner is the nucleophosmin (NPM) gene on chromosome 5q35, forming the NPM-ALK fusion gene [1]; other ALK translocation partners have also been identified. The presence of an ALK rearrangement in ALCL infers a better prognosis compared with ALK-negative ALCL.

ALK-positive ALCL can rarely relapse in the CNS, and this is historically associated with survival measured in short months. There is no standard treatment approach to CNS relapse of ALK-positive ALCL; however, the development of targeted treatment in the form of CNS-penetrating ALK inhibitors provides some hope. Alectinib is a CNS-penetrating, second-generation, oral ALK tyrosine kinase inhibitor used successfully to treat ALK-positive non-small cell lung cancer with CNS involvement [3]. To our knowledge, there have only been two published case reports of the use of alectinib monotherapy in patients with CNS involvement of ALK-positive ALCL [4, 5].

2. Case Presentation

A 20-year-old male presented to the emergency department with a one-month history of recurrent fevers, night sweats, pleuritic chest pain, and progressive multifocal lymphadenopathy. Routine blood tests revealed leuconeutrophilia, cholestatic derangement of liver enzymes, and elevated lactate dehydrogenase and C-reactive protein. He was commenced on antibiotics, and an infectious screen was performed. Chest X-ray revealed a widened superior mediastinum and prominent right hilum, suspicious for lymphadenopathy, along with a right-sided pleural effusion. Computed tomography (CT) scan confirmed mediastinal, hilar, and retroperitoneal lymphadenopathy with splenomegaly. It also demonstrated extranodal involvement in the form of pulmonary nodules and pleural enhancement with an associated right-sided effusion. A pleural fluid aspirate was obtained, along with a fine needle aspirate via endobronchial ultrasound; however, both were inconclusive. An open biopsy of a right neck nodal mass was then performed under general anaesthesia.

The histology showed sheets of intermediate-sized abnormal lymphoid cells with abundant cytoplasm and irregular nuclear membranes. The abnormal lymphocytes expressed CD30, BCL2, and EMA by immunohistochemistry (IHC) and had patchy expression of CD3. The cells also had strong nuclear expression of ALKp80 by IHC. The cells did not express CD10 or CD20. The morphological and immune-histochemical features of the biopsy were consistent with ALK-positive ALCL. Dedicated fluorescence in situ hybridisation studies for ALK gene rearrangement was not performed due to the strong IHC positivity. Additional workup included a bone marrow biopsy that was negative for lymphoma involvement. An upfront lumbar puncture was not performed. The patient was diagnosed with stage IVB ALK-positive ALCL, and the disease was classified as high-risk based on his international prognostic index score of 4 (>1 extranodal site, advanced stage, elevated LDH, and performance score on admission of 2).

The patient was commenced on high-dose prephase prednisone 80 mg daily for 3 days followed by CHOEP-14 systemic chemotherapy (cyclophosphamide 750 mg/m^2, doxorubicin 50 mg/m^2, vincristine 1.4 mg/m^2 (capped at 2 mg), etoposide 100 mg/m^2 on days 1–3 (days 2-3 given orally), and prednisone 100 mg/day days 1–5, with PEG-filgrastim support). He was planned for six cycles of CHOEP-14 and was not planned for upfront CNS prophylaxis.

The patient had a rapid clinical improvement on systemic chemotherapy. An interim CT scan performed after 3 cycles of chemotherapy confirmed a complete response with resolution of his lymphadenopathy and splenomegaly.

Three weeks after completing his 6th cycle of CHOEP systemic chemotherapy, the patient represented acutely to the emergency department with a 2 week history of fevers and severe headaches that were associated with vomiting and photophobia. An urgent CT brain with contrast revealed mild right parietal leptomeningeal enhancement. The CT scan was followed by dedicated magnetic resonance imaging (MRI) of his brain. The MRI demonstrated an abnormal 3.4 cm lesion with high T2 signal change in the right parietal cortex, along with associated leptomeningeal enhancement (Figure 1). A lumbar puncture was performed, and the CSF demonstrated large numbers of abnormal lymphocytes (Figure 2) that expressed CD30 by flow cytometry. They also had variable expression of CD7, coexpressed CD4/8, had reduced expression of CD3, and were negative for CD5. Dexamethasone was commenced. A CT of his neck, chest, abdomen, and pelvis excluded systemic relapse of disease, and the patient was confirmed as having an isolated CNS relapse of his ALK-positive ALCL.

The patient was commenced on salvage chemotherapy two days later as per the protocol developed by Korfel et al. [6] for CNS relapse of aggressive lymphomas (methotrexate 4 g/m^2 intravenously (IV) day 1, ifosfamide 2 g/m^2 IV days 3–5, and oral dexamethasone 4 mg bd on days 6–10. This induction course is repeated on day 22 in those patients without clinical progression) with a plan to proceed to autologous stem cell transplant. The salvage chemotherapy was to be administered along with concurrent twice weekly intrathecal (IT) chemotherapy (alternating IT methotrexate 12.5 mg and IT cytarabine 50 mg) for 2 weeks.

Two days into his salvage treatment, the patient developed an iatrogenic acute kidney injury following the administration of high-dose IV methotrexate, delaying the ifosfamide by several days. After review of the clinical situation, a decision was made to suspend the salvage chemotherapy and trial compassionate access alectinib (600 mg bd), a second-generation ALK inhibitor with good CNS penetration. Importantly, at the time of commencing alectinib monotherapy, the patient's CSF was still positive for disease by flow cytometry.

The patient's symptoms quickly resolved on the alectinib monotherapy, and multiple further CSF analyses were clear of lymphoma cells. A follow-up MRI brain 3 months after commencing alectinib confirmed that the patient was in complete radiological remission (Figure 1). The patient has had no recognised adverse effects to alectinib.

At a routine outpatient clinic appointment 12 months after commencing alectinib, the patient complained of intermittent headaches for the preceding 3 weeks. A repeat MRI brain and CSF analysis confirmed ongoing remission. The patient remains well on alectinib monotherapy, more than two years following his CNS relapse.

3. Discussion

We present a rare case of isolated CNS relapse of ALK-positive ALCL in a patient who had initially responded well to CHOEP systemic chemotherapy. CNS involvement of PTCL and ALK-positive ALCL is rare, with estimates between 2% and 6% [7, 8]. A Swedish population-based study found that 4.5% of patients (28/625) with PTCL had CNS relapse of disease [8]. Of the patients in the study with ALK-positive ALCL, 6% (3/48) experienced CNS relapse.

The outcomes of CNS relapse in PTCL are historically extremely poor, with survival estimates between 1 and 7 months [7]. The only risk factor for CNS involvement consistently identified in the limited studies available is ≥2 extranodal sites of disease [7–9]. ALK-positive ALCL with ≥2 extranodal sites of disease is considered high-risk for early CNS relapse [7]. Chihara et al. performed a retrospective analysis of CNS risk by PTCL subtype in 616 patients. They identified 18 patients that had both ALK-positive ALCL and ≥2 extranodal sites of disease. 4 of these 18 patients had CNS relapse, giving a one-year CNS relapse risk of 15% [7]. This in hindsight suggests that our patient should have had upfront CNS analysis and CNS prophylaxis therapy due to the lung and pleural involvement.

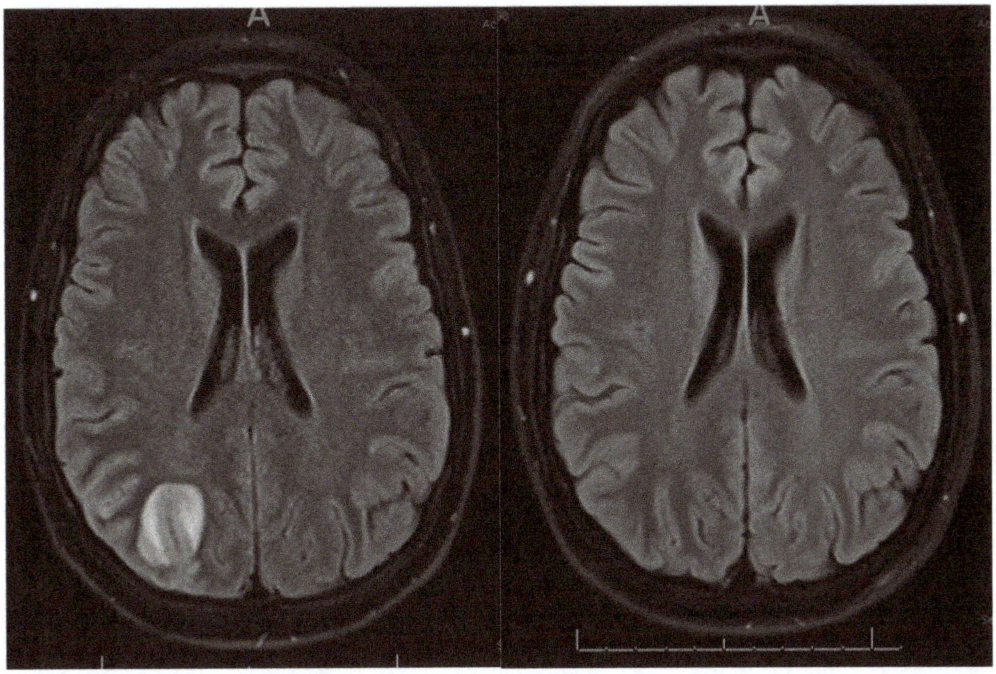

FIGURE 1: MRI brain at time of relapse (August 2019), on the left, demonstrating a 3.4 cm enhancing lesion within the parietal region with associated leptomeningeal enhancement. On the right, a repeat MRI brain (January 2020) after 3 months on alectinib monotherapy showing resolution of lesion and leptomeningeal enhancement.

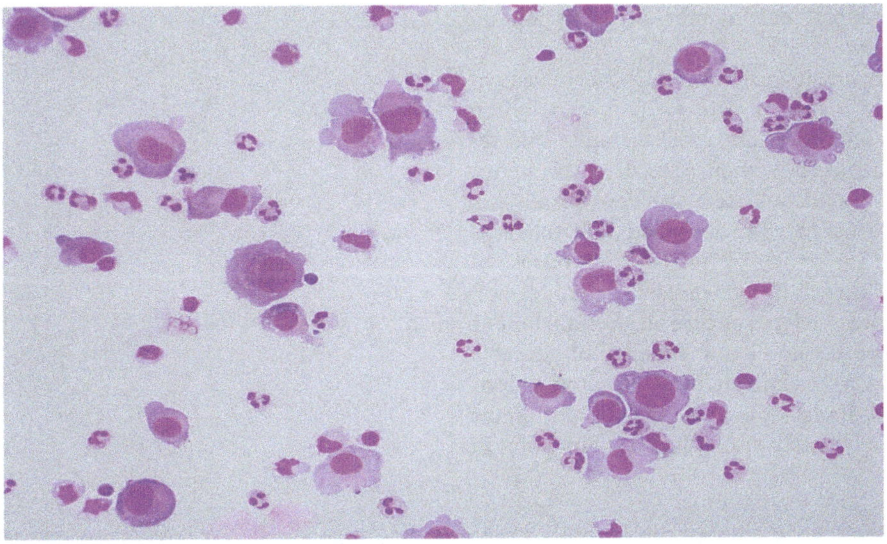

FIGURE 2: Cerebrospinal fluid analysis at time of isolated CNS relapse in August 2019 showing diffuse involvement by lymphoma cells.

When CNS relapse does occur in ALK-positive ALCL, there is no standard salvage approach. Given this lack of standard approach, we had initially planned to use a CNS-penetrating chemotherapy protocol developed by Korfel et al. [6], followed by a consolidative autologous stem cell transplant (ASCT). This protocol has shown reasonable results in treating CNS relapse of aggressive lymphomas with a 2-year OS of 63% for all patients and 68% for those completing an ASCT [6]. Of the patients included in the study, 10% (3/30) were PTCLs. Unfortunately, the development of an iatrogenic kidney injury in our patient precluded us completing the protocol.

Two potential targets for novel treatment in ALK-positive ALCL is the CD30 antigen and ALK tyrosine kinase. Brentuximab vedotin is used in relapsed/refractory systemic ALCL; however, there is no evidence to suggest it can penetrate the blood-brain barrier [10]. The constitutively activated ALK tyrosine kinase in ALK-positive ALCL was a logical alternative target, using the second-generation, CNS-penetrating, ALK tyrosine kinase inhibitor alectinib. Alectinib has demonstrated good efficacy in patients with CNS involvement of ALK-positive non-small cell lung cancer by averting the progression of baseline CNS metastases and preventing the development of new CNS lesions [3]. We were able to obtain alectinib on a compassionate access scheme for our patient.

To our knowledge, this is the third case report of a patient treated with alectinib monotherapy for CNS involvement of ALK-positive ALCL. In the first case, Reed et al. [5] presented a patient who had CNS involvement at presentation and was treated with CHOEP systemic chemotherapy and high-dose methotrexate (HD-MTX) for CNS involvement. The patient experienced disease progression whilst on this regimen and was subsequently commenced on alectinib. The patient completed 6 months of alectinib monotherapy, with imaging and CSF analysis showing complete response. The patient proceeded to a matched unrelated donor allogeneic stem cell transplant (allo-SCT), with the alectinib being discontinued at day of conditioning. The patient quickly relapsed on day 30 post-transplant. The patient was recommenced on alectinib with a quick clinical response.

In the second case, Tomlinson et al. [4] presented a patient that relapsed with cerebellar involvement of ALK-positive ALCL soon after completing systemic treatment with CHOEP chemotherapy. The patient completed 2 cycles of HD-MTX followed by alectinib monotherapy. Follow-up MRI confirmed radiological remission. The patient was planned for an allo-SCT and, however, had infectious complications that precluded this. At the time of publishing, the patient had endured >12 months of remission on alectinib monotherapy.

In summary, our patient with isolated CNS involvement of ALK-positive ALCL has to date (>24 months) been successfully treated with alectinib monotherapy. This remission has been achieved without concurrent systemic chemotherapy or consolidative stem cell transplantation. Alectinib appears to be an efficacious and well tolerated treatment option, in the setting of isolated CNS relapse of ALK-positive ALCL. There is no evidence base to guide us on long-term probabilities of relapse or cure on alectinib for our patient. We therefore do not know whether his durable remission should now be consolidated with an autologous or allogeneic stem cell transplant. We also do not know whether alectinib can be safely discontinued at any point in the future.

References

[1] G. Hapgood and K. J. Savage, "The biology and management of systemic anaplastic large cell lymphoma," *Blood*, vol. 126, no. 1, pp. 17–25, 2015.

[2] A. S. Freedman and J. C. Aster, *Clinical Manifestations, Pathologic Features, and Diagnosis of Systemic Anaplastic Large Cell Lymphoma*, UpToDate, Waltham, MA, USA, 2020.

[3] M. Nishio, K. Nakagawa, T. Mitsudomi et al., "Analysis of central nervous system efficacy in the J-ALEX study of alectinib versus crizotinib in ALK-positive non-small-cell lung cancer," *Lung Cancer*, vol. 121, pp. 37–40, 2018.

[4] S. B. Tomlinson, S. Sandwell, S. T. Chuang, M. D. Johnson, G. E. Vates, and P. M. Reagan, "Central nervous system relapse of systemic ALK-rearranged anaplastic large cell lymphoma treated with alectinib," *Leukemia Research*, vol. 83, Article ID 106164, 2019.

[5] D. R. Reed, R. D. Hall, R. D. Gentzler, L. Volodin, M. G. Douvas, and C. A. Portell, "Treatment of refractory ALK rearranged anaplastic large cell lymphoma with alectinib," *Clinical Lymphoma, Myeloma & Leukemia*, vol. 19, no. 6, pp. e247–e250, 2019.

[6] A. Korfel, T. Elter, E. Thiel et al., "Phase II study of central nervous system (CNS)-directed chemotherapy including high-dose chemotherapy with autologous stem cell transplantation for CNS relapse of aggressive lymphomas," *Haematologica*, vol. 98, no. 3, pp. 364–370, 2013.

[7] D. Chihara, M. A. Fanale, and R. N. Miranda, "The risk of central nervous system (CNS) relapses in patients with peripheral T-cell lymphoma," *PLoS One*, vol. 13, no. 3, pp. 1–9, 2018.

[8] F. Ellin, J. Landström, M. Jerkeman, and T. Relander, "Central nervous system relapse in peripheral T-cell lymphomas: a Swedish lymphoma registry study," *Blood*, vol. 126, no. 1, pp. 36–41, 2015.

[9] C. K. Chin and C. Y. Cheah, "How I treat patients with aggressive lymphoma at high risk of CNS relapse," *Blood*, vol. 130, no. 7, pp. 867–874, 2017.

[10] Y. Kim, A. Sudo, R. Oyama et al., "Isolated central nervous system progression during systemic treatment with brentuximab vedotin monotherapy in a pediatric patient with recurrent ALK-negative anaplastic large cell lymphoma," *Journal of Pediatric Hematology*, vol. 43, no. 6, pp. e864–e866, 2020.

2

Surgery in a Patient with Haemophilia A and Lymphoma

M. S. Cruz, J. Santillan, J. Lesser, J. Ortiz, L. Forzani, and P. Plaza

Fundación de la Hemofilia de Salta, Salta, Argentina

Correspondence should be addressed to M. S. Cruz; mariasolcruz@hotmail.com

Academic Editor: Masayuki Nagasawa

An increased incidence of haematologic malignancies and other cancer types among patients with haemophilia compared with matched controls has been reported in several longitudinal studies. Tumours initially misdiagnosed as haematomas and conversely haematomas mistaken for tumours have been reported. Here, we describe the case of a 43-year-old man with severe haemophilia A and a diffuse large B-cell lymphoma, originally diagnosed as a haematoma, who underwent a splenectomy and several associated surgeries as part of his lymphoma treatment. Perioperative treatment with octanate® (human coagulation factor VIII) enabled the successful performance of all surgical interventions required in the context of lymphoma treatment. Nevertheless, differential diagnosis of posttraumatic haematoma in patients with haemophilia should include the consideration of malignancy.

1. Introduction

Haemophilia A (HA) is an X-linked bleeding disorder that affects approximately 1 in 5000 male births [1]. It is characterised by spontaneous bleeding, mostly into muscles and joints. Severe bleeding episodes can be life-threatening [2], and repetitive bleeding into joints typically leads to irreversible joint damage and considerable morbidity (haemarthropathy) [3]. It is therefore important to prevent, or at least control, bleeding as effectively as possible. The standard of treatment for HA is administration of plasma-derived (pdFVIII) or recombinant coagulation factor VIII (rFVIII), either on-demand or prophylactically. For HA patients undergoing surgical procedures, maintaining adequate FVIII levels during and after the procedure is a crucial aspect of surgical management [2].

Here, we describe the case of a 43-year-old man with severe HA and a diffuse large B-cell lymphoma who underwent a splenectomy and several associated surgeries as part of his lymphoma treatment. All surgical procedures were successfully performed under FVIII cover.

2. Case Summary

A 43-year-old man with known HA presented with recurring back pain. He had been initially diagnosed with severe HA at 8 months of age and had received on-demand treatment with cryoprecipitate and transfusions until the age of 5 years and subsequently with pdFVIII. At age 6, he started intermittent prophylactic treatment using various pdFVIII concentrates at a dose of 25 international units (IU)/kg 3 times weekly. In the 1990s, the patient contracted hepatitis B and C as a result of treatment with a contaminated batch of Immunate®. For hepatitis C, a viral load of 2.3×10^6 was determined, and the virus strain was characterised as genotype 1, subtype 1b.

Prophylactic treatment was stopped at age 22, and the patient returned to on-demand treatment with various pdFVIII concentrates, depending on availability and product price—mostly Hemofil®, Immunate®, octanate®, and Beriate®—until age 34. The patient experienced approximately four joint bleeds a year on this regimen and developed chronic haemarthrosis in his knees and right elbow as a consequence. Stomach ulcer that occurred during this time, at age 32, was successfully treated with pdFVIII on-demand (Hemofil® 30–50 IU/kg) and a red blood cell transfusion. In 2010, at age 34, contact was established with the Hemophilia Foundation of Salta, Argentina. At age 35, the patient started prophylactic treatment with octanate®, a pdFVIII concentrate stabilised with von Willebrand factor with proven low immunogenicity [4], 25 IU/kg 3 times weekly, and has experienced only two haemarthroses in the right knee in 8 years since then.

In January 2015, at age 38, the patient had a fall, and a splenic haematoma was detected by echography. He received 100 IU/kg of octanate® 3 times weekly for 3 months and was advised to rest. As a second echography in April 2015 showed that the haematoma had decreased in size, the dose was reduced to the usual 25 IU/kg 3 times weekly, and the patient resumed his normal activities, including travelling; however, he experienced recurring back pain. The octanate® dose was again increased to 100 IU/kg 3 times weekly for a month, after which treatment was resumed with the usual 25 IU/kg 3 times weekly.

A physical examination produced no noticeable findings apart from abdominal pain. An echography in August 2015 indicated a re-expansion of the splenic haematoma, and the octanate® dose was again increased to 100 IU/kg 3 times weekly. However, in March 2016, the haematoma enlarged further despite the higher octanate® dose, and the patient reported severe pain. As the imaging results still pointed towards a haematoma of the spleen, which had persisted for 15 months at this point, it was decided to opt for a splenectomy under octanate® cover as the patient was already receiving this product and had generally responded well to treatment. Tests performed in preparation for the surgery showed normal FVIII recovery and no inhibitors to FVIII.

The patient was referred to hospital on 27 March 2016; splenectomy was performed on 1 April 2016 under general anaesthesia. He received perioperative treatment with octanate® consisting of a presurgery loading dose of 37.5 IU/kg and postsurgical cover of 100 IU/kg/day for the first 3 days and 75 IU/kg/day for the next 3 days. Due to decreased haemoglobin levels after surgery, he received a transfusion of one unit of red blood cells.

A biopsy of the excised spleen was performed on 4 April 2016 and revealed a neoplasm that occupied a large part of the splenic parenchyma. Based on histological and immunohistochemical findings, a diagnosis of diffuse large B-cell lymphoma was made.

Invasive surgery was performed on 7 April 2016 to drain the abscess and the haematoma that had formed postsurgery and also because the presence of malign cells at the excision site was suspected. octanate® was administered as a presurgery loading dose of 100 IU/kg and as postoperative treatment (100 IU/kg/day for 2 days and 37.5 IU/kg twice a day for 10 days). The patient was discharged from hospital one week after laparoscopy; ambulatory checkups were done for a week after discharge. Following the postoperative treatment phase, the octanate® dose was reduced to 37.5 IU/kg 3 times weekly.

In addition to the surgery, chemotherapy was planned as part of the lymphoma treatment. In preparation of this, the patient received a 12-week course of oral sofosbuvir and daclatasvir in November 2016 and has been seronegative for hepatitis C since then. In parallel, he started treatment with entecavir for hepatitis B in December 2016 which was continued until December 2017.

In January 2017, a tumour recurrence in the splenectomy bed was detected by ultrasound and tomography. The patient immediately received 8 cycles of chemotherapy with rituximab, cyclophosphamide, doxorubicin, vincristine, and prednisone every three weeks (R-CHOP) between January and June 2017; aciclovir was given as concomitant treatment to prevent viral reactivation. Shrinkage of the abdominal mass was confirmed by computed tomography (CT). A positron emission tomography/CT in August 2017 showed a persisting abdominal mass with a diameter of 57 mm in the left flank, in contact with the abdominal wall. Standardised uptake values suggested infectious or inflammatory changes; however, persistent disease could not be excluded. An exploratory laparotomy for an abdominal wall biopsy was performed in November 2017 with octanate® cover (36 IU/kg before and after the procedure) due to incomplete wound healing from the surgery. Afterwards, the patient returned to prophylaxis at an octanate® dose of 25–30 IU/kg 3 times weekly. The result of the biopsy was negative.

The patient continued to undergo twice yearly checkups to detect possible relapses but did not receive any further lymphoma treatment. He continued prophylactic treatment with octanate®, and analysis using the Web-Accessible Population Pharmacokinetic Service (WAPPS-Hemo; http://www.wapps-hemo.org) and an octanate®-specific population PK model confirmed the appropriateness of his current prophylaxis schedule. Treatment with octanate®, both prophylactic and perioperative, was well-tolerated. A transient low-titre inhibitor (2.3 Bethesda units) was detected in January 2017; however, this was not clinically relevant as the titre had returned to undetectable levels 7 months later, without a change in therapy.

3. Discussion

In this 43-year-old patient with severe HA and a diffuse large B-cell lymphoma, perioperative treatment with octanate® has enabled the successful performance of all surgical interventions required in the context of lymphoma treatment (Figure 1).

A total octanate® dose of 762.5 IU/kg, including a loading dose of 37.5 IU/kg followed by 10 days of postsurgical treatment with a total dose of 725 IU/kg, was planned to cover the splenectomy (the total dose administered was only 562.5 IU/kg because the treatment schedule was interrupted for another surgery). Guidelines for the management of HA recommend preoperative doses of 50–80 IU/kg for minor surgery and 80–100 IU/kg for major surgery. Recommended postprocedure dose for minor surgery is 30–80 IU/kg on postoperative days 1–3 and 60–80, 40–60 and 30–50 IU/kg on postoperative days 1–3, 4–6, and 7–14, respectively, for major surgery [2]. The core SmPC for FVIII products by the European Medicines Agency suggests the use of 30–60 IU/kg every day for a least 1 day for minor surgery and 60–80 IU/kg every 8–24 hours for major surgery until wound healing [5]. Planned dose and duration of treatment for the splenectomy are also in line with surgical procedures (both major and minor) performed under octanate® cover during clinical studies in previously treated patients (PTPs), where the duration of treatment ranged from 1–20 days and the mean dose per exposure day (ED) from 28.6–68.3 IU/kg (Octapharma, data on file). For other pdFVIII products, similar data have been reported: loading

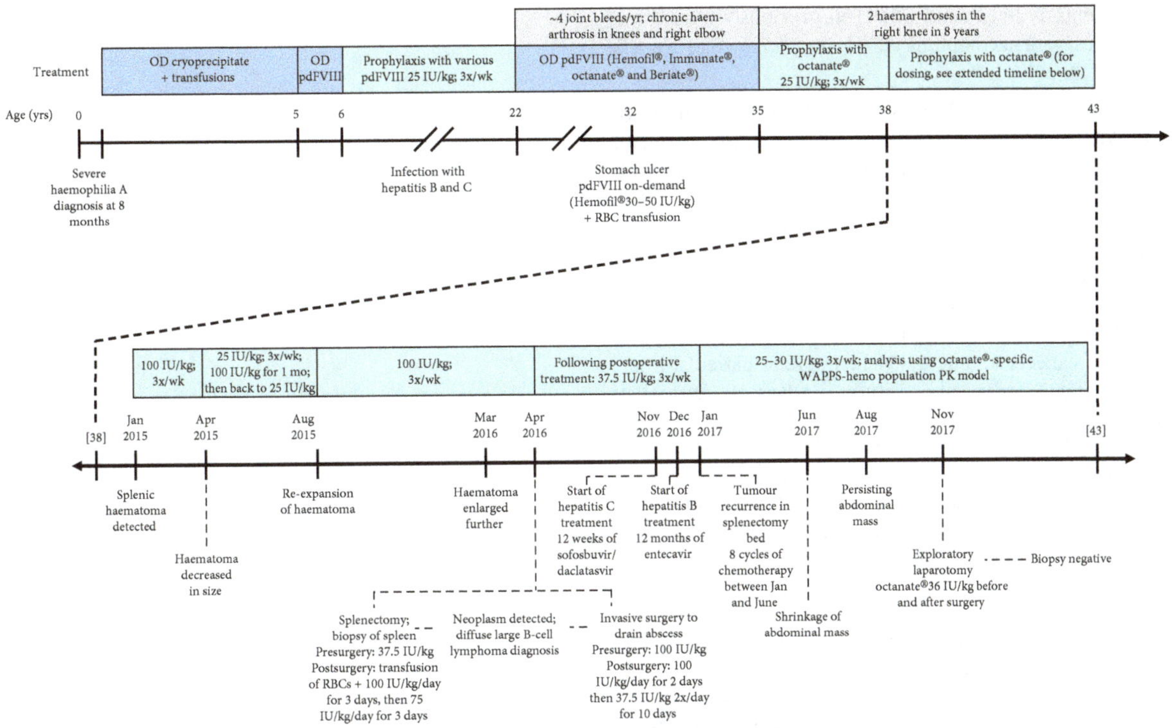

Figure 1: Timeline of key events.

doses ranged from 25–200 IU/kg, mean doses per ED were 50–70 IU/kg, and treatment for up to 10 days was common [6–9].

An increased incidence of haematologic malignancies and other cancer types among patients with haemophilia compared with matched controls has been reported in several longitudinal studies [10, 11]. Close follow-up for malignancies in these patients is therefore recommended [11]. In fact, several cases of haemophilia patients with tumours that were initially thought to be haematoma have been reported [12, 13]. Simple haematomas have also been mistaken for tumours [14–16]; nevertheless, differential diagnosis of posttraumatic haematoma in patients with haemophilia should include the consideration of malignancy [13].

In conclusion, this case report confirms the efficacy and tolerability of octanate® as surgical prophylaxis and provides further evidence showing that adequate FVIII cover enables major surgeries to be performed effectively in patients with severe HA.

Acknowledgments

Medical writing support was provided by nspm ltd., Meggen, Switzerland. Financial support for medical writing services and article processing charges was provided by Octapharma AG, Lachen, Switzerland.

References

[1] P. M. Mannucci and M. Franchini, "Haematology clinic: haemophilia A," *Hematology*, vol. 19, no. 3, pp. 181-182, 2014.

[2] A. Srivastava, A. K. Brewer, E. P. Mauser-Bunschoten et al., "Guidelines for the management of hemophilia," *Haemophilia*, vol. 19, no. 1, pp. e1–e47, 2013.

[3] A. Gringeri, B. Ewenstein, and A. Reininger, "The burden of bleeding in haemophilia: is one bleed too many?" *Haemophilia*, vol. 20, no. 4, pp. 459–463, 2014.

[4] A. Klukowska, V. Komrska, V. Vdovin et al., "Low incidence of factor VIII inhibitors in previously untreated patients with severe haemophilia A treated with octanate®: final report from a prospective study," *Haemophilia*, vol. 24, no. 2, pp. 221–228, 2018.

[5] Committee for Medicinal Products for Human Use (CHMP), *Guideline on Core SmPC for Human Plasma Derived and Recombinant Coagulation Factor VIII Products Rev. 3 (EMA/CHMP/BPWP/1619/1999 rev. 3)*, Committee for Medicinal Products for Human Use (CHMP), London, UK, 2018, https://www.ema.europa.eu/en/documents/scientific-guideline/guideline-core-smpc-human-plasma-derived-recombinant-coagulation-factor-viii-products-revision-3_en.pdf.

[6] V. Jiménez-Yuste, J. Oldenburg, S. Rangarajan, R. Peiró-Jordán, and E. Santagostino, "Long-term outcome of haemophilia A patients after successful immune tolerance induction therapy using a single plasma-derived FVIII/VWF product: the long-term ITI study," *Haemophilia*, vol. 22, no. 6, pp. 859–865, 2016.

[7] D. M. Wolf, R. Rokicka-Milewska, S. Lopaciuk et al., "Clinical efficacy, safety and pharmacokinetic properties of the factor

VIII concentrate haemoctin SDH in previously treated patients with severe haemophilia A," *Haemophilia*, vol. 10, no. 5, pp. 438–448, 2004.

[8] J. S. Powell, M. Bush, J. Harrison et al., "Safety and efficacy of solvent/detergent-treated antihaemophilic factor with an added 80°C terminal dry heat treatment in patients with haemophilia A," *Haemophilia*, vol. 6, no. 3, pp. 140–149, 2000.

[9] E. P. Mauser-Bunschoten, D. Posthouwer, K. Fischer, and H. M. van den Berg, "Safety and efficacy of a plasma-derived monoclonal purified factor VIII concentrate during 10 years of follow-up," *Haemophilia*, vol. 13, no. 6, pp. 697–700, 2007.

[10] Y.-C. Huang, Y.-T. Tsan, W.-C. Chan et al., "Incidence and survival of cancers among 1,054 hemophilia patients: a nationwide and 14-year cohort study," *American Journal of Hematology*, vol. 90, no. 4, pp. E55–E59, 2015.

[11] S. Lövdahl, K. M. Henriksson, F. Baghaei, M. Holmström, E. Berntorp, and J. Astermark, "Malignancies in Swedish persons with haemophilia: a longitudinal registry study," *Blood Coagulation & Fibrinolysis*, vol. 27, no. 6, pp. 631–636, 2016.

[12] Z. Liu, X. Yang, J. Liu, and J. Yang, "FDG PET/CT demonstrated precursor B-cell lymphoblastic lymphoma in a pediatric patient with hemophilia B," *Clinical Nuclear Medicine*, vol. 44, no. 8, pp. 683–685, 2019.

[13] N. Ozdemir, A. Yurt, E. Turkan, and T. Celkan, "Non-Hodgkin's lymphoma in a hemophilic patient with a traumatic hematoma," *Turkish Journal of Hematology*, vol. 28, no. 3, pp. 237-238, 2011.

[14] A. Rath, L. Nakamura, N. van der Werf-Grohmann, and B. Zieger, "Acute "tumour-like" tongue haematoma: the challenge to diagnose haemophilia A," *Klinische Pädiatrie*, vol. 227, no. 6-7, pp. 360–362, 2015.

[15] B. Abuzayed, S. A. Oğuzoğlu, R. Dashti, and E. Ozyurt, "Spinal chronic subdural hematoma mimicking intradural tumor in a patient with history of hemophilia A: case report," *Turkish Neurosurgery*, vol. 19, no. 2, pp. 189–191, 2009.

[16] M. Gothwal, J. Oldenburg, T. Woltering, L. Nakamura, J. Schelling, and B. Zieger, "A bladder hematoma mimicking a tumor in a newborn with severe hemophilia A," *Klinische Pädiatrie*, vol. 227, no. 6-7, pp. 358-359, 2015.

3

Chronic Benign CD8+ Proliferation: A Rare Affection that Can Mimic a Lymphoma Relapse

Marcela Osovská,[1] **Andrea Janíková**,[1] **Leoš Křen**,[2] **and Andrea Marečková**[3]

[1]*Department of Hematology and Oncology, University Hospital Brno, Faculty of Medicine, Masaryk University Brno, Brno, Czech Republic*
[2]*Department of Pathology, University Hospital Brno, Faculty of Medicine, Masaryk University Brno, Brno, Czech Republic*
[3]*Department of Molecular Biology and Genetics, University Hospital Brno, Faculty of Medicine, Masaryk University Brno, Brno, Czech Republic*

Correspondence should be addressed to Marcela Osovská; osovska.marcela@fnbrno.cz

Academic Editor: Tatsuharu Ohno

Chronic benign CD8+ proliferation is a rare syndrome that can take the form of a variety of other diseases. Peripheral adenopathy, cytopenia, and infiltration of the liver, kidneys, bowels, or other organs are the most common clinical presentations of the syndrome. CD8+ expansion can be clonal and nonclonal. It generally occurs in patients with innate or acquired immunodeficiency (HIV+) or in patients receiving immunosuppressive therapy. It has been found repeatedly in patients who developed severe hypogammaglobulinemia after treatment with rituximab. Diagnosis of the disease can be difficult because it can mimic relapse of a lymphoma, and a common biopsy examination cannot identify the problem at first. The authors describe a case of a patient pretreated with rituximab who developed agammaglobulinemia and peripheral adenopathy. Biopsy of an enlarged lymph node showed "reactive lymphadenitis." Additionally, a flow-cytometric examination revealed a pathological population of CD8+ lymphocytes. The treatment, which differed from treatments of lymphoma relapse, consisted of corticosteroids and IVIG substitutions and has led to a regression of clinical symptoms. With more frequent usage of rituximab, one can expect increased occurrence of a very rare CD8+ expansion that can reliably emulate the relapse of a lymphoma.

1. Introduction

Chronic CD8+ T-cell proliferation is a rare heterogeneous group of disorders which is characterized by an increased population of CD8+CD3+ cells in the tissues and organs, morphologically in the form of large granular lymphocytes. The expansion of CD8+ lymphocytes comprises a population of activated cytotoxic T-cells in the final phase of their development and can be of clonal (reactive) or nonclonal origin [1, 2]. The CD8+ expansion was previously documented in conditions connected to immunodeficiency (e.g., in patients with common variable immunodeficiency, in HIV-positive patients, and in patients undergoing immunosuppressive therapy).

CD8+ lymphoproliferation in HIV patients is thought to be a part of the immune system's reaction to HIV (although it is not present in all such patients) and can take two forms: (1) CD8+ lymphocytosis and (2) diffuse infiltrative lymphocytosis syndrome (DILS). DILS is typical of sequestration of CD8+ cells into the salivary glands, lymph nodes, lungs, kidneys, and other organs, displaying a clinical similarity to Sjögren's syndrome [3–6]. Furthermore, in patients with CVID, a cytotoxic T-lymphoproliferation can be sometimes associated with liver impairment reminiscent of a lymphoma (nodular regenerative liver hyperplasia) [7, 8].

Over the past two decades, rituximab has shown good effectiveness in the treatment of B-lymphomas, both as a single agent and in combination with conventional chemotherapy [9–11]. Rituximab is a chimerical monoclonal anti-CD20 antibody, of which the mechanism of the effect in humans is not fully known. The CD20 antigen is expressed on the surface of B-lymphatic cells (excluding lymphoblasts, pre-B-cells, and plasmacytes), both benign and malignant. In nonmalignant cells, the linkage to the CD20 antigen leads to the inhibition of cell activity, proliferation, differentiation, and lowering of immunoglobulin secretion. Compared with chemotherapy, rituximab appears to be practically nontoxic. However, the anti-CD20 antibody has affected the immune system of several patients. In certain cases, especially in repeated doses, it causes clinically apparent immunodeficiency. Infections and neutropenia, usually combined with severe hypogammaglobulinemia, are the most common long-term side effects [12–14].

In the following text, we present a case of the still rather rare chronic CD8+ lymphoproliferation in a patient with follicular lymphoma who had been treated repeatedly with rituximab. Only a few patients worldwide have been reported with a similar diagnosis. The authors assume that, with long-term and massive repeated use of the anti-CD20 antibodies for B-lymphoproliferation treatments, the number of patients with this secondary affection will increase. The diagnosis of the disease can be difficult because it can easily evoke a relapse of the former lymphoma and the development of CD8-lymphoproliferation can occur with a significant delay after the end of immunochemotherapy.

2. Case Report

A 78-year-old female with follicular lymphoma came to the hematology-oncology department for a routine checkup in May 2016. She had been suffering from intermittent fevers, tiredness, significant weight loss, and night sweats for several weeks. She was treated repeatedly with antibiotics with no clinical effect. Up to that point, the patient was still working and was an active woman with no other diseases or chronic medication.

Initially, the patient was diagnosed with a follicular lymphoma (FL) of stage IIIA in 1999 and underwent standard treatment consisting of 6 cycles of CHOP with the achievement of a complete remission. In 2003, the patient developed asymptomatic, low-burden, histology-proven relapse of indolent FL, but therapy was only started in October 2004, when bulky disease and symptoms were revealed. The patient was treated with 6 cycles of R-COPP immunochemotherapy, resulting in a complete remission.

Since 2015, PET/CT had shown mild lymphadenopathy (up to 25×15 mm; SUVmax up to 5.79), but the patient remained asymptomatic and no treatment was administered. In May 2016, the progression of cervical lymphadenopathy and systemic symptoms occurred, accompanied by a significant elevation of the liver enzymes, LDH, and CRP (ALT 6.01 μkat/l, AST 5.96 μkat/l, ALP 22.69 μkat/l, GGT 20.40 μkat/l, LDH 8.19 μkat/l, and CRP 27.6 mg/l). However, lymph biopsy showed no evidence of malignant cells; only reactive inflammatory infiltration with central coliquation was found. The patient's condition was deteriorating rapidly with continuous fevers, and she developed ascites. Serological and PCR tests (CMV, EBV, hepatitis A, B, C, HIV, HHV-8, chlamydia, and mycoplasma) gave negative results. The bone marrow and paracentesis were free of pathology. Flow cytometry identified an elevated count of T-lymphocytes and a nearly zero level of B-lymphocytes concordant with deep hypogammaglobulinemia (IgG < 0.4 g/l, IgA < 0.05 g/l, and IgM = 0.09 g/l). Thorough immunological analysis revealed a significant elevation of CD8+ cells in the blood up to 57% (normal 39%), mildly elevated CD3+ cells; conversely, the population of CD19+ was almost undetectable. The examination of the liver, portal system, and biliary tract by CT and ultrasound showed no pathology.

In conclusion, based on a finding of severe B-lymphocytopenia, agammaglobulinemia, and unusual CD8+ cell population, we assumed that our patient suffered from a rare CD8+ lymphoproliferation. We performed additional special (not routinely performed) staining of bone marrow and lymph node specimens targeted at the CD8+ cells, where an evident clonal CD8+ cell population was found. Corresponding T-cell clonality in the peripheral blood and bone marrow was also confirmed.

There is currently no standard treatment available for this disorder. Based on published case reports, we administered a combination of intravenous immunoglobulin (IVIG 0.3 g/kg—once every three weeks) and corticosteroids (initial dosage of prednisone 1 mg/kg/day) [1]. Within four weeks, the patient's condition had improved significantly, lymphadenopathy diminished, ascites and systemic symptoms disappeared, and liver enzymes decreased (ALT 1.71 μkat/l, AST 1.32 μkat/l, ALP 7.32 μkat/l, and GGT 11.41 μkat/l). Thus, we could slowly reduce the dosage of corticosteroids. Since April 2017, the patient has been asymptomatic with laboratory tests within the norm and now is on a small dose of prednisone (5 mg/day). Up to now, the patient is well without symptoms of lymphoma or CD8+ lymphoproliferation, but regular IVIG substitution is necessary.

3. Discussion

So far, only a few cases of chronic CD8+ T-lymphoproliferation have been described. One of the largest published studies, with 14 patients, reported only two cases of CD8+ proliferation after rituximab treatment. One patient received rituximab maintenance, and another was treated with rituximab plus a fludarabine-based regimen. At the time of the CD8+ lymphoproliferation diagnosis, both patients (similarly to our patient) were in complete remission and had developed significant hypogammaglobulinemia. The first patient developed CD8+ expansion one year after the rituximab maintenance; it was manifested by aseptic CD8+ lymphocytic meningitis with fever, diarrhea, and lymphocytosis, and with bone marrow CD8 lymphocyte infiltration. The patient was treated successfully with intravenous immunoglobulins (0.5 g/kg every 3 weeks for 6 months), and rituximab was discontinued. After this treatment, the neurological symptoms resolved completely and the CD8+ T-cell lymphocytes disappeared from the CSF. The second patient developed unusually severe pancytopenia during rituximab-containing therapy, associated with persistent diarrhea and portal hypertension with ascites because of regenerative nodular hyperplasia. The CD8+ T-cell lymphocytes were present in the ascites liquid, in the peripheral blood, and in the bone marrow. A colon biopsy showed mucosal CD8+ T-cell infiltration. The patient's condition improved dramatically, and the blood cell count recovered after intravenous immunoglobulin treatment (0.5 g/kg every 3 weeks for 6 months) [1].

Another case report discusses a patient with long-term hypogammaglobulinemia persisting for 6 years after the end of rituximab-based therapy. The patient developed severe hypogammaglobulinemia within 10 months after end of the treatment with zero levels of IgG, IgA, and IgM, and no clinical symptoms. Before the treatment, the patient's globulin level was within the normal limits, the level of IgG dropped below 1 g/l, and IgA and IgM became undetectable. The patient was HIV-negative, with no family history of immunodeficiency, and had maintained complete remission since 2009. The levels of immunoglobulins have shown no changes after intravenous treatment (dose 5 g/month) for 6 years despite the recovery of the peripheral B-cell counts [15].

In the mentioned cases, hypogammaglobulinemia developed within a maximum of 1 year after the rituximab treatment. However, our patient developed immunodeficiency 11 years after the end of the treatment. Therefore, it is necessary to consider the diagnosis of CD8+ lymphoproliferation as a possible diagnosis even in patients with long-term remission of lymphoma. A biopsy with focused staining for CD8+ should be recommended as part of the histological algorithm, especially in cases of nonspecific "inflammatory" changes in the sample. With the massive use of CD20 antibody, we expect to see more cases with CD8+ expansion in such patients in the future. It is difficult to identify CD8+ lymphoproliferation during a standard histology examination of the tissue.

According to several studies, rituximab combined with chemotherapy leads to a loss of cell differentiation, increase in B-cell apoptosis, and changes in the T-cell population, which results in panhypogammaglobulinemia. The mechanism of invocation of the CD8+ lymphoproliferation after rituximab is caused by the CD27+IgM-IgD memory cell reduction. The B-cells stop their differentiation into the memory cells or plasmocyte and they produce less IgG. There are also secondary changes in the T-cell population. The expanded CD8+ T-lymphocytes represent activated T-lymphocytes at a terminal stage of their differentiation, which have usually lost their cytotoxic properties to become effector memory T-lymphocytes. The CD8+ T-cell expansions can result in symptomatic organ infiltration including the blood and bone marrow. They can also manifest in a variety of symptoms such as cytopenia, autoimmune disease, hepatitis, colitis, or lymphadenitis.

4. Conclusion

Although chronic benign CD8+ proliferation is a rare syndrome, we have to consider this diagnosis with immunocompromised patients and patients after rituximab treatment. It can mimic a systemic relapse of lymphoma with its typical laboratory and clinical symptoms, but a misdiagnosis with the administration of chemotherapy in those cases may be fatal. The diagnosis of the disease can be difficult, and it is necessary to know about this possibility. A standard biopsy examination has to be performed, but it will not identify the problem at first, which is a problem of which we have to be aware.

Abbreviations

CNS: Central nervous system
CSF: Cerebral spinal fluid
CMV: Cytomegalovirus
CVID: Common variable immunodeficiency
DILS: Diffuse infiltrative lymphocytosis syndrome
EBV: Epstein–Barr virus
HAV: Hepatitis A virus
HHV-8: Human herpes virus
IVIG: Intravenous immunoglobulin
PET/CT: Positron emission tomography and computed tomography
R-COPP: Rituximab, cyclophosphamide, vincristine, procarbazine, and prednisone
R-CHOP: Rituximab, cyclophosphamide, vincristine, doxorubicin, and prednisone.

Acknowledgments

This work was supported by research grants from the Ministry of Education and Youth of the Czech Republic AZV CR 16-31092A on behalf of CLSG.

References

[1] E. Ghrenassia, L. Roulin, A. Aline-Fardin et al., "The spectrum of chronic CD8+ T-cell expansions: clinical features in 14 patients," *PLoS One*, vol. 9, no. 3, pp. 1–10, 2014.

[2] B. I. Pereira and A. N. Akbar, "Convergence of innate and adaptive immunity during human aging," *Frontiers in Immunology*, vol. 7, p. 445, 2016.

[3] D. Brugnoni, E. Prati, F. Malacarne, R. Gorla, P. Airò, and R. Cataneo, "The primary response to HIV infection is characterized by an expansion of activated CD8+ CD28– cells," *AIDS*, vol. 10, no. 1, pp. 104-105, 1996.

[4] J. C. Mudd and M. M. Lederman, "CD8 T cell persistence in treated HIV infection," *Current Opinion in HIV and AIDS*, vol. 9, no. 5, pp. 500–505, 2014.

[5] P. R. Smith, J. D. Cavenagh, T. Milne et al., "Benign monoclonal expansion of CD8+ lymphocytes in HIV infection," *Journal of Clinical Pathology*, vol. 53, no. 3, pp. 177–181, 2000.

[6] E. Ghrenassia, N. Martis, J. Boyer, F. Burel-Vandenbos, A. Mekinian, and P. Coppo, "The diffuse infiltrative lymphocytosis syndrome (DILS). A comprehensive review," *Journal of Autoimmunity*, vol. 59, pp. 19–25, 2015.

[7] J.-F. Viallard, C. Ruiz, M. Guillet, J.-L. Pellegrin, and J.-F. Moreau, "Perturbations of the CD8+ T-cell repertoire in CVID patients with complications," *Results in Immunology*, vol. 3, pp. 122–128, 2013.

[8] V. Szablewski, C. René, and V. Costes, "Indolent cytotoxic T cell lymphoproliferation associated with nodular

regenerative hyperplasia: a common liver lesion in the context of common variable immunodeficiency disorder," *Virchows Archiv*, vol. 467, no. 6, pp. 733–740, 2015.

[9] M. Ghielmini, U. Vitolo, E. Kimby et al., "ESMO Guidelines consensus conference on malignant lymphoma 2011 part 1: diffuse large B-cell lymphoma (DLBCL), follicular lymphoma (FL) and chronic lymphocytic leukemia (CLL)," *Annals of Oncology*, vol. 24, no. 3, pp. 561–576, 2013.

[10] M. M. Griffin and N. Morley, "Rituximab in the treatment of non-Hodgkin's lymphoma—a critical evaluation of randomized controlled trials," *Expert Opinion on Biological Therapy*, vol. 13, no. 5, pp. 803–811, 2013.

[11] P. L. Zinzani, M. Marchetti, A. Billio et al., "SIE, SIES, GITMO revised guidelines for the management of follicular lymphoma," *American Journal of Hematology*, vol. 88, no. 3, pp. 185–192, 2013.

[12] C. Casulo, J. Maragulia, and A. D. Zelenetz, "Incidence of hypogammaglobulinemia in patients receiving rituximab and the use of intravenous immunoglobulin for recurrent infections," *Clinical Lymphoma Myeloma and Leukemia*, vol. 13, no. 2, pp. 106–111, 2013.

[13] C. Cattaneo, P. Spedini, S. Casari et al., "Delayed-onset peripheral blood cytopenia after rituximab: frequency and risk factor assessment in a consecutive series of 77 treatments," *Leukemia & Lymphoma*, vol. 47, no. 6, pp. 1013–1017, 2006.

[14] C. Nabhan, N. J. Ollberding, D. Villines et al., "A systematic review of comparative schedule-related toxicities with maintenance rituximab in follicular and mantle cell lymphomas," *Leukemia & Lymphoma*, vol. 55, no. 6, pp. 1288–1294, 2014.

[15] E. Irie, Y. Shirota, C. Suzuki et al., "Severe hypogammaglobulinemia persisting for 6 years after treatment with rituximab combined chemotherapy due to arrest of B lymphocyte differentiation together with alteration of T lymphocyte homeostasis," *International Journal of Hematology*, vol. 91, no. 3, pp. 501–508, 2010.

4

First Report of Hereditary Lysozyme Amyloidosis in a South Asian Family

Madiha Iqbal, Prachi Jani, Salman Ahmed, and Taimur Sher

Department of Hematology and Oncology, Mayo Clinic, Jacksonville, FL, USA

Correspondence should be addressed to Taimur Sher; sher.taimur@mayo.edu

Academic Editor: Sylvain Choquet

Lysozyme amyloidosis (ALys) is an exceedingly rare autosomal dominant hereditary type of systemic amyloidosis that can be misdiagnosed as other common types of systemic amyloidosis. The gastrointestinal tract and the kidney are the most common sites of organ involvement. No specific treatment exists for ALys, and the management primarily consists of organ-directed supportive care. To our knowledge, this disorder has been previously reported only in European ancestries; here, we first report the occurrence of ALys in South Asian ancestry. This report highlights the need of awareness amongst physicians regarding the extension of this unique and challenging disorder to non-European ancestries.

1. Introduction

Amyloidosis is a fascinating group of disorders characterized by extracellular deposition of amyloid fibrils in tissues and organs. Amyloid fibrils are derived from misfolded proteins in beta-pleated sheets from a wide variety of protein precursors (over 30 precursor types known) that can cause diseases belonging to a wide spectrum of human disorders such as familial cardiomyopathy (transthyretin amyloidosis), neoplastic disorders of plasma cells (immunoglobulin light chain amyloidosis), neurodegenerative diseases (Alzheimer's disease), and infectious diseases (prion disease) among others. This systemic amyloidosis can be acquired or hereditary depending upon the type of protein and the site of mutation (germline vs. acquired). Lysozyme amyloidosis, noted as ALys in the latest amyloidosis nomenclature, is an extremely rare nonneuropathic hereditary type of amyloidosis. In its normal form, lysozyme, as part of the innate immune system, plays an important role in mucosal defenses at sites such as the mucosal lining of the aerodigestive tract and conjunctiva. In ALys-specific germline, mutation(s) render the mutant lysozyme prone to misfolding in beta-pleated configuration giving rise to lysozyme amyloidosis. Only a handful of mutations have been reported to cause ALys, and these predominantly affect the gastrointestinal tract, kidney, and lymph nodes. A high degree of penetrance is noted in affected families; however, clinical presentation is quite heterogeneous among affected family members. To the best of our knowledge, all families that have been reported in the literature belong to the European ancestry (Table 1). Here, we describe a novel mutation causing ALys in a South Asian pedigree.

2. Case Presentation

The proband is a 39-year-old South Asian female of Indian origin who was diagnosed with systemic amyloidosis of unknown type when she was 16 years of age. At the time of diagnosis, she was pregnant and was experiencing gastrointestinal symptoms of abdominal bloating, dyspepsia, heartburn, and nausea. These symptoms persisted postpartum, and the patient underwent an upper endoscopy with biopsy, which was consistent with the presence of amyloid material; however, the type could not be determined. Thereafter, the patient continued to live a fairly normal life and did not seek any further medical attention until her daughter who when turned 16 started experiencing similar symptoms and underwent an upper endoscopy with biopsy results consistent with the presence of amyloid. At that time, the family sought medical attention at our institute. The

TABLE 1: Families reported in the literature with Alys.

Family	Mutation	Ethnicity	Dominant clinical features
1	W64R/TGG/CGG	French [1]	Nephropathy/Sicca syndrome
2	W64R/TGG/AGG	Italian [2]	Gastrointestinal
3	W64R/TGG/AGG	Italian [3]	Gastrointestinal
4	W64R/TGG/AGG	French [4]	Internal organ bleeding
5	I56T	English [5]	Nephropathy/easy bruisability
6	F57I	Italian [6]	Nephropathy
7	D67H	English [7]	Internal organ bleeding
8	D67H	English [8]	Nephropathy/GI bleeding
9	pTyr54Asn	Swedish [9]	Gastrointestinal/Sicca syndrome
10	I56T (our case)	South Asian	Gastrointestinal/nephropathy/internal organ bleeding
11	p.Leu102Ser	English with mixed lineage [10]	Nephropathy/neuropathy/gastrointestinal/ cardiac
12	W64R/TGG/AGG	Italian [11]	Gastrointestinal
13	Mutation not specified; however, lysozyme C confirmed as amyloidogenic protein per LCMS	English [12]	Nephropathy/internal organ bleeding
14	D67H	English [13]	Internal organ bleeding

proband reported that, in spite of an overall normal life, she had continued to experience dyspeptic symptoms that worsened with stress. She also reported around 12–15 episodes of hematemesis since her initial diagnosis. Additional symptoms on close questioning included easy bruisability, periorbital purpura, and ecchymosis associated with activities such as retching and vomiting. An upper endoscopy was performed at the Mayo Clinic. No morphological abnormality was seen on the endoscopy; however, Congo red stain demonstrated the presence of amyloid material in the gastroesophageal junction, stomach, and duodenum. Serum and urine protein electrophoresis were normal. Proteomic assessment with laser capture mass spectrometry (LCMS) evaluation of the congophilic material detected an amino acid sequence abnormality in the lysozyme protein (I56T). Peripheral blood genotyping confirmed I56T mutation (DNA change c.221T > C) in exon 2 of the lysozyme gene, which replacing isoleucine with threonine at position 56. I56T mutation per human genome variation society (HGVS) nomenclature is now known as I74T. Patient's renal and hepatic functions were normal, and she did not have any adenopathy. Besides iron deficiency and mildly delayed gastric emptying, no other abnormality was noted. The patient continues with yearly follow-up in our amyloidosis clinic with periodic exacerbations of dyspeptic symptoms and a few episodes of small-volume hematemesis, which have responded to high-dose acid suppressive treatment.

3. Family History

Proband's daughter at 16 year of age started experiencing anxiety and upper abdominal pain along with dyspeptic symptoms, which lead to an upper GI tract endoscopy and biopsy confirming I56T mutant Alys via LCMS. Her most significant symptoms were indigestion, anorexia, altered bowel habits, and easy bruisability. She was also noted to have moderate iron deficiency anemia secondary to heavy menstruation. Her symptoms subsequently improved with change in dietary habits. At the time of most recent evaluation, which was a year ago, the patient has been doing relatively well with the exception of intermittent nausea and abdominal bloating.

Proband's only other child is a 12-year-old son who diagnosed with "Henoch–Schonlein Purpura (HSP)" at the age of ten. He is currently doing well, is without any symptoms, and is in the process of genetic counseling.

Proband's extended family is settled in India; however, various members of the family are suspected to be suffering from symptoms that are likely secondary to lysozyme amyloidosis. All the affected members belong to proband's paternal side of the family without any report of any member suspected to be affected from proband's maternal side.

Proband's father who expired at age 67 secondary to cardiac valvulopathy is suspected of having suffered from lysozyme amyloidosis due to the report of prolonged hemorrhage after a sports incident as well as report of hematemesis that occurred on a few instances without any clear etiology after evaluation. Proband's brother who is currently 39 years of age suffers from frequent bouts of gastritis and subconjunctival hemorrhage and is considered possibly affected. Proband's father had a total of six siblings including him with three sisters and two brothers.

Proband's eldest uncle is currently alive and in his eighties who is reported to be healthy and does not have any offsprings. Proband's second uncle is in his sixties and suffers from kidney dysfunction without any clear etiology explaining the dysfunction and is therefore considered possibly affected in our report. He has recently started undergoing hemodialysis. He has two female offsprings with one of them undergoing a renal transplant in 2009. She was diagnosed with renal failure in her teens and was on hemodialysis for a few years before her transplant. She is now doing well. No clear etiology has been found for her kidney dysfunction after extensive evaluation and is therefore considered possibly affected. The other female offspring is reported to be healthy.

One of the paternal aunts passed away in 1994 after childbirth. She was in her 30s then and underwent a

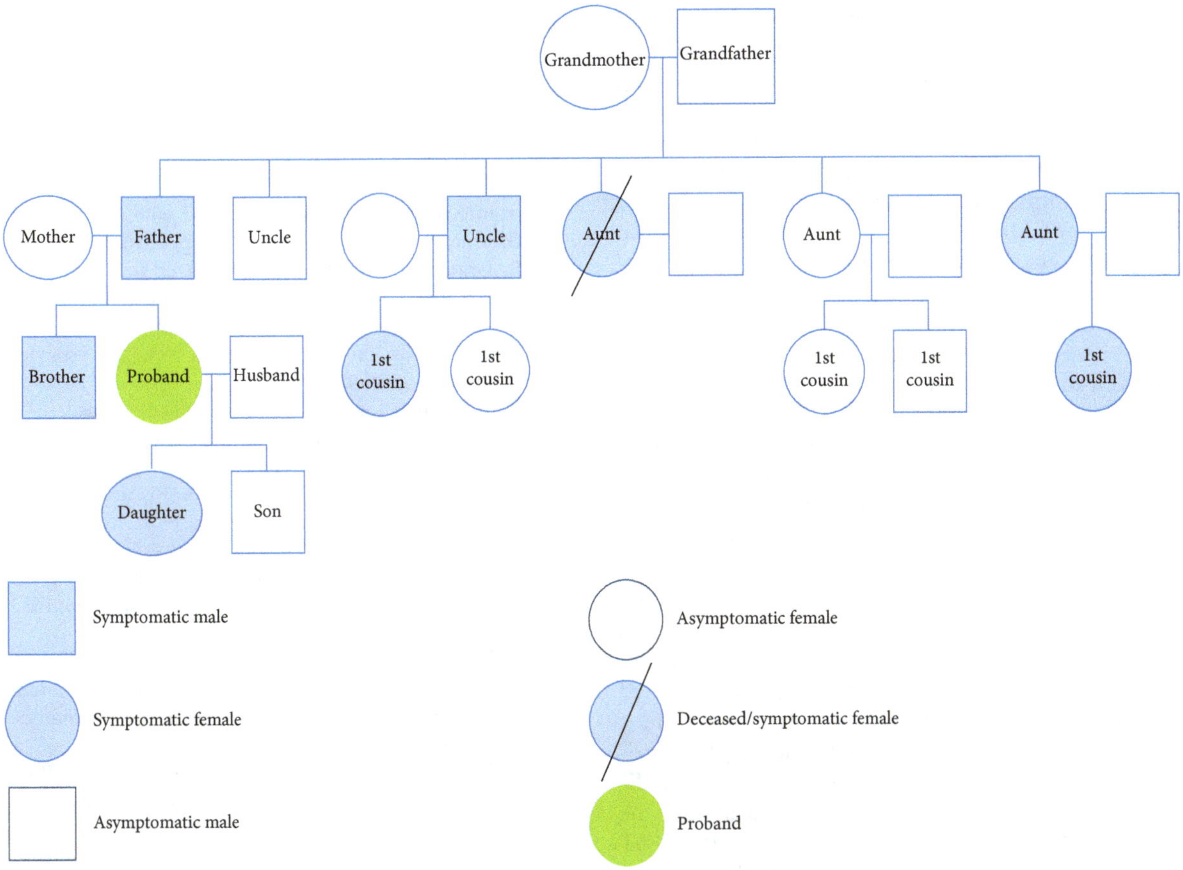

Figure 1: Family tree illustrating proband's paternal pedigree.

caesarean section; however, postoperatively, she had massive internal hemorrhage from her liver, which could not be explained by the local physicians. She is also reported to have suffered from bruising and gastritis prior to her death. She is considered as possibly affected.

Another aunt suffers from early stages of kidney dysfunction with reports of proteinuria. She was also evaluated as a possible kidney donor for her only daughter who is 30 years old and suffers from progressively worsening renal disease with significant amount of proteinuria and is currently being evaluated for renal transplant. However, as a part of evaluation as a potential kidney donor, a renal biopsy was done which was positive for the presence of amyloid deposition. Proband's cousin also suffers from frequent bouts of abdominal discomfort and dyspepsia.

A family tree of paternal pedigree is illustrated in Figure 1.

4. Discussion

Lysozyme amyloidosis has been reported in a handful of families belonging to the European ancestry [4, 9, 11, 12]. There are no reports of ALys in the South Asian ancestry. Our report is unique in being the only report of an affected family of the South Asian origin.

The diagnosis of ALys continues to be challenging due to the rarity of the disease and nonspecific presentation with regard to symptomology in most instances. In a study of 350 patients with systemic amyloidosis who had been given the presumptive diagnosis of AL (light chain) amyloidosis, 34 patients (10%) were found to have hereditary amyloidosis after undergoing testing for amyloidogenic mutations highlighting the importance of including hereditary types of amyloidosis in the differential of systemic amyloidosis. In this study, one patient was found to have ALys [14].

While suspecting a diagnosis of hereditary systemic amyloidosis, a through family history is of paramount importance. Various methods are employed to diagnose lysozyme amyloidosis with the most common being the histological analysis of the lysozyme protein via immunohistochemistry. Other methods, which are more specific compared to histological analysis, include testing for DNA mutations and conducting laser microdissection with mass spectrometry.

The association of mutations in the lysozyme gene with systemic amyloidosis was first described by Pepys et al. in 1993 [15]. Unlike familial transthyretin amyloidosis (which is the most common form of hereditary systemic amyloidosis) where more than 100 pathogenic mutations are known, only a handful of amyloidogenic mutations have been reported in the lysozyme gene (W64R, I56T, D67H, and F57I) [4, 15]. Recently, another mutation in exon 2 caused by the substitution of T by A leading to replacement of Tyr by Asn (pTyr54Asn) has also been reported in a family with Swedish ancestry [9].

A heterogeneous presentation is quite notable among members of the affected family with the gastrointestinal tract being most commonly affected [11, 12]. Symptoms attributable to gastrointestinal (GI) involvement can be quite varied ranging from mild abdominal discomfort, nausea, to bleeding from the GI tract [11, 12]. Renal involvement is also quite frequently encountered, and varied degrees of renal impairment are seen ranging from mild dysfunction to the need of hemodialysis. W64R and F571 mutations have been noted to be associated with renal dysfunction [1]. Hepatic involvement leading to spontaneous hepatic rupture has also been reported though defined coagulation abnormalities like factor X deficiency in AL amyloidosis have not been reported in lysozyme amyloidosis [13]. Other organs that have been reported in the literature to be involved by lysozyme amyloidosis include salivary glands [16], lymph nodes [5], spleen [5], heart [10], and the bone marrow [2]. There does not appear to be direct corelation between mutation type and symptomology; however, most families present with involvement of a predominant single organ system. Our reported family however uniquely presented with involvement of multiple organ systems in various members including renal, gastrointestinal, and a propensity towards hemorrhage. Interestingly, a bleeding diathesis has been mostly seen in families harboring the D67H mutation; whereas our family carried the I56T mutation, again illustrating the observation that mechanisms other than the mutation type are behind various clinical presentations.

Currently, there is no specific treatment that is available for this rare disease. The median survival rate for ALys has been reported to be 17.9 years from diagnosis [17]. Treatment options currently are focused on alleviating patient symptoms. Kidney transplantation can be considered in patients who suffer from progressive renal failure. In a series of 104 patients who underwent renal transplant for various types of systemic amyloidosis [18], only three patients had lysozyme amyloidosis. The reported median time from diagnosis of lysozyme amyloidosis to ESRD was at 10.6 years with all grafts functioning well without any evidence of amyloid recurrence. Liver transplantation has also been described in the literature; however, the procedure is not curative unlike TTR amyloidosis as cells other than the hepatocytes frequently produce lysozyme [13]. Immunotherapy-based options are in the early stages of evaluation for Alys [19].

This report highlights the need of awareness among physicians of this rare form of amyloidosis and, more importantly, that this is not limited to European ethnicities. Patients and family members who suffer from this disease require long-term follow-up. Genetic counseling and patient education about symptoms including the risk of bleeding is important, given the rarity of the disease and nonspecific symptomology. Multisite collaboration to identify patients and families with this rare disease to better understand the natural history and develop novel therapeutic approaches is critical.

References

[1] S. Valleix, S. Drunat, J.-B. Philit et al., "Hereditary renal amyloidosis caused by a new variant lysozyme W64R in a French family," *Kidney International*, vol. 61, no. 3, pp. 907–912, 2002.

[2] B. Granel, J. Serratrice, S. Valleix et al., "A family with gastrointestinal amyloidosis associated with variant lysozyme," *Gastroenterology*, vol. 123, no. 4, pp. 1346–1349, 2002.

[3] B. Granel, J. Serratrice, P. Disdier et al., "Underdiagnosed amyloidosis: amyloidosis of lysozyme variant," *American Journal of Medicine*, vol. 118, no. 3, pp. 321-322, 2005.

[4] B. Granel, S. Valleix, J. Serratrice et al., "Lysozyme amyloidosis," *Medicine*, vol. 85, no. 1, pp. 66–73, 2006.

[5] A. M. Zalin, S. Jones, N. J. Fitch, and D. B. Ramsden, "Familial nephropathic non-neuropathic amyloidosis: clinical features, immunohistochemistry and chemistry," *QJM: An International Journal of Medicine*, vol. 81, no. 2, pp. 945–956, 1991.

[6] M. Yazaki, S. A. Farrell, and M. D. Benson, "A novel lysozyme mutation Phe57Ile associated with hereditary renal amyloidosis," *Kidney International*, vol. 63, no. 5, pp. 1652–1657, 2003.

[7] R. F. Harrison, P. N. Hawkins, W. R. Roche, R. F. MacMahon, S. G. Hubscher, and J. A. Buckels, "'Fragile' liver and massive hepatic haemorrhage due to hereditary amyloidosis," *Gut*, vol. 38, no. 1, pp. 151-152, 1996.

[8] J. D. Gillmore, S. Madhooh, M. B. Pepyss, D. R. Booth, and P. N. Hawkins, "Hereditary renal amyloidosis associated with variant lysozyme in a large English family," *Nephrology Dialysis Transplantation*, vol. 14, no. 11, pp. 2639–2644, 1999.

[9] S. Girnius, M. Skinner, B. Spencer et al., "A new lysozyme tyr54asn mutation causing amyloidosis in a family of Swedish ancestry with gastrointestinal symptoms," *Amyloid*, vol. 19, no. 4, pp. 182–185, 2012.

[10] S. H. Nasr, S. Dasari, J. R. Mills et al., "Hereditary lysozyme amyloidosis variant p.Leu102Ser associates with unique phenotype," *Journal of the American Society of Nephrology*, vol. 28, no. 2, pp. 431–438, 2017.

[11] E. Jean et al., "A new family with hereditary lysozyme amyloidosis with gastritis and inflammatory bowel disease as prevailing symptoms," *BMC Gastroenterology*, vol. 14, p. 159, 2014.

[12] C. Pleyer, J. Flesche, and F. Saeed, "Lysozyme amyloidosis—a case report and review of the literature," *Clinical Nephrology Case Studies*, vol. 3, pp. 42–45, 2015.

[13] M. Loss, W. S. Ng, R. Z. Karim et al., "Hereditary lysozyme amyloidosis: spontaneous hepatic rupture (15 years apart) in mother and daughter. Role of emergency liver transplantation," *Liver Transplantation*, vol. 12, no. 7, pp. 1152–1155, 2006.

[14] H. J. Lachmann, D. R. Booth, S. E. Booth et al., "Misdiagnosis of hereditary amyloidosis as AL (primary) amyloidosis," *New England Journal of Medicine*, vol. 346, no. 23, pp. 1786–1791, 2002.

[15] M. B. Pepys, P. N. Hawkins, D. R. Booth et al., "Human lysozyme gene mutations cause hereditary systemic amyloidosis," *Nature*, vol. 362, no. 6420, pp. 553–557, 1993.

[16] J. Lanham, M. L. Meltzer, F. C. de Beer, G. R. V. Hughes, and M. B. Pepys, "Familial amyloidosis of Ostertag," *QJM: An International Journal of Medicine*, vol. 51, no. 1, pp. 25–32, 1982.

[17] P. T. Sattianayagam, S. D. J. Gibbs, D. Rowczenio et al., "Hereditary lysozyme amyloidosis—phenotypic heterogeneity

and the role of solid organ transplantation," *Journal of Internal Medicine*, vol. 272, no. 1, pp. 36–44, 2011.

[18] J. H. Pinney, H. J. Lachmann, P. T. Sattianayagam et al., "Renal transplantation in systemic amyloidosis-importance of amyloid fibril type and precursor protein abundance," *American Journal of Transplantation*, vol. 13, no. 2, pp. 433–441, 2012.

[19] M. Dumoulin, A. M. Last, A. Desmyter et al., "A camelid antibody fragment inhibits the formation of amyloid fibrils by human lysozyme," *Nature*, vol. 424, no. 6950, pp. 783–788, 2003.

5

The Development of Primary Effusion Lymphoma-Like Lymphoma in a Patient with Preexisting Essential Thrombocythemia

Yoshiki Uemura[1], **Marina Komoto**[2] **and Mitsuo Okada**[3]

[1]*Department of Hematology, Chikamori Hospital, 1-1-16, Okawasuzi, Kochi-shi, Kochi- ken 780-8522, Japan*
[2]*Department of Cardiology, Chikamori Hospital, 1-1-16, Okawasuzi, Kochi-shi, Kochi- ken 780-8522, Japan*
[3]*Department of Gastroenterology, Chikamori Hospital, 1-1-16, Okawasuzi, Kochi-shi, Kochi-ken 780-8522, Japan*

Correspondence should be addressed to Yoshiki Uemura; khs1040@chikamori.com

Academic Editor: Kostas Konstantopoulos

A 71-year-old Japanese male was diagnosed with essential thrombocythemia (ET) with the JAK2 V617F mutation variation, in April 2011. He was mainly treated with hydroxyurea following which the number of platelets was maintained within the normal limit. At age 80, he was hospitalized due to cardiac tamponade. Computed tomography showed no evidence of tumor masses or lymphadenopathy. Pericardial drainage was performed, and cytopathologic examination of the fluid revealed atypical lymphoid cells consistent with an effusion lymphoma of B cell lineage. The pericardial effusion was completely drained, and complete remission was achieved. Ultimately, the patient was diagnosed with primary effusion lymphoma-like lymphoma (PEL-LL). To the best of our knowledge, this is the first report of PEL-LL following ET.

1. Introduction

The incidence of solid cancer is 1.5–3.0 times higher in patients with myeloproliferative tumor (MPN) than in the general population. Particularly, the onset of lymphoid hematological cancer, such as non-Hodgkin lymphoma (NHL), Hodgkin lymphoma, chronic lymphocytic leukemia, and multiple myeloma, is 2.5–3.5 times higher [1].

Primary effusion lymphoma (PEL) is a rare type of high-grade B cell lymphoma localized only in body cavities, without forming masses [2]. It is caused by human herpes virus Type 8 (HHV-8) in HIV-infected patients [3]. The median overall survival for the disease course is 6–9 months [4]. On the other hand, most elderly patients with PEL are HHV-8 negative and are often administered chemotherapy. They are often cured only by body cavity drainage and generally have a good prognosis. Patients with these characteristics are distinguished from those with PEL-like lymphoma (PEL-LL) [5, 6].

We encountered a case of PEL-LL that developed during the course of treatment for the essential thrombocythemia (ET). A case of PEL-LL secondary to MPN has not been reported yet. We report this case along with a literature review.

2. Case Presentation

A 71-year-old Japanese male was diagnosed with ET, with a JAK2 V617F mutation variation, at another hospital in April 2011. The number of platelets (PLT) was maintained at approximately $50 \times 10^4/\mu l$ following 500 mg–1000 mg of hydroxyurea (HU). He was transferred to our hospital in March 2016 and was continued on the same treatment. The progression of anemia and increased number of PLT were detected afterwards. We added 0.5 mg–1.0 mg of anagrelide to the 500 mg–1000 mg of HU from June 2017 and planned to stabilize the hemoglobin (Hb) level and the number of PLT. However, we could not suppress the progression of anemia by regulating the dosage of each drug. The bone marrow histology showed bone marrow hyperplasia with an increase in megakaryocytes and a significant decrease in erythroblasts in November 2018. The bone marrow chromosome analysis showed normal variation of inv(9) (p12q13) in all analyzed cells. We considered that he might have concomitant, acquired pure red cell aplasia (PRCA) without human parvovirus B19 infection and thymoma. He received 200 mg of cyclosporine (CyA) for PRCA in place of anagrelide from December 2018. The chest X-ray taken in December 2018 showed mild cardiomegaly in comparison to that of May 2017. Echocardiography revealed a large pericardial effusion. We did not perform the pericardiocentesis because he had no symptoms, such as dyspnea. He was followed up on furosemide alone. Echocardiography showed a slight decrease in pericardial effusion in January 2019. (Figure 1).

The change from anagrelide to CyA resulted in a slight improvement in anemia. However, the PLT and white blood cell count (WBC) increased, and myeloblasts began to appear in the peripheral blood (PB). Then, we considered that he might have secondary myelofibrosis (MF), although we were unable to obtain a histopathological diagnosis because of insufficient material in the bone marrow biopsy. He was started on 10 mg ruxolitinib in place of CyA in January 2019. However, he discontinued ruxolitinib because it induced interstitial pneumonitis on the ninth day. Interstitial pneumonitis was relieved by immediate steroid therapy. He was then commenced on 10 mg metenolone acetate from February 2019 because the WBC and PLT gradually decreased. After that, WBC, PLT, and Hb levels increased rapidly. He received 2.5 mg of busulfan (BU) for cell reduction from mid-February 2019. However, he also discontinued BU because of interstitial pneumonitis on the seventh day. He then commenced HU because the WBC and PLT levels increased again after BU was discontinued. HU decreased the WBC count and the PLT; however, the anemia worsened. Therefore, the frequency of blood transfusions was increased. Afterwards, he recommenced BU from May 2019; then, the WBC count and PLT were normalized, the Hb level increased to around 8 g/dl, and then, the blast cells in peripheral blood disappeared. This time, while taking BU, there was no interstitial pneumonitis. He stopped taking BU in August 2019 due to a decrease in the WBC count and PLT. He cancelled metenolone acetate in November, 2019, because of the increase of the WBC and the PLT. After that, the WBC, the Hb level, and the PLT were kept without remarkable change. However, the WBC and the PLT soared from April, 2020. He was admitted to our hospital in April, 2020, because of severe dyspnea. He was diagnosed with cardiac tamponade caused by a large pericardial effusion (Figure 2). The examination results at the time of hospitalization are presented in Table 1. Dyspnea improved soon after the cardiac drainage. He had a class IV pericardial fluid cytodiagnosis. Immunohistochemical staining of the cell block was positive for CD20, EBER, and MUM-1, and 50% of MIB-1 (Figure 3); HHV-8 DNA was negative, and we diagnosed the patient with PEL-LL. After the drainage, the WBC count, Hb level, and PLT decreased slowly. He had a steady progression of the leg edema and showed a precipitous increase in the PB WBC and blast cell counts, from August 2020. The PLT decreased precipitously in October 2020. The bone marrow biopsy in October 2020 showed bone marrow hyperplasia with an increase in megakaryocytes and blast cells, followed by myelofibrosis of grade two or three. The blast cells occupied 32% of the bone marrow. Peroxidase staining was positive in more than 3% of the samples. Chromosomal analysis of PB demonstrated inv(3) (q21,3q26.2) in addition to inv(9) (p12q13). He was then diagnosed with acute myeloid leukemia (AML). Computed tomography (CT) showed no body cavity retention on October 1, 2020. However, massive ascites was observed on October 31, 2020 (Figure 4). Although the possibility of PEL-LL in the abdominal cavity was suggested, cytologic examination of ascitic fluid showed no malignancy. The levels of M2BPGi, type IV collagen, hyaluronic acid, and ammonia were high, and the levels of coagulation factors, albumin, and cholinesterase, from the liver, were low. Furthermore, CT and ultrasonography showed no features of cirrhosis. The CT value of the liver increased because of iron overload caused by the frequent blood transfusion. Although 5.1 L of ascites was drained at once, it reaccumulated immediately. Even after cell-free and concentrated ascites reinfusion therapy (CART), the ascites reaccumulated immediately. Subsequently, he worsened renal dysfunction and hyperammonemia and finally died of pneumonia in November 2020.

3. Discussion

Patients with MPN such as polycythemia vera (PV) or ET are at a high risk of solid carcinoma. Brabrand and Frederiksen demonstrated that the incidence of a new malignant tumor is 1.5–3.0 times higher in patients with MPNs [1]. The frequency of malignant lymphoma, skin cancer, lung cancer, renal cancer, and thyroid cancer is relatively high in new malignant tumors. The frequency of lymphoid hematological cancer is 2.5–3.5 times higher than those of other cancers [1]. The cause of the high frequency of secondary cancers in MPN is still unclear. The participation of shared risk factors, inherent tendency to cancer, and antitumor treatment are suspect [7–14]. Antitumor agents for treating MPN influence the risk of transformation to AML [10, 15]; however, it is unknown whether these agents influence the risk of solid carcinoma and lymphoid tumor. Two cohort studies recently reported that the incidence of aggressive B cell lymphoma in the MPN patients who received JAK1/2 inhibitor is approximately 15 times that of healthy persons [16]. Because the occurrence of pericardial effusion was detected before ruxolitinib and the dosing period was short (nine days), we excluded ruxolitinib as a cause of PEL-LL. However, ruxolitinib may promote the development of pericardial fluid. Generally, most patients treated with JAK inhibitors have previously received HU or alkylating agents. This suggests that the cumulative phenomenon of immunosuppression or insufficiency of immune surveillance could also be a cause of lymphoproliferative neoplasm (LPN). Our patient had also received HU long-term and BU and CyA short-term, prior

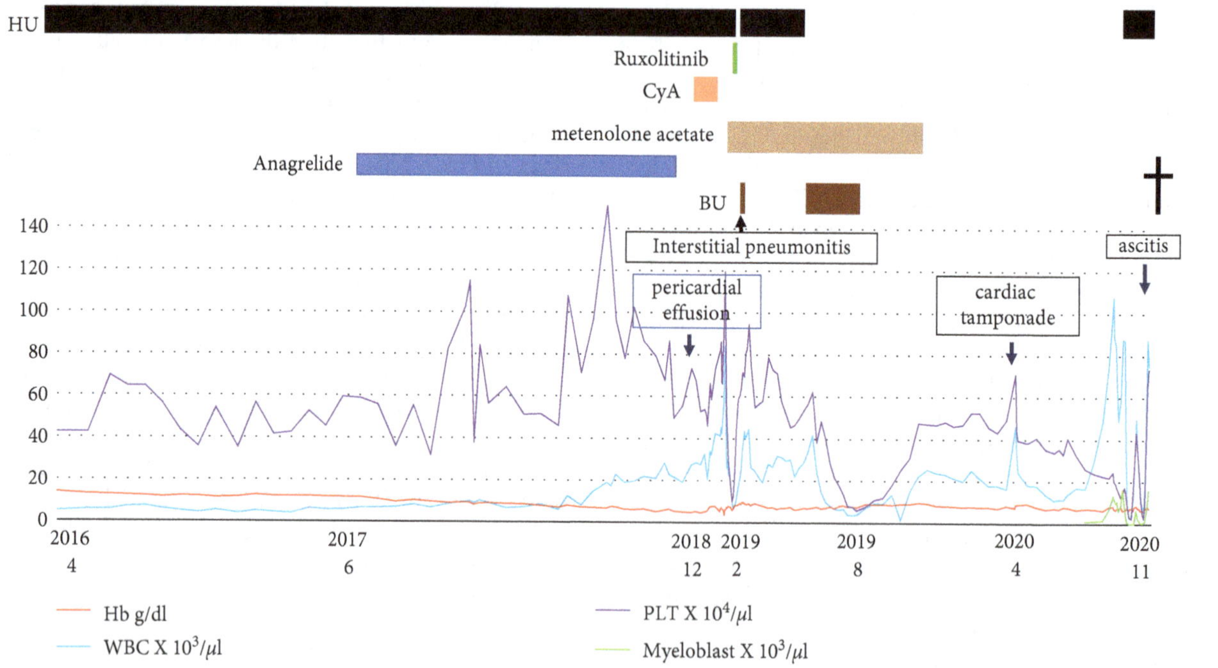

Figure 1: Clinical course. HU, hydroxyurea; CyA, cyclosporine; BU, busulfan; Hb, hemoglobin; WBC, white blood cell; PLT, platelets.

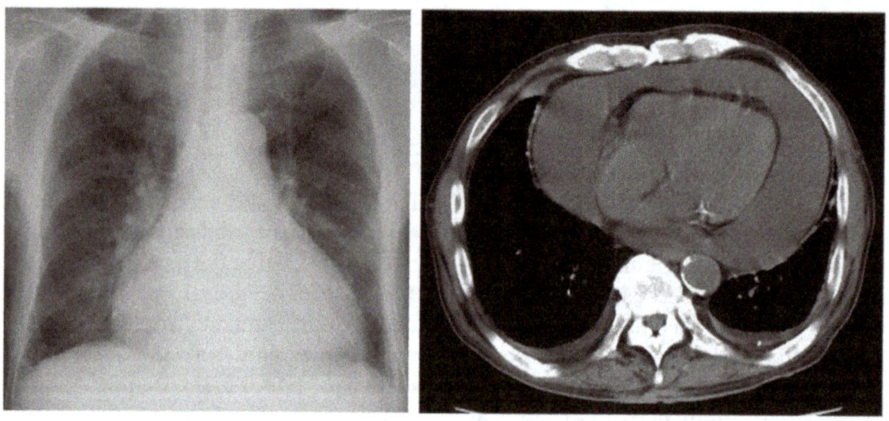

Figure 2: Imaging revealed heart enlargement, massive pericardial fluid, and a small amount of pleural fluid retention.

Table 1: Laboratory findings.

Complete blood		Count biochemistry		Test serological test	
WBC	46,100/μl	TP	7.1 g/dl	C3	66 mg/dl
Myeloblast	(+)H	Alb	3.8 g/dl	C4	19 mg/dl
Myelocyte	2.0%	AST	15 U/l	ANA	<40
Metamyelocyte	0.5%	ALT	23 U/l	RF	<5 IU/ml
Banded neutrophil	7.0%	ALP	281 IU/ml	BNP	125 pg/ml
Segmented neutrophil	78.5%	γ-GTP	31 IU/l	CK-MB	mg/dl
Lymphocyte	3.0%	LDH	208 U/l	MB/CK	52%
Monocyte	6.5%	T-bil	1.0 mg/dl	Troponin T	0.012
Eosinophil	1.5%	BUN	65.1 mg/dl	HCV ab	(−)
Basophilic	1.0%	Cr	2.36 mg/dl	HBs Ag	(−)
RBC	227 × 104/μl	UA	16.9 mg/dl	IgG	1316 mg/dl
Hb	7.3 g/dl	T-CHO	104 mg/dl	IgA	255 mg/dl
Ht	22.5%	TG	60 mg/dl	IgM	114 mg/dl
MCV	99.1 fl	Glu	220 mg/dl	sIL-2R	1920 U/ml
Plt	70.8 × 104/μl	HbA1c	6.4%		

Table 1: Continued.

Complete blood		Count biochemistry		Test serological test	
		Na	128 mEq/l	*Coagulation*	
Urinalysis		K	4.8 mEq/l	PT-INR	1.52
Color	Yellow	Cl	95 mEq/l	APTT	57.9 sec
Protein	1(+)	CRP	3.73 mg/dl	Fibrinogen	272.3 mg/dl
Glucose	(−)	ESR	2 mm/h	FDP	3.0 μg/ml
Occult blood	1(+)			D-dimer	1.5 μg/ml
				Quantitation of viral DNA	
				HHV-8 DNA < 100 copy/ml	

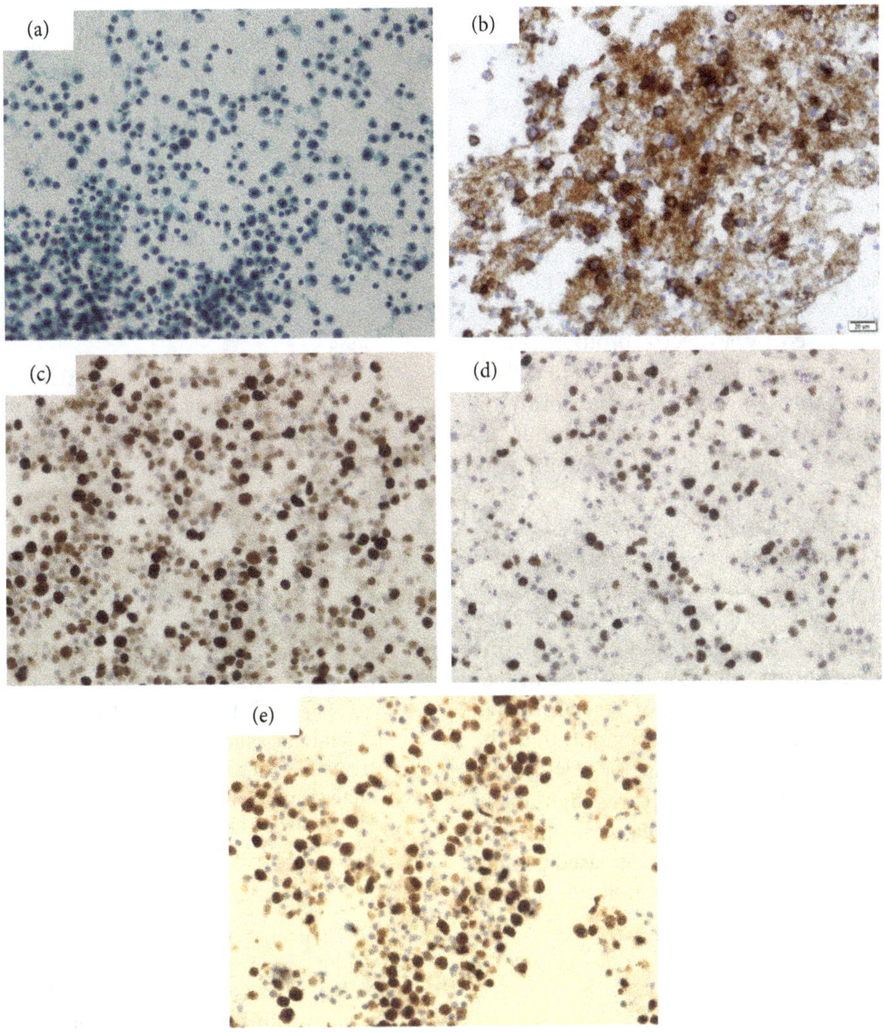

Figure 3: Cytological pericardial effusion findings. (a) Pap staining (×40). Cell block with ((b)–(e)) immunocytochemical findings. (b) CD20. (c) Ki-67 (MIB-1 index 50%). (d) EBER. (e) MUM-1 ((b)–(e) ×40).

to the administration of ruxolitinib. These preceding agents could exacerbate the risk of LPN. MPN is recognized as a model of inflammatory disease in which cytokines play an important role in the onset and progression of the disease [17]. The mechanism of NHL by JAK2 inhibitors is largely still unknown in MPN. JAK2 inhibitors damage the natural killer cells and dendritic cells quantitatively and functionally and decreases the regulatory T cells (Tregs), resulting in the suppression of inflammatory cytokine secretion mediated by CD4-positive T lymphocyte [18–20]. Thus, ruxolitinib is antagonistic towards immunological surveillance. Generally, the PLT in ET can be controlled well by HU.

The management of PLT by HU was difficult because of the progression of anemia in our case. As previously shown, erythroblasts decrease while granulocytic cells and megakaryocytes increase at the early stage of myelofibrosis [21]. Bone marrow fibrosis was not observed when the bone marrow fluid was aspirated. Although he was commenced

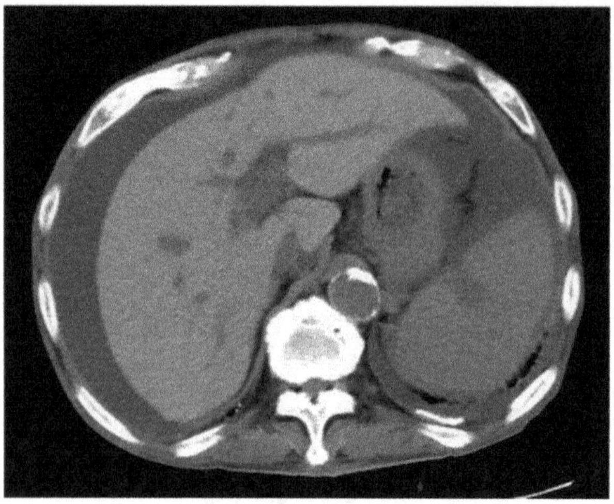

FIGURE 4: Image of plain computed tomography. Massive ascites and increased liver density.

on CyA in consideration of PRCA, the anemia did not improve. We reported that PRCA developed as ET progressed [22]. As previously considered, the onset of PRCA in patients with MPN is caused by a diverse proliferation of MPN stem cells and a diverse reaction of MPN stem cells to growth factors; however, this is not based on an immunological foundation. Therefore, the previous study finding did not support the efficacy of CyA for PRCA in patients with MPN.

We first speculated that the acute development of ascites might indicate the possibility of PEL-LL. However, cytodiagnosis of ascites showed no malignancy. Papanicolaou staining did not reveal any lymphoma cell. May–Grünwald–Giemsa (May–Giemsa) staining could not prove any lymphoma cells. Flow cytometry did not reveal the monoclonality of B cell. In addition, the ascites reaccumulated promptly after drainage. Therefore, we thought that the ascites were not derived from PEL-LL. Since CT showed a smooth liver surface, although the CT value was high due to transfusional iron overload, we rejected liver cirrhosis as the cause of the ascites. We hypothesized that decreased protein synthesis due to liver fibrosis or hepatic infiltration with leukemia cells might cause ascites.

4. Conclusion

We encountered a case of PEL-LL with severe cardiac tamponade throughout the progression of ET. If an unidentified pericardial effusion is detected during the course of MPN, it is important to consider PEL-LL as a differential diagnosis.

Acknowledgments

The authors thank Editage (http://www.editage.com) for English language editing.

References

[1] M. Brabrand and H. Frederiksen, "Risks of solid and lymphoid malignancies in patients with myeloproliferative neoplasms: clinical implications," *Cancers*, vol. 12, no. 10, p. 3061, 2020.

[2] E. Campo, S. H. Swerdlow, N. L. Harris, S. Pileri, H. Stein, and E. S. Jaffe, "The 2008 WHO classification of lymphoid neoplasms and beyond: evolving concepts and practical applications," *Blood*, vol. 117, no. 19, pp. 5019–5032, 2011.

[3] A. Carbone and A. Gloghini, "KSHV/HHV8-associated lymphomas," *British Journal of Haematology*, vol. 140, no. 1, pp. 13–24, 2008.

[4] C. Aguilar, C. Laberiano, B. Beltran, C. Diaz, A. Taype-Rondan, and J. J. Castillo, "Clinicopathologic characteristics and survival of patients with primary effusion lymphoma," *Leukemia and Lymphoma*, vol. 61, no. 9, pp. 2093–2102, 2020.

[5] Y. Kobayashi, Y. Kamitsuji, J. Kuroda et al., "Comparison of human herpes virus 8 related primary effusion lymphoma with human herpes virus 8 unrelated primary effusion lymphoma-like lymphoma on the basis of HIV: report of 2 cases and review of 212 cases in the literature," *Acta Haematologica*, vol. 117, no. 3, pp. 132–144, 2007.

[6] A. Carbone and A. Gloghini, "PEL and HHV8-unrelated effusion lymphomas," *Cancer*, vol. 114, no. 4, pp. 225–227, 2008.

[7] J. Grinfeld, J. Nangalia, E. J. Baxter et al., "Classification and personalized prognosis in myeloproliferative neoplasms," *New England Journal of Medicine*, vol. 379, no. 15, pp. 1416–1430, 2018.

[8] P. D. Berk, J. D. Goldberg, M. N. Silverstein et al., "Increased incidence of acute leukemia in polycythemia vera associated with chlorambucil therapy," *New England Journal of Medicine*, vol. 304, no. 8, pp. 441–447, 1981.

[9] G. Finazzi, V. Caruso, and R. Marchioli, "Acute leukemia in polycythemia vera: an analysis of 1638 patients enrolled in a prospective observational study," *Blood*, vol. 105, no. 7, pp. 2664–2670, 2005.

[10] Y. Najean, J. D. Rain, and C. Dresch, "Risk of leukaemia, carcinoma, and myelofibrosis in 32P- or chemotherapy-treated patients with polycythaemia vera: a prospective analysis of 682 cases," *The "French Cooperative Group for the Study of Polycythaemias," Leuk Lymphoma*, vol. 22, no. S1, pp. 111–119, 1996.

[11] C. Nielsen, H. S. Birgens, B. G. Nordestgaard, L. Kjaer, and S. E. Bojesen, "The JAK2 V617F somatic mutation, mortality and cancer risk in the general population," *Haematologica*, vol. 96, no. 3, pp. 450–453, 2011.

[12] N. H. Thoennissen, U. O. Krug, D. H. T. Lee et al., "Prevalence and prognostic impact of allelic imbalances associated with leukemic transformation of Philadelphia chromosome-negative myeloproliferative neoplasms," *Blood*, vol. 115, no. 14, pp. 2882–2890, 2010.

[13] T. Barbui, A. Ghirardi, A. Masciulli et al., "Second cancer in Philadelphia negative myeloproliferative neoplasms (MPN-K). A nested case-control study," *Leukemia*, vol. 33, no. 8, pp. 1996–2005, 2019.

[14] F. Radaelli, F. Onida, F. G. Rossi et al., "Second malignancies in essential thrombocythemia (ET): a retrospective analysis of 331 patients with long-term follow-up from a single institution," *Hematology*, vol. 13, no. 4, pp. 195–202, 2008.

[15] Y. Najean and J.-D. Rain, "Treatment of polycythemia vera: use of 32P alone or in combination with maintenance therapy using hydroxyurea in 461 patients greater than 65 years of age," *Blood*, vol. 89, no. 7, pp. 2319–2327, 1997.

[16] E. Porpaczy, S. Tripolt, A. Hoelbl-Kovacic et al., "Aggressive B-cell lymphomas in patients with myelofibrosis receiving JAK1/2 inhibitor therapy," *Blood*, vol. 132, no. 7, pp. 694–706, 2018.

[17] L. F. Mendez Luque, A. L. Blackmon, G. Ramanathan, and A. G. Fleischman, "Key role of inflammation in myeloproliferative neoplasms: instigator of disease initiation, progression. And symptoms," *Current Hematologic Malignancy Reports*, vol. 14, no. 3, pp. 145–153, 2019.

[18] K. Schönberg, J. Rudolph, M. Vonnahme et al., "JAK inhibition impairs NK cell function in myeloproliferative neoplasms," *Cancer Research*, vol. 75, no. 11, pp. 2187–2199, 2015.

[19] A. Heine, S. A. E. Held, S. N. Daecke et al., "The JAK-inhibitor ruxolitinib impairs dendritic cell function in vitro and in vivo," *Blood*, vol. 122, no. 7, pp. 1192–1202, 2013.

[20] S. Parampalli Yajnanarayana, T. Stübig, I. Cornez et al., "JAK1/2 inhibition impairs T cell function in vitro and in patients with myeloproliferative neoplasms," *British Journal of Haematology*, vol. 169, no. 6, pp. 824–833, 2015.

[21] S. H. Swerdlow, E. Campo, N. L. Harris et al., "Reviced WHO classification of tumours of haematopoietic and lymphoid tissues," in *WHO Classification of Tumours*, LARC Press, Lyon, France, 4th edition, 2017.

[22] R. Sarode, P. Bambery, N. Marwaha, A. Gupta, G. Garewal, and S. D. Deodhar, "Pure red cell aplasia associated with essential thrombocythemia (a case report)," *Indian Journal of Cancer*, vol. 27, no. 3, pp. 138–142, 1990.

6

The Combination of Interferon-Alpha and Ponatinib Enables Faster and Deeper Molecular Responses in Patient with De Novo Blast Crisis of CML: Interferon-Alpha May Return as a CML Treatment

Kunio Hayashi,[1] **Kazuhiro Ikegame**,[2] **and Naoto Takahashi**[3]

[1]*Division of Hematology, Meiwa General Hospital, 4-31 Agenaruocho, Nishinomiya, Hyogo 663-8186, Japan*
[2]*Division of Hematology, Hyogo College of Medicine, Mukogawacho, Nishinomiya, Hyogo 663-8501, Japan*
[3]*Department of Hematology Nephrology and Rheumatology, Akita University, 1-1 Hondo 1-Chome, Akita 010-8543, Japan*

Correspondence should be addressed to Naoto Takahashi; naotot@doc.med.akita-u.ac.jp

Academic Editor: Pier Paolo Piccaluga

In the era of tyrosine kinase inhibitor (TKI) treatment, its effectiveness in treating chronic myelogenous leukemia (CML) has been improved, ensuring the same prognosis as that of healthy people of the same age. However, there are some patients with de novo blast crisis that undergoes acute conversion from the time of diagnosis and does not respond to TKI treatment, especially in the older patients. Here, we present a case of an older patient with de novo lymphoid crisis who was first treated with a combination of TKI and chemotherapy, but it was difficult to maintain a durable deep molecular response (DMR). After he achieved major molecular response (MMR) or less, it was possible to suppress IS% to DMR by performing a combined treatment with interferon-α (IFN-α) and ponatinib. It is considered that DMR can be maintained by the combination of the two-way action of IFN-α, that is, the transfer of dormant CML stem cells to the cellcycle and the activation of a specific immune response to CML cells. This clinical result suggests the possibility of the re-emergence of IFN-α, which has been used a therapeutic drug in the past.

1. Introduction

Long-term survival in patients with chronic myelogenous leukemia (CML) was not possible to achieve until the introduction of tyrosine kinase inhibitor (TKI) therapy. Until the era of TKI treatment, allogeneic hematopoietic stem cell transplantation (allo-SCT) and interferon-α (IFN-α) therapy were the available treatment options; however, they were successful only in a limited number of people. TKIs have significantly improved survival outcomes in CML patients [1], and the possibility to discontinue TKI treatment for successful cases without recurrence has been recently explored [2, 3]. However, there are some CML patients who do not achieve a deep molecular response (DMR) and they have to continue TKI therapy in spite of various side effects. In the case of de novo blast crisis, it is much more difficult to achieve MRD [4]. Although allo-SCT can be selected as a treatment mode, it is associated with high risks and is generally not indicated for older patients. For patients with chronic phase CML (CML-CP) who cannot obtain optimal response, some investigators were using a combination of IFN-α and TKI for treatment [5, 6]. Through this combination treatment, they have succeeded in obtaining a durable DMR [7]. In this report, we present a case of a patient with de novo blast crisis treated with the same combination after the chemotherapy to obtain early DMR and maintain a stable condition. This combination of IFN-α and TKI suggests the possibility of a resurgence of IFN-α in the treatment of CML.

2. Case Presentation

A 68-year-old man was referred to our hospital, who presented with fever and loss of appetite. His routine annual

TABLE 1: Laboratory findings on admission.

Peripheral blood	
WBC	25, 200/μl
Blast	78%
Stab	0%
Seg	1%
Lymph	20%
Mono	0%
Eo	1%
Baso	0%
RBC	220 × 10e4/μl
Hb	7.1 g/dl
Ht	20.90%
Plt	2.2 × 10e4/μl
NAP-R	89% (61~99)
NAP-S	381 (170~355)
Coagulation	
PT	13.3 sec
APTT	34.8 sec
Fibrinogen	321 mg/dl
FDP	3.5 μg/μl
D-dimer	1.2 μg/ml
AT-III	110%
Biochemistry	
TP	7.0 g/dl
Alb	3.9 g/dl
Tbili	0.4 mg/dl
Dbili	0.1 mg/dl
AST	21 U/l
ALT	23 U/l
LDH	248 U/l
γGTP	75 U/l
BUN	14.7 mg/dl
Cr	0.93 mg/dl
UA	5.4 mg/dl
eGFR	62.5 ml/min
Glu	71 mg/dl
CRP	1.8 mg/dl
Ferritin	1011.6 ng/ml
Bone marrow	
NCC	28.8 × 10e4/μl
Mgk	+
Blast	98.80%
M/E	165
G-Band karyotype of bone marrow	
46, XY, t(9; 22) (q34; q11.2) [16]	
46, XY [4]	
BCR-ABL1 transcripts	
Major BCR-ABL1 18 × 10e5, HLA-DR+	
Immunophenotype of blasts in bone marrow	
CD34+, HLA = DR+, MPO−, CD3−, TdT+, CD19+, CD79a+, CD13±	

Abbreviation: WBC, white blood cells; blast, myeloblast; myelo, myelocytes; meta, metamyelocytes; stab, stab cells; seg, segmented cells; lym, lymphocytes; mono, monocytes; eo, eosinophiles; baso, basophiles; Hb, hemoglobin; Ht, hematocrit; Plt, platelet; NAP-rate, neutrophil alkaline phosphatase activities-rate; NAT-score, neutrophil alkaline phosphatase activities-score; NCC, nuclear cell counts; Mgk, megakaryocytes; M/E, myeloid erythroid ratio; PT, prothrombin time; APTT, activated partial thromboplastin time; FDP, fibrin/fibrinogen degradation product; AT-III, antithrombin-III.

health checkup results were normal and he had no history of an illness that required hospitalization. He had developed fever and cough approximately 10 days previously and had been treated by a doctor nearby. However, a blood test revealed a high white blood cell count of 25, 000/μl and he was advised to visit our hospital. Laboratory test results on admission are shown in Table 1. Although he was suspected of having Philadelphia chromosome-positive acute lymphoid leukemia, the diagnosis of de novo lymphoid blast crisis CML was confirmed based on the results of the

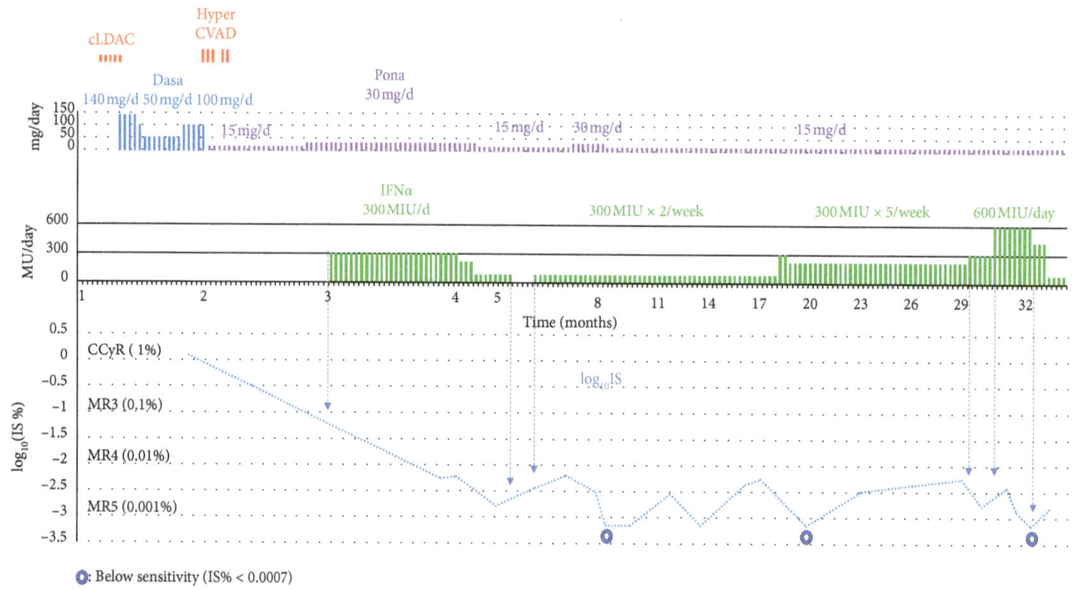

Figure 1: Clinical course of de novo blast crisis. Abbreviation: Nilo, nilotinib; Dasa, dasatinib; Pona, ponatinib; cLDAC, continuous infusion of low dose cytarabine (AraC); Hyper CVAD, hyperfractionated cyclophosphamide, vincristine, doxorubicin (adriacin), and dexamethasone.

examinations. In the immunophenotypic data, blasts strongly expressed HLA-DR, CD34, CD19, CD10, and CD79a. The breakpoint was found in the major BCR, and the minor breakpoint region associated with Ph chromosome positive acute lymphoblastic leukemia was not detected. Dasatinib was initiated as the first-line therapy with a continuous low-dose cytarabine, but there was no hematological effect. The chemotherapy regimen was changed to the reduced doses of cyclophosphamide, vincristine, doxorubicin (adriacin), and dexamethasone (Hyper CVAD) with ponatinib 15 mg/day [6, 8]. Hematological remission was obtained on day 40 of this treatment. At that time, the bone marrow nucleated cell count was $1.1 \times 10^4/\mu l$ and the proportion of blast cells was 1.4%, while the major BCR-ABL1 mRNA was 94×10^3 copies/μg. After the chemotherapy with Hyper CVAD, white blood cells were less than 1000/μl for 20 days and neutrocytes were less than 500/μl for 22 days during which time endogenous infection was complicated even under antibiotic treatment. In order to avoid worsening infectious diseases of febrile neutropenia, the chemotherapy was discontinued and treatment was changed to a combination of ponatinib 30 mg/day and IFN-α (300 MIU/day). In one month, the IS-PCR value was decreased to 0.0056% (MR4). The dose of ponatinib was reduced to 15 mg/day and IFN-α was continued at 300 MIU/day twice a week; after that, the IS-PCR value was decreased further to 0.0016%. When IFN-α was discontinued, the IS-PCR value was increased to 0.0064%. When IFN-α 300 MIU/day was restarted twice a week, the IS-PCR value was decreased to 0.0007% after 4.5 months and it fell below the detection sensitivity limit after another 4 months. The IS-PCR value was not stable and was increased again to 0.0055% after 3 months. When the dose of IFN-α was increased to 300 MIU/day five days a week, the IS-PCR value fell below the detection sensitivity in 2 months. Frequent measurements of the BCR-ABL1 transcript revealed fluctuations in its values, and IFN-α suppressed it and reduced the width of fluctuations in a dose-dependent manner. The course of treatment and the transition of IS% are shown in Figure 1. Because the de novo blast crises in older patients are maladapted for stem cell transplantation, such a deep molecular genetic response of BCR-ABL1 to INF-α is a great way to obtain a better prognosis.

3. Discussion

In the present case of the de novo lymphoid crisis in older patient, we succeeded to suppress the fluctuations in IS values and maintain DMR using the treatment of ponatinib combined with IFN-α. IFN-α therapy has become less commonly used with the advent of TKIs, but some studies suggested the possible effective use of IFN-α. In the Stop Imatinib (STIM) study, which first investigated the discontinuation of TKIs, having a history of IFN-α treatment was one of the prognostic factors that enhanced treatment-free response (TFR) [9]. The German CML and Scandinavian CML research groups have shown that a mode of combination treatment with IFN-α could elicit a faster and deeper response in high-risk CML patients than treatment with imatinib alone. These studies suggested that IFN-α provided clinical benefits [10].

TKIs have the effect of inactivating Ph-positive leukemia cells and inducing apoptosis but cannot eliminate these cells directly [3]. IFN-α acts on dormant leukemia stem cells, which cause the relapse, and recruits them into the cell cycle to be affected by TKI and further regulates gene expression in CML cells or induces cytotoxic T cells and natural killer cells [11]. Due to the synergistic effect of these various actions, the combined treatment of ponatinib and IFN-α is thought to suppress the progression of the disease. As observed in our case, the efficacy of IFN-α appears to be dose-dependent, but detailed studies to establish the optimal dosage and treatment duration of IFN-α are needed in the future.

Consent

IFN-α and ponatinib have been approved for the treatment of CML. Since no direct study of this combination treatment has been conducted, we obtained the approval of the ethics committee in our hospital and explained the need for this treatment to the patient and received his consent.

References

[1] B. J. Druker, F. Guilhot, S. G. O'Brien et al., "Five-year follow-up of patients receiving imatinib for chronic myeloid leukemia," *New England Journal of Medicine*, vol. 355, no. 23, pp. 2408–2417, 2006.

[2] E. Jabbour, "Chronic myeloid leukemia: first-line drug of choice," *American Journal of Hematology*, vol. 91, no. 1, pp. 59–66, 2016.

[3] A. Hochhaus, M. Baccarani, R. T. Silver et al., "European leukemianet 2020 recommendations for treating chronic myeloid leukemia," *Leukemia*, vol. 34, no. 4, pp. 966–984, 2020.

[4] P. Jain, H. M. Kantarjian, A. Ghorab et al., "Prognostic factors and survival outcomes in patients with chronic myeloid leukemia in blast phase in the tyrosine kinase inhibitor era: cohort study of 477 patients," *Cancer*, vol. 123, no. 22, pp. 4391–4402, 2017.

[5] V. Polivkova, P. Rohon, H. Klamova et al., "Interferon-α revisited: individualized treatment management eased the selective pressure of tyrosine kinase inhibitors on BCR-ABL1 mutations resulting in a molecular response in high-risk CML patients," *PLoS One*, vol. 11, no. 5, Article ID e0155959, 2016.

[6] Y. Motomura, K. Arai, K. Yoshifuji et al., "Chronic myeloid leukemia harboring T315I and F317L mutations successfully treated with interferon-α and ponatinib," *Rinsho Ketsueki*, vol. 60, no. 1, pp. 33–38, 2019.

[7] C. Cumbo, L. Anelli, G. Specchia, and F. Albano, "Monitoring of minimal residual disease (MRD) in chronic myeloid leukemia: recent advances," *Cancer Management and Research*, vol. 12, pp. 3175–3189, 2020.

[8] K. Sasaki, E. J. Jabbour, F. Ravandi et al., "Hyper-CVAD plus ponatinib versus hyper-CVAD plus dasatinib as frontline therapy for patients with Philadelphia chromosome-positive acute lymphoblastic leukemia: a propensity score analysis," *Cancer*, vol. 122, no. 23, pp. 3650–3656, 2016.

[9] F.-X. Mahon, D. Réa, J. Guilhot et al., "Discontinuation of imatinib in patients with chronic myeloid leukaemia who have maintained complete molecular remission for at least 2 years: the prospective, multicentre stop imatinib (STIM) trial," *The Lancet Oncology*, vol. 11, no. 11, pp. 1029–1035, 2010.

[10] P. E. Westerweel and P. A. W. te Boekhorst, "New approaches and treatment combinations for the management of chronic myeloid leukemia," *Frontiers in Oncology*, vol. 9, pp. 1–7, 2019.

[11] M. Talpaz, R. Hehlmann, A. Quintás-Cardama, J. Mercer, and J. Cortes, "Re-emergence of interferon-α in the treatment of chronic myeloid leukemia," *Leukemia*, vol. 27, no. 4, pp. 803–812, 2013.

7

Sézary Syndrome with CD4/CD8 Double-Negative Neoplastic T Cells in Peripheral Blood

Yuki Kageyama[1,2] **Kenshiro Tsuda,**[3] **Yuma Nato,**[1] **Keiki Nagaharu**[2] **Kazutaka Suzuki,**[1] **Akihiko Sawaki,**[1] **and Hiroyuki Miyashita**[1]

[1]*Department of Hematology, Yokkaichi Municipal Hospital, 2-2-37 Shibata, Yokkaichi 510-8567, Japan*
[2]*Department of Hematology and Oncology, Mie University Graduate School of Medicine, 2-174 Edobashi, Tsu 514-8507, Japan*
[3]*Department of Dermatology, Yokkaichi Municipal Hospital, 2-2-37 Shibata, Yokkaichi 510-8567, Japan*

Correspondence should be addressed to Yuki Kageyama; ykageyama@clin.medic.mie-u.ac.jp

Academic Editor: Kostas Konstantopoulos

Sézary syndrome is a rare leukemic type of cutaneous T-cell lymphoma characterized by the presence of neoplastic T cells with cerebriform nuclei (Sézary cells) in the skin, lymph nodes, and peripheral blood. Typical Sézary cells have a $CD3^+CD4^+CD8^-$ phenotype; however, in cases of the aberrant loss of antigens on Sézary cells, especially the loss of critically important T-cell antigens such as CD4, there is a possibility of misdiagnosing the disease or underestimating the tumor burden of the disease. Here, we report a rare case of Sézary syndrome with CD4/CD8 double-negative Sézary cells in the peripheral blood. Most of the Sézary cells in the peripheral blood had lost CD4 expression, and we diagnosed the disease and evaluated the tumor burden by multicolor flow cytometry. Intriguingly, the Sézary cells showed a typical $CD4^+CD8^-CD7^-$ phenotype in the skin even though the cells in the peripheral blood lacked CD4. The patient responded well to treatment with bexarotene and narrow-band ultraviolet B therapy. Analysis by multicolor flow cytometry is essential to diagnose this rare type of Sézary syndrome and evaluate the tumor burden.

1. Introduction

Sézary syndrome (SS) is a rare leukemic type of cutaneous T-cell lymphoma defined by erythroderma, generalized lymphadenopathy, and the presence of neoplastic T cells with cerebriform nuclei (Sézary cells) in the skin, lymph nodes, and peripheral blood (PB) [1]. In addition to demonstrating clonally related neoplastic T cells in the skin and PB, one or more of the following criteria are required to diagnose SS: an absolute Sézary cell count $\geq 1{,}000/\mu L$; an expanded $CD4^+$ T-cell population resulting in a CD4 : CD8 ratio of ≥10; or the loss of one or more T-cell antigens. Because of the morphologic heterogeneity of Sézary cells, flow cytometric analysis of PB is essential for diagnostic purposes and tumor burden monitoring during follow-up [2, 3]. Typical Sézary cells have a $CD3^+CD4^+CD8^-$ phenotype and characteristically lack CD7 and CD26 [4]. In cases with an aberrant loss of CD4 on Sézary cells, it is difficult to diagnose the disease and to evaluate the tumor burden using routine flow cytometric analysis. In this article, we report a rare case of SS with $CD4^-CD8^-$ Sézary cells in PB detected by multicolor flow cytometry.

2. Case Presentation

An 82-year-old woman presented to our hospital because of erythroderma with scattered invasive erythemas, nodules, and tumors on the face, trunk, and extremities (Figure 1). PB analysis revealed a white blood cell count of $14{,}730/\mu L$ (reference range, $3.3–8.6 \times 10^3/\mu L$), with 28% abnormal cells containing cerebriform nuclei (Figure 2), a hemoglobin level of 12.2 g/dL (11.6–14.8 g/dL), and a platelet count of $311 \times 10^3/\mu L$ ($158–348 \times 10^3/\mu L$). The blood levels of lactate dehydrogenase and soluble interleukin-2 receptor were 362 IU/L (124–224 IU/L) and 2,139 U/mL (122–496 U/mL), respectively. A serologic test for human T-cell leukemia

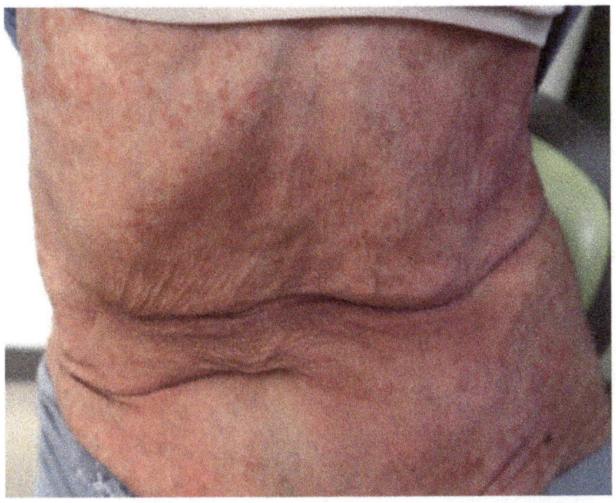

Figure 1: Image of the patient's chest and abdomen with erythroderma.

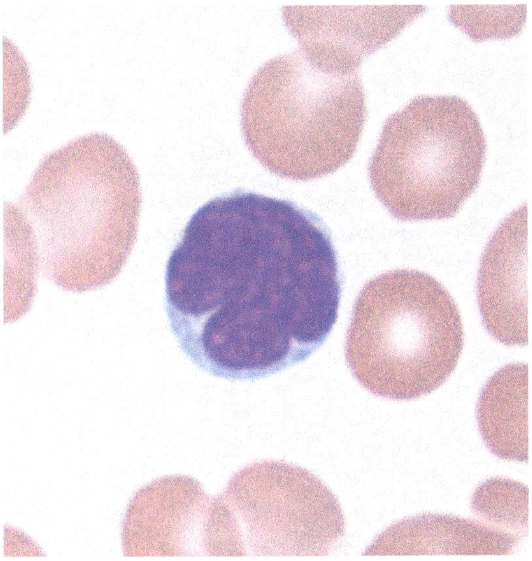

Figure 2: May–Giemsa staining of a blood smear showing abnormal cells with cerebriform nuclei (×1,000).

virus type 1 was negative. Computed tomography revealed no lymphadenopathy or hepatosplenomegaly. Skin biopsy specimens from a tumor on the left arm showed the infiltration of abnormal lymphocytes with medium- to large-sized nuclei containing convolutions in the superficial dermis (Figure 3). Immunohistochemical staining of skin biopsy specimens revealed abnormal lymphocytes expressing CD3 and CD4, but not CD7, CD8, CD20, or CD30. Despite approximately 30% of leukocytes in PB being morphologically abnormal, a small percentage of PB cells expressed CD4, and the CD4 : CD8 ratio analyzed by conventional two-color flow cytometry was 1.7.

Next, we performed a detailed phenotypical analysis by multicolor flow cytometry using a BD LSRFortessa™ cell analyzer (BD Biosciences, Franklin Lakes, NJ, USA). Among $CD3^+$ T cells, 84.0% were $CD4^-CD8^-$, 10.8% were $CD4^+CD8^-$, and 4.8% were $CD4^-CD8^+$ (Figure 4). $CD4^+CD8^-$ T cells expressed CD7 and/or CD26 similar to normal helper T cells, whereas $CD4^-CD8^-$ T cells had a diminished expression of CD7 and lacked CD26 expression, consistent with the Sézary cell phenotype. T-cell receptor (TCR) β-chain gene clonality assays were performed in the PB and skin samples in accordance with the BIOMED-2 guidelines of polymerase chain reaction- (PCR-) based immunoglobulin/TCR clonality testing (performed by SRL, Inc., Tokyo, Japan) [5]. Both PB and skin samples showed a clonal peak in $V\beta + J\beta 1/2$ and $D\beta + J\beta 1/2$, and the size of those PCR products was completely matched between both specimens as 273 bp in $V\beta + J\beta 1/2$ and 296 bp in $D\beta + J\beta 1/2$ (Figure 5). The results suggested that tumor cells in PB and skin were clonally identical, consistent with the pathological definition of SS.

Based on these clinical, histopathological, immunohistochemical, and genetic features, this case was diagnosed as stage IVA1 (T4N0M0B2) SS according to the International Society for Cutaneous Lymphoma/European Organization for Research and Treatment of Cancer system. The patient was treated with bexarotene and narrow-band ultraviolet B therapy, which effectively reduced the cutaneous lesions and PB involvement. The best global response of the disease was a partial response based on the proposed response criteria [6]. The patient has been under this treatment for more than 9 months.

3. Discussion

In SS, the aberrant loss of T-cell antigens is frequently observed. The loss of CD7 and/or CD26 on neoplastic T cells is sensitive and highly specific for SS [7]. The slightly dim expression of CD4 on Sézary cells was reported in a case series [3]; however, $CD4^-$ Sézary cells have rarely been described. A previous study reported a case of SS where 66% of the $CD3^+$ fraction was $CD4^-CD8^-$ Sézary cells [3]. Unlike our case, the Sézary cells expressed CD7 and partially lacked CD26. Because the criteria for blood involvement including an absolute Sézary cell count ≥1,000/μL and a CD4 : CD8 ratio of ≥10 are greatly affected in cases where CD4 molecules are lost in the PB, it is difficult to diagnose SS using conventional flow cytometry. In such cases, the analysis of Sézary cells using multicolor flow cytometry is essential. Intriguingly, our case showed typical $CD4^+CD8^-CD7^-$ neoplastic cell invasion of the skin even though Sézary cells in PB lacked CD4. In addition, the results of PCR-based TCR β-chain gene rearrangement analyses suggested that tumor cells in skin and PB were clonally identical. Based on these findings, we were able to make a reliable diagnosis.

SS is an aggressive disease, with a 5-year overall survival rate of less than 40% [1,8]. Combination therapies with skin-directed and systemic therapies have been suggested as treatment regimens. We selected narrow-band ultraviolet B therapy as a skin-directed therapy and bexarotene, an oral retinoid, as systemic therapy. Although the patient responded well to the treatments, the potential relationship between the $CD4^-CD8^-$ phenotype and a good response to the treatment is unclear because of the scarcity of the disease. In mycosis fungoides, another subtype of cutaneous T-cell lymphoma, it was reported that patients with $CD4^-CD8^-$

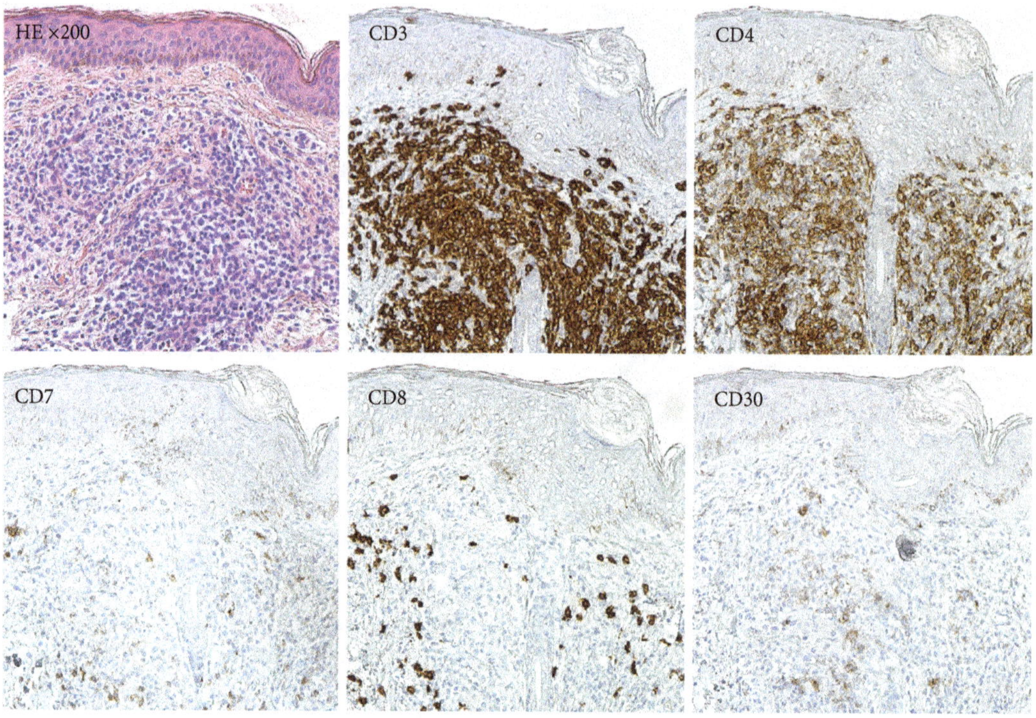

Figure 3: Hematoxylin-eosin (HE) staining and immunohistochemical staining of skin biopsy specimens (×200). HE staining shows the infiltration of abnormal lymphocytes in the superficial dermis (upper left). Immunohistochemical staining shows abnormal lymphocytes are positive for CD3 (upper middle) and CD4 (upper right), but negative for CD7 (lower left), CD8 (lower middle), and CD30 (lower right).

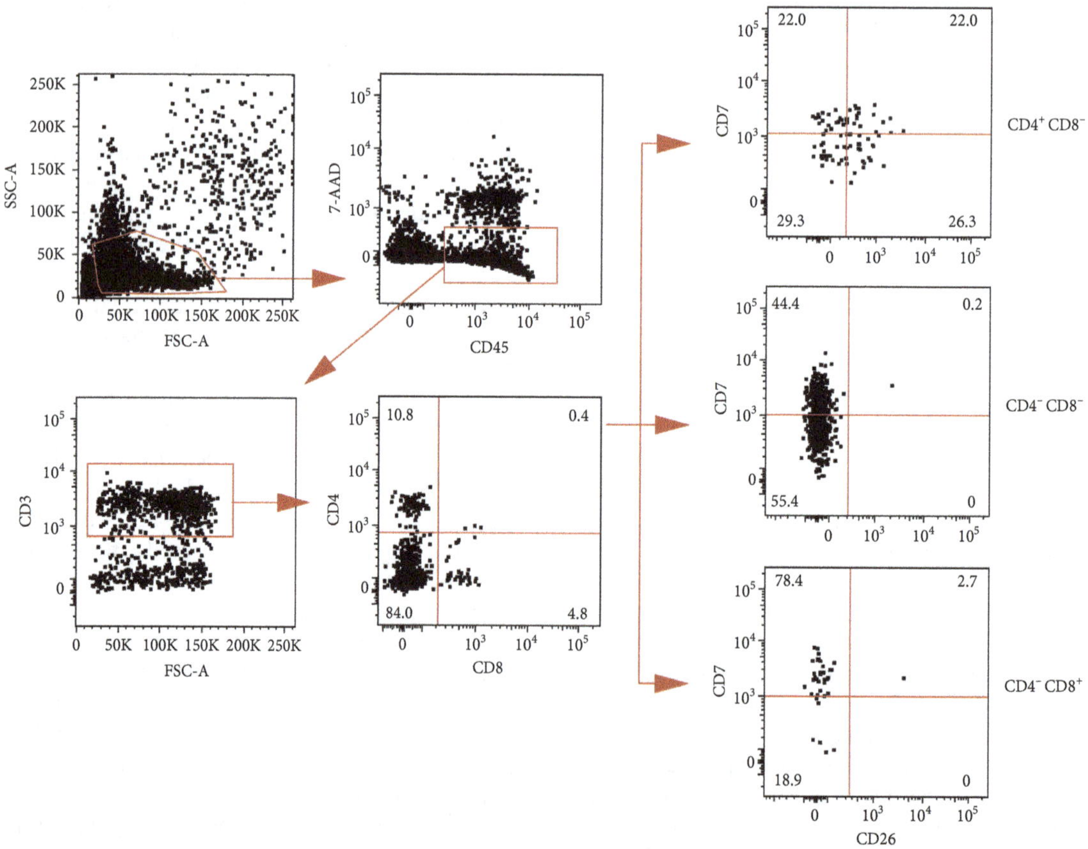

Figure 4: Results of multicolor flow cytometry of PB cells. After discriminating for dead cells and $CD45^-$ cells, the remaining cells were gated on $CD3^+$, and then three T-lymphocyte fractions, $CD4^+CD8^-$, $CD4^-CD8^-$, and $CD4^-CD8^+$, were analyzed for CD7 and CD26 expression. Percentages of each cell fraction are indicated in the plot areas. Abbreviations: FSC-A, forward scatter area; SSC-A, side scatter area; 7-AAD, 7-aminoactinomycin D.

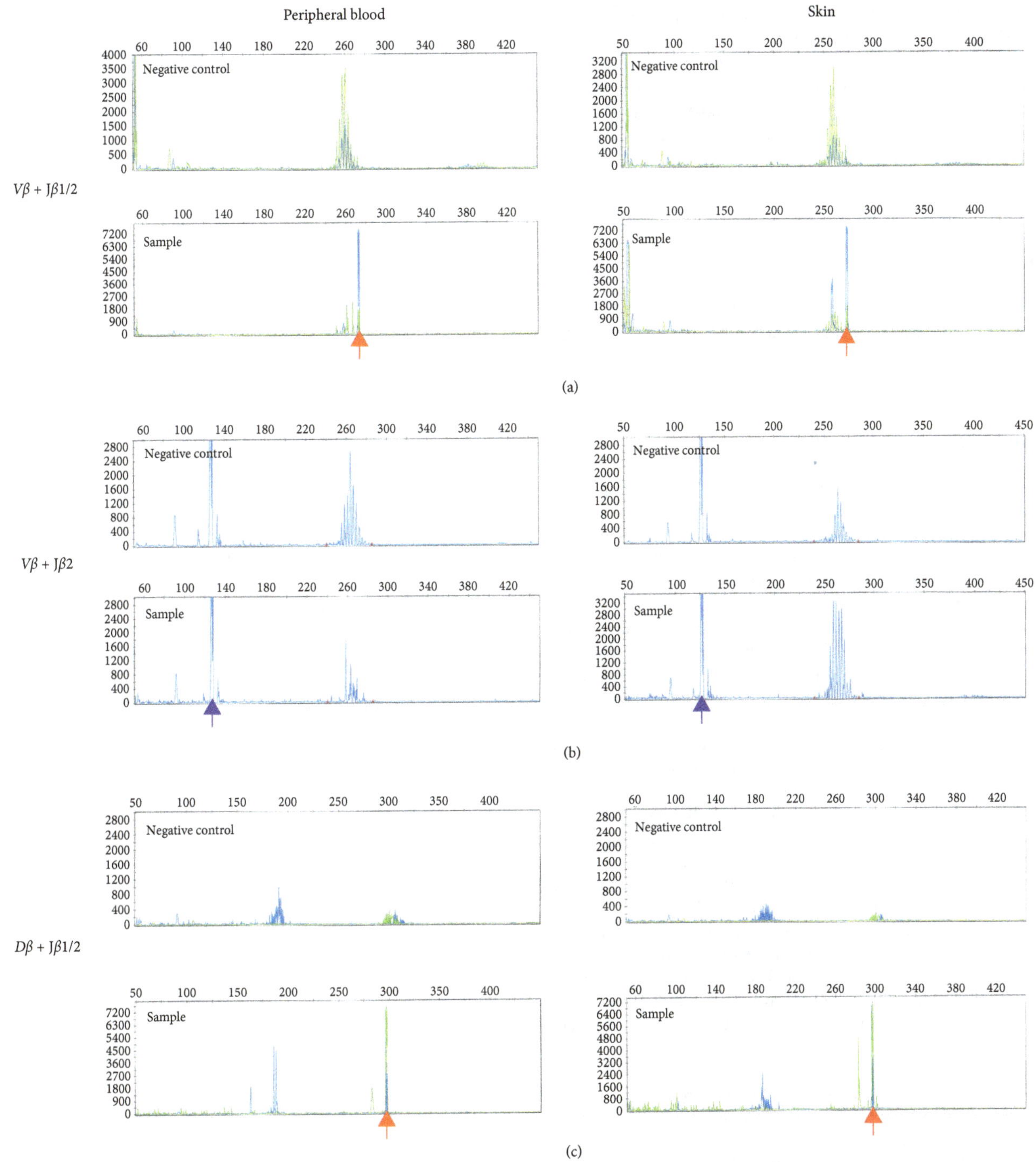

Figure 5: Results of TCR β-chain gene clonality assays. PCR products were produced and analyzed in accordance with the BIOMED-2 guidelines. The results of capillary electrophoresis of PCR products derived from PB (left) and skin (right) samples are shown. (a), (b), and (c) indicate the data of $V\beta + J\beta 1/2$, $V\beta + J\beta 2$, and $D\beta + J\beta 1/2$, respectively. In each figure, an upper figure shows data from negative control and a lower shows data from sample. The vertical line shows fluorescence intensity, the horizontal line shows fragment size, red arrows show clonal peak, and blue arrows show non-specific peak.

tumor cells had an indolent clinical course typical of patients harboring $CD4^+$ tumor cells [9].

In conclusion, $CD4^-CD8^-$ SS is a rare immunophenotype of SS. Analysis by multicolor flow cytometry was essential to diagnose the disease and evaluate the tumor burden. Further studies are needed to clarify the pathogenesis and prognosis of $CD4^-CD8^-$ SS.

Acknowledgments

We thank J. Ludovic Croxford, PhD, from Edanz Group (https://en-author-services.edanz.com/ac) for editing a draft of this manuscript.

References

[1] R. Willemze, L. Cerroni, W. Kempf et al., "The 2018 update of the WHO-EORTC classification for primary cutaneous lymphomas," *Blood*, vol. 133, no. 16, pp. 1703–1714, 2019.

[2] M. Novelli, P. Fava, C. Sarda et al., "Blood flow cytometry in Sézary syndrome," *American Journal of Clinical Pathology*, vol. 143, no. 1, pp. 57–69, 2015.

[3] P. Horna, S. A. Wang, K. L. Wolniak et al., "Flow cytometric evaluation of peripheral blood for suspected Sézary syndrome or mycosis fungoides: International guidelines for assay characteristics," *Cytometry Part B: Clinical Cytometry*, 2020.

[4] A. C. Hristov, E. C. Vonderheid, and M. J. Borowitz, "Simplified flow cytometric assessment in mycosis fungoides and Sézary syndrome," *American Journal of Clinical Pathology*, vol. 136, no. 6, pp. 944–953, 2011.

[5] A. W. Langerak, P. J. T. A. Groenen, M. Brüggemann et al., "EuroClonality/BIOMED-2 guidelines for interpretation and reporting of Ig/TCR clonality testing in suspected lymphoproliferations," *Leukemia*, vol. 26, no. 10, pp. 2159–2171, 2012.

[6] E. A. Olsen, S. Whittaker, Y. H. Kim et al., "Clinical end points and response criteria in mycosis fungoides and Sézary syndrome: a consensus statement of the international society for cutaneous lymphomas, the United States cutaneous lymphoma consortium, and the cutaneous lymphoma task force of the European organisation for Research and treatment of cancer," *Journal of Clinical Oncology*, vol. 29, no. 18, pp. 2598–2607, 2011.

[7] S. E. Boonk, W. H. Zoutman, A. Marie-Cardine et al., "Evaluation of immunophenotypic and molecular biomarkers for Sézary syndrome using standard operating procedures: a multicenter study of 59 patients," *Journal of Investigative Dermatology*, vol. 136, no. 7, pp. 1364–1372, 2016.

[8] J. J. Scarisbrick, H. M. Prince, M. H. Vermeer et al., "Cutaneous lymphoma international consortium study of outcome in advanced stages of mycosis fungoides and Sézary syndrome: effect of specific prognostic markers on survival and development of a prognostic model," *Journal of Clinical Oncology*, vol. 33, pp. 3766–3773, 2015.

[9] E. Hodak, M. David, L. Maron, A. Aviram, E. Kaganovsky, and M. Feinmesser, "CD4/CD8 double-negative epidermotropic cutaneous T-cell lymphoma: an immunohistochemical variant of mycosis fungoides," *Journal of the American Academy of Dermatology*, vol. 55, no. 2, pp. 276–284, 2006.

8

Autoimmune Hemolytic Anemia as Presenting Symptom of Hodgkin Lymphoma

Nicholas B. Burley,[1] Paul S. Dy,[1] Suraj Hande,[1] Shreyas Kalantri,[1] Chirayu Mohindroo,[1] and Kenneth Miller[2]

[1]*Department of Internal Medicine, Sinai Hospital of Baltimore, Baltimore, MD, USA*
[2]*Department of Hematology/Oncology, Sinai Hospital of Baltimore, Baltimore, MD, USA*

Correspondence should be addressed to Nicholas B. Burley; nburley@lifebridgehealth.org

Academic Editor: Saveria Capria

Autoimmune hemolytic anemia (AIHA) is related to an underlying condition in an estimated 50 to 60%, while the remaining is idiopathic, as a result of a combination of immune activation, deficiency, or dysregulation. AIHA is associated with viral infections, autoimmune disorders, immunodeficiencies, lymphoproliferative disorders, and pregnancy. AIHA has predictive properties and may be a harbinger of future lymphoproliferative disorders in up to 20% of AIHA cases. Autoimmune hemolytic anemia (AIHA) has been associated with lymphoproliferative disorders particularly chronic lymphocytic leukemia and non-Hodgkin lymphoma. Rarely is it seen in Hodgkin disease. In the following report, we describe the presentation of AIHA, ultimately resulting in the diagnosis of nodular sclerosis Hodgkin lymphoma (stage III). From the limited reports and reviews available, it is understood that advanced Hodgkin (stage III or IV) of nodular sclerosis (NS) or mixed cellularity (MC) types portend a stronger affiliation to AIHA. The majority of AIHA-associated Hodgkin lymphoma presents as stage III or IV disease with the hemolysis being the presenting symptom, as in this case. The mainstay of AIHA therapy has been corticosteroids; however, this first-line regimen appears to be less effective when treating AIHA in the setting of HL. The exact mechanism of AIHA related to HL is unclear, and it may be thought to be that tumor cell produced autoantibodies. Other hypotheses include paraneoplastic phenomena or more, perhaps immunity to tumor cells may cross-react with antigens on the red cells. Although these mechanisms require further investigation, the relationship of the AIHA and HL represents a piece to a larger puzzle between autoimmune disorders and lymphoproliferative conditions.

1. Introduction

The etiology of autoimmune hemolytic anemia (AIHA) is related to an underlying condition in an estimated 50 to 60%, while the remaining is idiopathic, as a result of a combination of immune activation, deficiency, or dysregulation [1]. AIHA is associated with viral infections, autoimmune disorders, immunodeficiencies, lymphoproliferative disorders, and pregnancy. This group of AIHA disorders can be related to autoimmune lymphoproliferative syndrome (ALPS), chronic lymphocytic leukemia (CLL), lymphoma, and clot agglutinin-related disease. AIHA has predictive properties and may be a harbinger of future lymphoproliferative disorders in AIHA cases [2]. While AIHA has well-known associations with non-Hodgkin lymphoma, its relationship to Hodgkin lymphoma is rare and potentially less recognized. Limited reports and reviews suggest that NS, MC, and stages III and IV HL are more commonly associated with AIHA [3]. AIHA may be the presenting symptom leading to the diagnosis of Hodgkin lymphoma

(HL). In the following report, we describe the presentation of AIHA ultimately resulting in the diagnosis of nodular sclerosis Hodgkin lymphoma (stage III).

1.1. Case Summary. A 20-year-old female college student with no medical comorbidities presented to the hospital with progressive presyncopal symptoms, exertional dyspnea, and fatigue that was worsening over the course of several months. She noted increased difficulty with exertion, particularly climbing several flights of stairs requiring several breaks to recover. At the time of presentation, she had worsened presyncope, diaphoresis, and severe generalized weakness. She reported no recent illness, travel, sick contacts, or high-risk behavior (i.e., sexual activity and intravenous drug use), except for occasional nonbinge drinking alcohol use.

On initial examination, she was found to have conjunctival pallor, left supraclavicular lymphadenopathy (measured 3-4 cm width), lower anterior cervical firm adenopathy (measured 3-4 cm width), left axillary fullness without discrete masses, and a palpable spleen tip below the costal margin.

Preliminary laboratory results revealed white blood cell count 1.73 K/mm^3, hemoglobin 4.6 mg/dL, hematocrit 15.7%, reticulocyte 9.9%, haptoglobin <20 mg/dL, total bilirubin 1.3 mg/dL, direct bilirubin 0.30 mg/dL, and lactate dehydrogenase 312 unit/L. White blood cell differentiation revealed reduced absolute lymphocyte count of 0.74 K/mm^3 although relatively increased differential of 44%. Additional laboratory studies included a positive direct Coombs test for warm A plasma, IgG and C3, and cold agglutinin positivity. Further autoimmune antibody screening tests were not pursued. Her erythropoietin level was elevated erythropoietin 579.1 milli units/ml. Folate and B12 levels were within normal limits. Free light chains kappa and lambda showed no monoclonal gammopathy. Serum protein electrophoresis showed no evidence of monoclonal protein in the gamma region. Urine protein electrophoresis was negative for monoclonal protein in the gamma region.

Computed tomography of thorax, abdomen, and pelvis demonstrated diffuse bulky adenopathy (see Figure 1), as well as splenomegaly and retroperitoneal adenopathy.

A core needle biopsy of the supraclavicular lymph node was performed, and pathologic evaluation demonstrated classical Hodgkin lymphoma with Reed–Sternberg cells expressing CD15 and CD30. Evaluation of the bone marrow demonstrated no evidence of Hodgkin lymphoma. After further imaging and biopsies, the patient was diagnosed with stage III classic Hodgkin lymphoma (nodular sclerosing) after the presenting symptom of warm autoimmune hemolytic anemia.

This patient's anemia was highly symptomatic. Multiple units of red cells were ordered but were delayed due to her multiple antibodies. After receiving blood, her symptoms significantly improved with repeat hemoglobin greater than 9.0 mg/dL. Patient's hemolysis was managed with intravenous methylprednisolone 1 mg/kg every 6 hours during her hospital stay lasting several days which was then tapered to oral prednisone 40 mg daily until the initiation of her chemotherapy regimen of Adriamycin, brentuximab-vedotin, vinblastine, and dacarbazine (A(BV)VD).

In the oncology clinic, after completing two cycles with A(BV)VD of a planned six cycles, the PET scan showed good response to treatment with a marked decrease in size and FDG uptake in the left neck and mediastinal nodes SUV max of 1.58 compared to pretreatment SUV max of 15.6. There were residual nodes in these regions having very low-level FDG activity equal to that of the mediastinal blood pool. No new site of disease was seen. With chemotherapy patient's hemolysis resolved, steroids were tapered and discontinued. Further re-evaluation of plasma IgG, C3, and cold agglutinin statuses were not pursued after chemotherapy given patient's excellent recovery.

At this time, the patient has completed six cycles of A(BV)VD with complete metabolic resolution and PET avidity resolution and is not recommended for radiation therapy. She is planned for ongoing surveillance.

2. Discussion

The majority of AIHA is related to an underlying etiology that alters immune system activity such infectious, autoimmune disorders, immunodeficiencies, lymphoproliferative disorders, and pregnancy. The lymphoproliferative disorders are comprised of diseases such as ALPS, CLL, non-Hodgkin lymphoma, and Hodgkin lymphoma [3–6]. While AIHA has well-known associations with non-Hodgkin lymphoma and CLL, its relationship to Hodgkin lymphoma is rarer and potentially less well recognized. In one German study, the incidence of AIHA in Hodgkin disease is 0.2% [7].

From the limited reviews, it is understood that advanced Hodgkin (stage III or IV) of nodular sclerosis (NS) or mixed cellularity (MC) types portend a stronger affiliation to AIHA [8, 9]. In these limited studies, some demographic associations have been identified including advanced age, male sex, and laboratory findings such as high reticulocyte count, high ESR, and low absolute lymphocyte count [10]. The most identified HL subtypes were nodular sclerosing and mixed cellularity subtypes [11]. Notably, there are been cases that indicate that tumor burden may not necessarily relate to the onset of AIHA [12]

In the limited reports of AIHA in HL, there is a potential for worsened prognostication although this may coincide with the typically late-presenting stage of the disease rather than the AIHA itself [13].

While anemia is commonly present in HL, approximately a third of cases, which is typically related to chronic inflammation, further investigation for other etiologies should be considered, especially in the setting of hemolysis.

The exact mechanism of AIHA related to HL is unclear, and it may be thought to be that tumor cell produced autoantibodies as the majority are direct antibodies testing positive [7]. Other hypotheses include paraneoplastic pathways or autoimmunity of antibodies targeting the tumor cells that also affect the red blood cells. Although these mechanisms require further investigation, the relationship of the AIHA and HL represents a piece to a larger puzzle

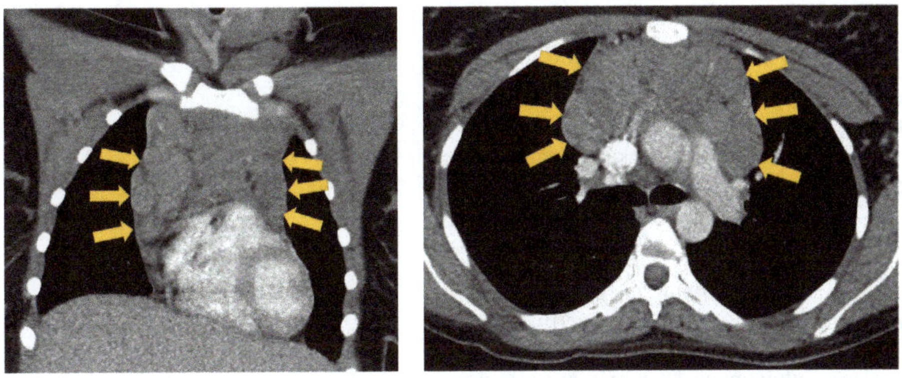

(a) (b)

Figure 1: CT thorax demonstrating multiple pathologically enlarged left supraclavicular lymph nodes associated with enlarged partially visualized left cervical lymph nodes. Mass effect on the left lobe of the thyroid gland and the trachea from the pathologically enlarged left supraclavicular lymph nodes. Pathologically enlarged lymph nodes throughout the anterior mediastinum. Enlarged right paratracheal lymph nodes as well. Pathologically enlarged left axillary and subpectoral lymph nodes as well.

between autoimmune disorders and lymphoproliferative conditions [3, 6, 14].

In very rare cases, HL-related AIHA may be direct antiglobulin test negative which may be attributed to undetectably low levels of IgG, low-affinity bound IgG antibodies are washed away during pretest processing, or non-IgG antibodies are the cause of the AIHA (e.g., IgA and IgM) [15].

The mainstay of AIHA has been corticosteroids; however, this first-line regimen appears to be less effective when treating AIHA in the setting of HL [10, 16]. In one single-center study, the use of rituximab, traditionally a second-line therapy, had significantly improved mortality rates compared to corticosteroids in those with warm AIHA and lymphoproliferative disease [16]. As seen in this case, treatment of the primary disease with combination chemotherapy led to treatment of AIHA. In very rare cases, splenectomy may be advocated as an effective therapy [17].

While there is much to be elucidated about the relationship between AIHA and HL, it is clear that further study must be done into the interactions of lymphoproliferative diseases, their effects on the immune system, and the development of autoimmune disorders. As we continue to develop foundational knowledge of these interactions, greater understanding of best treatments for AIHA in the setting of HL will aid in management of this complication and potentially reveal further mechanisms to research.

References

[1] W. Barcellini, B. Fattizzo, A. Zaninoni et al., "Clinical heterogeneity and predictors of outcome in primary autoimmune hemolytic anemia: a GIMEMA study of 308 patients," *Blood*, vol. 124, no. 19, pp. 2930–2936, 2014.

[2] S. Sallah, J. Y. Wan, and L. R. Hanrahan, "Future development of lymphoproliferative disorders in patients with autoimmune hemolytic anemia," *Clinical Cancer Research: An Official Journal of the American Association for Cancer Research*, vol. 7, no. 4, pp. 791–794, 2001.

[3] M. Ehrenfeld, M. Abu-Shakra, D. Buskila, and Y. Shoenfeld, "The dual association between lymphoma and autoimmunity," *Blood Cells, Molecules, and Diseases*, vol. 27, no. 4, pp. 750–756, 2001.

[4] A. J. Bowdler and I. W. Glick, "Autoimmune hemolytic anemia as the herald state of hodgkin's disease," *Annals of Internal Medicine*, vol. 65, no. 4, pp. 761-767, 1966.

[5] S. S. Shah, S. R. Khubchandani, R. S. Parikh et al., "Autoimmune hemolytic anemia IN hodgkin's lymphoma: a case report," *Hematology & Transfusion International Journal*, vol. 4, no. 6, pp. 145–147, 2017.

[6] Q. Feng, D. Zak, and R. Daya, "Autoimmune hemolytic anemia and classical Hodgkin lymphoma: a case report and literature review," *Clinical Advances in Hematology & Oncology: H&O*, vol. 10, no. 4, pp. 270–276, 2012.

[7] F. Ozdemir, M. Yilmaz, R. Akdogan et al., "Hodgkin's disease and autoimmune hemolytic anemia: a case report," *Medical Principles and Practice*, vol. 14, no. 3, pp. 205–207, 2005.

[8] M. B. Shah, V. Nanjapp, H. S. Devaraj, and K. S. Sindhu, "Autoimmune hemolytic anaemia in Hodgkin's lymphoma," *The Journal of the Association of Physicians of India*, vol. 61, no. 7, pp. 492–494, 2013.

[9] R. D. Sierra, "Coombs-positive hemolytic anemia in Hodgkin's disease: case presentation and review of the literature," *Military Medicine*, vol. 156, no. 12, pp. 691-692, 1991.

[10] M. Dimou, M. K. Angelopoulou, G. A. Pangalis et al., "Autoimmune hemolytic anemia and autoimmune thrombocytopenia at diagnosis and during follow-up of Hodgkin lymphoma," *Leukemia & Lymphoma*, vol. 53, no. 8, pp. 1481–1487, 2012.

[11] G. Majumdar, "Unremitting severe autoimmune haemolytic anaemia as a presenting feature of Hodgkin's disease with minimum tumour load," *Leuk Lymphoma*, vol. 20, no. 1-2, pp. 169–172, 1995.

[12] J. M. Andrieu, P. Youinou, and A. Marcelli, "Anémie hémolytique auto-immune associée à la maladie de Hodgkin. Caractéristiques, pronostic et incidence [Autoimmune haemolytic anaemia associated with Hodgkin's disease. Characteristics, prognosis and incidence (author's transl)]," *Nouv Presse Med*, vol. 10, no. 36, pp. 2951–2954, 1981, French. PMID: 7290949.

[13] S. Sallah, J. Y. Wan, and L. R. Hanrahan, "Future development of lymphoproliferative disorders in patients with autoimmune hemolytic anemia," *Clinical Cancer Research*, vol. 1, no. 7, pp. 791–794, 2001.

[14] J. Kühböck, P. Aiginger, P. Pötzi, and J. Smolen, "Hämolytische Anämie bei Morbus Hodgkin [Hemolytic anemia in Hodgkin's disease]," *Acta Med Austriaca*, vol. 6, no. 5, pp. 186–189, 1979.

[15] N. Siddiqui and A. Aleem, "Autoimmune haemolytic anaemia preceding the diagnosis of Hodgkin's disease: a report of two cases and review of the literature," *JPMA. The Journal of the Pakistan Medical Association*, vol. 59, no. 5, pp. 316–319, 2009.

[16] M. Roumier, V. Loustau, C. Guillaud et al., "Characteristics and outcome of warm autoimmune hemolytic anemia in adults: new insights based on a single-center experience with 60 patients," *American Journal of Hematology*, vol. 89, no. 9, pp. E150–E155, 2014 Sep.

[17] A. Bajpayee, A. Dubey, A. Verma, and R. K. Chaudhary, "A report of a rare case of autoimmune haemolytic anaemia in a patient with Hodgkin's disease in whom routine serology was negative," *Blood Transfusion*, vol. 12, pp. s299–301, 2014.

9

An Unusual Cause of Bleeding in a Patient with Chronic Myeloid Leukemia Chronic Phase

S. Kartthik,[1] Prakas K. Mandal,[2] and Saleh Mohammed Abdullah[3]

[1]*Department of Haematology-Oncology, GKNM Hospital, Coimbatore, Tamilnadu, India*
[2]*Department of Haematology, NRS Medical College and Hospital, Kolkata, West Bengal, India*
[3]*Department of Medical Laboratory, Faculty of Applied Medical Sciences, Jazan University, Jazan, Saudi Arabia*

Correspondence should be addressed to S. Kartthik; kartthiks@gmail.com

Academic Editor: Masayuki Nagasawa

Chronic myelogenous leukemia (CML) is a clonal myeloproliferative neoplasm (MPN) characterized by dysregulated and uncontrolled proliferation of mature and maturing granulocytes with normal differentiation. A genetic hallmark of CML is the presence of the fusion gene product BCR-ABL. Bleeding diathesis in CML patients is rare (<10%) and primarily caused by acquired platelet dysfunction. We report a rare case of an adult CML chronic phase patient who presented with spontaneous muscle hematoma due to acquired Glanzmann's thrombasthenia (GT). On laboratory workup, a GT was confirmed along with the diagnosis of CML in chronic phase. The muscle hematoma was completely resolved following imatinib therapy. The present case demonstrates that bleeding is a complication of MPNs and highlights the importance of both acquired GT diagnosis to determine the cause of bleeding in CML and of prompt treatment with imatinib to reverse this condition.

1. Introduction

Chronic myeloid leukemia (CML) is a clonal hematopoietic stem cell disorder driven by the BCR-ABL1 chimeric gene product and resulting from a reciprocal balanced translocation between the long arms of chromosomes 9 and 22, t(9;22), cytogenetically detected as the Philadelphia chromosome (Ph). Hemorrhagic manifestations are not uncommon in CML patients. Platelet dysfunction appears to be the primary cause of bleeding in patients with CML. Hemorrhagic manifestations typically resolve with treatment, suggesting that the platelet dysfunction is related to disease activity [1]. Acquired Glanzmann's thrombasthenia (GT) is a rare bleeding disorder characterized by abrupt onset of moderate-to-severe bleeding tendency and prolonged bleeding time but with normal platelet count and normal or reduced platelet glycoprotein (GP) expression. Acquired GT is an uncommon event in association with CML, and it may be caused by the formation of autoantibodies against the GPIIb/IIIa complex [2]. Nurden has reported that platelet glycoprotein dysfunction and signaling defects may occur in myeloproliferative neoplasms (MPNs), including CML [3].

We report a rare case of adult CML chronic phase in a patient who presented with spontaneous muscle hematoma due to acquired GT; however, due to constraints, glycoprotein expression was not measured. The present case demonstrates that bleeding is a complication of MPNs and emphasizes the importance of acquired GT diagnosis to identify the cause of bleeding in CML; furthermore, prompt treatment with imatinib can achieve a reversal of this condition.

2. Case Presentation

A 45-year-old married female patient presented with swelling in the right thigh and low-grade intermittent fever for the past month with no history of trauma. The patient had a history of two small hematomas in the right and left thigh region in the preceding 3 months that had resolved spontaneously. There was no family history of bleeding disorder, and she was not taking any prior medication. On

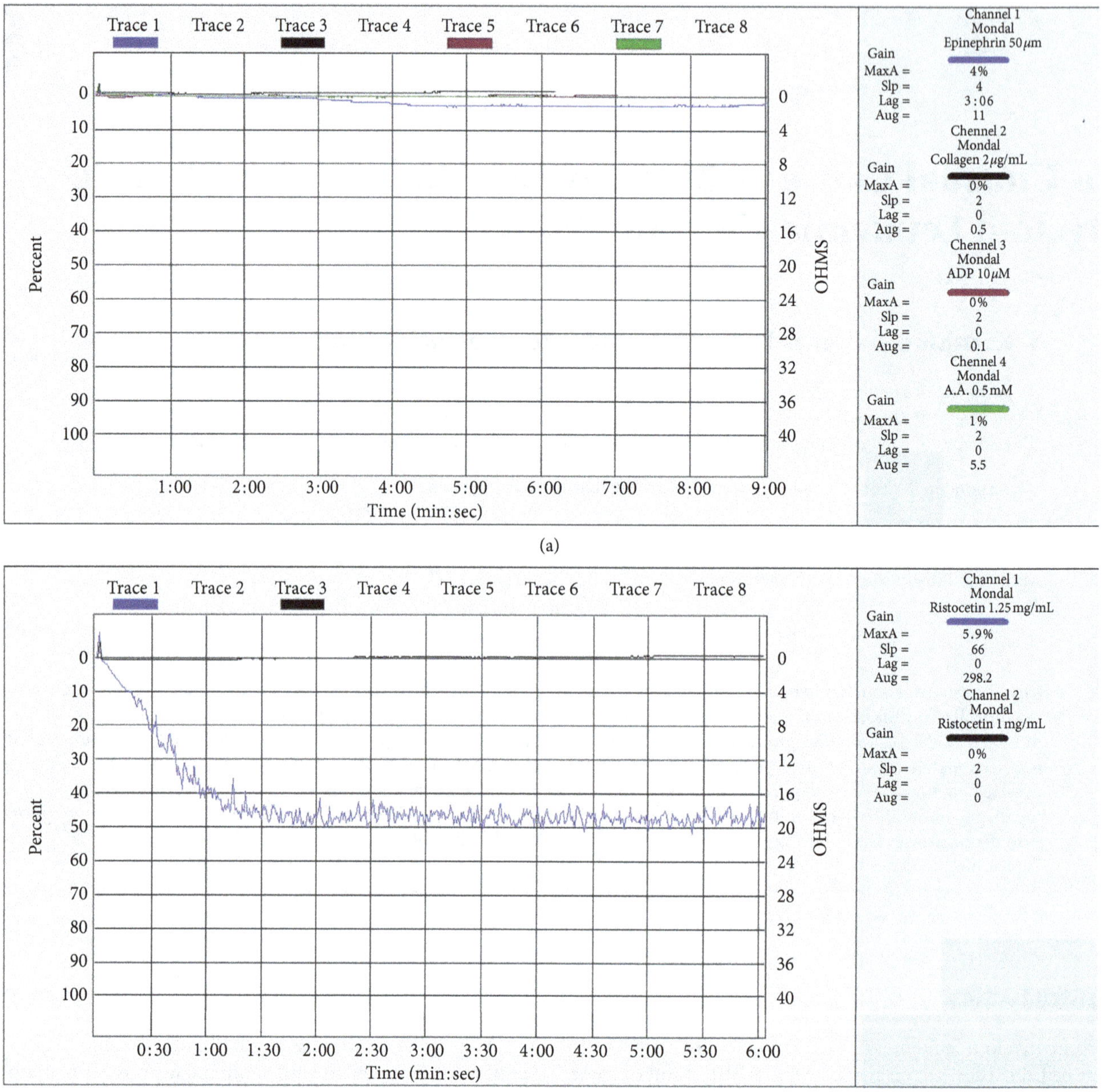

FIGURE 1: Platelet aggregation test by LTA at the time diagnosis. (a) Platelet aggregation test with collagen, ADP, thrombin, and arachidonic acid shows a complete absence of platelet aggregation. (b) Platelet aggregation test with ristocetin shows a normal response.

examination, she had normal vital status with mild pallor, mild hepatomegaly, and moderate splenomegaly. Ultrasonography of the abdomen showed hepatomegaly with a liver span of 16.1 cm and massive splenomegaly of 14 cm below the left costal margin, while ultrasonography of the right thigh showed extensive hematoma on the anterolateral aspect limited in the upper-mid region of both intramuscular and fascial planes.

Complete hemogram with peripheral blood smear showed Hb 8.5 gm/dl, hematocrit 20.0%, MCV 82.3 fl, MCH 35.0 pg, MCHC 42.5 gm/dl, platelet count $303 \times 10^3/\mu l$, and a very high leukocyte count of $193 \times 10^9/l$ with neutrophil 41%, lymphocyte 1%, basophil 2%, myelocyte 37%, metamyelocyte 14%, blast cell 5%, 4 nRBC/100 WBC, and reticulocyte count 4.9%. Bone marrow aspiration (BMA) revealed hypercellular marrow spaces with increased granulocytic precursors, basophils, and eosinophils. Chromosomal analysis of the BMA specimen showed 46 XX t(9; 22) (q34;q11.2) in 100% of the 20 metaphase cells examined. Reverse transcription real-time multiplex PCR was positive for the BCR-ABL1 fusion transcript p210. Based on the peripheral blood film, BMA findings, and molecular studies, a diagnosis of CML chronic phase was established.

Considering a bleeding diathesis in a CML patient, we then attempted to identify the etiology. The screening coagulation tests included bleeding time (BT) 14 min;

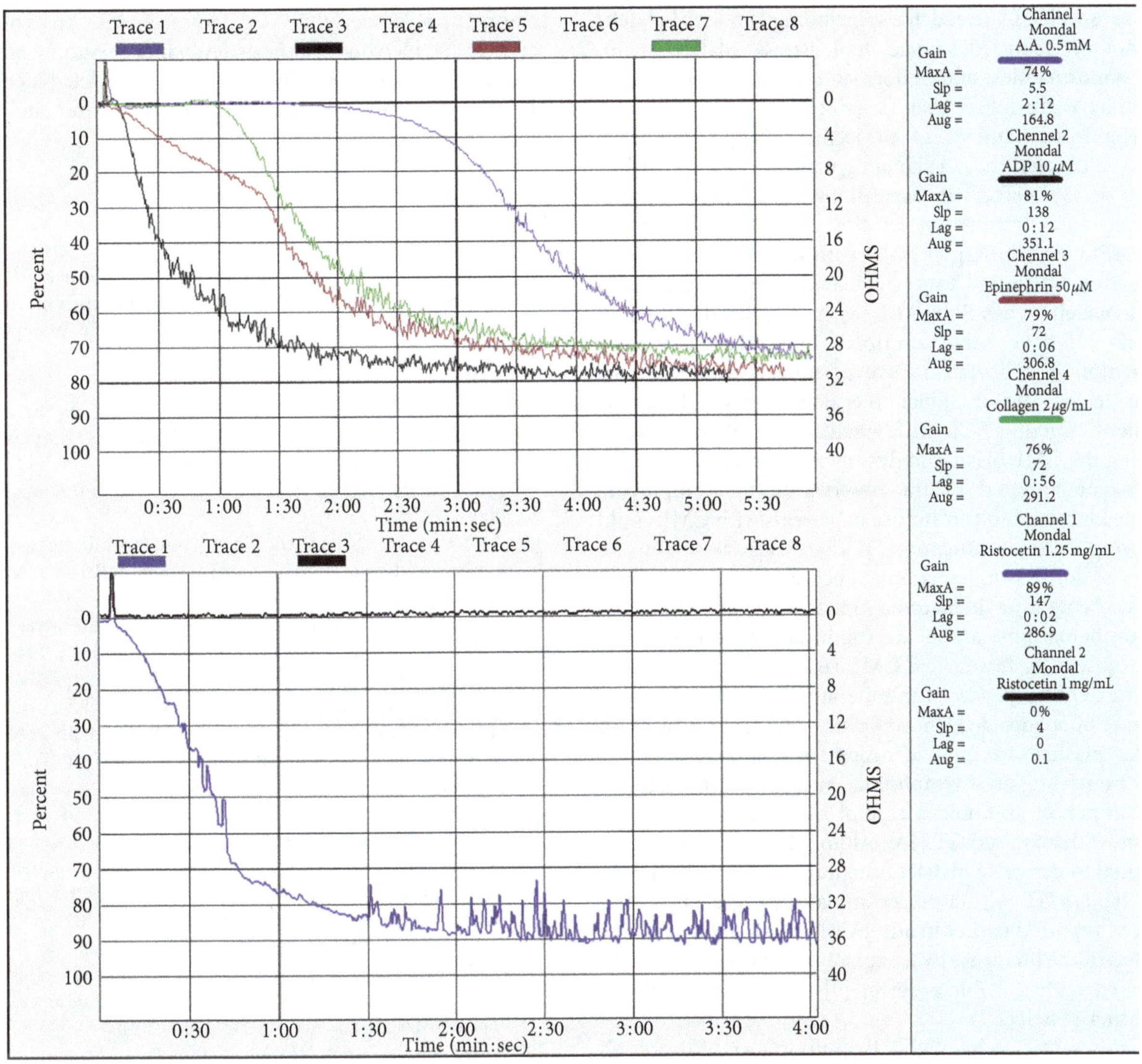

Figure 2: Platelet aggregation study by LTA at 3 months follow-up showing a normal response to all of the agonists.

prothrombin time (PT) 13 sec; activated partial thromboplastin time (aPTT) 29 sec, and fibrinogen level 260 mg/dl. She had normal PT, aPTT, and fibrinogen levels. The clot was insoluble at 37°C in 24 hr incubation, but her bleeding time was prolonged. A von Willebrand factor (vWF) assay was performed and showed a value >120%. Platelet function testing revealed no platelet aggregation with ADP (10 μM), epinephrine (50 μM), collagen (2 μg/mL), arachidonic acid (0.5 mM), and normal ristocetin aggregation (1.25 mg/mL and 0.5 mg/mL; Figure 1). The pattern of platelet aggregation response was suggestive of an acquired GT, such as a defect in a case of CML chronic phase. However, an ELISA (AssayMax™ Human GPIIb/IIIa ELISA Kit, Assaypro, St. Charles, MO) for anti-GPIIb/IIIa antibody titer was negative.

The patient was started on imatinib mesylate 400 mg once daily after obtaining the BCR-ABL report. Bleeding was managed initially with tranexamic acid and intranasal desmopressin. Detection of a GT-like condition did not change the course of management in this patient. Clinical reversal of bleeding was noted following imatinib therapy. After 1 month of therapy, the swelling completely disappeared. Her platelet function test, repeated after 3 months, showed normalization of response to all of the agonists (Figure 2). The patient attained major molecular response (MMR) at 3 months. This patient did not show any bleeding manifestation until the most recent follow-up (i.e., 18 months after MMR).

3. Discussion

A qualitative or quantitative defect—either congenital or acquired—of either GPIIb or GPIIIa is the essential biochemical basis for GT. GPIIb/IIIa is a calcium-dependent heterodimer that binds preferentially to fibrinogen or vWF, but it also binds to fibronectin or vitronectin. Consequently, GT is characterized by defective *in vitro* platelet aggregation and a lifelong bleeding tendency. Platelet dysfunction, whether in the form of platelet hypofunction or hyperfunction, in chronic myeloproliferative disorder is multifactorial in cause. Specific platelet defects, including abnormal platelet morphology, acquired storage pool disease, platelet membrane abnormalities, and abnormal arachidonic acid metabolism, have previously been described [4].

Several mechanisms of projecting GT phenotype in CML, such as defects in a signaling pathway vital for $\alpha IIb\beta 3$ activation [5], defects in activation-dependent inside-out signaling [6], dysfunction in the phosphatidylinositol-3 kinase (PI3 kinase)/Rap1/$\alpha IIb\beta 3$ pathway [7], poor platelet aggregation attributed to dysregulated tyrosine kinase activity associated with BCR-ABL [8], and reduced $\alpha IIb\beta 3$ on platelets [9] have been described. In CML, the platelet dysfunction is believed to have originated from a clonal expansion of dysfunctional megakaryocytes. Thus, the treatment targeting BCR-ABL would be equally effective in reducing the CML blasts and dysfunctional megakaryocytes. This is corroborated by the observation that employing tyrosine kinase inhibitors for use in patients with CML could improve platelet dysfunction [5]. There exist very few case reports of soft tissue hematoma, such as spontaneous mediastinal hematoma, hematoma in iliac psoas muscle, spinal epidural hematoma, and acute subdural hematoma, as the initial presenting features of CML [10–12].

An extensive review of the literature revealed that very few cases of acquired GT have been reported in association with neoplasms of lymphoid origin such as multiple myeloma, non-Hodgkin's lymphoma, and Hodgkin's disease [13]. Kannan et al. found a case of hairy cell leukemia associated with acquired GT [14]. Although bleeding diathesis attributed to defective platelet function is not uncommon in CML, typical GT (e.g., a defect in platelet aggregation) has not been reported earlier in adult CML. A singular case was reported in the literature by Chauhan et al. of pediatric CML associated with a GT-like defect [9] due to dysfunctional circulating platelets.

The present case highlights the importance of thorough investigation in a CML patient who presents with muscle hematoma and of using appropriate coagulation studies since acquired GT as a cause often remains underdiagnosed. Caution is warranted because imatinib itself has been reported to have a negative effect on platelet aggregation; it has been associated with bleeding diathesis. Hence, regular follow-up is needed after imatinib therapy to examine any clinical evidence of bleeding and monitor platelet function. This patient is on regular follow-up and did not manifest any bleeding until this visit.

In conclusion, our report demonstrates that soft tissue hematoma may be a presenting feature of CML due to platelet dysfunction. Poor platelet aggregation in this case is possibly attributed to dysregulated tyrosine kinase activity associated with BCR-ABL; treatment with imatinib, which targets this kinase, restored the aggregation response. Bleeding manifestation can occur in <10% of CML patients with or without imatinib therapy. The concordance of hematoma formation with signs and symptoms of MPN suggests bleeding secondary to MPN. Moreover, basic coagulation profile, platelet aggregation studies, and autoantibodies to platelet glycoprotein are recommended to identify the cause of bleeding in CML patients [9]. Successful treatment of underlying CML reduces the risk of life-threatening bleeding diathesis. Advanced studies and research would further help to identify platelet, blood cell, plasma, and vascular gene variants that may influence bleeding in MPN.

References

[1] D. G. Savage, R. M. Szydlo, and J. M. Goldman, "Clinical features at diagnosis in 430 patients with chronic myeloid leukaemia seen at a referral centre over a 16-year period," *British Journal of Haematology*, vol. 96, no. 1, pp. 111–116, 1997.

[2] A. J. C. Bloor, G. A. Smith, M. Jaswon, N. E. Parker, W. H. Ouwehand, and R. Liesner, "Acquired thrombasthenia due to GPIIbIIIa platelet autoantibodies in a 4-yr-old child," *European Journal of Haematology*, vol. 76, no. 1, pp. 89-90, 2006.

[3] A. T. Nurden, "Acquired Glanzmann thrombasthenia: from antibodies to anti-platelet drugs," *Blood Reviews*, vol. 36, pp. 10–22, 2019.

[4] A. I. Schafer, "Bleeding and thrombosis in the myeloproliferative disorders," *Blood*, vol. 64, no. 1, pp. 1–12, 1984.

[5] M. H. Ginsberg, A. L. Frelinger, S. C.-T. Lam et al., "Analysis of platelet aggregation disorders based on flow cytometric analysis of membrane glycoprotein IIb–IIIa with conformation-specific monoclonal antibodies," *Blood*, vol. 76, no. 10, pp. 2017–2023, 1990.

[6] R. Kaplan, J. Gabbeta, L. Sun, G. F. Mao, and A. K. Rao, "Combined defect in membrane expression and activation of platelet GPIIb–IIIa complex without primary sequence abnormalities in myeloproliferative disease," *British Journal of Haematology*, vol. 111, no. 3, pp. 954–964, 2000.

[7] S. F. Moore, R. W. Hunter, M. T. Harper et al., "Dysfunction of the PI3 kinase/Rap1/integrin IIb 3 pathway underlies ex vivo platelet hypoactivity in essential thrombocythemia," *Blood*, vol. 121, no. 7, pp. 1209–1219, 2013.

[8] A. P. Ng, P. Servadei, A. Tuckfield, A. Friedhuber, and A. Grigg, "Resolution of platelet function defects with imatinib therapy in a patient with chronic myeloid leukaemia in chronic phase," *Blood Coagulation & Fibrinolysis*, vol. 20, no. 1, pp. 81–83, 2009.

[9] R. Chauhan, S. Sazawal, K. Singh et al., "Reversal of Glanzmann thrombasthenia platelet phenotype after imatinib treatment in a pediatric chronic myeloid leukemia patient," *Platelets*, vol. 29, no. 2, pp. 203–206, 2018.

[10] A. Shimabukuro-Vornhagen, A. Rothe, L. Nogova, M. Kochanek, C. Scheid, and M. von Bergwelt-Baildon, "Improvement of platelet dysfunction in chronic myelogenous leukemia following treatment with imatinib: a case report," *Journal of Medical Case Reports*, vol. 5, no. 1, p. 215, 2011.

[11] Y. C. Kuo, H. C. Wang, K. A. Chu, and J. Y. Lu, "Chronic myeloid leukemia initially presenting with spontaneous mediastinal hematoma and hemothorax," *Zhonghua Yi Xue Za Zhi*, vol. 63, no. 2, pp. 170–174, 2000.

[12] O. Bauduceau, T. De Revel, J. Fogelman, S. Amadou, B. Souleau, and G. Nedellec, "Spontaneous hematoma of the iliac psoas muscle in chronic myeloid leukemia," *Annales de Médecine Interne*, vol. 154, no. 3, pp. 183–186, 2003.

[13] U. Malik, J. P. Dutcher, and L. Oleksowicz, "Acquired Glanzmann's thrombasthenia associated with Hodgkin's lymphoma," *Cancer*, vol. 82, no. 9, pp. 1764–1768, 1998.

[14] M. Kannan, T. Chatterjee, F. Ahmad, R. Kumar, V. P. Choudhry, and R. Saxena, "Acquired Glanzmann's thrombasthenia associated with Hairy cell leukaemia," *European Journal of Clinical Investigation*, vol. 39, no. 12, pp. 1110-1111, 2009.

10

A Case with Hepatic Involvement Mimicking Metastatic Disease in Multiple Myeloma

Mert Erciyestepe,[1] **Tarık Onur Tiryaki**,[2] **İpek Yönal Hindilerden**,[2] **Gülçin Yeğen**,[3] **and Meliha Nalçacı**[2]

[1]*Istanbul University, Istanbul Medical Faculty, Department of Internal Medicine, Istanbul, Turkey*
[2]*Istanbul University, Istanbul Medical Faculty, Department of Internal Medicine, Division of Hematology, Istanbul, Turkey*
[3]*Istanbul University, Istanbul Medical Faculty, Department of Pathology, Istanbul, Turkey*

Correspondence should be addressed to Mert Erciyestepe; merterciyestepe@gmail.com

Academic Editor: Kostas Konstantopoulos

Multiple myeloma is a type of plasma cell disorder and can be seen in different forms. According to current knowledge, it is not a curable disease. Smoldering multiple myeloma (SMM) is an asymptomatic clonal plasma cell disorder and distinguished from monoclonal gammopathy of undetermined significance by a much higher risk of progression to multiple myeloma. We present a 53-year-old female patient who started with SMM which turned into multiple myeloma after four years. Despite 26 cycles of lenalidomide treatment, we performed the second autologous stem transplantation. After 12 years from the diagnosis of the disease, it was transformed into plasma cell leukemia and widespread nodular lesions were seen in the liver. Different presentations could be seen due to malignant plasma cell infiltrations or primary amyloidosis. Liver involvement is one of them and is less common than other organ involvement. We report a case of myeloma presenting with extensive nodular involvement in the liver and misdiagnosed as metastatic disease. It is important because of its rarity and change of the treatment approach.

1. Introduction

Different presentation forms and different treatment regimens are available in multiple myeloma. Liver involvement is one of the different presentation forms, and it can mimic metastatic disease.

2. Case

A 53-year-old female patient presented with gastrointestinal complaints in June 2006. The general medical examination is unremarkable. She was with no significant medical history. The laboratory findings were within normal limits. A serum protein electrophoresis was performed that demonstrated a monoclonal IgG protein of 1.52 g/dL, and the free kappa/lambda light chain ratio was 12 : 5. There were no bone lesions in bone radiographs or skeletal x-rays. Bone marrow biopsy showed normocellular marrow with 20% plasmositosis. Conventional cytogenetics were normal. So, the patient was diagnosed as IgG kappa smoldering myeloma and had started to follow-up without treatment.

After 4 years, in January 2010, the patient progressed to multiple myeloma with anemia, and a bortezomib-based regimen (bortezomib, cyclophosphamide, and dexamethasone) (CyBorD) was given. After achieving a very good partial response, peripheral stem cells were collected with a filgrastim-alone mobilization regimen. Then, autologous stem cell transplantation was performed with high-dose melphalan (200 mg/m^2) in December 2010. Maintenance therapy was not given due to the country's reimbursement.

In the fourth year after transplantation, in May 2014, she experienced first nonaggressive relapse and received a lenalidomide and dexamethasone regimen. Anemia and monocytosis occurred during the second year of the lenalidomid treatment. On peripheral blood, the plasma cell count was 2000/mm^3. Bone marrow biopsy showed a

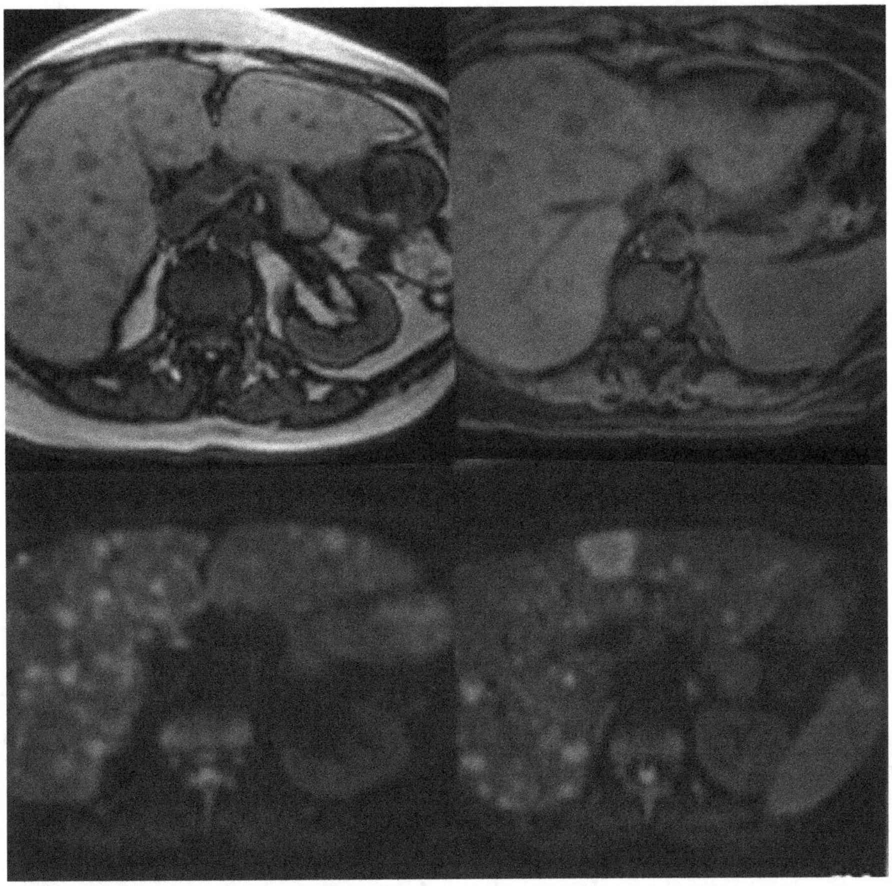

FIGURE 1: Increased liver size and multiple diffusely distributed lesions which are hyperintense in T2A series and hypointense lesions in T1A series are seen.

hypocellular marrow with 30% plasmositosis. At this stage, conventional cytogenetic and FISH studies (*t* (14; 20), *t* (6; 14), *t* (4; 14), *t* (14; 16), *t* (11; 14), 11q13, and 17p13) were evaluated as normal. In June 2016, CyBorD therapy was initiated again due to the complete response with the bortezomib-based regimen previously and relapses more than 5 years after initial treatment, and the patient's performance was not compatible with high-dose combined regimens (VDT-PACE, DICEP).

After achieving a very good partial response again, although she received 26 cycles of lenalidomid, peripheral blood stem cell harvesting was tried with high doses of cyclophosphamide and etoposide plus filgrastim. Stem cells were collected, and transplantation was performed with 140 mg/m^2 melphalan for the second time, in March 2017. Posttransplant maintenance therapy was not given due to unresponsiveness to previous lenalidomide therapy.

About 1 year after the second transplantation, the patient was admitted to the hospital with right upper quadrant pain over the last two days. On the physical examination, she was pale and had painful hepatomegaly. The complete blood count values were similar with the last one. But, some biochemical tests were abnormal. Aspartate aminotransferase 26 U/L (5–42), alanine aminotransferase 35 U/L (5–42), alkaline phosphatase 122 U/L (35–104), and gama glutamintransferase 234 U/L (5–85) were detected. Tumor markers were evaluated: CA 125 (cancer antigen 125) was 2096 U/ml (<35), and CA 15-3 value was 374 U/ml (<25). There were multiple hypodense lesions on the liver, the largest one being 3 cm length, on the images of the abdomen, Figure 1. Biopsy was taken from the liver lesions and pathological evaluation of the lesion biopsy revealed CD38 (+) Kappa (+) Lambda (−) plasma cell infiltration. There were big patchy grouped atypical cells infiltrations Figure 2. These findings were related with the diagnosis of kappa light chain neoplastic plasma cell infiltration. The patient was dead in the following 2 months, although the chemotherapeutic regimens and supportive cares were given.

3. Discussion

Liver involvement is uncommon in the course of multiple myeloma. This involvement is usually due to plasma cell infiltration or concomitant amyloidosis. In one study, Talamo et al. found that gastrointestinal system involvement was present in 24 of 2584 myeloma patients. Liver involvement was seen in 11 of them [1]. However, microscopic plasma cell infiltration is observed more frequently. Thomas et al. reported that, in an autopsy series including 64 patients, 40% had plasma cell infiltration of the liver [2, 3]. Liver involvement may be nodular, sinusoidal, or diffuse or may be in a mixed pattern [4]. Soft tissue involvement may

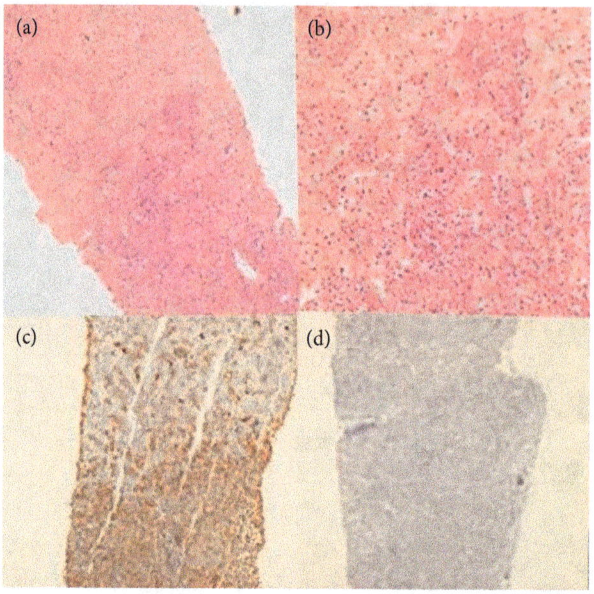

FIGURE 2: (a, b) Liver paranchyme is infiltrated by plasma cells and full of atypical cells. (c) Kappa (+) neoplastic plasma cells infiltrations are seen. (d) Lambda (–) neoplastic plasma cells infiltrations.

be seen due to decreased expression of adhesion molecules, downregulation of chemokine receptors, downregulation of tetraspanins, increased heparanase-1 expression, angiogenesis, and mutations in alternative or classical nuclear factor-kB pathways [4, 5]. Liver involvement in extramedullary myeloma is found as hypoechoic nodules on the CT scan. Rarely, it may present as hyperechoic nodules and hypervascular lesions [6–8]. It is sometimes confused with metastatic tumors due to the involvement pattern. The fact that the disease is seen in the course of the disease usually plays an important role in revealing the etiology. However, multiple lesions may be seen in the liver in the first diagnosis of the disease, rarely. Definitive diagnosis is made by biopsy from the existing lesions.

Another important feature of this case is that stem cells could be collected after 26 cycles of lenalidomide treatment. It is known in the literature that lenalidomide treatment, especially 4 cycles and above, is a risk factor for mobilization failure [9]. However, this is not a rule, and stem cell harvesting may be attempted in patients who have received 4 cycles and above with lenalidomide therapy.

4. Conclusions

Although extramedullary/soft tissue involvement is a rare form of multiple myeloma, it has become more common with the development of imaging techniques. It is not clear whether extramedullary involvement is poor cytogenetic and has negative prognostic features. When the first presentation is with extramedullary involvement, it may cause a delay in diagnosis. New treatment modalities are required, since there is no known treatment method that can provide complete remission, except for allogeneic stem cell transplantation. In selected patients whose treatment options have been exhausted, the autologous transplantation option may be considered once again, despite the number of lenalidomide cycles.

Consent

Informed consent was obtained.

Authors' Contributions

ME and TOT wrote the manuscript. İYH and MN edited and provided expertise. GY contributed to the pathological evaluation. All authors have read and approved the manuscript.

References

[1] G. Talamo, F. Cavallo, M. Zangari et al., "Clinical and biological features of multiple myeloma involving the gastrointestinal system," *Haematologica*, vol. 91, no. 7, pp. 964–967, 2006.

[2] F. B. Thomas, K. P. Clausen, and N. J. Greenberger, "Liver disease in multiple myeloma," *Archives of Internal Medicine*, vol. 132, no. 2, pp. 195–202, 1973.

[3] K. Oshima, Y. Kanda, Y. Nannya et al., "Clinical and pathologic findings in 52 consecutively autopsied cases with multiple myeloma," *American Journal of Hematology*, vol. 67, no. 1, pp. 1–5, 2001.

[4] A. C. Tiu, R. Potdar, V. Arguello-Gerra, and M. Morginstin, "Multiple liver nodules mimicking metastatic disease as initial presentation of multiple myeloma," *Case Reports in Hematology*, vol. 2018, Article ID 7954816, 6 pages, 2018.

[5] J. Bladé, C. Fernández de Larrea, L. Rosiñol, M. T. Cibeira, R. Jiménez, and R. Powles, "Soft-tissue plasmacytomas in

multiple myeloma: incidence, mechanisms of extramedullary spread, and treatment approach," *Journal of Clinical Oncology*, vol. 29, no. 28, pp. 3805–3812, 2011.

[6] H. Huang, F. Bazerbachi, H. Mesa, and P. Gupta, "Asymptomatic multiple myeloma presenting as a nodular hepatic lesion: a case report and review of the literature," *The Ochsner Journal*, vol. 15, no. 4, pp. 457–467, 2015.

[7] J. Bladé, C. F. de Larrea, and L. Rosiñol, "Extramedullary involvement in multiple myeloma," *Haematologica*, vol. 97, no. 11, pp. 1618-1619, 2012.

[8] C. H. Tan, M. Wang, W. J. Fu, and R. Vikram, "Nodular extramedullary multiple myeloma: hepatic involvement presenting as hypervascular lesions on CT," *Annals of the Academy of Medicine, Singapore*, vol. 40, no. 7, pp. 329–331, 2011.

[9] W. D. Wallis and M. H. Qazilbash, "Peripheral blood stem cell mobilization in multiple myeloma: growth factors or chemotherapy?" *World Journal of Transplantation*, vol. 7, no. 5, pp. 250–259, 2017.

11

Diagnosis and Management of Atypical Chronic Myeloid Leukemia with a t(2;13)(q33;q12) Translocation

John S. Wang, Omar Elghawy, Brett R. Kurpiel, and Michael G. Douvas

School of Medicine, University of Virginia, Charlottesville, Virginia, USA

Correspondence should be addressed to Michael G. Douvas; mgd9a@hscmail.mcc.virginia.edu

Academic Editor: Sudhir Tauro

Atypical chronic myeloid leukemia (aCML) is a rare myeloproliferative disorder that shares clinical features with chronic myeloid leukemia but lacks the classic t(9;22) *BCR-ABL1* translocation and features prominent dysgranulopoiesis and granulocytic dysplasia. Challenges of this diagnosis include clinical and biologic heterogeneity, the high risk of transformation to acute myeloid leukemia, and the lack of standard treatment options. Allogeneic hematopoietic stem cell transplant is likely the preferred treatment, but this can be limited by patient psychosocial support, age, concomitant medical conditions, and availability of an appropriate donor. We report the case of a 61-year-old male with no significant past medical history diagnosed with aCML with a rare t(2;13)(q33;q12). He presented with weight loss, night sweats, splenomegaly, hyperleukocytosis, a leukoerythroblastic differential with a predominant neutrophilia, anemia, and thrombocytopenia. Subsequent peripheral blood and bone marrow studies lead to the diagnosis of aCML. He was recommended to undergo an allogeneic stem cell transplant evaluation and declined. He was initially treated with hydroxyurea and imatinib to which he responded for approximately three years. After clinical progression, he was treated with sorafenib, a multiprotein kinase inhibitor more commonly used in the treatment of hepatocellular and renal cell carcinoma due to its off target FLT3 inhibition. The patient achieved complete hematologic response which has been sustained for 7 years with tolerable side effects.

1. Introduction

Atypical chronic myeloid leukemia (aCML) is a myeloproliferative neoplasm with a poor prognosis due to its clinical and biologic heterogeneity, its high risk of transformation to acute myeloid leukemia, and its lack of a standardized treatment protocol [1]. aCML is characterized by marked leukocytosis/granulocytosis but unlike classic CML, shows no evidence of the classic t(9;22) *BCR-ABL1* translocation by cytogenetic studies, polymerase chain reaction (PCR), or fluorescence situ hybridization (FISH) [1, 2]. The morphologic features of aCML share similarities with CML and include leukocytosis, granulocytosis, and a spectrum of immature granulocytes in peripheral blood. aCML, however, is unique in that patients also exhibit features of prominent dysgranulopoiesis and granulocytic dysplasia. Patients often present with signs and symptoms of anemia and hepatosplenomegaly on physical exam. The disease is extremely rare with an estimated incidence of less than one in a million people per year [3]. In this case report, we present an older man presenting with aCML with a t(2;13)(q33;q12) who attained a complete clinical and hematologic remission when treated with the protein kinase inhibitor sorafenib after previously having a partial response to imatinib.

2. Case Report

An otherwise healthy 61-year-old male presented for evaluation of weight loss, night sweats, and left upper quadrant discomfort. He had no significant medical history, and his family history was significant only for hypothyroidism. Physical exam revealed a well appearing man with palpable splenomegaly to 5 fingerbreadths below the left costal margin in the midclavicular line. A complete blood count with differential revealed mild thrombocytopenia (103 K), borderline elevated hemoglobin (17.4), and leukocytosis to 93 k with a leukoerythroblastic differential (PMN 44%, bands 8%, myelocytes/metamyelocytes 14%, promyelocytes 8%, blasts 2%, eosinophils 17%, and basophils 2%). Review of his peripheral blood smear showed significant dysgranulopoiesis with a leukoerythroblastic differential felt to be most consistent with aCML (Figure 1(a)). Routine laboratory workup revealed no significant abnormalities, except a moderately elevated lactate dehydrogenase of 755 (ULN 250) and a mildly elevated uric acid of 8.8 (ULN 7.2). A bone marrow aspiration was performed and showed findings similar to peripheral blood with 57% neutrophils and bands, 17% eosinophils, and no elevation in blasts. The bone marrow core biopsy showed marked hypercellularity of 100%, notable granulocytic dysplasia, and myeloid hyperplasia with a markedly elevated myeloid: erythroid ratio of 30 : 1 (Figure 1(b)). Cytogenetic analysis was negative for *BCR-ABL1* translocation by FISH but revealed a balanced reciprocal translocation between chromosomes 2 and 13 t(2; 13)(q33;q12) in all 19 cells analyzed by karyotype (Figure 2(a)). FISH analysis for translocations involving *PDGFRA* and *PDGFRB* was negative as was a quantitative PCR for p210 *BCR-ABL1*. FISH using the CytoCell 13q14.3/ 13q34 break-apart probe for 13q showed no evidence of disruption but did demonstrate that this probe had been translocated to chromosome 2 (Figure 2(b)). The diagnosis of aCML was made in concordance with the WHO diagnostic criteria for aCML [4]. Due to the lack of a standard medical regimen for a diagnosis of aCML with a t(2;13) translocation, a stem cell transplant evaluation was recommended, but ultimately declined by the patient. He was started initially on both hydroxyurea and in the process of evaluation on imatinib, given the strikingly similar presentation to CML and lack of other available treatment modalities. Hydroxyurea was stopped after 5 months after significant improvement in leukocytosis. Somewhat unexpectedly, the patient continued to clinically respond to imatinib for approximately three years with normalization of white blood cell count and decrease of LDH (Figure 3), regression of splenomegaly, and overall increased quality of life. After three years, however, the patient developed worsening thrombocytopenia and anemia despite subsequent dose reductions of imatinib. He also developed severe right-hand pain that was unresponsive to NSAIDs and prednisone. A plain film of the hand revealed diffuse severe lucency of the entire hamate bone with a thin peripheral cortex visible, and a subsequent MRI revealed severe bone marrow replacement throughout the distal radius and ulna, carpal bones, and metacarpals with complete abnormal marrow replacement of the trapezoid, capitate, and hamate (Figure 4). There was a strong concern for possible transformation to acute myeloid leukemia (AML), but the patient did not have peripheral blasts on the routine blood smear. The patient declined a repeat bone marrow biopsy, next-generation sequencing, and recommended transfusions for platelets of 11 K/μL and Hgb of 5.3 g/dL. Given a previous case report of a patient with a similar presentation and a t(2; 13)(q33,q12) involving the *FLT3* locus, a search of tyrosine kinase inhibitors with activity on the FLT3 protein ensued [5]. Due to the patient's worsening blood counts and a lack of alternative treatments options, the patient was started on sorafenib therapy as it was the only commercially available FLT3 inhibitor at the time. The patient had rapid clinical improvement of both blood counts and pain and swelling of his right hand after initiation of sorafenib. He ultimately normalized his WBC count and differential, hemoglobin, and LDH with a resolution of splenomegaly on exam, normalization of his hand exam, resolution of bone pain, and improvement in his platelet count to mild stable thrombocytopenia of approximately 100 K/μL (Figure 3). He has now been on sorafenib for over seven years with mild and manageable side effects of peripheral edema, hypertension requiring single-agent antihypertensive medication, and intermittent loose stools.

3. Discussion

Our patient presented with atypical CML defined by his *BCR-ABL1*(-) status in the setting of marked leukocytosis/ granulocytosis and prominent dysgranulopoiesis, and granulocytic dysplasia. This is the first case reported in the literature of a patient with myeloproliferative neoplasm with t(2;13)(q33;q12) being successfully treated with sorafenib. This case complements the atypical CML case described by Grand et al. [6]. Their patient had a similar presentation with elevated white blood cells, anemia, thrombocytopenia, and splenomegaly [6]. They confirmed via molecular testing that their patient with a t(2;13)(p13;q12) translocation had a fusion of *SPTBN1-FLT3* with fluorescent in-situ hybridization and PCR confirming the fusion of the two genes. The *SPTBN1* gene encodes a nonerythrocytic beta-spectrin that is a tetrameric cytoskeletal protein with characteristic two coiled-coil domains that are preserved when fused with the entire tyrosine kinase domain of FLT3. The chimeric fusion was described to result in a constitutively active *FLT3* mutant that phosphorylates *STAT5* protein [7–9] which has been implicated in upregulating proliferative pathways in the myeloid lineage, particularly in AML patients [10, 11]. While the patient in Grant et al. was treated with an allogeneic stem cell transplant and with donor lymphocyte infusion after cytogenetic relapse years later, patient-derived cell growth was shown to be inhibited in vitro by *FLT3* inhibitors in a dose-dependent manner [6]. We posit that a similar pathway via a chimeric *FLT3* mutant is responsible for the atypical CML observed in our patient and his subsequent response to tyrosine kinase inhibitor (TKI) therapy [12]. Unfortunately, molecular studies were not performed on our patient at the time of his presentation or at time of progression due in part to the patient's wishes.

Conventional treatment for classical CML with the t(9; 22) *BCR-ABL* translocation is therapy with tyrosine kinase inhibitors such as imatinib which are very effective [13, 14]. Interestingly, in our case, we observed the patient to respond initially to imatinib therapy in the absence of the t(9;22) translocation for nearly three years. There are two potential explanations for our patient's partial response to imatinib. One possibility is that our patient developed a myeloid or lymphoid neoplasm with

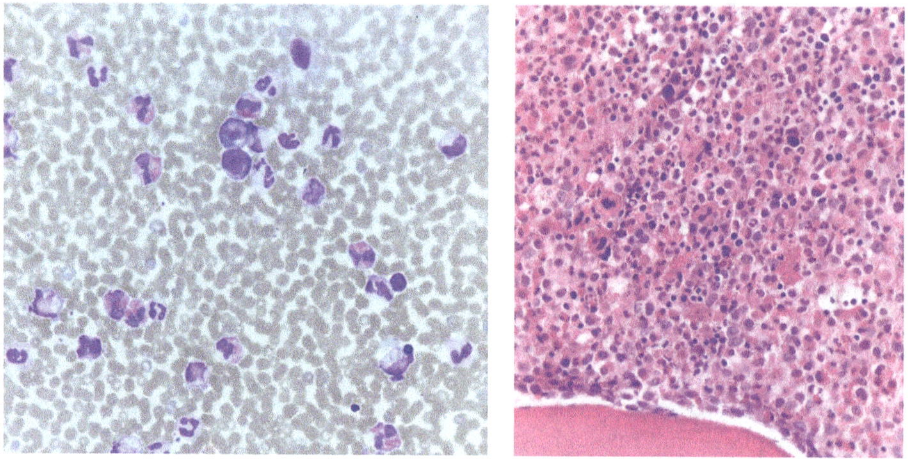

(a) (b)

Figure 1: (a) Peripheral blood smear demonstrating a leukocytosis with myeloid left shift, basophilia, eosinophilia, polycythemia, and thrombocytopenia; Wright-Giemsa, original image ×1,000, oil immersion. (b) High-power image of the bone marrow biopsy highlighting the dramatic myeloid predominance with only few, rare erythroid precursors and small, hypolobated megakaryocytes; hematoxylin-eosin, original image ×500, oil immersion.

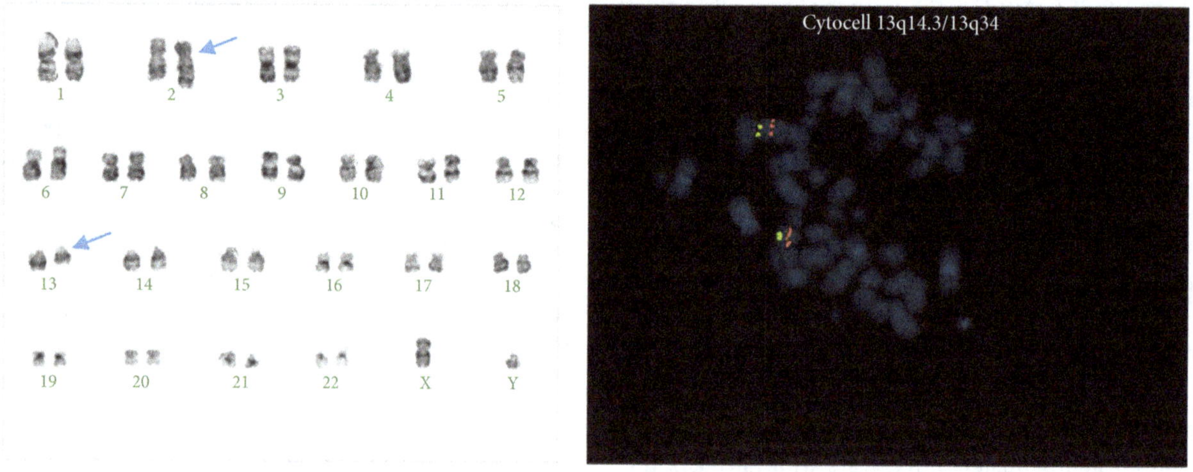

(a) (b)

Figure 2: (a) Karyotype images showing t(2;13). (b) FISH image demonstrating the probes for chromosome 13 hybridizing to the normal chromosome 13 (small chromosome) and chromosome 2 (large chromosome), demonstrating the translocation of chromosome 13 material to chromosome 2.

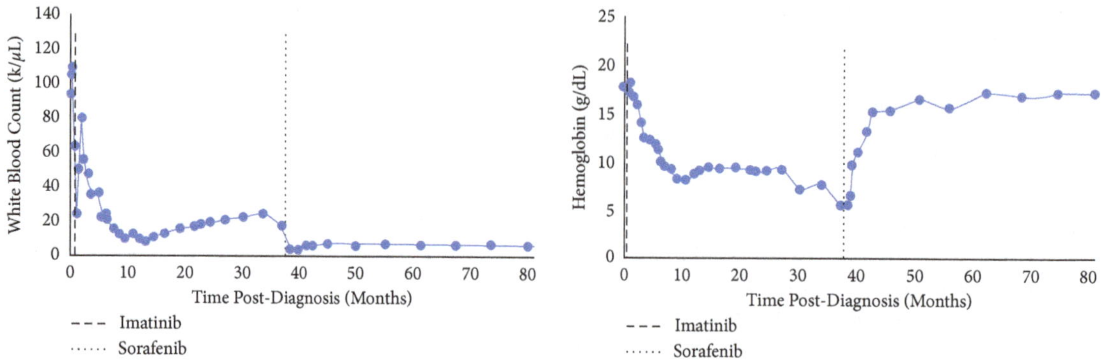

(a) (b)

Figure 3: Continued.

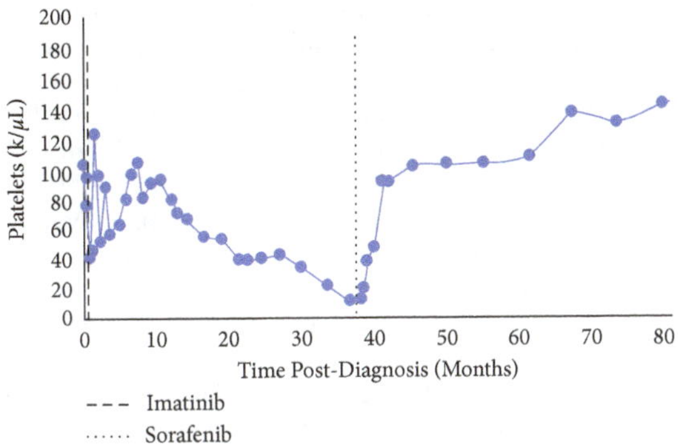

(c)

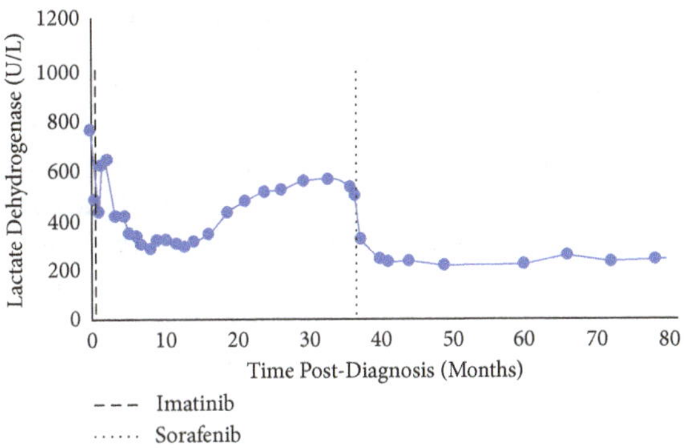

(d)

FIGURE 3: (a) WBC count. (b) Hemoglobin. (c) Platelets. (d) LDH for the patient over time from date of presentation to current. The thick dashed line represents the time of imatinib administration while the thin dashed line represents the time of therapy conversion to sorafenib.

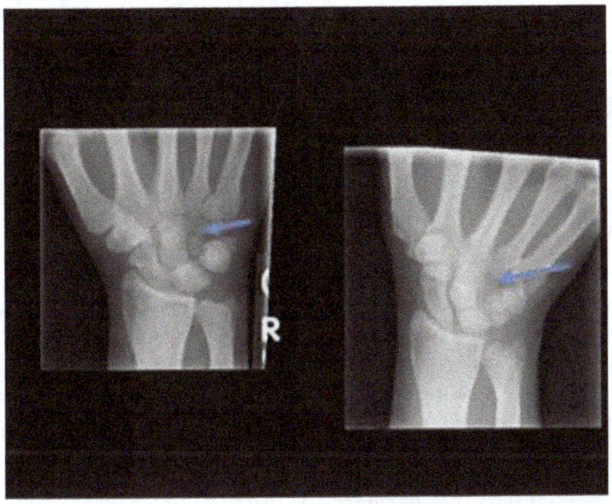

(a)

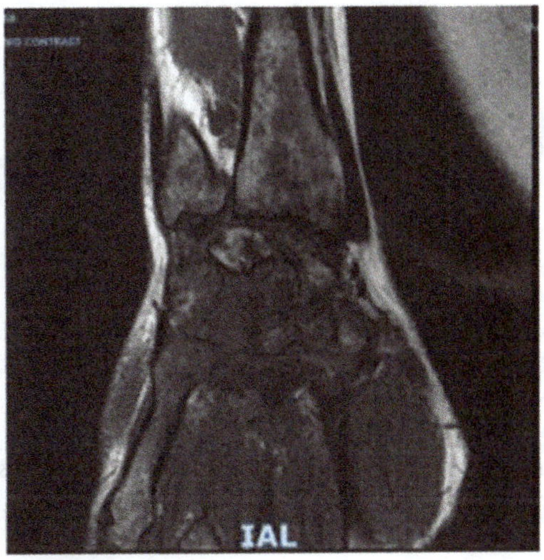

(b)

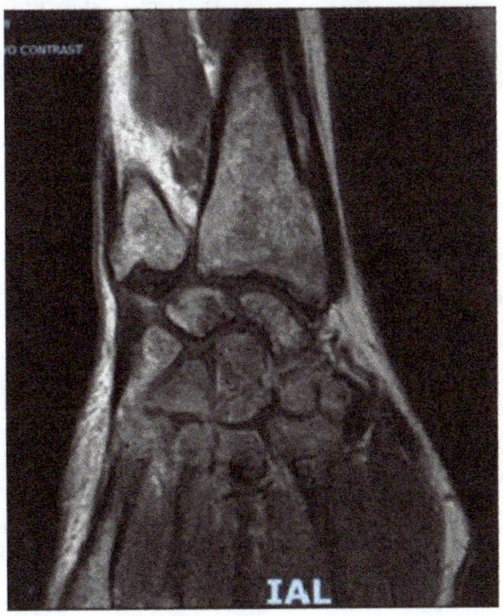

(c)

FIGURE 4: (a) Plain film X-ray of the right hand reveals diffuse severe lucency of the entire hamate bone (blue arrows) with a thin peripheral cortex visible. (b) T1 MRI. (c) T2-weighted MRI with contrast of the right hand reveals severe bone marrow replacement throughout the distal radius and ulna, carpal bones, and metacarpals with complete replacement of the trapezoid, capitate, and hamate.

eosinophilia and rearrangement of the PDGFRA, PDGFRB, FGFR1, or PCM1-JAK2 genes leading to a partial response to imatinib [15]. Assessment with FISH for the most common PDGFRA/B gene translocations in our patient was negative, and while the presence of a cryptic rearrangement could explain our patient's partial response to imatinib, it would not explain his full response to sorafenib. More likely, we speculate that imatinib had some efficacy, albeit temporary and less complete, in inhibiting the t(2;13)(q33;q12) chimeric *FLT3* kinase in our case.

In light of our patient's clinical course, it is noted to be important to both report rare clinical presentations for the potential benefit of other similar patients and to attempt to perform appropriate molecular testing whenever possible to advance understanding of the pathophysiology of rare diseases. Sorafenib, a drug most often used in the treatment of hepatocellular and renal cell carcinoma, would not have been chosen as the treatment modality for this patient if not for the previous case report detailing in vitro response to various TKIs [16–18]. As demonstrated in the case presented here, the recognition of the t(2;13)(q33;q12) translocation and the prior case report were the keys to the successful treatment for our patient.

Additional Points

(1) Atypical CML is a rare variant of CML that shares many clinical characteristics of CML but lacks the *BCR-ABL1* t(9; 22) of CML and features prominent dysgranulopoiesis and granulocytic dysplasia. (2) Atypical CML involving the (q33; q12) locus (that includes *FLT3*) may respond well to sorafenib or other more potent FLT3 inhibitors now commercially available.

Disclosure

This article has not been published or presented previously.

Acknowledgments

The authors would like to acknowledge the Genetics and Pathology departments of the University of Virginia Medical Center for their technical assistance in the workup of this case and to Dr. Mark Anderson of the Department of Radiology and Ms. Amy Radigan, PA-C of the Department of Orthopedic Surgery at the University of Virginia for their help in selection of the MRI images used in Figure 4.

References

[1] A. Marumo, T. Mizuki, and S. Tanosaki, "Atypical chronic myeloid leukemia achieving good response with azacitidine," *Indian Journal of Cancer*, vol. 56, no. 4, p. 354, 2019.

[2] J. M. Bennett, D. Catovsky, M. T. Daniel et al., "The chronic myeloid leukaemias: guidelines for distinguishing chronic granulocytic, atypical chronic myeloid, and chronic myelomonocytic leukaemia: proposals by the French-American-British Cooperative Leukaemia Group," *British Journal of Haematology*, vol. 87, no. 4, pp. 746–754, 1994.

[3] M. Cazzola, L. Malcovati, and R. Invernizzi, "Myelodysplastic/myeloproliferative neoplasms," *Hematology*, vol. 2011, no. 1, pp. 264–272, 2011.

[4] J. Gotlib, "How I treat atypical chronic myeloid leukemia," *Blood*, vol. 129, no. 7, pp. 838–845, 2017.

[5] A. Antar, Z. K. Otrock, J. El-Cheikh et al., "Inhibition of FLT3 in AML: a focus on sorafenib," *Bone Marrow Transplantation*, vol. 52, no. 3, pp. 344–351, 2017.

[6] F. H. Grand, S. Iqbal, L. Zhang, N. H. Russell, A. Chase, and N. C. P. Cross, "A constitutively active SPTBN1-FLT3 fusion in atypical chronic myeloid leukemia is sensitive to tyrosine kinase inhibitors and immunotherapy," *Experimental Hematology*, vol. 35, no. 11, pp. 1723–1727, 2007.

[7] M. A. S. Moore, D. C. Dorn, J. J. Schuringa, K. Y. Chung, and G. Morrone, "Constitutive activation of Flt3 and STAT5A enhances self-renewal and alters differentiation of hematopoietic stem cells," *Experimental Hematology*, vol. 35, no. 4, pp. 105–116, 2007.

[8] C. Choudhary, C. Brandts, J. Schwable et al., "Activation mechanisms of STAT5 by oncogenic Flt3-ITD," *Blood*, vol. 110, no. 1, pp. 370–374, 2007.

[9] R. Grundler, C. Thiede, C. Miething, C. Steudel, C. Peschel, and J. Duyster, "Sensitivity toward tyrosine kinase inhibitors varies between different activating mutations of the FLT3 receptor," *Blood*, vol. 102, no. 2, pp. 646–651, 2003.

[10] B. Wingelhofer, B. Maurer, E. C. Heyes et al., "Pharmacologic inhibition of STAT5 in acute myeloid leukemia," *Leukemia*, vol. 32, no. 5, pp. 1135–1146, 2018.

[11] B. Wingelhofer, H. A. Neubauer, P. Valent et al., "Implications of STAT3 and STAT5 signaling on gene regulation and chromatin remodeling in hematopoietic cancer," *Leukemia*, vol. 32, no. 8, pp. 1713–1726, 2018.

[12] D. Small, "Targeting FLT3 for the treatment of leukemia," *Seminars in Hematology*, vol. 45, no. 3 Suppl 2, pp. S17–S21, 2008.

[13] T. Sacha, "Imatinib in chronic myeloid leukemia: an overview," *Mediterranean Journal of Hematology and Infectious Diseases*, vol. 6, no. 1, Article ID e2014007, 2013.

[14] A. Hochhaus, R. A. Larson, F. Guilhot et al., "Long-term outcomes of imatinib treatment for chronic myeloid leukemia," *New England Journal of Medicine*, vol. 376, no. 10, pp. 917–927, 2017.

[15] A. Reiter and J. Gotlib, "Myeloid neoplasms with eosinophilia," *Blood*, vol. 129, no. 6, pp. 704–714, 2017.

[16] Y. j Zhu, B. Zheng, H. y Wang, and L. Chen, "New knowledge of the mechanisms of sorafenib resistance in liver cancer," *Acta Pharmacologica Sinica*, vol. 38, no. 5, pp. 614–622, 2017.

[17] M. Cervello, D. Bachvarov, N. Lampiasi et al., "Molecular mechanisms of sorafenib action in liver cancer cells," *Cell Cycle*, vol. 11, no. 15, pp. 2843–2855, 2012.

[18] P.-Y. Dumas, C. Naudin, S. Martin-Lannerée et al., "Hematopoietic niche drives FLT3-ITD acute myeloid leukemia resistance to quizartinib via STAT5-and hypoxia-dependent upregulation of AXL," *Haematologica*, vol. 104, no. 10, pp. 2017–2027, 2019.

12

A Rare Case of Ixazomib-Induced Cutaneous Necrotizing Vasculitis in a Patient with Relapsed Myeloma

Heather Katz,[1] Mina Shenouda,[2] Deena Dahshan,[3] George Sonnier,[4] and Yehuda Lebowicz[5]

[1]*Department of Hematology/Oncology, Donald and Barbara Zucker School of Medicine at Hofstra/Northwell, 500 Hofstra Blvd, Hempstead, NY 11549, USA*
[2]*Department of Hematology/Oncology, Joan C. Edwards School of Medicine, Marshall University, 1600 Medical Center Dr., Huntington, WV 25701, USA*
[3]*Joan C. Edwards School of Medicine, Marshall University, 1600 Medical Center Dr., Huntington, WV 25701, USA*
[4]*Department of Dermatology, University of Louisville School of Medicine, Louisville, KY 40203, USA*
[5]*Department of Hematology/Oncology, UPMC Hillman Cancer Center, 1030 Beaver Hollow Rd., Beaver, PA 15009, USA*

Correspondence should be addressed to Heather Katz; dockatz0211@gmail.com

Academic Editor: Sylvain Choquet

Ixazomib is the only oral proteasome inhibitor used in relapsed/refractory myeloma. Cutaneous side effects due to ixazomib have been documented in the literature; however, cutaneous necrotizing vasculitis is extremely rare. We describe a case of a 74-year-old man with relapsed multiple myeloma who was started on ixazomib, lenalidomide, and dexamethasone. He developed several skin lesions that were biopsied and revealed cutaneous necrotizing vasculitis. Ixazomib was held with resolution of the vasculitic lesions and restarted with dexamethasone to 20 mg on the day of treatment and 20 mg dose the day after treatment.

1. Introduction

There are several approved treatments for relapsed/refractory multiple myeloma; however, only one completely oral triplet regimen is approved. The combination of ixazomib, a proteasome inhibitor, lenalidomide, an immunomodulatory medication, and dexamethasone, a steroid, IRd, is the only triplet regimen in which all of the medications can be taken by mouth providing convenience to the patient as they do not need to come to the clinic as frequently for treatment. Typically, IRd is well tolerated with common toxicities including gastrointestinal issues, rash, thrombocytopenia, peripheral edema, and peripheral neuropathy. Cutaneous adverse events should be monitored with ixazomib and rash, and urticaria and dry skin have been discussed in the literature. Necrotizing cutaneous vasculitis due to treatment from ixazomib is extremely rare and has only been reported once in the literature. We report a case of ixazomib-induced necrotizing cutaneous vasculitis in a 74-year-old-male treated with ixazomib for relapsed myeloma that resolved by holding the medication. He was restarted on ixazomib plus steroids with no recurrence of cutaneous vasculitis and no complications of increased steroid dose.

2. Case Report

A 74-year-old-male with a past medical history of bronchitis, carpal tunnel, COPD, depression, gout, and hypertension was initially diagnosed with IgG Kappa smoldering myeloma in 2006. He was monitored with close surveillance until 2014 when he developed back pain. MRI of his spine showed a T-9 vertebral fracture which was biopsied. Final pathology was consistent with plasma cell neoplasm. In June 2014, he had a bone marrow biopsy which revealed 21% plasma cells. Myeloma FISH analysis showed monosomy 13 and gain of chromosomes 7, 9, and 15. Cytogenetics was normal. He received palliative radiation to T-9 and was started on lenalidomide 25 mg, days 1–21 of a 28-day cycle and dexamethasone 20 mg weekly. He was also started on zolendronic acid 4 mg IV every 3 months. Lenalidomide and dexamethasone were discontinued after 18 months due to patient preference. In February 2018, a PET-CT scan was performed and showed bilateral rib uptake associated with healing and nondisplaced fractures as well as left femur greater trochanter uptake secondary to a nondisplaced fracture. Repeat bone marrow biopsy in March 2018 showed 30% involvement with plasma cells. He was started on lenalidomide, bortezomib, and dexamethasone (RVd) without side effects. About 6 months after starting RVd, due to difficulty getting to the clinic, he was started on oral triplet therapy including lenalidomide 25 mg days 1–21, ixazomib 4 mg days 1, 8, and 15, and dexamethasone 20 mg days 1, 8, 15, and 22. After one week of being on this regimen, he developed multiple small lesions on his neck and chest (Figures 1 and 2).

The patient was told to hold the ixazomib and presented to the dermatologist for a biopsy. Biopsy revealed intense dermal and pannicular infiltrate that is neutrophil rich and demonstrates overlapping features between Sweet's syndrome and the necrotizing vasculitis process (Figure 3).

Vascular destruction was seen confirming the concept of leukocytoclastic vasculitis (Figure 4).

Ixazomib was held and the lesions resolved completely. After complete resolution of the lesions, he was restarted on ixazomib with decadron 20 mg on the day of and 20 mg day after Ixazomib treatment and has not had further skin lesions. Workup for systemic vasculitis was also negative. Three-month follow-up revealed no further cutaneous manifestations and no other complications due to increased steroid dose.

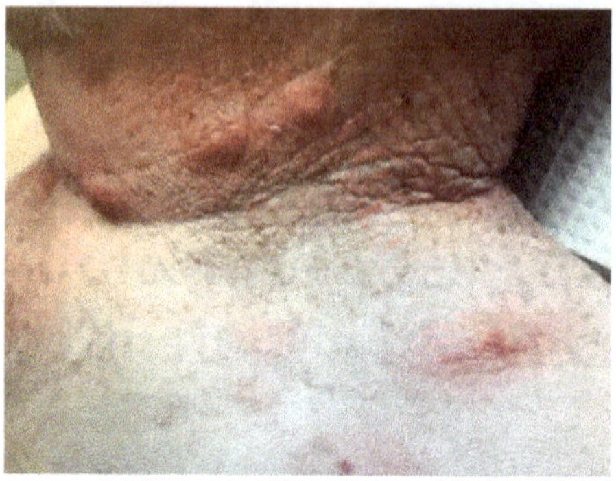

FIGURE 1: Multiple small lesions on his neck and chest.

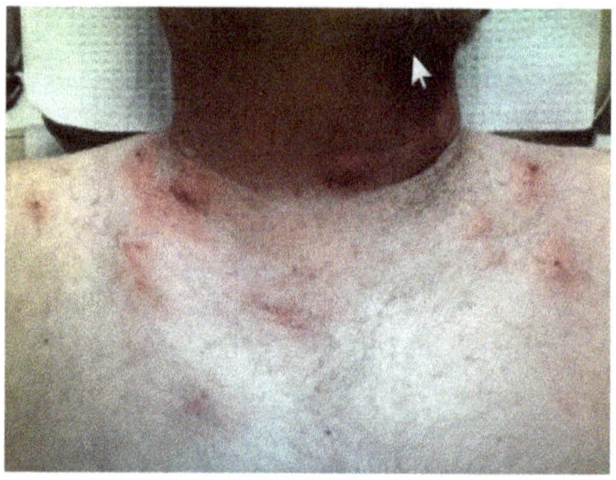

FIGURE 2: Multiple small lesions on neck and chest.

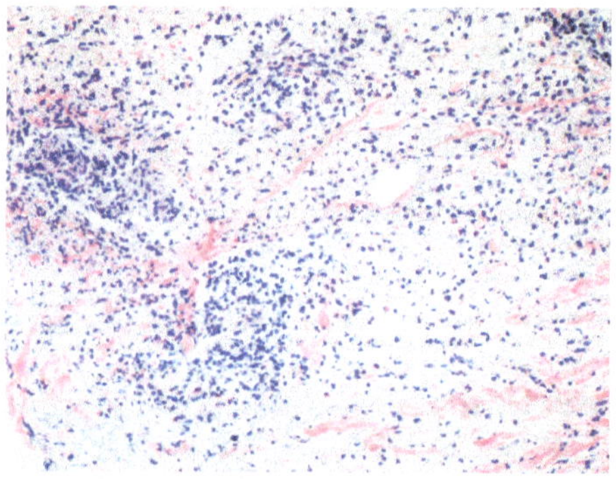

FIGURE 3: Prominent neutrophilic component of intense mixed dermal inflammation and vascular destruction from vasculitis (200x).

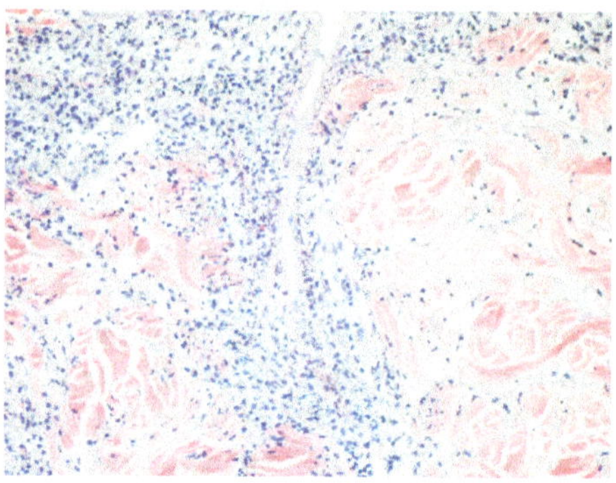

FIGURE 4: Deep dermal inflammation with leukocytoclastic vasculitis (200x).

3. Discussion

Multiple myeloma is a clonal plasma cell hematologic malignancy [1]. Despite initial treatment, patients with multiple myeloma often relapse or become refractory to treatment requiring a change in treatment [1]. The current preferred treatment regimens for patients with initial relapse receiving at least one prior therapy include proteasome inhibitors, immunomodulatory drugs, steroids, and monoclonal antibodies, commonly administered as a combination of 2 or 3 drugs [1]. Although there are several combinations approved in the setting of relapsed/refractory myeloma, the only orally available regimen for patients is the combination of ixazomib, lenalidomide, and dexamethasone (IRd). This oral regimen offers convenience to patients and clinicians as patients only need to return to clinic monthly for clinical assessment and review of laboratory data.

Ixazomib, or Ninlaro, is the first and only FDA-approved oral proteasome inhibitor. It is used in combination with lenalidomide and dexamethasone for multiple myeloma patients who received at least one prior treatment [2]. Ixazomib is an oral proteasome inhibitor alternative that may be preferred to bortezomib or carfilzomib based on its side effect profile, especially in patients with significant preexisting neuropathy or relapse to bortezomib; however, efficacy of ixazomib compared with carfilzomib or bortezomib is unknown as trials approving ixazomib were compared regimens without a proteasome inhibitor [1]. Moreau et al. [3] and Hou et al. [4] discussed the safety and efficacy of ixazomib in patients with refractory or recurring myeloma, and further studies are evaluating the role of ixazomib as a maintenance therapy for multiple myeloma [5]. The combination of ixazomib, lenalidomide, and dexamethasone demonstrated significantly longer progression-free survival rates when compared with placebo, lenalidomide, and dexamethasone [3], as well as overall survival, which favored the IRd group [4]. Ixazomib with lenalidomide and dexamethasone treatment also revealed a manageable tolerability profile, with data reporting gastrointestinal issues, rash, thrombocytopenia, peripheral edema, and peripheral neuropathy as common toxicities [3–6]. Cutaneous adverse events of rash, dry skin, and urticaria have been identified in association with ixazomib. In the phase III trial that led to ixazomib's approval for relapsed myeloma, 36% of the ixazomib group experienced rash (grade 1 and 2) and 21% resolved without intervention compared to 23% in the placebo group with 12% resolving without intervention [3]. Cutaneous necrotizing vasculitis is extremely rare, and its pathogenesis is unknown [7, 8].

Guidelines for ixazomib-induced cutaneous necrotizing vasculitis are currently ambiguous, and little characterization is available as it is not a commonly reported adverse event [1, 7, 8]. Recognizing cutaneous toxicities secondary to myeloma therapies is critical for early intervention [8]. Vasculitic skin lesions may manifest due to vasculitis also involving internal organs, requiring systemic workup to rule out other possible causes, making diagnosing cutaneous vasculitis a diagnosis of exclusion [9]. A single case report of cutaneous necrotizing vasculitis secondary to ixazomib documents two cases of ixazomib-induced vasculitis in a myeloma patient and a patient with Waldenstrom's macroglobulinemia. Both patients had negative systemic vasculitis workup and presented with rashes involving plaques with a single central purpuric macula. Skin biopsies demonstrated interface dermatitis, lymphocytic vasculitis, and mixed, acute, and chronic granulomatous necrotizing vasculitis involving small- and medium-sized vessels with a lot of eosinophils. Both patients received treatment for their respective diseases; however, dose reductions and low dose steroids were needed [8].

Eruption and spreading of the rash can be managed by administering a corticosteroid on nontreatment days, holding treatment for a week and reducing ixazomib dosage [8]. Topical steroids will only provide symptomatic relief, and in trials with bortezomib-induced cutaneous vasculitis, recurrence is prevented by premedication before treatments [10].

It is important for clinicians to recognize that cutaneous vasculitis with other myeloma treatments other than ixazomib exist, especially as treatment plans continue to evolve and often include multiple medications that can cause cutaneous manifestations. Both lenolidamide and bortezimib, which our patient was on prior to ixazomib for approximately 6 months without issue, can also cause cutaneous vasculitis [11, 12] Vasculitis due to bortezomib typically appear after 2 cycles although they can erupt within cycles 1–4 [11] Although possibly induced by one of the other medications he was previously exposed to, our patient's cutaneous vasculitic presentation was most likely due to ixazomib as that was the only new medication prior to his skin manifestations.

4. Conclusions

Close monitoring for skin reactions is important following treatment with ixazomib. Recognizing and identifying cutaneous adverse events, especially in rare cases of necrotizing vasculitis, allow for early intervention and management while allowing for a continued effective treatment for relapsed myeloma. Cutaneous necrotizing vasculitis should be recognized and understood by clinicians and considered as a differential diagnosis when following relapse/refractory myeloma on ixazomib.

References

[1] P. Sonneveld and A. Broijl, "Treatment of relapsed and refractory multiple myeloma," *Haematologica*, vol. 101, no. 4, pp. 396–406, 2016.

[2] G. Varga, Z. Nagy, J. Demeter et al., "Real world efficacy and safety results of ixazomib lenalidomide and dexamethasone combination in relapsed/refractory multiple myeloma: data collected from the Hungarian ixazomib named patient program," *Pathology & Oncology Research*, pp. 1–6, 2019.

[3] P. Moreau, T. Masszi, N. Grzasko et al., "Oral ixazomib, lenalidomide, and dexamethasone for multiple myeloma," *New England Journal of Medicine*, vol. 374, no. 17, pp. 1621–1634, 2016.

[4] J. Hou, J. Jin, Y. Xu et al., "Randomized, double-blind, placebo-controlled phase III study of ixazomib plus lenalidomide-dexamethasone in patients with relapsed/refractory multiple myeloma: China continuation study," *Journal of Hematology & Oncology*, vol. 10, no. 1, p. 137, 2017.

[5] N. Gupta, R. Labotka, G. Liu, A.-M. Hui, and K. Venkatakrishnan, "Exposure-safety-efficacy analysis of single-agent ixazomib, an oral proteasome inhibitor, in relapsed/refractory multiple myeloma: dose selection for a phase 3 maintenance study," *Investigational New Drugs*, vol. 34, no. 3, pp. 338–346, 2016.

[6] D. C. Smith, T. Kalebic, J. R. Infante et al., "Phase 1 study of ixazomib, an investigational proteasome inhibitor, in advanced non-hematologic malignancies," *Investigational New Drugs*, vol. 33, no. 3, pp. 652–663, 2015.

[7] G. Campanile, G. Hautmann, and T. M. Lotti, "The etiology of cutaneous necrotizing vasculitis," *Clinics in Dermatology*, vol. 17, no. 5, pp. 505–508, 1999.

[8] A. Alloo, H. Khosravi, S. R. Granter et al., "Ixazomib-induced cutaneous necrotizing vasculitis," *Supportive Care in Cancer*, vol. 26, no. 7, pp. 2247–2250, 2018.

[9] A. V. Marzano, P. Vezzoli, and E. Berti, "Skin involvement in cutaneous and systemic vasculitis," *Autoimmunity Reviews*, vol. 12, no. 4, pp. 467–476, 2013.

[10] J. D. Ransohoff and B. Y. Kwong, "Cutaneous adverse events of targeted therapies for hematolymphoid malignancies,"

Clinical Lymphoma Myeloma and Leukemia, vol. 17, no. 12, pp. 834–851, 2017.

[11] M. Rodriguez-Martin, M. Sáez-Rodríguez, M. García-Bustínduy et al., "Bortezomib-induced cutaneous lesions in multiple myeloma patients: a case report," *Dermatology Online Journal*, vol. 14, no. 11, 2008.

[12] J. M. Loree, E. Cai, B. S. Sheffield et al., "Leukocytoclastic vasculitis following lenalidomide during the treatment of follicular lymphoma," *Leukemia & Lymphoma*, vol. 58, no. 3, pp. 711–714, 2017.

13

Plasma Cell Leukemia: A Review of 3 Cases Managed in Kenya

Matilda Ong'ondi[1] **and Elizabeth Kagotho**[2]

[1]*Department of Internal Medicine; Hemato-oncology Unit, Kenyatta National Hospital, Nairobi, Kenya*
[2]*Department of Pathology and Laboratory Medicine, Aga Khan University hospital, Nairobi, Kenya*

Correspondence should be addressed to Matilda Ong'ondi; mongondi@gmail.com

Academic Editor: Pier Paolo Piccaluga

Plasma Cell Leukemia (PCL) is a rare and aggressive form of plasma cell dyscrasia that can arise either de novo (primary plasma cell leukemia) or evolve from previously diagnosed and treated multiple myeloma (secondary PCL). We highlight three clinical cases with very different presentations as a reminder of this diagnosis. The cases also highlight the diversity and variability that cover a patient's journey that is highly dependent on accessibility based on financial capability and social support. The clinical presentation is more aggressive due to the higher tumour burden and more proliferative tumor cells with cytopenias being profound and more organomegaly. The diagnosis is made based on at least 20% of total white blood cells being circulating plasma cells with a peripheral blood absolute plasma cell count of at least 2×10^9/l. Treatment with novel agents followed by autologous stem cell transplant in those who are transplant eligible leads to better outcomes.

1. Introduction

Plasma Cell Leukemia (PCL) is a rare and aggressive form of plasma cell dyscrasia that can arise either de novo (primary plasma cell leukemia) or evolve from previously diagnosed and treated multiple myeloma (secondary PCL) [1]. These are seen as distinct entities that vary in clinical presentation and survival. Due to the rarity of this clinical entity, most of the data are case reviews and retrospective studies. We report 3 clinical cases recently managed and discuss briefly the available data around this condition.

2. Case Discussions

2.1. Case 1. A 51-year-old female with no comorbidities was diagnosed with primary plasma cell leukemia in July 2018 after presenting with symptomatic anemia. She also reported headaches with no focal neurological deficits and had right lower limb swelling not associated with trauma or skin lesions. On physical examination, the only remarkable finding was pallor and right calf swelling with no signs of cellulitis. A complete blood count revealed a leucocytosis of 99,000/ul, normocytic anemia of 7.9 g/dl, and thrombocytopenia of 68,000/ul. A peripheral blood film revealed 79% plasma cells, and bone marrow aspirate showed plasmacytosis of 89% with serum protein electrophoresis having an M protein of 6 g/l. The serum creatinine was slightly elevated at 158 umol/l, and calcium levels were normal with an elevation of lactate dehydrogenase at 469 U/l. A Doppler ultrasound of the right lower limb ruled out deep venous thrombosis but found a fluid collection suspected to be a hematoma. A few days into her first admission at the referral hospital, she complained of worsening headaches with associated blurring of vision and vomiting. Computed Tomography (CT) of the brain performed showed bilateral frontoparietal and temporal region subacute subdural hematomas. She was managed conservatively for the hematomas and prophylactic low-molecular-weight heparin (enoxaparin) held.

Initial definitive treatment was commenced with cyclophosphamide, thalidomide, and dexamethasone based on the available medications; she received 5 cycles. On reassessment, there was clearance of peripheral blood plasmacytosis on the peripheral smear; however, bone marrow biopsy had persistent bone marrow plasmacytosis of 90% with immunohistochemistry stains being positive for CD138, CD 20, MUM 1, and BCL 2 with negative CD56, as shown in Figure 1.

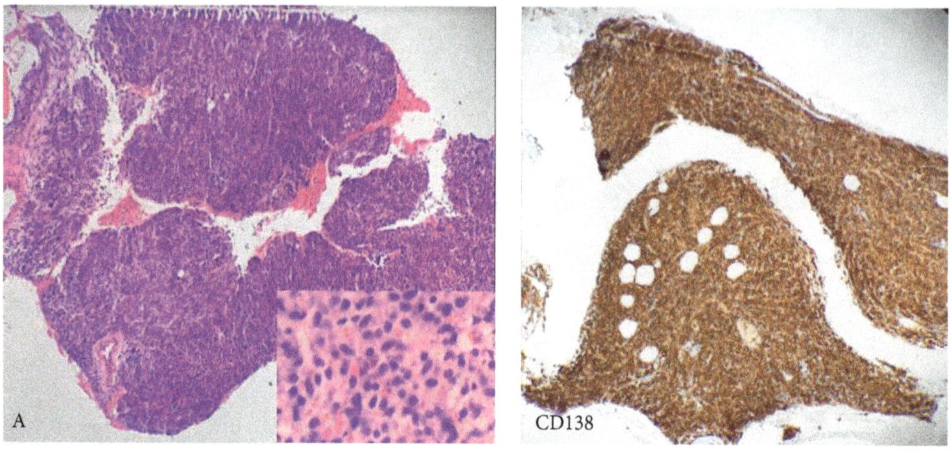

(a) (b)

Figure 1: Representative micrograph of the bone marrow biopsy (a, b); original magnification ×20 haematoxylin eosin (H&E) stain shows a diffuse infiltration by plasma cells with suppressed trilineage haematopoiesis. These plasma cells are positive for CD138 and negative for CD56.

Her treatment regimen was changed to bortezomib, lenalidomide, and dexamethasone with complete response after 4 cycles, no M protein, and normal serum free light chains with bone marrow biopsy with immunohistochemistry showing a plasmacytosis of less than 5%. She proceeded to go for autologous stem cell transplant out of country in May 2019.

Evaluation at the transplant facility included a bone marrow aspirate and trephine that revealed a plasmacytosis of 2% with no peripheral blood plasma cells. Other blood parameters such as total blood count and liver and kidney tests were normal, and a PET CT showed extensive lytic lesions. She received 2 more doses of bortezomib and dexamethasone as she awaited pretransplant work up.

She was mobilized with plerixafor after unsuccessful attempts with Granulocyte Colony-Stimulating Factor (GCSF), and conditioning was with melphalan at 200 mg/m2 followed by infusion of stem cells 24 hours later. Her posttransplant period was complicated by mucositis and febrile neutropenia that responded well to broad-spectrum antibiotics. She had minimal signs of engraftment syndrome managed with steroids and achieved engraftment of white cells and platelets by day 11. After normalization of counts and full recovery, she was discharged back home to have consolidation chemotherapy after 60days after transplant (twice weekly bortezomib and dexamethasone with 21 days of lenalidomide 10 mg) and then proceed to maintenance with lenalidomide and dexamethasone. The patient did well and remained in remission for 1 year.

2.2. Case 2. A 48-year-old male patient presented with generalized body weakness and unintentional weight loss with no fever or bleeding diathesis. Upon admission, he was found to have pallor but no palpable peripheral adenopathy or hepatosplenomegaly. A total blood count revealed a macrocytic anemia (Hb 7.9 g/dl, MCV 106 fl) with a leucocytosis of 36,290/ul (neutrophils 26%, lymphocytes 20%, and monocytes 51%) with a platelet count of 141,000/ul. Reticulocyte count was low at 1% with normal serum B12 and folate levels. A peripheral smear revealed anisocytosis, normochromic red cells, left shift of white blood cells, and large mononuclear plasmacytoid cells which were more than 20%. A diagnosis of plasma cell leukemia was made after bone marrow aspiration that showed infiltration with plasma cells and increase in small mature lymphocytes; however, there was no trephine with immunohistochemistry. In addition, flow cytometry on peripheral blood showed that the abnormal cell population expressed CD38, CD138 and they were lambda restricted; however, B- and T-cell markers were negative as well as CD56. Serum protein electrophoresis showed an M band of 4.2 g/l, as shown in Figure 2, with elevated lambda free light chains of 461 mg/l. Serum immunofixation was not performed in this case. CT scans of the chest and abdomen were unremarkable with no adenopathy and normal-size spleen and liver. Serology for HIV, hepatitis B, and hepatitis C was negative.

He was transfused during his first admission, discharged home, but was readmitted one week later with worsening generalized body weakness, dyspnea, and diarrhoea. He was sick looking and markedly dehydrated with bilateral pitting edema to the level of the knee but clear chest exam. He was hypotensive with a blood pressure of 84/37 mmHg with hypoxia of 87% room air but afebrile at 36.7°C, and a diagnosis of severe sepsis due to gastroenteritis was made and he transferred from the emergency unit to the high-dependency unit. His haemoglobin level was 11 g/dl given recent transfusion but worsening of leucocytosis (60,000/ul) and thrombocytopenia of 43,000/ul. He had acute kidney injury with low total protein and serum albumin (Table 1 outlines a summary of a few selected results during his hospital stay).

The second admission was more protracted lasting 30 days with a predominant time being spent in the high-dependency unit (HDU). Due to lack of blood pressure response to fluid resuscitation, he was initiated on inotropic support. Hypoalbuminemia resulted in third spacing of fluid, but this improved with administration of intravenous albumin. Given the aggressiveness of disease with declining haemoglobin and

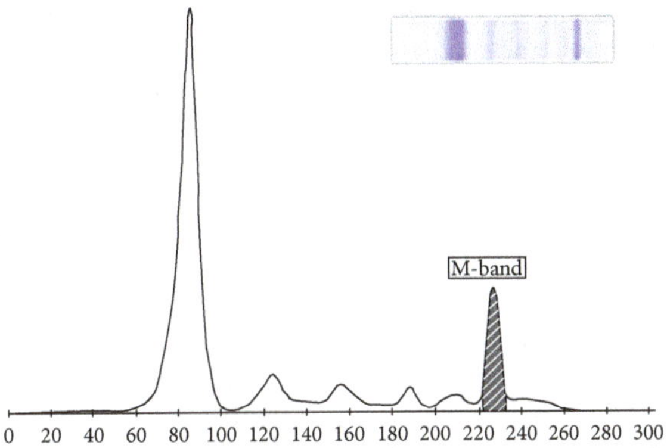

Fractions	%	Ref. %		g/dl	Ref. g/dl
Albumin	63.1	55.8 - 66.1		2.52	3.97 - 4.95
Alpha 1	7.8	2.9 - 4.9	>	0.31	0.21 - 0.35
Alpha 2	7.4	7.1 - 11.8		0.30	0.51 - 0.85
Beta 1	3.5	4.7 - 7.2	<	0.14	0.34 - 0.52
Beta 2	3.2	3.2 - 6.5		0.13	0.23 - 0.47
Gamma	15.0	11.1 - 18.8		0.60	0.80 - 1.35

Peaks	%	g/dl
M-band	10.6	0.42

Figure 2: Serum protein electrophoresis showing an M protein of 4.2 g/l.

Table 1: Selected lab investigations during his hospital stay.

Investigations	Baseline	Day 4	Day 9	Day 13	Day 15	Day 16
Hemoglobin (g/dl)	11.3	9.9	9.3	11.6	12.9	12.3
White cell count	60.2	44.98	25.35	12.13	13.48	17.34
Platelet	43	36	31	76	86	161
Urea (1.5–8.5 mmol/l)	8.95	6.97	5.41	3.88	4.09	3.6
Creatinine (40–133 umol/l)	154	148	80	58	53	60
K (3.5–5.5 mmol/l)	4.15	4.25	3.48	3.23	3.8	4.18
T protein (60–83 gm/l)	39.8	41.9	46.8	57.3	53.8	—
Albumin (35–52 g/l)	24.27	27	27.6	43.56	37.8	—
ALT (0–41 u/l)	30.6	40.9	53.6	31.5	21	—
Total bilirubin(2–21 umol/l)	37	33	45	45	23	—
LDH (90–244 u/l)	1116	—	—	738	—	—
Uric acid (202–416 umol/l)	399	122	119	220		
Calcium (2.02–2.6 mmol/l)	2.2	—	2.2	—	—	—

platelet count, he received adjusted-dose chemotherapy: 1 gram of intravenous cyclophosphamide and weekly dexamethasone 40 mg with bortezomib being held due to low platelets. He tolerated his chemotherapy well. However, on hospital day 10, he developed worsening respiratory symptoms with a new oxygen requirement, and chest radiograph revealed features of pneumonia for which he was commenced on broad-spectrum antibiotics with piperacillin-tazobactam. Subsequently, on hospital day 15, he further desaturated with clinical signs of a right-sided pleural effusion. This was hemorrhagic and drained with a pigtail catheter with the fluid analysis showing an exudate, normal adenine deaminase levels, negative Zielh Niessen stain, and no malignant cells on cytology. This was, therefore, managed as a parapneumonic effusion and drain removed after having no more output. He required transfusions whenever his haemoglobin dropped but did not need platelet transfusion.

He slowly improved initially getting off inotropes, weaning off oxygen successfully to the point of discharge after 30 days in the hospital.

Two weeks after discharge, the patient was more stable with good rehabilitation given prolonged hospitalization that was associated with significant weight loss and reduced level of activity. He was commenced on a bortezomib-based regimen (bortezomib, lenalidomide, and dexamethasone) and has achieved complete response with a plan for autologous stem cell transplant to consolidate the response.

2.3. Case 3. A 53-year-old female referred with a 9-month history of easy fatigability. She had associated bone pains, predominantly back and knee pain, which were previously managed as arthritis. She had no bleeding diathesis, hematemesis, or melena. There was no known family history of malignancy or haematological condition, and she had no history of tobacco use or exposure to chemicals and reported no underlying comorbidities.

She presented to a health facility with palpitations and worsening general body weakness. There, she was found to have severe anemia (haemoglobin of 4.5 g/dl), thrombocytopenia, and acute kidney injury with high serum calcium levels. Her record of actual values was not available. She was transfused both packed red blood cells and pooled platelets. In addition, she received intravenous fluids which resulted in improvement of her renal function. Other laboratory investigations revealed normal serum folate and B12 levels, elevated uric acid, and lactate dehydrogenase (LDH) and a total protein of 100 gm/dl with a monoclonal protein of 54 g/l. An abdominal ultrasound revealed splenomegaly but no intra-abdominal adenopathy. A peripheral blood film showed a leucoerythroblastic picture with atypical mononuclear cells with plasmacytoid appearance at 45% and bone marrow aspirate and trephine revealed infiltration with 74% atypical plasmacytoid cells with a limited immunohistochemistry stains being positive for CD38 and negative for CD20, CD3, MUM1/IRF4, and Tdt.

Her initial treatment course comprised steroids and allopurinol while receiving transfusions of blood products and later was started on bortezomib, lenalidomide, and dexamethasone. Bortezomib was held after a few treatments due to low platelet counts and challenges of platelet transfusions; she, therefore, continued with low-dose lenalidomide and dexamethasone. Two months into her treatment, she developed congestive heart failure with preserved ejection fraction on echocardiography and symptoms improved on diuretics. She had treatment interruptions due to congestive hepatopathy resulting in transaminitis, and medications were restarted when this improved. She also continued to fluctuate in her transfusion requirements which would be carried out at remote facilities due to financial constraints. Initially, she did well; however, during her third cycle, she was reported to have easy fatiguability and shortness of breath and taken to a nearby hospital for urgent care; however, she succumbed in a few days. The cause of death at this point was not clear given lack of access to records from the admitting hospital.

This case highlights the challenges that clinicians in sub-Saharan Africa face in managing patients where cost affects choices patients make in seeking care, especially with regard to hospital admissions. As a result, in the clinical journey, they receive part of care at a facility away from their primary doctor, especially in-patient.

3. Epidemiology and Clinical Presentation

PCL is not common with various studies reporting incidence of less than 1% to 4% [2–4]. The median age is younger than for MM patients, between 50 and 60 years with a slight male predominance [5, 6]. Studies conducted in China revealed a younger population below 50 years [7, 8]. Our patients were all less than 60 years with the youngest being 48 years.

Unlike MM, patients with plasma cell leukemia have a more aggressive clinical presentation due to a higher tumour burden. The symptoms may range from profound cytopenias, mainly anemia and thrombocytopenia resulting in bleeding diathesis. They can also present with bone pain, symptoms due to hypercalcemia, or acute kidney injury [5, 9, 10].

On physical examination, these patients have a higher prevalence of organomegaly with involvement of the liver and spleen [11]. Other patients may have pleural effusion, neurological deficits due to CNS involvement, or palpable extramedullary soft tissue plasmacytomas. This is reflected by cases discussed.

Lytic lesions on imaging is reported to be lower than in MM; however, it may be found in approximately half of the patients more so those with sPCL [11]. This is illustrated in the first case where the patient had extensive lytic disease, hence the question whether she had sPCL as opposed to pPCL.

4. Diagnosis

Kyles' criteria described in 1974 required at least 20% of total white blood cells be circulating plasma cells with a peripheral blood absolute plasma cell count of at least 2×10^9/l [12]. There is debate on whether both criteria need to be met as per Kyle et al.'s recommendation, and many reports have used the presence of at least one criteria, although there is no consensus as to threshold for diagnosis, with the increasing studies showing that patients with circulating plasma cells between 5 and 20% had shorter median overall survival of approximately 6 months, similar to those with >20% PCs.

Advances in flow cytometry have allowed for better characterization and clonal assessment of plasma cell population. Clonality is important to establish to rule out reactive plasma cells in context of infection or inflammation which are polyclonal or exclude other lymphoproliferative diseases such as lymphoplasmacytic lymphoma [9]. The International Myeloma Working Group (IMWG) and the World Health Organization (WHO) have accepted that either one of the criteria is sufficient.

CD138 and CD38 are expressed in plasma cells in multiple myeloma and plasma cell leukemia. CD56, a neuronal cell adhesion molecule, seems to be more prevalent in MM as opposed to B-cell marker CD 20 which are more positive in PCL. CD56 which facilitates interactions with the bone marrow microenvironment and prevents circulation from the bone marrow to the blood tends to be absent in PCL [13]. In addition, there is lower expression of CD9, CD117, and HLA DR. There is higher CD28 expression in secondary PCL which correlates with a rise in plasma cell proliferation and disease progression. Increased expression of CD27 has been associated with activation of the antiapoptotic pathway. The IMWG consensus on PCL is that measurement of immunophenotypic residual disease is needed when there is no evidence of plasma cell infiltration on routine morphology evaluation.

A majority of patients will have markedly elevated serum lactate dehydrogenase (LDH) levels and B_2 macroglobulin [1, 14].

Most patients with PCL tend to have hypodiploidy or pseudodiploidy and high risk or complex cytogenetic abnormalities [5, 8, 15]. Majority of the PCL cases had translocation involving the immunoglobulin heavy-chain locus (IgH) on 14q32 such as t (11, 14), t (4; 14), and t (14; 16). TP53 inactivation, MYC translocations, and mutations in K-RAS and N-RAS were among those documented with PTEN deletion which cause Akt activation being more in sPCL.

Imaging either by whole-body MRI or PET CT scan is important to check for any extramedullary component [1].

5. Management

Management includes adequate supportive care as well as definitive therapy that depends on the transplant eligibility. Choice of regimen will depend on patient performance status, existing comorbidities, and availability of drugs, as well as the centres' ability to administer the regimen.

Supportive treatment includes, but is not limited to, transfusions, treating hypercalcemia, renal insufficiency, and infections. It is important to watch out for tumour lysis given the high tumour burden in this patient population. This would require the managing team to monitor uric acid, potassium, calcium, phosphorous, and creatinine levels at the time of instituting definitive therapy.

Studies have shown that use of drug combinations involving novel agents has better responses and median overall survival than use of single agents or conventional chemotherapy [16]. The use of novel agents (immunomodulators and proteasome inhibitors) has been associated with a higher response rate which is consolidated to an even deeper response by autologous stem cell transplant resulting in improved overall survival [17]. Some examples of regimes in transplant candidates are VTD-PACE (bortezomib, thalidomide, dexamethasone, cisplatin, doxorubicin, cyclophosphamide, and etoposide), HyperCVAD-VTD (hyperfractionated cyclophosphamide, vincristine, adriamycin, dexamethasone, bortezomib, thalidomide, and dexamethasone), PAD (Bortezomib, Adriamycin, and Dexamethasone), and VCD (bortezomib, cyclophosphamide, and dexamethasone). After transplant, it is highly recommended that these patients receive consolidation therapy with bortezomib-based combinations followed by maintenance.

Nontransplant candidates also receive bortezomib-based regimens so as to achieve a rapid response and improve outcome. These include CyBorD (cyclophosphamide, bortezomib, and dexamethasone), VTD (bortezomib, thalidomide, and dexamethasone), and MPV (melphalan, bortezomib, and prednisone) among others [18].

Many studies have demonstrated the effectiveness of bortezomib in clearing plasma cell leukemia, normalizing platelet count, and better overall survival compared to conventional therapies [13, 19, 20]. Musto et al. showed 92% overall response with the use of bortezomib which was also replicated by the Greek Myeloma group that looked at a larger patient population [16, 19]. It is, therefore, important that where patients have no contraindications, bortezomib-based regimens be used.

Lenalidomide-based therapies have reported overall responses of 60% with clear lack of benefit with thalidomide. The later should, therefore, be avoided as initial therapy and especially as monotherapy [19, 21–23].

An Italian multicentre retrospective review of 128 PCL patients showed that hematopoietic stem cell transplant improves overall survival and duration of response by 69% and 88%, respectively [6]. Results from the Center for International Blood and Marrow Transplant Research showed that autologous stem cell transplant is better than allogeneic stem cell transplant due to higher nonrelapse mortality with no benefit in overall survival [21]. The current challenge is the short duration of response as demonstrated by a large cohort of 272 pPCL patients in the European Group for Blood and Marrow Transplantation when compared to myeloma [24]. Newer agents have also been used in plasma cell leukemia such as carfilzomib, ixazomib, monoclonal antibodies to CD38 such as daratumumab, and novel therapies such as Bcl-2 inhibitor, venetoclax in those with t(11; 14) [25, 26].

6. Prognosis

Plasma cell leukemia has a poor prognosis in comparison to multiple myeloma [11, 14, 26]. In addition, the outcome for sPCL is much worse and most studies report survival of few months in comparison to pPCL [9, 12, 14, 27]. Talamo et al. who studied the outcome of PCL in the era of novel agents found a median survival of 21 months for pPCL in comparison to 4 months for sPCL which was statistically significant ($p = 0.015$) [27].

The Center for International Blood and Marrow Transplant Research documented an overall survival of 51% at 5 years after pPCL treatment had been consolidated with autologous stem cell transplant [21].

Studies have demonstrated some factors such as age more than 60 yrs, platelet count less than 100,000/ul, and peripheral blood plasma cells more than 20% to be predictors of worse survival [17]. Others reported include poor performance status (ECOG >2) and elevated serum LDH, as well as B2 microglobulin and cytogenetics such as 17 p deletion [7].

7. Conclusions

Plasma cell leukemia is a rare aggressive form of plasma cell dysrasia that needs to be diagnosed early and managed aggressively before patients get complications. Given poor prognosis, it is important to use novel agents as part of the induction regimen followed by autologous transplant in those who are transplant eligible. Despite the improvement in diagnostics and treatment, sub-Saharan Africa faces challenges where the patients' treatment journey depends on what they are able to afford and accessibility to those services.

References

[1] M. T. Gundesen, T. Lund, H. E. H. Moeller, and N. Abildgaard, "Plasma cell leukemia: definition, presentation, and treatment," *Current Oncology Reports*, vol. 21, no. 1, p. 8, 2019.

[2] G. Ramsingh, P. Mehan, J. Luo, R. Vij, and D. Morgensztern, "Plasma cell leukemia: a SEER database analysis," *Journal of Clinical Oncology*, vol. 27, no. 15_suppl, p. 8605, 2009.

[3] M. Sant, C. Allemani, C. Tereanu et al., "Incidence of hematologic malignancies in Europe by morphologic subtype: results of the HAEMACARE project," *Blood*, vol. 116, no. 19, pp. 3724–3734, 2010.

[4] P. Gimsing, M. Holmstrøm, T. Wirenfelt Klausen et al., "The Danish national multiple myeloma registry," *Clinical Epidemiology*, vol. 8, pp. 583–587, 2016.

[5] M. Čolović, G. Janković, N. Suvajdžić, N. Milić, V. Dordević, and S. Janković, "Thirty patients with primary plasma cell leukemia: a single center experience," *Medical Oncology*, vol. 25, no. 2, pp. 154–160, 2008.

[6] L. Pagano, C. G. Valentini, V. de Stefano et al., "Primary plasma cell leukemia: a retrospective multicenter study of 73 patients," *Annals of Oncology*, vol. 22, no. 7, pp. 1628–1635, 2011.

[7] C. Zeji and Z. Guozhen, "Primary plasma cell leukemia," *Chinese Journal of Cancer Research*, vol. 3, no. 2, pp. 71–74, 1991.

[8] Q. Peijing, X. Yan, W. Yafei et al., "A retrospective analysis of thirty-one cases of plasma cell leukemia from a single center in China," *Acta Haematologica*, vol. 121, no. 1, pp. 47–51, 2009.

[9] C. Fernández de Larrea, R. A. Kyle, R. A. Kyle et al., "Plasma cell leukemia: consensus statement on diagnostic requirements, response criteria and treatment recommendations by the International Myeloma Working Group," *Leukemia*, vol. 27, no. 4, pp. 780–791, 2013.

[10] R. Costello, D. Sainty, R. Bouabdallah et al., "Primary plasma cell leukaemia: a report of 18 cases," *Leukemia Research*, vol. 25, no. 2, pp. 103–107, 2001.

[11] N. Yadav, M. Aggarwal, P. Mehta et al., "Primary plasma cell leukemia: a retrospective study of a rare disease from tertiary cancer centre from India," *Indian Journal of Hematology and Blood Transfusion*, vol. 35, no. 4, pp. 649–654, 2019.

[12] R. A. Kyle, J. E. Maldonado, and E. D. Bayrd, "Plasma cell leukemia. Report on 17 cases," *Archives of Internal Medicine*, vol. 133, no. 5, pp. 813–818, 1974.

[13] C. Al-Nawakil, J. Tamburini, V. Bardet et al., "Bortezomib, doxorubicin and dexamethasone association is an effective option for plasma cell leukemia induction therapy," *Leukemia & Lymphoma*, vol. 49, no. 10, pp. 2012–2014, 2008.

[14] G. Talamo, N. G. Dolloff, K. Sharma, J. Zhu, and J. Malysz, "Clinical features and outcomes of plasma cell leukemia: a single-institution experience in the era of novel agents," *Rare Tumors*, vol. 4, no. 3, p. e39, 2012.

[15] R. E. Tiedemann, N. Gonzalez-Paz, R. A. Kyle et al., "Genetic aberrations and survival in plasma cell leukemia," *Leukemia*, vol. 22, no. 5, pp. 1044–1052, 2008.

[16] E. Katodritou, E. Terpos, C. Kelaidi et al., "Treatment with bortezomib-based regimens improves overall response and predicts for survival in patients with primary or secondary plasma cell leukemia: analysis of the Greek myeloma study group," *American Journal of Hematology*, vol. 89, no. 2, pp. 145–150, 2014.

[17] A. Jurczyszyn, J. Radocha, J. Davila et al., "Prognostic indicators in primary plasma cell leukaemia: a multicentre retrospective study of 117 patients," *British Journal of Haematology*, vol. 180, no. 6, pp. 831–839, 2018.

[18] A. Suska, D. H. Vesole, J. J. Castillo et al., "Plasma cell leukemia - facts and controversies: more questions than answers?" *Clinical Hematology International*, vol. 2, no. 4, p. 133, 2020.

[19] P. Musto, F. Rossini, F. Gay et al., "Efficacy and safety of bortezomib in patients with plasma cell leukemia," *Cancer*, vol. 109, no. 11, pp. 2285–2290, 2007.

[20] D. Lebovic, L. Zhang, M. Alsina et al., "Clinical outcomes of patients with plasma cell leukemia in the era of novel therapies and hematopoietic stem cell transplantation strategies: a single-institution experience," *Clinical Lymphoma Myeloma and Leukemia*, vol. 11, no. 6, pp. 507–511, 2011.

[21] A. Mahindra, M. E. Kalaycio, J. Vela-Ojeda et al., "Hematopoietic cell transplantation for primary plasma cell leukemia: results from the center for international blood and marrow transplant research," *Leukemia*, vol. 26, no. 5, pp. 1091–1097, 2012.

[22] M. T. Petrucci, V. Martini, A. Levi et al., "Thalidomide does not modify the prognosis of plasma cell leukemia patients: experience of a single center," *Leukemia & Lymphoma*, vol. 48, no. 1, pp. 180–182, 2007.

[23] D. M. Benson and M. K. Smith, "Effectiveness of lenalidomide (Revlimid) for the treatment of plasma cell leukemia," *Leukemia & Lymphoma*, vol. 48, no. 7, pp. 1423–1425, 2007.

[24] M. B. Drake, S. Iacobelli, A. van Biezen et al., "Primary plasma cell leukemia and autologous stem cell transplantation," *Haematologica*, vol. 95, no. 5, pp. 804–809, 2010.

[25] S. Ngu, D. Asti, G. Valecha, N. Thumallapally, M. Pant, and A. Bershadskiy, "Primary plasma cell leukemia: a case report and review of the literature," *Clinical Case Reports*, vol. 7, no. 9, pp. 1702–1708, 2019.

[26] W. I. Gonsalves, F. K. Buadi, and S. K. Kumar, "Combination therapy incorporating Bcl-2 inhibition with Venetoclax for the treatment of refractory primary plasma cell leukemia with t (11; 14)," *European Journal of Haematology*, vol. 100, no. 2, pp. 215–217, 2018.

[27] H. Wang, H. Zhou, Z. Zhang, C. Geng, and W. Chen, "Bortezomib-based regimens improve the outcome of patients with primary or secondary plasma cell leukemia: a retrospective cohort study," *Turkish Journal of Hematology*, vol. 37, no. 2, pp. 91–97, 2020.

14

A Rare Case of Extracavitary Primary Effusion Lymphoma in the Bladder and Ureter

Jiankun Tong[1] **Sana Jadallah,**[1] **William H. Rodgers,**[1,2] **Gabriel Jung,**[3] **Malvina Fulman,**[3] **and Abhisek Swaika**[3]

[1]*Department of Pathology, New York–Presbyterian Queens, 56-45 Main Street, Flushing, NY 11355, USA*
[2]*Weill Cornell Medical College, 525 East 68th Street, Box 130, New York, NY 10065, USA*
[3]*Hematology & Medical Oncology, Queens Medical Associates, 176-60 Union Tpke # 360, Fresh Meadows, NY 11366, USA*

Correspondence should be addressed to Jiankun Tong; jtong90@hotmail.com

Academic Editor: Sylvain Choquet

Primary effusion lymphoma (PEL) is a rare and very aggressive large B-cell lymphoma usually presenting as serous effusions without a tumor mass. It is universally associated with human herpesvirus type-8 (HHV-8) infection. It most commonly occurs in the body cavities and rarely develops as solid tumor masses in the wall of cavity and other organs, and it has been termed as extracavitary PEL. Extracavitary PEL has been reported in the lymph nodes and extranodal sites. Here we report a rare case of extracavitary PEL occurring in the bladder and ureter of a human immunodeficiency virus (HIV)-negative 76-year-old Chinese male, presenting with right leg swelling, erythema, and pain. To the best of our knowledge, this is the first case of extracavitary PEL presenting in the bladder and ureter.

1. Case Presentation

A 76-year-old Chinese male, former smoker, with no other significant past medical history or other high-risk behavior and not on medications presented to the hospital for worsening right lower extremity swelling, erythema, and pain. The swelling suddenly started 3 days ago, with occasional cough and dyspnea on exertion. He denied trauma or injury to the area, fever, chills, chest pain, nausea, vomiting, abdominal pain, and dysuria. He did mention some unintentional weight loss. Physical exam was pertinent for right leg swelling, decreased breath sounds on right side, and abdominal distension.

Laboratory analysis revealed mild leukocytosis with normal differentials, mild anemia (Hb 10.6 g/dl), and a normal platelet count of 386 K/μl. His creatinine was elevated. HIV and hepatitis testing were negative. Epstein–Barr virus (EBV) serology signified a past infection. HHV-8 serology testing was not available. Bilateral Doppler ultrasound results were negative for deep vein thrombosis, and a ventilation-perfusion (VQ) scan revealed a low probability for pulmonary embolism.

Renal ultrasound demonstrated moderate hydronephrosis on the right and mild hydronephrosis on the left, with no evidence of calculi in the kidney, ureters, and bladder. Computed tomography (CT) and a following positron emission tomography (PET) scan revealed a mass like encasement of the proximal right ureter and bladder (Figures 1(a) and 1(b)), along with retroperitoneal lymphadenopathy on the right side. Moderate to large pleural effusion was noted on the chest CT scan. Subcutaneous lymphedema was seen on magnetic resonance imaging (MRI) of the right lower extremity. His ejection fraction was normal on echocardiogram. Patient refused a lumbar puncture. He did not have any neurological symptoms.

Urine cytology revealed atypical urothelial cells. Patient underwent cystoscopy and right ureteroscopy, demonstrating bullous edema and erosion at the bilateral trigone areas and in the right mid-distal ureter. Bladder biopsy was taken and a right ureteral stent was placed. The patient also underwent a diagnostic and therapeutic thoracentesis.

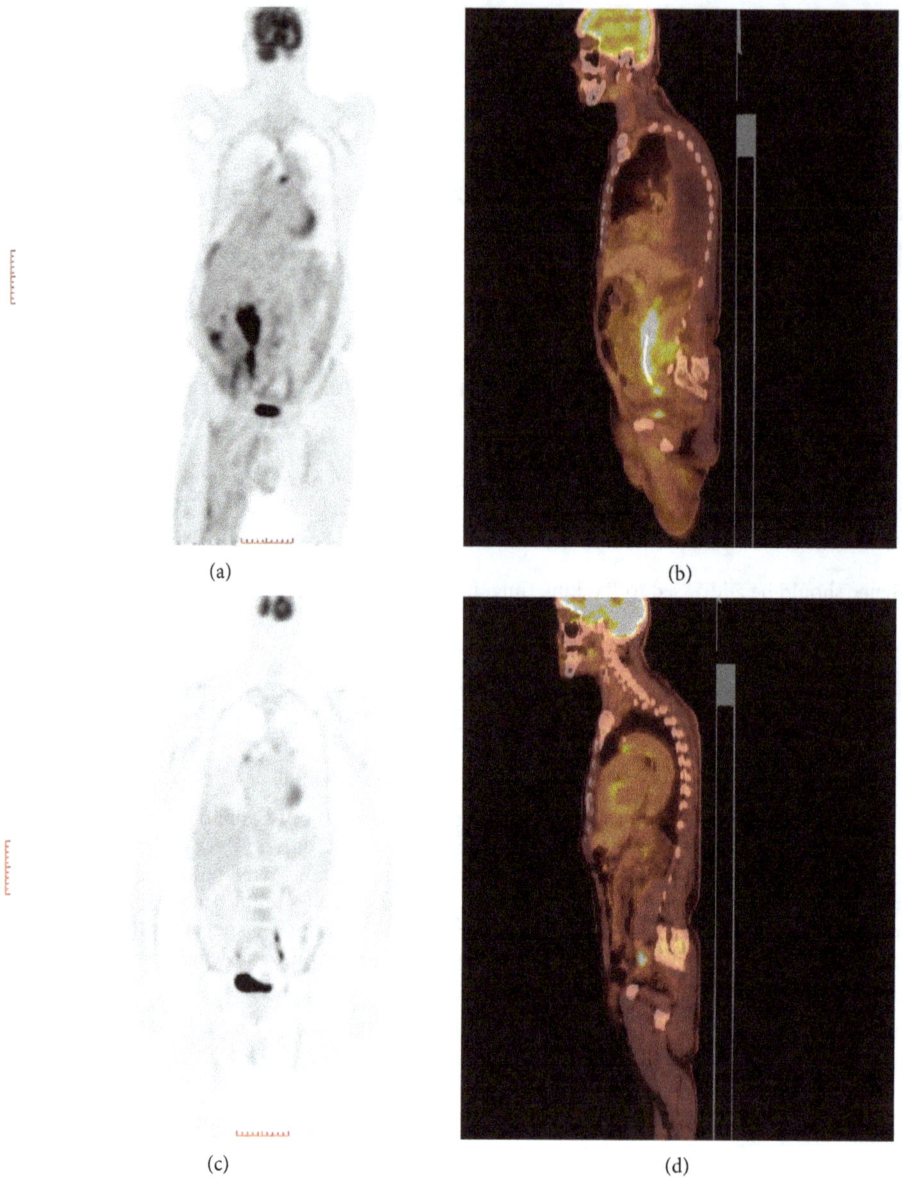

Figure 1: Initial diagnostic PET-CT scan with soft tissue mass encasing the right proximal ureter (a and b). Complete resolution of right periureteral mass on treatment completion PET-CT scan (c and d).

2. Diagnosis

Microscopic examination of the histologic sections showed sheets of medium-sized to large neoplastic cells in the suburothelium (Figures 2(a) and 2(b)) with scant cytoplasm, a high nuclear/cytoplasmic (N/C) ratio, round or oval nuclei with fine or vesicular chromatin, and indistinct nucleoli (Figure 2(c)). Mitotic figures and apoptotic bodies were frequently seen. The urothelial mucosa demonstrated focal erosion and hemorrhage (Figure 2(b)).

An extensive immunohistochemistry (IHC) panel was performed which found the neoplastic cells to be positive for CD30 (Figure 2(d)), CD45 (weak), CD138 (Figure 2(e)), EMA (Figure 2(f)), MUM-1 (Figure 2(g)), EBER (Figure 2(h)), and human herpesvirus 8 (HHV-8) (Figure 2(i)), while being negative for AE1/3, ALK-1, BCL-1, BCL-6, CAM 5.2, CD3, CD5, CD10, CD20, CD34, CD68, CD79a, CD99, chromogranin, desmin, HMB-45, kappa and lambda, Mart-1, PAX-5, S100, synaptophysin, TdT, and WT-1.

The thin-prep and cell block analysis on the pleural fluid also demonstrated the large atypical hematopoietic cells (Figure 3(a)) and had a similar immunophenotype profile to that of the bladder biopsy, also being positive for HHV-8 (Figure 3(b)).

The consistent morphology and immunophenotypic characteristics along with the clinical presentation led to the diagnosis of an extracavitary PEL of the bladder and ureter.

3. Treatment

Due to the aggressive nature of this subtype of lymphoma, International Prognostic Index (IPI) score 5, the patient was

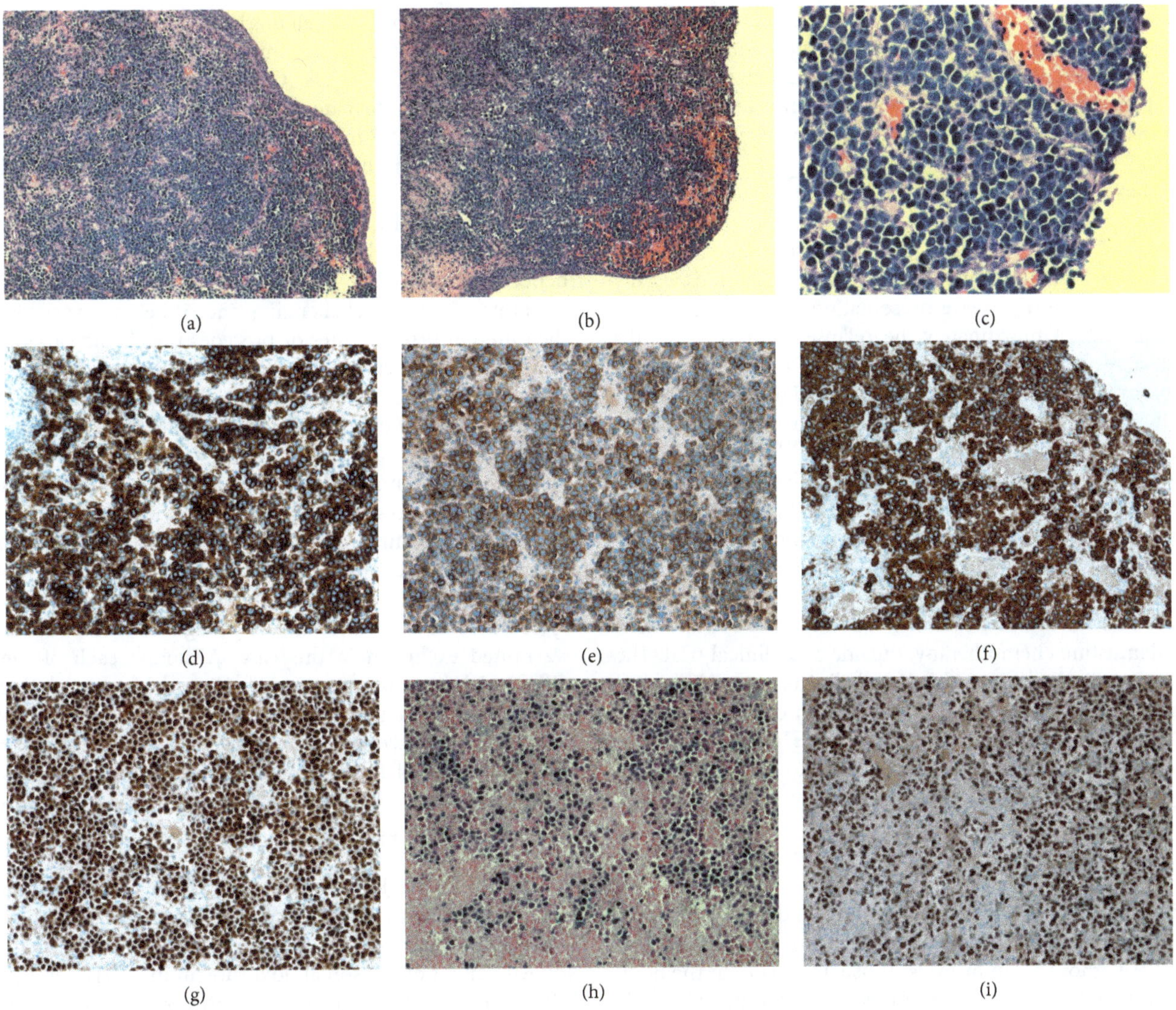

FIGURE 2: HE section shows the neoplastic cells in the suburothelium (×2) (a). Urothelial mucosa in bladder shows focal mucosal erosion and ulceration (×2) (b). HE section shows medium-sized to large neoplastic cells (×40) (c). The neoplastic cells are positive for CD30 (d), CD138 (e), EMA (f), MUM-1 (g), EBER (h), and HHV-8 (i).

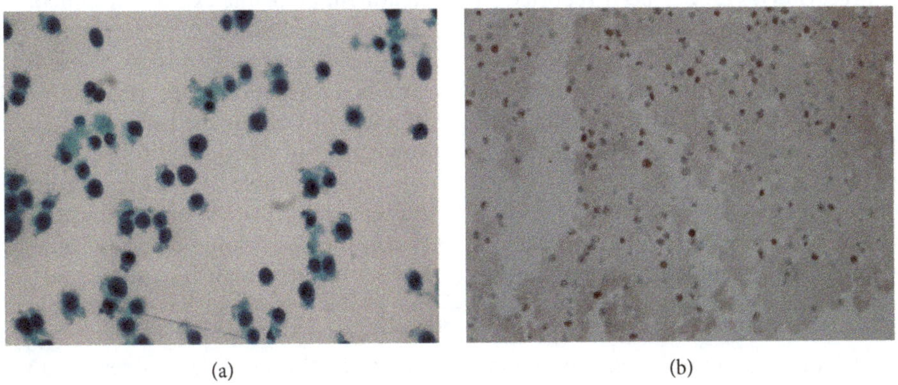

FIGURE 3: The thin-prep shows large atypical hematopoietic cells in the pleural fluid (×40) (a). The neoplastic cells are positive for HHV-8 (b).

promptly started on chemotherapy with cyclophosphamide, Adriamycin, vincristine, and prednisone (CHOP), outside of a clinical trial. He tolerated the treatment well and had a continued significant clinical and radiological response to chemotherapy. His breathing improved, and he did not require any further thoracentesis. He gained weight, and his creatinine also normalized, undergoing an interim stent exchange. An interim PET scan after 2 cycles demonstrated decreasing bladder wall thickness and size of the periureteral mass and lymphadenopathy, along with reduced pleural effusion. He continued on the CHOP chemotherapy and completed 6 cycles attaining almost complete radiological remission on the following PET-CT scan (Figures 1(c) and 1(d)).

He was started on active surveillance. Due to the initial advanced stage presentation (lymphomatous pleural effusion) and complete radiological response to systemic chemotherapy, radiation therapy was not considered especially due to the site of disease presentation and the paucity of clinical data. Unfortunately, he relapsed within 3 months with a recurrent periureteral mass, abdominal lymphadenopathy, and neck lesions. Repeat biopsy of the neck lesion confirmed the extracavitary PEL diagnosis with the same IHC profile as prior (HHV-8+, CD 30+, EBER+, MUM-1+, and CD 20−). Kaposi sarcoma and multicentric Castleman disease were again ruled out given the HHV-8 positivity. He was deemed to not be a transplant candidate. With the paucity of available and accessible appropriate clinical trial for an HIV-negative rare PEL presentation, the patient was started on salvage brentuximab vedotin (CD-30+) and then bendamustine chemotherapy, outside of a clinical trial. The patient again had very abbreviated clinical and radiological responses to the treatments, but thereafter could not tolerate any further antineoplastic treatments. He was placed in hospice, and he passed away due to this aggressive lymphoma.

4. Discussion

Primary effusion lymphoma is a rare and very aggressive large B-cell lymphoma usually presenting as malignant effusions without a tumor mass. It usually occurs in the body cavities, and the most common sites are the pleural, pericardial, and peritoneal cavities [1–3]. Most cases are limited to the body cavities of origin, but subsequent dissemination can happen. It rarely develops as solid tumor masses in the wall of cavity and other organs and has been termed as extracavitary PEL. Extracavitary PEL has been reported in the lymph nodes, the most frequent site, and few extranodal sites, such as the central nervous system, intestinal tract, lungs, and skin [1–7], similar to the other extranodal noncavitary non-Hodgkin lymphoma (NHL) presentations.

PEL accounts for approximately 4% of HIV-associated non-Hodgkin lymphoma and <1% of non-HIV-related lymphomas [8]. There is a frequent coinfection of EBV, accounting for 60%–90% of cases [9–11]. PEL and extracavitary PEL are universally associated with human herpesvirus type-8 (HHV-8) infection [9, 12].

Diagnosis of PEL and extracavitary PEL is based on the clinical manifestation along with morphology, immunohistochemistry, and molecular studies.

On histopathological analysis, the lymphoma cells exhibit a variety of appearances, ranging from large immunoblastic/plasmablastic cells to cells with anaplastic morphology [13]. The IHC is typically positive for CD30, CD38, CD45, VS38c, CD138, HHV-8, and MUM-1. EMA is variably expressed on the lymphoma cells, but they usually lack the expression of B-cell markers (CD19, CD20, CD79a, surface and cytoplasmic immunoglobulin) and T-cell markers (CD2, CD3, CD4, CD5, CD7, and CD8) [13–17]. The definitive/confirmatory diagnosis of PEL requires the detection of HHV-8 infection in lymphoma cells, which can be performed by immunohistochemistry, PCR, or molecular studies [14].

PEL is clinically unique as it predominantly presents as a lymphomatous malignant effusion within body cavities, hence confirming the diagnosis, whereas the diagnosis of extracavitary PEL is challenging since it behaves variably at the different primary sites or precedes the classic variant of PEL. By no difference, the histopathological feature of extracavitary PEL is similar to PEL thereby aiding with the diagnosis [13], though other differentials need to be diligently excluded.

The most common differential diagnosis includes other subtypes of aggressive non-Hodgkin lymphoma such as plasmablastic lymphoma, anaplastic large-cell lymphoma, diffuse large B-cell lymphoma, and plasmacytoma with anaplastic variant. Other malignant tumors such plasmacytoid urothelial carcinoma, and malignant melanoma also warranted exclusion in this case. Although each of these differential diagnoses mentioned above shares morphologic features and some immunophenotypic profile with PEL and extracavitary PEL, each can be easily distinguished from PEL by the absence of HHV-8 antigen within neoplastic cells.

PEL is most commonly seen in immunocompromised patients, such as patients with concomitant HIV infection, organ transplant, etc. As in other lymphomas, active treatment of the HIV infection, reversal of the immune suppression, takes precedence along with antilymphoma treatment as demonstrated in a recent case study of prolonged benefit of liposomal doxorubicin in an HIV infected PEL patient [18]. PEL can, however, rarely present in patients with an intact immune function, like in our patient. Due to the rarity of this malignancy, treatment recommendations are generally based on expert opinions, retrospective case series, reports, etc., and hence no consensus treatment guideline exists. Enrollment in well designed and prospective clinical trial is understandably challenging.

Initial treatment consists of use of standard aggressive lymphoma chemotherapy regimens such as dose adjusted EPOCH or CHOP. The lack of CD-20 expression precludes any benefit of rituximab use. Patients with relapsed disease are treated similar to other aggressive lymphomas and should be evaluated for autologous stem cell transplant. More emphasis should be placed on an expedited diagnosis and early enrollment in clinical trials.

To the best of our knowledge, this is the first case of an extracavitary PEL which occurred in the bladder and ureter, along with the more classical serosal involvement of the right pleural cavity.

In summary, extracavitary PEL can clinically present as an aggressive lymphoma at any unexpected location, even in the absence of HIV infection or other forms of immune suppression. A diligent diagnostic suspicion should promptly lead to a HHV-8 antigen testing to avoid a diagnostic pitfall, and help initiate an expedited antilymphoma treatment. PEL is associated with a very poor prognosis, and clinical trial enrollment should be strongly encouraged.

References

[1] M. W. Beaty, S. Kumar, L. Sorbara, K. Miller, M. Raffeld, and E. S. Jaffe, "A biphenotypic human herpesvirus 8–associated primary bowel lymphoma," *The American Journal of Surgical Pathology*, vol. 23, no. 8, pp. 992–994, 1999.

[2] W. DePond, J. W. Said, T. Tasaka et al., "Kaposi's sarcoma-associated herpesvirus and human herpesvirus 8 (KSHV/HHV8)-associated lymphoma of the bowel," *The American Journal of Surgical Pathology*, vol. 21, no. 6, pp. 719–724, 1997.

[3] T. Otsuki, S. Kumar, B. Ensoli et al., "Detection of HHV-8/KSHV DNA sequences in AIDS-associated extranodal lymphoid malignancies," *Leukemia*, vol. 10, no. 8, pp. 1358–1362, 1996.

[4] A. Chadburn, E. Hyjek, S. Mathew, E. Cesarman, J. Said, and D. M. Knowles, "KSHV-positive solid lymphomas represent an extra-cavitary variant of primary effusion lymphoma," *The American Journal of Surgical Pathology*, vol. 28, no. 11, pp. 1401–1416, 2004.

[5] S. E. Coupland, F. Charlotte, G. Mansour, K. Maloum, M. Hummel, and H. Stein, "HHV-8-associated T-cell lymphoma in a lymph node with concurrent peritoneal effusion in an HIV-positive man," *The American Journal of Surgical Pathology*, vol. 29, no. 5, pp. 647–652, 2005.

[6] O. E. Kabiawu-Ajise, J. Harris, N. Ismaili, E. Amorosi, and S. Ibrahim, "Primary effusion lymphoma with central nervous system involvement in an HIV-negative homosexual male," *Acta Haematologica*, vol. 128, no. 2, pp. 77–82, 2012.

[7] U. Pielasinski, C. Santonja, S. M. Rodríguez-Pinilla, and L. Requena, "Extracavitary primary effusion lymphoma presenting as a cutaneous tumor: a case report and literature review," *Journal of Cutaneous Pathology*, vol. 41, no. 9, pp. 745–753, 2014.

[8] L. D. Kaplan, "Human herpesvirus-8: kaposi sarcoma, multicentric Castleman disease, and primary effusion lymphoma," *Hematology*, vol. 2013, no. 1, pp. 103–108, 2013.

[9] E. Cesarman, Y. Chang, P. S. Moore, J. W. Said, and D. M. Knowles, "Kaposi's sarcoma-associated herpesvirus-like DNA sequences in AIDS-related body-cavity-based lymphomas," *New England Journal of Medicine*, vol. 332, no. 18, pp. 1186–1191, 1995.

[10] R. G. Nador, E. Cesarman, A. Chadburn et al., "Primary effusion lymphoma: a distinct clinicopathologic entity associated with the Kaposi's sarcoma-associated herpes virus," *Blood*, vol. 88, no. 2, pp. 645–656, 1996.

[11] K. Dunleavy and W. H. Wilson, "How I treat HIV-associated lymphoma," *Blood*, vol. 119, no. 14, pp. 3245–3255, 2012.

[12] Y. Chang, E. Cesarman, M. Pessin et al., "Identification of herpesvirus-like DNA sequences in AIDS-associated Kaposi's sarcoma," *Science*, vol. 266, no. 5192, pp. 1865–1869, 1994.

[13] S. H. Swerdlow, E. Campo, N. L. Harris et al., *WHO Classification of Tumor of Haematopoietic and Lymphoid Tissue* WHO Press, Geneva, Switzerland, 5th edition, 2017.

[14] M. Narkhede, S. Arora, and C. Ujjani, "Primary effusion lymphoma: current perspectives," *OncoTargets and Therapy* vol. 11, pp. 3747–3754, 2018. ,

[15] Y. Kim, C. J. Park, J. Roh, and J. Huh, "Current concepts in primary effusion lymphoma and other effusion-based lymphomas," *Korean Journal of Pathology*, vol. 48, no. 2,, pp. 81–90, 2014.

[16] S. Okada, H. Goto, and M. Yotsumoto, "Current status of treatment for primary effusion lymphoma," *Intractable & Rare Diseases Research*, vol. 3, no. 3, pp. 65–74, 2014.

[17] H. Stein, D. Mason, J. Gerdes et al., "The expression of the Hodgkin's disease associated antigen Ki-1 in reactive and neoplastic lymphoid tissue: evidence that Reed-Sternberg cells and histiocytic malignancies are derived from activated lymphoid cells," *Blood*, vol. 66, no. 4, pp. 848–858, 1985.

[18] J. Chen, V. Mehraj, J. Szabo, B. Routy, R. P. Michel, and J. P. Routy, "Multiple remissions of extracavitary primary effusion lymphoma treated with a single cycle of liposomal doxorubicin in a patient infected with HIV," *Current Oncology*, vol. 25, no. 6, pp. e592–e596, 2018.

15

Central Nervous System Double Relapse of Acute Promyelocytic Leukemia and Acute Myelomonocytic Leukemia

Laura M. Stanko,[1] Vishnu Reddy,[2] Fady M. Mikhail,[3] and Nikolaos Papadantonakis[4]

[1]*Internal Medicine Program, University of Alabama at Birmingham, Birmingham, AL, USA*
[2]*Division of Anatomic Pathology and Neuropathology, University of Alabama at Birmingham, Birmingham, AL, USA*
[3]*Department of Genetics, University of Alabama at Birmingham, Birmingham, AL, USA*
[4]*Division of Hematology/Oncology, University of Alabama at Birmingham, Birmingham, AL, USA*

Correspondence should be addressed to Nikolaos Papadantonakis; papadan@uab.edu

Academic Editor: Tomás J. González-López

Relapse of acute promyelocytic leukemia (APL) and non-M3-acute myeloid leukemia in the central nervous system (CNS) are rare events. Here, we describe a case of simultaneous relapses of APL and acute myelomonocytic leukemia on the CNS of a patient after allogeneic bone marrow transplant. This extremely unusual case highlights the difficulties that CNS leukemia relapses pose in the post-transplant setting.

1. Introduction

Central nervous system (CNS) recurrence in adults with either acute promyelocytic leukemia (APL) or other subtypes of acute myeloid leukemia (AML) is uncommon, with previous studies reporting occurrences of 3–5% in APL and 1–2.5% in AML [1, 2]. These recurrences are typically associated with poor prognosis, and there is no consensus as to optimal treatment regimens [2, 3].

We present here a case of simultaneous, double relapse, of acute myelomonocytic leukemia (AMML) and APL in the CNS of a patient with concurrent molecular relapse of APL in the bone marrow (BM).

2. Case Presentation

2.1. Diagnosis of APL. The patient was 62 years old at the time of initial diagnosis of APL. She was hospitalized with bruising and malaise and found to have a white blood cell count (WBC) of $0.46 \times 10^3/\text{cm}^3$, hemoglobin of 8.6 gr/dl, and platelets of $13 \times 10^3/\text{cm}^3$. Based on the Sanz schema, she had intermediate risk APL [4]. Bone marrow (BM) biopsy was consistent with APL (Table 1). FISH analysis of peripheral blood demonstrated the presence of *PML/RARA* fusion in 95.5% of cells. The patient underwent induction chemotherapy with all-trans retinoic acid (ATRA) and idarubicin. A BM biopsy performed on day 35 was without morphological evidence of APL, but FISH analysis revealed 5.5% of interphase cells were still positive for the *PML/RARA* fusion. The karyotype was normal. The *PML/RARA* RT-PCR assay was positive (0.009).

The patient underwent consolidation with three cycles of ATRA and anthracycline (idarubicin and mitoxantrone were used). Repeat BM biopsy on day 50 was without morphological evidence of APL, and FISH analysis was negative.

BM biopsy on day 133 of APL diagnosis was consistent with molecular complete remission (mCR) (*PML/RARA* fusion RT-PCR product was undetectable). The patient then received two years of maintenance therapy with ATRA, 6-mercaptopurine, and methotrexate. A repeat BM biopsy at 37 months from diagnosis of APL was consistent with ongoing molecular CR (mCR).

2.2. Diagnosis of AMML. The patient presented 39 months after APL diagnosis with fatigue, dyspnea on exertion, and epistaxis. Laboratory workup revealed a hemoglobin 6.1 gr/

dl, WBC $300 \times 10^3/cm^3$ with 86% blasts, and platelets $18 \times 10^3/cm^3$. The renal and liver function was within normal limits. The BM core biopsy revealed involvement by blasts. Karyotype was normal. FISH analysis for AML/MDS cytogenetic aberrations was normal. FISH analysis for *PML/RARA* translocation was negative. The *PML/RARA* fusion RT-PCR was also negative. Further analysis revealed that *CEBPA*, *FLT3-ITD*, and *C-Kit* mutations were not present; *FLT3-TKD* assay was positive. Flow cytometry identified two distinct populations (one showing CD34±, CD117+, CD13+, CD33+, CD15±, CD64±, CD14−, CD7−, CD2−, CD56−, and HLA-DRlo and a second population CD64+, CD14±, CD33+, and HLA-DRlo). Overall, the BM biopsy studies were consistent with AMML (Table 1).

Following a session of emergent leukapheresis, the patient underwent induction chemotherapy with FLAG regimen [fludarabine, high-dose cytarabine, and granulocyte colony-stimulating factor (G-CSF)]. Repeat BM biopsy one month after AMML diagnosis demonstrated CR. She then underwent consolidation with high-dose cytarabine (Ara-C), followed by haploidentical allogeneic bone marrow transplantation (alloHSCT) three months after diagnosis of AMML. The conditioning regimen included fludarabine, cyclophosphamide, and total body irradiation. She developed skin graft versus host disease (GVHD) controlled with topical steroids. She remained in CR for approximately 27 months following alloHSCT.

2.3. First Simultaneous Relapse of APL and AMML. The patient presented to the emergency department approximately 70 months after initial APL diagnosis and 30 months after AMML diagnosis with headache, nausea, and vomiting. CBC on presentation showed WBC $7.9 \times 10^3/cm^3$, hemoglobin 14.2 gr/dl, and platelets $146 \times 10^3/cm^3$. An MRI brain showed abnormal leptomeningeal enhancement in the posterior fossa as well as over both cerebral convexities with abnormal signal within the calvaria and upper cervical vertebra worrisome for leukemic infiltration of the marrow. Lumbar puncture was performed which revealed protein 217 mg/dl, glucose 73 mg/dl, and WBC 1,004 cm^3. CSF studies were positive for the presence of both myelomonocytic and APL blasts (Figures 1 and 2; Table 2). The FISH analysis performed on CSF cells showed that cells harbored the *PML/RARA* translocation (Figure 3). BM biopsy did not reveal dysplasia or increased blasts by morphology or flow cytometry. The karyotype was normal. FISH analysis was negative for *PML/RARA* translocation. However, *PML/RARA* fusion RT-PCR was detected in the BM biopsy sample (with a value of 28.692); notably, the *PML/RARA* fusion RT-PCR was undetectable in a peripheral blood sample. The CT scan of the chest/abdomen/pelvis with contrast was without suspicious findings for extramedullary disease. Overall, the findings were compatible with CNS relapse of APL and AMML and molecular relapse of APL in the BM.

The patient received IT triple therapy (cytarabine, methotrexate, and hydrocortisone) and high-dose Ara-C while hospitalized (2.0 gr/m^2 every 12 hours for a total of 8 doses). Repeat CSF studies six days after chemotherapy initiation showed a decrease in WBC to 48/cm^3. Repeat MRI brain 14 days after presentation showed interval resolution of the leptomeningeal enhancement with persistent BM heterogenicity. A repeat BM biopsy, at count recovery, remained without morphological or immunophenotypic evidence of AMML or APL. The *PML/RARA* fusion RT-PCR was negative.

We then formulated a treatment plan based on the European guidelines for APL (2007) including ATO and ATRA. She received a course of ATRA (45 mg/m^2 in two divided doses) and 28 doses of ATO (0.15 mg/kgr) in a 28-day cycle. Repeat BM biopsy after this course confirmed that the patient remained in mCR. We then proceeded to two weeks of ATO/ATRA administration that were repeated every four weeks. She completed six cycles, and BM biopsy confirmed ongoing mCR. The patient received ATRA for two weeks every three months for 2 cycles (5 months total).

2.4. Second Simultaneous Relapse of APL and AMML. Approximately 17 months after CNS relapse of APL and AMML and 87 months after initial APL diagnosis, the patient began experiencing headaches.

The CSF studies revealed WBC of 483 cm^3 and protein was 91 mg/dl (Table 2). Flow cytometry and FISH analysis for *PML/RARA* translocation in the CSF supported second simultaneous relapse of AMML and APL (Table 2). A BM biopsy was without morphological or immunophenotypic evidence of APL or AMML. PML/RARA fusion was again detected (level was 12.327), but FISH analysis for PML/RARA translocation and the karyotype were normal.

The patient completed 6 IT triple therapy treatments with clearance of her CSF. The patient also concurrently began ATRA 45 mg/m^2 in two divided doses and ATO (0.15 mg/kgr) for 28 doses. Repeat BM biopsy was without evidence of APL (mCR).

Despite the multiple treatments, our patient has not required hospitalizations after the high-dose cytarabine and did not experience significant toxicities.

3. Discussion

Recurrence of APL or non-M3-AML in the CNS is rare [5]. Here, we describe the simultaneous recurrence of both APL and AMML in the CNS of a patient. The rarity of non-M3-AML CNS involvement was highlighted in a study of 3,261 patients; 21 patients were identified at diagnosis and 34 at relapse [6]. In the study of Oshima et al. [7], CNS relapse in patients with leukemia that had underwent alloHSCT was described. They identified nine relapses in 533 patients with AML. In multivariate analysis, active disease at transplantation and history of CNS involvement were associated with CNS relapse.

In another report, outcomes of AML-isolated CNS recurrence of 34 patients, of which 18 had meningeal involvement, were described [3]. These patients underwent IT chemotherapy with methotrexate and dexamethasone plus cytarabine twice weekly until CR achieved; they were then given at least five additional monthly IT doses. Ultimately, 14

Table 1: Key studies at APL and AMML diagnosis.

BM studies	APL diagnosis	AMML diagnosis
Flow cytometry	CD34+, CD33+, CD117+, CD38+, and HLA-DR in majority of blasts.	Flow cytometry analysis of the peripheral blood revealed a population of immature myeloid and monocytic lineage cells accounting for 28% of the total cells with the following immunophenotypes: CD34±, CD117+, CD13+, CD33+, CD15 heterogeneous, CD64 heterogeneous, CD14−, CD7−, CD2−, CD56−, and HLA-DRlo. The monocytic lineage showed an increased population of immature cells (48% of cells CD64+, CD14±, CD33+, and HLA-DRlo, with heterogeneous expression of CD117, CD13, and CD15).
Morphological description	(i) Hypercellular marrow, >95% cellularity, and mostly replaced by leukemic infiltrates. Cytoplasmic granules were noticed in subsets of blasts. A small subset of blasts had cytoplasmic hypergranulation with rare Auer rods present. Scattered blasts also show bilobed nuclear morphology. Examination of the clot section and core biopsy showed hypercellular marrow (near 100%), replaced by sheets of immature cells. Subsets of the immature cells showed morphologic features of promyelocytes. No residual hematopoiesis was noted. (ii) These findings were consisted with APL, hypogranular type.	(i) Hypercellular (90%) marrow with blasts occupying in excess of 90% of the marrow space. The cellular elements were almost exclusively made up of blasts (>90%). No blasts with APL morphology were noted. Some of the blasts had round nucleus with fine chromatin and moderate cytoplasm (myeloid blasts) and others with more irregular and folded nuclei, fine chromatin, and abundant cytoplasm. Some blasts contained Auer rods. (ii) Overall, the BM biopsy was consistent with acute myeloid leukemia with myelomonocytic phenotype.
Cytogenetics	The t (15;17) was detected in 95.5% of analyzed cells.	Karyotype: 46, XY[20]. FISH analysis for *PML/RARA* translocation was normal.

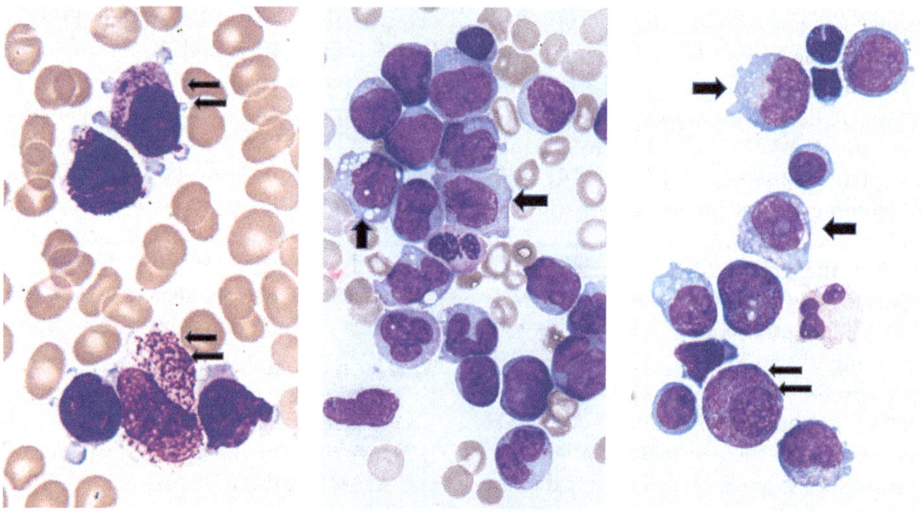

(a) (b) (c)

Figure 1: Initial APL blasts in the marrow (a). AMML occurrence in the bone marrow (b). CSF relapse showing myeloid/monoblasts (thick arrows) and APL blasts (small double arrows) (c).

out of the 18 patients achieved CNS-CR but unfortunately, the median overall survival of the 34 patients was 6.64 months [3]. Cheng et al. also conducted a retrospective study of AML patients (excluding FAB M3), demonstrating 5.1% of the 395 patients developed CNS disease with only 1% (four patients) having an isolated CNS relapse [1]. This study showed three out of the four patients also developed subsequent BM relapses and died. The median overall survival was 8.5 months from relapse [1]. Taken together, the involvement of CNS by non-M3-AML is rare and is associated with poor outcomes.

APL CNS relapse has been reported in cohort studies and in case series [8–10]. Eleven patients out of the 739 enrolled in PETHEMA LPA96 and LPA99 trials had documented CNS APL relapse [11]. The median time of CNS relapse was 16 months, and authors reported leukocytosis at diagnosis and

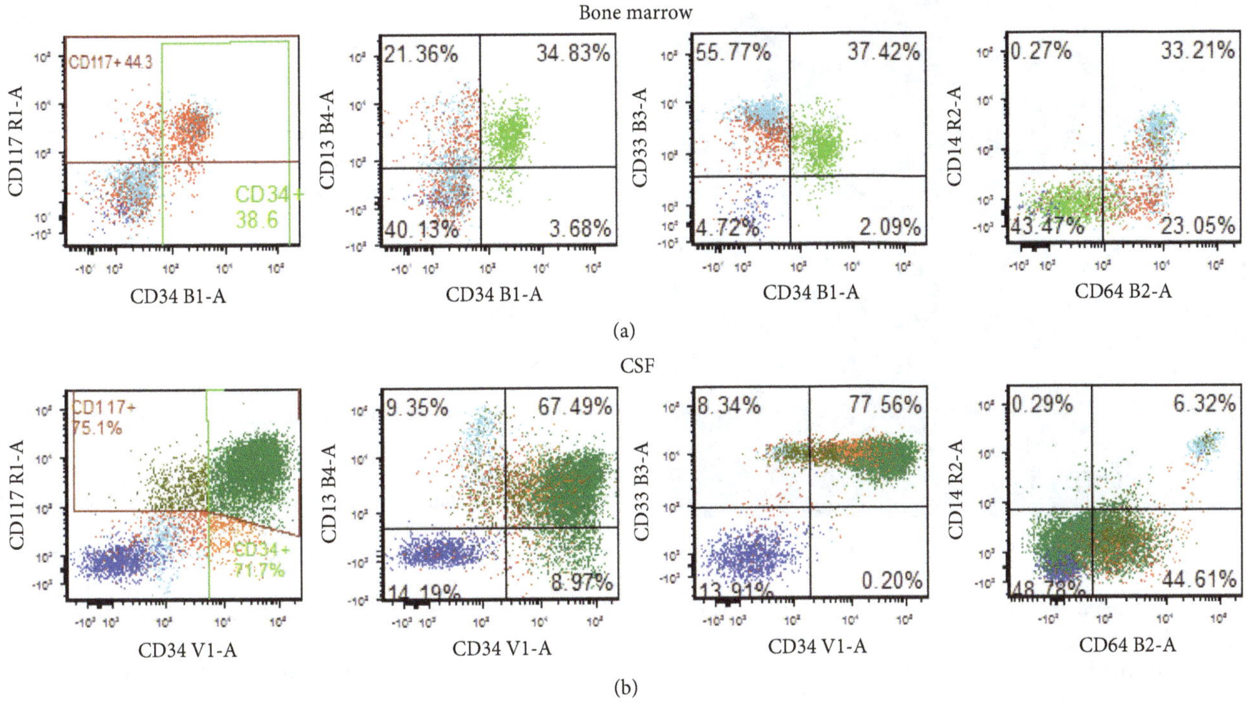

Figure 2: Flow cytometry: immunophenotypic similarity to AMML in the bone marrow at initial diagnosis (a) and CSF at relapse (b). Leukemic cells express of CD34, CD117, CD13, and CD64.

Table 2: Key CBC and CSF studies during patient course.

	CSF WBC (cm^3)	CSF RBC (cm^3)	CSF protein (mg/dl)	Flow cytometry analysis	FISH analysis	WBC ($\times 10^3/cm^3$)	Hgb (gr/dl)	Platelets ($\times 10^3/cm^3$)
First APL/ AMML double relapse	1,0004 (normal range: 0–5)	0 (normal range: 0-1)	217 (normal range: 18–53)	Flow cytometric analysis revealed a dysplastic population of myeloblasts comprising 19% of the total cells that are CD34+, CD117+, CD13+, CD33+, CD15–, CD64–, and CD14–	30% of the cells had the t (15;17)(q22;q21) translocation. Only 50 interphase cells were evaluated	7.9 (normal range: 4–11)	14.2 (normal range: 11.3–15.2)	146 (normal range: 150–440)
Second APL/ AMML double relapse	483 (normal range: 0–5)	0 (normal range: 0-1)	91 (normal range: 18–53)	Wright-stained cytospin revealed numerous blasts. Many had abundant cytoplasm, and rare blasts contain cytoplasmic granules. No definite abnormal promyelocytes noted. Flow cytometric analysis revealed an aberrant population of myeloblasts comprising 72% of the total cells that are CD34+, CD117+, CD38–, CD13+, CD33+ (96.7), CD15–, CD64–, CD14–, CD7+, CD56 heterogenous, HLA-DRlo/+, and CD123+ (92.5%)	60% of the cells had the t (15;17)(q22;q21) resulting in *PML/ RARA* fusion	7.42 (normal range: 4–11)	13.3 (normal range: 11.3–15.2)	227 (normal range: 150–440)

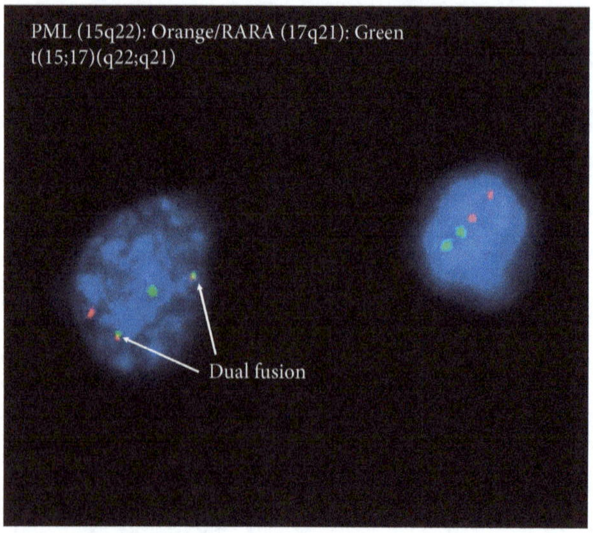

Figure 3: FISH analysis of CSF at double relapse.

CNS hemorrhage as risk factors. Notably, from the seven patients with CNS involvement without morphological involvement of the bone marrow, 5 patients experienced relapse (CNS or BM). Few case reports have reported CNS relapse after alloHSCT [11, 12]. In our patient, the relapse of APL in the CNS was also accompanied by BM molecular relapse given the presence of *PML/RARA* fusion RT-PCR product. Notably, it has been previously reported that CNS relapse of APL can be accompanied by systemic relapse [13]. There are no consensus guidelines for the treatment of CNS APL with systemic relapse [14], and different strategies can be employed.

For example, in the report of Vega-Ruiz et al. [2], seven patients with recurrence of APL in the CNS were described. CNS relapse was typically accompanied by or preceded by systemic relapse. All seven patients were treated with intrathecal chemotherapy and systemic chemotherapy (six out of the seven patients died within four months of development relapse) [2].

Our patient was treated for both APL and M4-AML relapse with a treatment regimen that includes intrathecal chemotherapy, high-dose ARA-C, and consolidation and postconsolidation phase based on ATO and ATRA. Prolonged maintenance was initiated and was based on ATRA. Unfortunately, the patient experienced a second simultaneous relapse in CNS as well as molecular relapse in the bone marrow.

For patients with relapsed APL, autologous transplantation is recommended, but our patient relapsed after alloHSCT. Given her recent relapse, she will be evaluated for possible donor lymphocyte infusion.

It is intriguing that this patient developed two acute leukemias that relapsed simultaneously. The CNS may escape from the graft versus leukemia effect, but the optimal strategy to avoid relapse in CNS has not been identified.

4. Conclusion

This case describes a double recurrence of APL and M4-AML in the CNS of the patient after alloHSCT, accompanied by APL molecular relapse in the bone marrow. Our patient responded transiently to combined schema of IT chemotherapy and ATO/ATRA for more than a year. Our case highlights the difficulty that relapsed APL and CNS recurrence of leukemia can pose. In addition, it highlights that a combination of treatments may lead to remissions with meaningful duration and without significant toxicities.

References

[1] C. L. Cheng, C. C. Li, H. A. Hou et al., "Risk factors and clinical outcomes of acute myeloid leukaemia with central nervous system involvement in adults," *BMC Cancer*, vol. 15, p. 344, 2015.

[2] A. Vega-Ruiz, S. Faderl, Z. Estrov et al., "Incidence of extramedullary disease in patients with acute promyelocytic leukemia: a single-institution experience," *International Journal of Hematology*, vol. 89, no. 4, pp. 489–496, 2009.

[3] C. Zheng, X. Liu, W. Zhu, X. Cai, J. Wu, and Z. Sun, "Tailored central nervous system-directed treatment strategy for isolated CNS recurrence of adult acute myeloid leukemia," *Hematology*, vol. 19, no. 4, pp. 208–212, 2014.

[4] M. A. Sanz, F. Lo Coco, G. Martín et al., "Definition of relapse risk and role of nonanthracycline drugs for consolidation in patients with acute promyelocytic leukemia: a joint study of the PETHEMA and GIMEMA cooperative groups," *Blood*, vol. 96, no. 4, pp. 1247–1253, 2000.

[5] F. Albano and G. Specchia, "Extramedullary disease in acute promyelocytic leukemia: two-in-one disease," *Mediterranean Journal of Hematology and Infectious Diseases*, vol. 3, no. 1, Article ID e2011066, 2011.

[6] N. Alakel, F. Stölzel, B. Mohr et al., "Symptomatic central nervous system involvement in adult patients with acute myeloid leukemia," *Cancer Management and Research*, vol. 9, pp. 97–102, 2017.

[7] K. Oshima, Y. Kanda, T. Yamashita et al., "Central nervous system relapse of leukemia after allogeneic hematopoietic stem cell transplantation," *Biology of Blood and Marrow Transplantation*, vol. 14, no. 10, pp. 1100–1107, 2008.

[8] G. Evans, D. Grimwade, H. G. Prentice, and N. Simpson, "Central nervous system relapse in acute promyelocytic leukaemia in patients treated with all-trans retinoic acid," *British Journal of Haematology*, vol. 98, no. 2, pp. 437–439, 1997.

[9] L. D. Burry and J. T. Seki, "CNS relapses of acute promyelocytic leukemia after all-trans retinoic acid," *The Annals of Pharmacotherapy*, vol. 36, no. 12, pp. 1900–1906, 2002.

[10] S. H. Seki, H. M. Ryoo, H. S. Cho, J. L. Lee, K. H. Lee, and M. S. Hyun, "Meningeal relapse in a patient with acute promyelocytic leukemia: a case report and review of the literature," *Journal of Korean Medical Science*, vol. 19, no. 2, pp. 311–314, 2004.

[11] P. Montesinos, J. Diaz-Mediavilla, G. Deben et al., "Central nervous system involvement at first relapse in patients with acute promyelocytic leukemia treated with all-trans retinoic acid and anthracycline monochemotherapy without intrathecal prophylaxis," *Haematologica*, vol. 94, no. 9, pp. 1242–1249, 2009.

[12] C. F. Classen, K.-M. Debatin, W. Friedrich, and A. S. Schulz, "Long-term remission of APL with a second allogeneic BMT

after CNS relapse following HLA-identical allogeneic BMT," *Bone Marrow Transplantation*, vol. 32, no. 8, pp. 843–846, 2003.
[13] H. Y. Lee, K. M. Kim, M.-H. Kang, J. H. Kang, K.-M. Kang, and G.-W. Lee, "Concurrent craniospinal radiotherapy and intrathecal chemotherapy in patient with acute promyelocytic leukemia second relapsed in central nervous system (CNS) following allogeneic stem cell transplantation," *Journal of Neuro-Oncology*, vol. 79, no. 1, pp. 73–75, 2006.
[14] M. S. Tallman and J. K. Altman, "How I treat acute promyelocytic leukemia," *Blood*, vol. 114, no. 25, pp. 5126–5135, 2009.

16

Idiopathic Multicentric Hyaline Vascular-Type Castleman Disease

Adelaide Moutinho, Rita Gamboa Cunha, Sheila Koch Jamal, Marta Meleiro Lisboa, and Sandra Tavares

Department of Internal Medicine, Hospital de Chaves—Centro Hospitalar de Trás-os-Montes e Alto Douro, Vila Real, Portugal

Correspondence should be addressed to Adelaide Moutinho; m.adelaide.moutinho@gmail.com

Academic Editor: Håkon Reikvam

Castleman disease is a rare lymphoproliferative disorder presenting with localized or disseminated lymphadenopathy and systemic symptoms. It can be categorized clinically as unicentric or multicentric, histopathologically as hyaline vascular, plasma cell, or mixed variant, and etiologically, considering the subtypes based on causative viral agents and associated syndromes. The multicentric type can mimic other haematological malignancies, ranging from asymptomatic to multiple organ involvement. Although its pathophysiology is not well known, the current approved treatments are directed towards interleukin-6, CD-20, and viral agents. The authors present an 82-year-old leucodermic man presented with a 2-week history of constitutional symptoms. Examination revealed pallor, hepatosplenomegaly, and palpable left axillary lymphadenopathy. Investigation showed anaemia, thrombocytopenia, polyclonal hypergammaglobulinemia, hypoalbuminemia, and high acute phase reactants, with image study revealing multiple axillary, mediastinal, inguinal, and pelvic lymphadenopathies. The lymph node biopsy was consistent with hyaline vascular-type Castleman disease without human herpersvirus-8 markers. He started prednisolone with initial improvement evolved poorly on a short term. Castleman disease has a broad spectrum of clinical manifestations, associations, and complications that bring a diagnostic challenge, requiring a multidisciplinary approach. Clinicians should be familiar with its features because proper diagnosis and aggressive targeted treatment are the pillars of proper management of these patients.

1. Introduction

Castleman disease (CD) is a heterogeneous group of lymphoproliferative diseases affecting single or generalized lymph nodes which can be classified clinically as unicentric or multicentric and histologically as hyaline vascular, plasma cell variant, or mixed type [1–4]. The hyaline variant, the most frequent one, is characterized by capillary proliferation with small hyaline vascular follicles and usually has a benign clinical course. The multicentric presentation can be linked to human herpesvirus-8 (HHV-8) infection, associated with POEMS, or be idiopathic, the latter recently subclassified in TAFRO-associated idiopathic multicentric Castleman Disease (iMCD) [1, 3, 5–7]. The authors report a case of a Portuguese patient with iMCD presenting with a two-week history of constitutional symptoms, hepatosplenomegaly, and a single palpable left axillary lymphadenopathy, with histology confirming hyaline vascular variant.

2. Case Presentation

An 82-year-old leucodermic man, with arterial hypertension with hypertensive cardiopathy and no other known end-organ damage, controlled with olmesartan 20 mg id, heart failure with preserved ejection fraction, class II New York Heart Association (NYHA), benign prostate hyperplasia medicated with *Serenoa repens* 160 mg id, and hyperuricemia controlled with allopurinol 300 mg id, presented to our emergency care unit. He had a 2-week history of low fever (axillary temperature 38°C), shivers, night sweats, fatigue, dry cough, and weight loss of 4 kg, with no response to paracetamol 1000 mg that he took three times a day for 3 days. His physical examination revealed a pale skin, a nontender, dull, 4 cm-diameter left axillary lymphadenopathy, nontender hepatomegaly palpable 8 cm below the right costal margin, and nontender palpable splenomegaly. He had stable vitals and normal pulmonary and cardiac examination, with no signs or symptoms of peripheral neuropathy. Laboratory findings revealed anaemia with haemoglobin of 9 g/dL, normocytic (mean corpuscular volume 87,0 fL; normal range (87–103)), normochromic (mean corpuscular haemoglobin 29,8 pg; normal range (27–33)), thrombocytopenia 129.000/μL, and a normal white cell count of 5.000/μL. His reticulocyte count was 1.21% with a reticulocyte index of 0.49 indicating medullary hypoproliferation, and his blood smear confirmed the normochromic normocytic red cells and thrombocytopenia with no further morphological changes. Regarding the coagulation study, he had a prothrombin time of 16.9 seconds, with an international normalized ration of 1.21, a partial thromboplastin time of 31.1 seconds, and normal-range fibrinogen (205 mg/dL) and d-dimer (0,48 μg/mL). There was no deficit of B12 vitamin, folic acid, or iron, with high acute phase reactants: ferritin 762 ng/mL, sedimentation rate 132 mm/1st hour, and C-reactive protein 6.87 mg/dL. His serum creatinine level was 1.3 mg/dL with a creatinine clearance of 63 mL/min, with 399 mg of protein in the 24-hour urine and normal urine sediment. The protein electrophoresis showed a polyclonal hypergammaglobulinemia with an albumin of 2.3 g/dL and total proteins of 4.3 g/dL. The electrolytes, hepatic enzymes, alkaline phosphatase, lactic dehydrogenase, and bilirubin were within the normal range. He had negative human immunodeficiency virus (HIV) 1 and 2 antibodies, negative anti-hepatitis C virus, and was not immune to hepatitis B virus. The immunologic study with antinuclear antibodies (ANAs) and anti-cytoplasm antibodies and angiotensin-converting enzyme was negative. The image findings obtained by the computerized tomography (CT) scan revealed homogeneous hepatomegaly with a bipolar diameter of 180 mm and splenomegaly with 146 mm of diameter without focal lesions and numerous lymphadenopathies located in multiple lymph node groups: left axillary, with the largest measuring 21.5 mm in diameter, mediastinum, supraclavicular, pelvic, and inguinal (Figure 1). There were no pleural or peritoneal effusions.

The bone marrow biopsy and myelogram revealed normocellularity, with hyperplasia of all series without lymphoproliferative involvement, with increased reticulin staining. The axillary lymph node biopsy (Figure 2) revealed numerous small follicular structures, with small centres containing CD21-positive follicular dendritic-type cells, endothelial cells, and CD20-positive small mantle lymphocytes arranged in concentric rings. The interfollicular areas contained rare well-differentiated CD138-positive plasmocytes. There was not any positivity for HHV-8 in any of the identified cells. Blood vessels with some hyaline walls were seen in the germinative centres. This appearance is highly suggestive of Castleman disease hyaline vascular type, and a diagnosis of iMCD hyaline vascular variant was made. Regarding the recent classification accepted by the Castleman Disease Collaborative Network, we can retrospectively assume the diagnosis of iMCD-TAFRO type, by compiling all histopathological criteria (typical lymph node pathology and negativity for HHV-8), three major criteria (fever >38°C, reticulin fibrosis, and organomegaly), and one minor criteria (hyperplasia of megakaryocytes within bone marrow biopsy) [1].

The patient started treatment with prednisolone 1 mg/kg/day with clinical, biochemical, and haematological improvement, as a bridge to improve clinical and hematologic status, waiting to start immunotherapy which was planned with anti-interleukin-6 (IL-6) therapy, namely, tocilizumab. However, he evolved with pulmonary oedema secondary to acute heart failure, pancytopenia, and end-organ damage without haemorrhage, coagulopathy, or intravascular disseminated coagulation criteria, without any response to the therapy imposed, deceasing 20 days after the final diagnosis.

3. Discussion

Since the first case report published by Dr. Benjamin Castleman in 1954, the term Castleman disease has been applied to several different lymphoproliferative disorders. This case report presents an elder man with CD classified clinically as multicentric, etiologically as idiopathic, and histologically as hyaline vascular variant.

The multicentric CD occurs normally in patients in the sixth decade of life, and it can occur in association with HHV-8 in HIV-positive and -negative patients and POEMS syndrome, or it can be idiopathic, subclassified in TAFRO associated or NOS, the latter when the criteria for TAFRO are not met [1–3, 6, 7]. Like the HHV-8-associated multicentric CD, the idiopathic variant shows histological features of both hyaline vascular and plasma cell variant CD. However, contrary to the case presented where the hyaline vascular type stands out, the idiopathic multicentric CD generally presents with marked plasmacytosis and a lesser degree of vascular proliferation and hyalination [5, 8], which are the typical histological patterns of plasma cell variant CD.

The similarity of the presentation of idiopathic multicentric CD with other lymphoproliferative disorders allied to the rarity of CD, the age of the patient, the clinical symptoms and signs, and laboratory findings induced the initial investigation of haematological malignancies with a main focus on lymphomas. On the other hand, the analysis of the lymph node biopsy had to be reviewed after the consideration of CD as a possible diagnosis, reminding us that the pathological findings with hematoxylin and eosin (HE) coloration are not entirely specific, since they can be seen in other reactive and neoplastic conditions [2], making the diagnosis even more challenging and, in this particular case, delaying it.

On the contrary that unicentric CD in which surgical treatment with or without radiotherapy is usually curative with a good prognosis, the optimal management of multicentric CD has not been well established and the outcome is clearly less favourable [1, 3, 7]. The latter guidelines for idiopathic Castleman disease presume the evaluation of the severity of the disease to decide the best treatment approach, being anti-IL6 monoclonal antibody the first line of treatment, with siltuximab or, as an alternative, tocilizumab [1, 3, 6, 9]. Rituximab, a monoclonal anti-CD20 antibody, is proven to be highly effective in HIV-positive multicentric

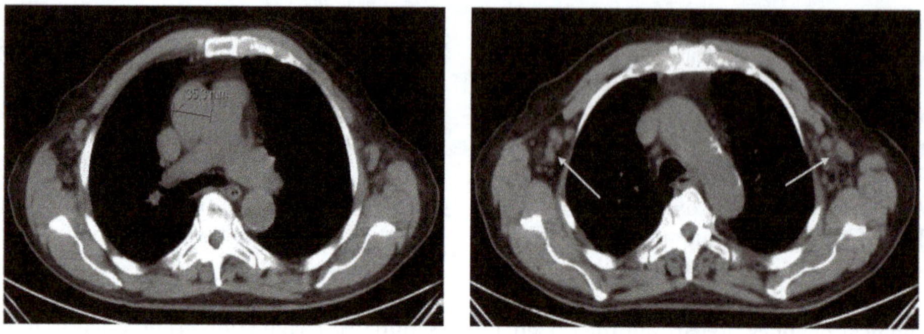

(a) (b)

Figure 1: (a) CT scan showing mediastinal lymphadenopathy measuring 35.3 mm (marker); (b) CT scan showing bilateral axillary lymphadenopathies (arrows).

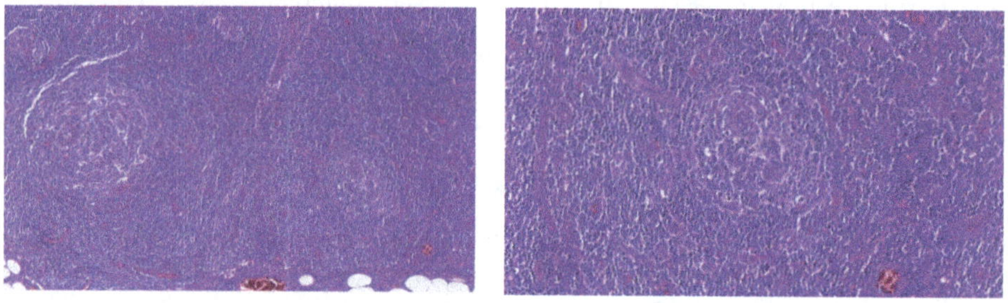

(a) (b)

Figure 2: Lymph node biopsy showing features of Castleman disease, hyaline vascular type. (a) HE coloration, 10x amplification. Numerous small follicular structures, follicular dendritic type cells, and blood vessels, some with hyaline walls. (b) HE coloration, 20x amplification. Concentric layers of lymphocytes around the follicles, the mantle zone.

CD, but it can be used as well in HIV negative patients [3], as an alternative to anti-IL6 monoclonal antibodies. Corticosteroids may be used as monotherapy in patients with more indolent diseases or as a symptom controller, but as well combined with immunotherapy with anti-IL6 or anti-CD20 monoclonal antibodies [1, 3, 9], this latter option being the one chosen to treat the patient presented. However, the immediate unavailability of the immunotherapy and the poor evolution of our patient made it impossible to perform.

The prognostic factors regarding CD are not well known. However, as it happens with other lymphoproliferative disorders, older age is associated with poorer prognosis [3]. Likewise, some studies report splenomegaly and low albumin levels as factors with worse prognosis [3]. POEMS syndrome and renal involvement with reduced creatinine clearance are independent prognostic factors [10]. The TAFRO subtype of iMCD is an aggressive clinical entity associated with multiorgan involvement, with quick and unfavourable evolution without proper treatment [1]. Considering this, and reviewing our case, there were some obvious indicators of a bad outcome.

In conclusion, although idiopathic multifocal CD currently has evidence-based consensus diagnostic and treatment guidelines, it should be considered as a differential diagnosis more often when patients who present with generalized lymphadenopathy and systemic symptoms, and the diagnosis must be properly made. Initiatives such as the unique Castleman Disease Collaborative Network are crucial to maximize the endeavours of research and data sharing of this rare disease, promoting its understanding and proper management of similar cases, and the expansion of knowledge of this entity.

References

[1] A. Dispenzieri and D. C. Fajgenbaum, "Overview of castleman disease," *Blood*, vol. 135, no. 16, pp. 1353–1364, 2020.

[2] D. B. Sevilla-Lizcano, C. L. Frias-Soria, C. Ortiz-Hidalgo et al., "Castleman disease. Histopathological and immunohistochemical analysis of thirty-nine cases," *Gaceta Médica de México*, vol. 153, no. 5, pp. 559–565, 2017.

[3] X. Zhang, H. Rao, X. Xu et al., "Clinical characteristics and outcomes of castleman disease: a multicenter study of 185 Chinese patients," *Cancer Science*, vol. 109, no. 1, pp. 199–206, 2018.

[4] S. Zhao, Y. Wan, Z. Huang, B. Song, and J. Yu, "Imaging and clinical features of castleman disease," *Cancer Imaging*, vol. 19, no. 1, pp. 1–8, 2019.

[5] M. Kojima, N. Nakamura, N. Tsukamoto et al., "Clinical implications of idiopathic Japanese : a report of 28 cases," *International Journal of Surgical Pathology*, vol. 16, no. 4, pp. 391–398, 2008.
[6] E. Oksenhendler, D. Boutboul, D. Fajgenbaum et al., "The full spectrum of castleman disease: 273 patients studied over 20 years," *British Journal of Haematology*, vol. 180, no. 2, pp. 206–216, 2018.
[7] D. Wu, M. S. Lim, and E. Jaffe, "Pathology of castleman disease," *Hematology/Oncology Clinics of North America*, vol. 32, no. 1, pp. 37–52, 2018.
[8] H.-W. Wang, S. Pittaluga, and E. S. Jaffe, "Multicentric castleman disease: where are we now?" *Seminars in Diagnostic Pathology*, vol. 33, no. 5, pp. 294–306, 2017.
[9] F. V. Rhee, P. Voorhees, A. Dispenzieri et al., "International, evidence-based consensus treatment guidelines for idiopathic multicentric castleman disease," *Blood*, vol. 132, no. 20, pp. 2115–2124, 2018.
[10] L. Zhang, Z. Li, X. Cao et al., "Clinical spectrum and survival analysis of 145 cases of HIV-negative castleman's disease: renal function is an important prognostic factor," *Scientific Reports*, vol. 6, Article ID 23831, 2016.

17

An Unusual Case of Breast Implant-Associated Anaplastic Large Cell Lymphoma

Sarah Premji,[1] Andreia Barbieri,[2] Christine Roth,[2] Eric M. Rohren,[3] Gustavo Rivero,[4,5] and Sravanti P Teegavarapu[4,5]

[1]*Department of Medicine, Baylor College of Medicine, Houston 77030, TX, USA*
[2]*Department of Pathology and Immunology, Baylor College of Medicine, Baylor St. Luke's Medical Center, Houston 77030, TX, USA*
[3]*Department of Radiology, Baylor College of Medicine, Houston 77030, TX, USA*
[4]*Department of Medicine, Section of Hematology-Oncology, Baylor College of Medicine, Houston 77030, TX, USA*
[5]*Dan L Duncan Comprehensive Cancer Center, Baylor College of Medicine, Houston, TX 77030, USA*

Correspondence should be addressed to Sravanti P Teegavarapu; teegavar@bcm.edu

Academic Editor: Kostas Konstantopoulos

Introduction. Breast implant-associated anaplastic large cell lymphoma (BIA-ALCL) is a rare disease entity associated with textured breast implants. Though the clinical course is typically indolent, BIA-ALCL can occasionally invade through the capsule into the breast parenchyma with spread to the regional lymph nodes and beyond including chest wall invasive disease. *Case.* We present the case of a 51-year-old female with a history of bilateral silicone breast implants placed approximately twenty years ago who presented with two months of progressively enlarging right breast mass. Ultrasound-guided biopsy of right breast mass and right axillary lymph node showed CD 30-positive *ALK*-negative anaplastic large cell lymphoma, and staging work up showed extension of the tumor to chest wall and ribs consistent with advanced disease. She received CHP-BV (cyclophosphamide, doxorubicin, prednisone, and brentuximab vedotin) for six cycles with complete metabolic response. This was followed by extensive surgical extirpation and reconstruction, radiation for residual disease and consolidation with autologous stem cell transplant. She is currently on maintenance brentuximab vedotin with no evidence of active disease post autologous stem cell transplant. *Conclusion.* Treatment guidelines for advanced chest wall invasive BIA-ALCL are not well defined. Lack of predictive factors warrants mutation analysis and genetic sequencing to identify those at highest risk of progression to chest wall invasive disease. This rare case highlights the need for definitive consensus on the optimal management of chest wall invasive BIA-ALCL.

1. Introduction

Breast implant-associated anaplastic large cell lymphoma (BIA-ALCL), an ALK-negative ALCL associated with textured breast implants, was first recognized in 1997 [1]. The lifetime prevalence of BIA-ALCL is 33 per 1 million persons with textured breast implants [2]. Most patients have excellent outcomes following surgical resection alone. However, in rare cases, BIA-ALCL invades through the capsule and spreads beyond the breast parenchyma to regional lymph nodes requiring systemic chemotherapy [3]. Here, we report a case of aggressive chest wall invasive BIA-ALCL which was successfully treated with a combination of surgery, chemotherapy, radiation, and stem cell transplant. The ideal treatment approach to chest wall invasive BIA-ALCL remains unclear, and this case highlights the need for consensus to optimally manage chest wall invasive BIA-ALCL.

2. Case Presentation

A 51-year-old female with history of bilateral retropectoral silicone breast implants placed in 1996 presented with a two-month history of progressively enlarging right breast.

Imaging including ultrasound and MRI showed a large infiltrative mass involving the right medial chest wall musculature with right axillary adenopathy along with a peri-implant fluid collection. Ultrasound guided biopsy of right chest wall mass in November 2019 showed a CD30-positive, *ALK*-negative ALCL which was negative for *DUSP22* and *TP63* gene rearrangements (Figure 1). Staging PET-CT showed a dominant, coalescent, and infiltrative $13 \times 10 \times 20$ centimeter mass centered in the right anterior chest wall with extension into the pleural/extrapleural compartment along with involvement of regional lymph nodes and osseous invasion of the ribs consistent with advanced disease (Figure 2(a)). She was started on neo-adjuvant chemotherapy with CHP-BV (cyclophosphamide, doxorubicin, prednisone, and brentuximab vedotin) and completed 6 cycles in May 2020 achieving a complete metabolic response. In July 2020, she underwent an anterior thoracotomy with resection of the right chest wall tumor, as well as ribs 3–5, partial sternectomy, en bloc removal of the right breast implant, right chest wall reconstruction with mesh/bone cement, thymectomy, serratus advancement flap, and adjacent tissue transfer. Her postoperative course was complicated by chest wall incision necrosis requiring debridement, washout and tissue transfer. Pathologic evaluation revealed viable residual tumor in the sternum, thymus, right anterior chest wall and lymph node samples. She went on to receive 36 Gy of radiation in 1.8 Gy fractions which she completed in November 2020. Restaging PET showed a complete metabolic response with SUVmax 3.9 and a Deauville score of 3 (Figure 2(b)). This was followed by consolidative auto-SCT in February 2021 with abbreviated BEAM where she received 50% of the conditioning regimen (carmustine 300 mg/m2 × 1 day, etoposide 200 mg/m2 × 2 days, cytarabine 200 mg/m2 × 2 days, and no melphalan) due to compliance issues. She engrafted well with no complications post auto-SCT. Three months post auto-SCT, she was started on maintenance BV which was stopped after 12 cycles due to worsening neuropathy. She is currently doing well about a year post auto-SCT with no evidence of active disease.

3. Discussion

ALCL is a rare *T*-cell lymphoma accounting for only 6% of all breast lymphomas [4]. The pathogenesis of BIA-ALCL is not well defined. It has been postulated *T*-cell activation due to sustained chronic inflammation mediated by a higher bacterial load associated with highly textured implants may be associated with development of *T*-cell malignancies [5]; however, no specific bacterial species have been found to predispose to BIA-ALCL [6]. In contrast to other ALCLs, BIA-ALCL are typically triple negative, negative for underlying *ALK, DUSP 22,* and *TP63* mutations. Activating mutations such as *JAK1* and *STAT3* have been implicated in excess expression of *T*-cell associated cytokines, notably, IL-6, TGF-β, and IL-10 along with activation of the JAK/STAT signaling pathways leading to accelerated division of lymphocytes predisposing to malignant changes. Further studies are being performed to determine if biomarkers such as SATB1 and JunB could be precursors to development of BIA-ALCL in an effort to identify these patients earlier to initiate treatment [7]. The median time to development of BIA-ALCL is 9 years with a wide range from 2 to 32 years [8]. Although the most common presentation is a peri-implant effusion, 30% of patients present with a palpable breast mass and up to 20% develop lymphadenopathy. 83% of BIA-ALCL patients are diagnosed at stage I and only 7% present with stage IV disease. The majority of patients with BIA-ALCL presenting with early-stage disease are known to have excellent prognosis. Complete capsulectomy along with removal of implant and all evidence of disease has shown improved event free and overall survival in BIA-ALCL [9]. On the other hand, those presenting with a mass tend to have lower survival and increased risk of death. In patients with advanced disease, NCCN guidelines recommend using a combination of chemotherapy (anthracycline-based chemotherapy regimens such as CHOP or CHOEP)$^{+/-}$ radiation. BV in combination with frontline chemotherapy has shown complete response rate of 92% with overall response rate of 100% [10] in CD30-positive peripheral *T*-cell lymphomas. In fact, BV in combination with systemic chemotherapy was approved for frontline treatment of systemic ALCL and CD30 positive peripheral *T*-cell lymphomas following an overall survival benefit when compared to chemotherapy alone [11]. Case reports of BV as monotherapy has also shown durable response in both limited and advanced stage BIA-ALCL in those unable to receive anthracycline based therapy. [12, 13].

However, the optimal management approach to advanced disease remains yet to be determined. There are no prospective trials to guide the management of patients with disseminated disease. Most therapies have been extrapolated from the treatment experience of primary cutaneous and systemic ALCL. In a recent review, 39 patients diagnosed with advanced BIA-ALCL showed higher frequency of limited surgery, chemotherapy, salvage chemotherapy, external beam radiation therapy, and autologous stem cell transplantation when compared with a control group of early-stage BIA-ALCL. The rate of definitive surgery was lower as well as the time to surgery prolonged in advanced disease [14]. While delay in surgery is associated with inferior outcomes, the precise timing of surgery is unclear especially in those with aggressive chest wall invasive disease who may require neoadjuvant chemotherapy to help achieve improved surgical margins and better response rates. Coombs et al. [15] reported two such aggressive chest wall invasive BIA-ALCL cases who were successfully treated with a combination of neoadjuvant chemotherapy followed by chest wall resection and composite reconstruction for residual disease after systemic treatment. This data suggests that chest wall invasive disease may warrant a multimodality approach for improved response rate including use of neoadjuvant chemotherapy prior to definitive surgery. In fact, chest wall infiltration is a critical prognostic factor in BIA-ALCL influencing the possibility of performing a surgical radical tumor extirpation [16]. These uncommon neoplasms also represent a clinical challenge for surgeons as incorrect diagnosis, incomplete resection and unsuccessful

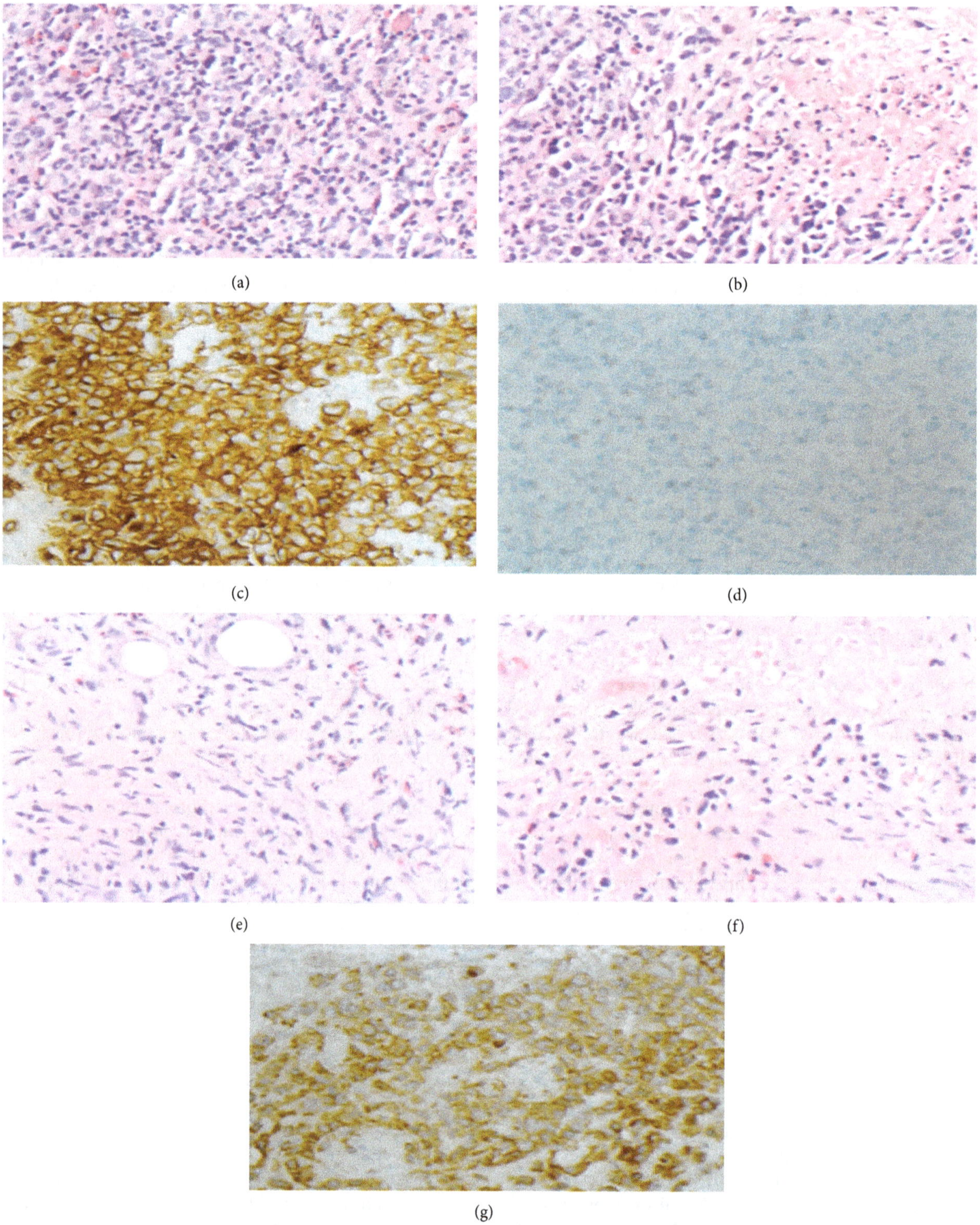

Figure 1: Right axillary lymph node biopsy. (a) Proliferation of large, atypical cells with irregular nuclear contours, vesicular chromatin, and moderately abundant eosinophilic cytoplasm, with background small lymphocytes and eosinophils. (b) Proliferation of large, atypical cells alternating with areas of necrosis. (c) Lymphoma cells stain positive for CD30. (d) Lymphoma cells stain negative for ALK. Right chest wall mass biopsy with (e) large lymphoma cells within background fibrosis, small lymphocytes, and eosinophils (f) with associated adjacent necrosis (g) with lymphoma cells staining positive for CD30.

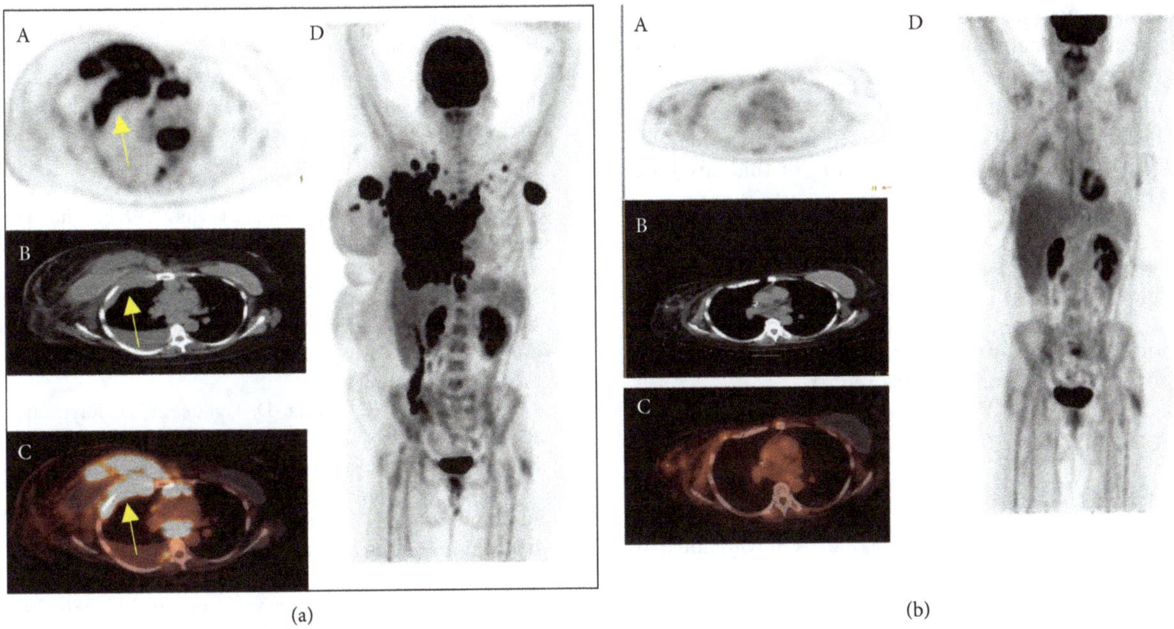

FIGURE 2: (a) Baseline: (A) axial PET, (B) CT, and (C) fused images from an FDG-PET/CT scan performed at baseline demonstrate a large, infiltrative mass in the right chest wall measuring approximately 13 x 10 x 20 cm. The mass spans the subcutaneous, muscular, and chest wall compartments with extension into the pleural/extrapleural compartments (arrows). (D) A maximum intensity projection (MIP) image shows the large extent of disease. (b) Post treatment: (A) Axial PET after treatment with 6 cycles of CHP/BV, Surgery and XRT, (B) CT, and (C) fused images with stable postsurgical changes showing (d) overall significant positive response with slight interval increase in interstitial opacity in the central right breast with low-grade FDG uptake thought to be related to inflammation post radiation.

reconstruction of thoracic wall defects have resulted in high rates of perioperative morbidity and mortality [17]. Globally, this highlights the need for definitive consensus regarding surgery and systemic therapy. Radiation for BIA-ALCL is mostly recommended for incomplete resection or residual disease though long-term toxicity to heart and lungs is unknown. Data on stem cell transplant in BIA-ALCL are limited. Collins et al. [14] reported that 8/39 (20.5%) advanced BIA-ALCL patients underwent an auto-SCT. Most of them had relapsed or refractory cases. 7/8 (87.5%) who underwent auto-SCT remain in CR, the longest follow-up to date being 120 months.

There are some limitations in our case report. Firstly, the factors contributing to extensive chest wall involvement in our patient are unknown. It would be interesting to coalesce larger number of advanced disease cases to determine whether lactate dehydrogenase (LDH) and other potential biomarkers such as beta-2-microglobulin (B2M) retain predictably for chest wall expansion. Secondly, the lack of genomic sequencing restricts our ability to correlate our patient presentation with aggressive genomic features. Despite this, our case demonstrates remarkable benefit of neoadjuvant chemotherapy prior to surgery, upfront consolidation with stem cell transplant followed by CD30 monoclonal antibody maintenance for advanced chest wall invasive BIA-ALCL. This observation is particularly of interest given the known hyper-progression phenomena previously associated with rapid chest wall involvement in the context of indolent disease when partially excised although that was not our patient's case. In near future, investigation of disease predictors and mutational signature for aggressive BIA-ALCL could assist in identification of hyper-progression cases. Most of screening continues to rely on routine mammogram in asymptomatic patients. Additionally, there is no known intervention to reduce the risk of aggressive disease. It is important to detect early seroma development to perform ultrasound/MRIs to guide aspiration of effusion. *T*-cell hyperplasia linked with bacterial biofilms is associated with BIA-ALCL suggesting that reducing infection risk, early detection of capsular contraction can reduce the activation of lymphocytes and possible conversion to BIA-ALCL [18]. Our case highlights the need to determine the optimal timing for surgical intervention as well as consensus regarding treatment paradigm for this uncommon group of patients with aggressive chest wall invasive BIA-ALCL. To date, several unresolved questions remain, which include as follows: (1) would aggressive chest wall invasive cases benefit from consolidation with auto-SCT upfront? (2) Is there a role for maintenance therapy in BIA-ALCL? Finally, our case reinforces the concept that maintenance BV after auto-SCT may improve the outcome of patients diagnosed with *T*-cell lymphomas [19] and should be considered in aggressive chest wall invasive disease to reduce recurrence. Ultimately, cooperative large-scale studies may assist in determining best therapy for aggressive chest wall invasive BIA-ALCL.

4. Conclusion

The treatment paradigm for chest wall invasive BIA-ALCL is not well delineated. Our case here supports the use of a multimodality approach including use of neoadjuvant chemotherapy, surgery, radiation, consolidation with stem cell transplant, and maintenance therapy post transplant for this aggressive variety of BIA-ALCL. Further research looking into the predictors of aggressive disease is much needed. Future studies with randomized control trials will help develop an evidence-based algorithm for this rare type of BIA-ALCL.

Acknowledgments

The authors would like to thank the patient for providing consent for publication of this case report.

References

[1] J. A. Keech and B. J. Creech, "Anaplastic *T*-cell lymphoma in proximity to a saline-filled breast implant," *Plastic Reconstructive Surgery*, vol. 100, no. 2, 1997.

[2] E. L. Doren, R. N. Miranda, J. C. Selber et al., "U.S. Epidemiology of breast implant–associated anaplastic large cell lymphoma," *Plastic and Reconstructive Surgery*, vol. 139, no. 5, pp. 1042–1050, 2017.

[3] A. E. Quesada, L. J. Medeiros, M. W. Clemens, M. C. Ferrufino-Schmidt, S. Pina-Oviedo, and R. N. Miranda, "Breast implant-associated anaplastic large cell lymphoma: a review," *Modern Pathology*, vol. 32, no. 2, pp. 166–188, 2019.

[4] S. S. Talwalkar, R. N. Miranda, J. R. Valbuena, M. J. Routbort, A. W. Martin, and L. J. Medeiros, "Lymphomas involving the breast: a study of 106 cases comparing localized and disseminated neoplasms," *The American Journal of Surgical Pathology*, vol. 32, no. 9, pp. 1299–1309, 2008.

[5] J. L. Jones, A. M. Hanby, C. Wells et al., "Breast implant-associated anaplastic large cell lymphoma (BIA-ALCL): an overview of presentation and pathogenesis and guidelines for pathological diagnosis and management," *Histopathology*, vol. 75, no. 6, pp. 787–796, 2019.

[6] J. N. Walker, B. M. Hanson, C. L. Pinkner et al., "Insights into the microbiome of breast implants and periprosthetic tissue in breast implant-associated anaplastic large cell lymphoma," *Scientific Reports*, vol. 9, no. 1, Article ID 10393, 2019.

[7] M. E. Kadin, A. Deva, H. Xu et al., "Biomarkers provide clues to early events in the pathogenesis of breast implant-associated anaplastic large cell lymphoma," *Aesthetic Surgery Journal*, vol. 36, no. 7, pp. 773–781, 2016.

[8] R. N. Miranda, T. N. Aladily, H. M. Prince et al., "Breast implant-associated anaplastic large-cell lymphoma: long-term follow-up of 60 patients," *Journal of Clinical Oncology*, vol. 32, no. 2, pp. 114–120, 2014.

[9] M. W. Clemens, L. J. Medeiros, C. E. Butler et al., "Complete surgical excision is essential for the management of patients with breast implant-associated anaplastic large-cell lymphoma," *Journal of Clinical Oncology*, vol. 34, no. 2, pp. 160–168, 2016.

[10] M. A. Fanale, S. M. Horwitz, A. Forero-Torres et al., "Five-year outcomes for frontline brentuximab vedotin with CHP for CD30-expressing peripheral *T*-cell lymphomas," *Blood*, vol. 131, no. 19, pp. 2120–2124, 2018.

[11] S. Horwitz, O. A. O'Connor, B. Pro et al., "Brentuximab vedotin with chemotherapy for CD30-positive peripheral *T*-cell lymphoma (ECHELON-2): a global, double-blind, randomised, phase 3 trial," *Lancet*, vol. 393, no. 10168, pp. 229–240, 2019.

[12] J. P. Alderuccio, A. Desai, M. M. Yepes, J. R. Chapman, F. Vega, and I. S. Lossos, "Frontline brentuximab vedotin in breast implant-associated anaplastic large-cell lymphoma," *Clinical Case Reports*, vol. 6, no. 4, pp. 634–637, 2018.

[13] A. Stack, N. Ali, and N. Khan, "Breast implant-associated anaplastic large cell lymphoma: a review with emphasis on the role of brentuximab vedotin," *Journal of Cell Immunology*, vol. 2, no. 3, pp. 80–89, 2020.

[14] M. S. Collins, R. N. Miranda, L. J. Medeiros et al., "Characteristics and treatment of advanced breast implant-associated anaplastic large cell lymphoma," *Plastic and Reconstructive Surgery*, vol. 143, 2019.

[15] D. M. Coombs, R. Aliotta, D. Jagadeesh, D. Raymond, and R. Isakov, "Breast implant-associated anaplastic large cell lymphoma with invasive chest wall masses," *Annals of Plastic Surgery*, vol. 87, no. 4, pp. 409–414, 2021.

[16] A. Campanale, A. Di Napoli, M. Ventimiglia et al., "Chest wall infiltration is a critical prognostic factor in breast implant-associated anaplastic large-cell lymphoma affected patients," *European Journal of Cancer*, vol. 148, pp. 277–286, 2021.

[17] G. Q. Lin, Y. Q. Li, L. J. Huang, F. Y. Luo, H. H. Jiang, and W. J. Luo, "Chest wall tumors: diagnosis, treatment and reconstruction," *Experimental and Therapeutic Medicine*, vol. 9, no. 5, pp. 1807–1812, 2015.

[18] P. A. Thompson and H. M. Prince, "Breast implant-associated anaplastic large cell lymphoma: a systematic review of the literature and mini-meta analysis," *Curr Hematol Malig Rep*, vol. 8, no. 3, pp. 196–210, 2013.

[19] J. M. Vose, "Outcomes for PTCL: which pathway to success?" *Blood*, vol. 137, no. 19, pp. 2570-2571, 2021.

18

A Case of Acute Eosinophilic Leukemia with a Novel *PHF6* Mutation

J. J. Lipof,[1] E. J. Huselton,[1] C. S. Zent,[1] A. Evans,[2] B. Zhang,[2] P. G. Rothberg,[2] and J. M. Bennett[1,2]

[1]*Division of Hematology/Oncology, University of Rochester Medical Center, James P. Wilmot Cancer Institute, Rochester, NY, USA*
[2]*Department of Pathology and Laboratory Medicine, University of Rochester Medical Center, Rochester, NY, USA*

Correspondence should be addressed to J. J. Lipof; jodi_lipof@urmc.rochester.edu

Academic Editor: Tatsuharu Ohno

Acute eosinophilic leukemia (AEL) is a rare form of acute myeloid leukemia (AML) that requires prompt exclusion of reactive etiologies of eosinophilia and identification of an underlying acute myeloid neoplasm. Myeloid neoplasms with prominent eosinophilia often have rearrangements in the platelet-derived growth factor receptor α (*PDGFRA*) or β (*PDGFRB*) or are associated with core-binding factor AML. In this report, we describe a 35-year-old male presenting with chest discomfort and altered mental status, found to have marked leukocytosis with eosinophilic predominance and an elevated blast count. Bone marrow aspirate and biopsy findings were morphologically consistent with AEL. Fluorescence in situ hybridization (FISH) and standard karyotype analysis did not reveal any abnormalities, and mutation analysis using next generation sequencing (NGS) revealed a pathogenic mutation in *PHF6*. Cardiac work-up revealed findings suggestive of eosinophilic myocarditis. High-dose glucocorticoid therapy was initiated followed by standard intensive induction chemotherapy with cytarabine and idarubicin. He experienced a rapid reduction in peripheral blood eosinophil and blast count and was found to be in a complete remission at the time of his postinduction bone marrow examination. He underwent allogeneic stem cell transplantation with a matched sibling donor after consolidative high-dose cytarabine and remains in remission at the time of this report, 6 months following his initial diagnosis. The rarity of this condition has resulted in a paucity of data to guide management. Additional studies are needed to better characterize this entity and inform optimal management strategies to attain a long-term sustained remission in these patients.

1. Introduction

The differential diagnosis of peripheral blood eosinophilia is broad and includes both malignant and reactive etiologies. Triggers for reactive eosinophilia include drugs, infections (commonly parasitic), and allergies. Patients are diagnosed with hypereosinophilic syndrome (HES) when there is persistent eosinophilia ($>1.5\times10^9$/L) for greater than 6 months, absence of a clear cause, and clinical manifestations with evidence of organ involvement [1]. Most of these cases are determined to be reactive, resulting from cytokines released in the setting of a known trigger. Rarely, a clonal aberration is identified, and the eosinophilia is found to be related to a myeloproliferative neoplasm (MPN) such as chronic eosinophilic leukemia (CEL), acute myeloid leukemia (AML), or acute lymphoblastic leukemia (ALL). Here, we present a case of acute myeloid leukemia with minimal differentiation and prominent eosinophilia, with a pathogenic mutation involving plant homeodomain finger 6 (*PHF6*) with a variant allele frequency (VAF) of 13%, as well as a mutation in *ZRSR2* (VAF: 73%).

2. Case Presentation

A 35-year-old male with no significant past medical history presented to an outside hospital with fever to 38.9 C, altered mental status, headache, and chest pain. EKG showed normal sinus rhythm with diffuse ST segment depression in leads II, aVF, and V3–V6. He was found to have leukocytosis with a white blood cell (WBC) count of 55.45×10^9/L (normal range: 4.2 to 9.1×10^9/L), thrombocytopenia with a platelet count of 102×10^9/L (150 to 330×10^9/L), and hemoglobin of 15.7 g/dL (13.7 to 17.5 g/dL). The leukocyte differential count revealed marked eosinophilia with an absolute eosinophil count of 16.64×10^9/L (0.0 to 0.5×10^9/L), representing 30% of the total WBC count. The remainder of the differential was significant for 44% neutrophils, 5% lymphocytes, 4% monocytes, 2% basophils, and 13% blasts (Figure 1). A transthoracic echocardiogram showed a low normal systolic function with an estimated left ventricular ejection fraction of approximately 55% and concern for a left ventricular (LV) apical thrombus versus endomyocardial fibrosis. He subsequently underwent cardiac magnetic resonance imaging (MRI) which revealed large areas of subendocardial and midmyocardial delayed enhancement most prominent in the LV apex, suggestive of eosinophilic myocarditis, and confirmed the LV apical thrombus. A left heart catheterization revealed no evidence of coronary artery disease. He was transferred to our institution for further care.

Bone marrow aspirate and biopsy showed acute myeloid leukemia, minimally differentiated, with prominent eosinophilia and 28% blasts (Figure 2). Flow cytometry on the aspirate specimen revealed a prominent and discrete low side scatter, dim CD45 blast gate comprising approximately 30% of total events, expressing CD34 (partial, 50%), CD33, CD38, HLA-DR, CD7 (bright), CD123, and CD71, while negative for cytoplasmic TdT, myeloperoxidase (MPO), and all other lymphoid and monocytic markers (25 additional antigens tested). Bone marrow core biopsy was hypercellular (95%) with abundant immature mononuclear blast forms and eosinophils present. Immunohistochemistry was negative for CD34, CD117, MPO, TdT, and PAX5.

Chromosome analysis and fluorescence in situ hybridization (FISH) analysis were performed using standard cytogenetic methods by the Cytogenetics Laboratory at the University of Rochester Medical Center. Twenty metaphase spreads were analyzed, and no clonal aberrations were detected. FISH analysis was performed on 200 interphase nuclei and revealed a normal pattern for each of the following probes: *PDGFRA* (4q12), *PDGFRB*, *BCR/ABL*1, *RUNX*1*T*1/*RUNX*1, *KMT*2*A*, and *CBFB*. Additional FISH analysis performed at a reference laboratory found no evidence of JAK2 and FGFR1 rearrangements. Taken together, cytogenetic analysis did not detect any recurrent gene rearrangements associated with eosinophilic myeloid neoplasms.

Mutation analysis was performed using next-generation sequencing on the Illumina (San Diego CA) MiSeqDx after library preparation using the Illumina TruSight Myeloid Sequencing Panel. Data analysis was performed using the Illumina MiSeq Reporter and VariantStudio programs, as well as custom software. Analysis revealed a pathogenic mutation in plant homeodomain finger 6 (*PFH*6) with VAF of 13%. The *PHF*6 mutation c.684_705delinsCCC causes a shift in the reading frame and premature termination of translation (p.His229ProfsTer44), thus deemed pathogenic as a chain-terminating mutation. Additionally, a mutation was found in ZRSR2 with VAF 73%. The ZRSR2 mutation c.1332_1343dup is an in-frame duplication of 4 amino acids (p.Ser445_Arg448dup). It has been reported in the gnomAD exomes database at about 0.2% and is likely not pathogenic.

Therapy was initiated with intravenous methylprednisolone 125 mg daily for 3 days followed by oral prednisone 1 mg/kg for 4 days. His symptoms improved, and his peripheral blood blast count was reduced to 1%, while the absolute peripheral blood eosinophil count was reduced to 10.6×10^9/L. This was followed by standard chemotherapy for AML with cytarabine (100 mg/m^2 by intravenous continuous infusion on days 1–7) and idarubicin (12 mg/m^2 intravenously on days 1–3). His day 14 bone marrow biopsy was hypocellular and consistent with chemotherapy-induced ablation, with no morphologic evidence of leukemia. A postinduction biopsy on day 39 was consistent with complete remission with complete hematologic recovery. He had one cycle of consolidative high-dose cytarabine followed by matched sibling donor allogeneic stem cell transplantation. He is in a sustained complete remission at the time of this report, with no evidence of relapse at 6 months after initial diagnosis.

3. Discussion

The majority of myeloid neoplasms that present with prominent eosinophilia are associated with rearrangements in the platelet-derived growth factor receptor α (*PDGFRA*) or β (*PDGFRB*), and fibroblast growth factor receptor 1 (*FGFR*1), which lead to constitutively active tyrosine kinase fusion genes, and often manifest as MPNs [2]. It is important to assess whether an underlying *PDGFR* rearrangement is present because even upon transition to a blast phase disease, these can remain sensitive to tyrosine kinase inhibition [3, 4]. Bone marrow eosinophilia is a feature of core-binding factor AML with t(8; 21) (q22; q22.1) or inv(16) (p13.1q22), which is associated with a favorable prognosis due to a high degree of chemosensitivity [5]. Marrow eosinophilia has also been described in rare forms of myelomonocytic leukemia. ETV6 fusions with different tyrosine kinase proteins including *ABL*1, *FLT*3, *JAK*2, and *FGFR*3 are associated with leukemogenesis and hypereosinophilia [6]. In these cases, prognosis has largely been determined by the fusion partner and responsiveness to different targeted therapies.

In this report, we describe a patient presenting with acute myeloid leukemia with minimal differentiation and prominent eosinophilia, with a pathogenic mutation in *PHF*6 at low variant allele frequency. *PHF*6 is a tumor suppressor gene with its locus on the X-chromosome (Xq26.2). It is recurrently mutated in T-cell acute lymphoblastic lymphoma (ALL) and occurs in about 3% of all AML cases, much more commonly in males than females [7]. Little is known about the exact mechanisms by which *PHF*6 mutations may contribute to the pathogenesis of AML or eosinophilia. The majority of these mutations are loss of function mutations, as it was in our case. They are commonly seen without evidence of cytogenetic abnormalities but with

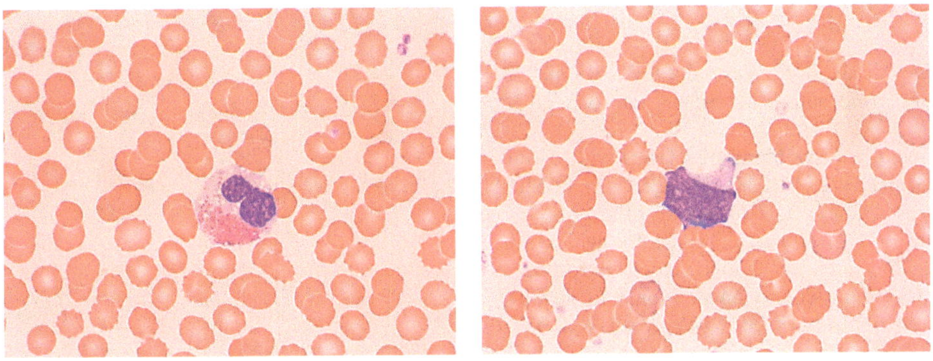

(a) (b)

FIGURE 1: Peripheral blood smear: (a) mature eosinophil with hypogranulation and prominent vacuoles and (b) a blast with rare azurophil granules. Wright–Giemsa stain: 1000x.

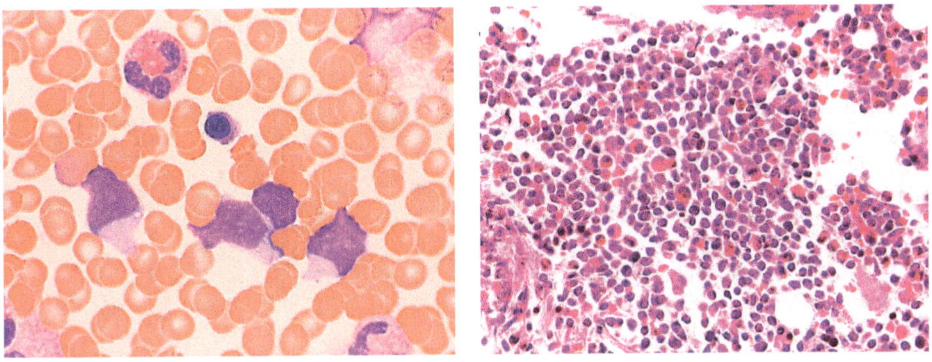

(a) (b)

FIGURE 2: Bone marrow aspirate (BMA) and bone marrow biopsy (BMB): hematoxylin and eosin; 400x: (a) several agranular blasts and (b) numerous eosinophils and immature myeloid precursors.

additional mutations in *ASXL*1, *RUNX*1, *TET*2, and *DNMT*3*A*. In this case, the patient had a normal karyotype analysis and a mutation in an additional gene located on the X-chromosome, *ZRSR*2, which has been detected in 1–3% of AML cases and has no known prognostic or therapeutic implications [8, 9]. To our knowledge, this is the first reported case of *PHF*6-mutated acute myeloid leukemia that presented with prominent eosinophilia, with clinical and radiographic evidence of associated organ involvement. Previous reports have been called either acute eosinophilic leukemia (AEL) or acute myeloid leukemia with eosinophilia [10, 11]. Eosinophil dysplasia has been noted in both benign and neoplastic disorders but may be helpful in the differential diagnosis of potential myeloid neoplasms [12]. We prefer the term AEL as being consistent with other AML subtypes.

There are limited data to guide the management of these patients due to the rarity of the condition. Our report highlights that, in cases of AEL, it is important to initiate the standard cytogenetic and molecular analysis that is performed in new cases of AML, in addition to evaluation for aberrations that are associated with eosinophilia. In the absence of targetable mutations or chromosomal rearrangements that may inform management, one reasonable approach is the use of high-dose glucocorticoids for symptomatic hypereosinophilia with organ involvement, as well as standard induction chemotherapy followed by allogeneic stem cell transplant for the treatment of AEL. Additional studies are required for better characterization of these patients and determination of the optimal treatment strategies to result in long-term remission.

Authors' Contributions

J.J. Lipof drafted the initial manuscript and provided critical revisions. E.J. Huselton and C.S. Zent contributed to data analysis and provided critical revisions. A. Evans contributed to data analysis and interpretation and provided critical revisions. B. Zhang performed chromosome analysis and fluorescence in situ hybridization and provided critical revisions. P.G. Rothberg performed mutational analysis, contributed to data analysis and interpretation, and provided critical revisions. J.M. Bennett contributed to data analysis and interpretation, drafted the manuscript, provided critical revisions, and approved the final version.

References

[1] M. J. Chusid, D. C. Dale, B. C. West, and S. M. Wolff, "The hypereosinophilic syndrome," *Medicine*, vol. 54, no. 1, pp. 1–27, 1975.

[2] B. J. Bain, "Myeloid and lymphoid neoplasms with eosinophilia and abnormalities of PDGFRA, PDGFRB or FGFR1," *Haematologica*, vol. 95, no. 5, pp. 696–698, 2010.

[3] P. U. Ogbogu, B. S. Bochner, J. H. Butterfield et al., "Hypereosinophilic syndrome: a multicenter, retrospective analysis of clinical characteristics and response to therapy," *Journal of Allergy and Clinical Immunology*, vol. 124, no. 6, pp. 1319–1325, 2009.

[4] J. Cools, D. J. DeAngelo, J. Gotlib et al., "A tyrosine kinase created by fusion of thePDGFRAandFIP1L1Genes as a therapeutic target of imatinib in idiopathic hypereosinophilic syndrome," *New England Journal of Medicine*, vol. 348, no. 13, pp. 1201–1214, 2003.

[5] M. A. Bitter, M. M. Le Beau, R. A. Larson et al., "A morphologic and cytochemical study of acute myelomonocytic leukemia with abnormal marrow eosinophils associated with inv(16)(p13q22)," *American Journal of Clinical Pathology*, vol. 81, no. 6, pp. 733–741, 1984.

[6] F. Zhou and B. Chen, "Acute myeloid leukemia carrying ETV6 mutations: biologic and clinical features," *Hematology*, vol. 23, no. 9, pp. 608–612, 2018.

[7] P. Van Vlierberghe, J. Patel, O. Abdel-Wahab et al., "PHF6 mutations in adult acute myeloid leukemia," *Leukemia*, vol. 25, no. 1, pp. 130–134, 2011.

[8] K. H. Metzeler, T. Herold, M. Rothenberg-Thurley et al., "Spectrum and prognostic relevance of driver gene mutations in acute myeloid leukemia," *Blood*, vol. 128, no. 5, pp. 686–698, 2016.

[9] F. Thol, S. Kade, C. Schlarmann et al., "Frequency and prognostic impact of mutations in SRSF2, U2AF1, and ZRSR2 in patients with myelodysplastic syndromes," *Blood*, vol. 119, no. 15, pp. 3578–3584, 2012.

[10] R. S. Weinger, J. André-Schwartz, J. F. Desforges, and M. Baker, "Acute leukaemia with eosinophilia or acute eosinophilic leukaemia: a dilemma," *British Journal of Haematology*, vol. 30, no. 1, pp. 65–70, 1975.

[11] M. A. Lichtman and G. B. Segel, "Uncommon phenotypes of acute myelogenous leukemia: basophilic, mast cell, eosinophilic, and myeloid dendritic cell subtypes: a review," *Blood Cells, Molecules, and Diseases*, vol. 35, no. 3, pp. 370–383, 2005.

[12] J. E. Goasguen, J. M. Bennett, B. J. Bain et al., "The role of eosinophil morphology in distinguishing between reactive eosinophilia and eosinophilia as a feature of a myeloid neoplasm," *British Journal of Haematology*, vol. 191, no. 3, pp. 497–504, 2020.

19

Case of a CD3 Negative Hepatosplenic T-Cell Lymphoma: Diagnostic and Therapeutic Challenges

Laura Alder,[1] **Scott Graupner**,[2] **Guanhua Lai**,[3] **and Victor Yazbeck**[2]

[1]*Department of Medicine, VCU Health, 1201 E Marshall St, Richmond, VA 23298, USA*
[2]*Department of Hematology Oncology, Massey Cancer Center, VCU Health, 401 College St, Richmond, VA 23298, USA*
[3]*Department of Pathology, VCU Health, 1201 E Marshall St, Richmond, VA 23298, USA*

Correspondence should be addressed to Laura Alder; laura.alder@vcuhealth.org

Academic Editor: Pier P. Piccaluga

Hepatosplenic T-cell lymphomas (TCLs) are a rare, aggressive subset of TCLs, accounting for less than 5% of all peripheral T-cell and natural killer (NK) cell lymphomas. We report the case of a CD3 negative hepatosplenic T-cell lymphoma in a 42-year-old female, who presented with left-sided abdominal pain. She underwent a liver biopsy that showed marked abnormal sinusoidal lymphoid infiltration. PET scan revealed increased splenic and pharyngeal lymph node uptake. Immunophenotype was remarkable for negative CD3, gamma delta T-cell receptor, and alpha beta-T-cell receptor expression. She received 6 cycles of DA-EPOCH, had primary refractory disease and then underwent palliative splenectomy secondary to painful necrosis. Then, she was started on pralatrexate as a single agent and then in combination with romidepsin as a potential bridge to an allogeneic stem cell transplantation from her sibling.

1. Background

Hepatosplenic T-cell lymphomas (HSTCLs) are a rare subtype, accounting for less than 5% of all peripheral T-cell and NK cell lymphomas. They have a very poor prognosis, with median survival less than 5 years and rare complete remissions [1]. They are characterized by cytotoxic T-cells infiltrating hepatosplenic sinus leading to hepatosplenomegaly as the most common clinical presentation. While the bone marrow is involved in two-thirds of cases, minimal nodal involvement is typical. Cytopenias, especially thrombocytopenia, are common with a predilection for developing hemophagocytic syndrome [2]. HSTCLs are predominantly seen in males with a median age of onset of 35 years [3]. Diagnosis is made by histologic examination and immunohistochemistry of a bone marrow biopsy and/or liver biopsy or splenectomy vs spleen biopsy. Tumors involve cytotoxic T-cells frequently expressing the gamma/delta T-cell receptor and the immunophenotype CD2+, CD3+, CD56+, and TIA1+ by flow cytometry analysis. Genetic features commonly detected by FISH analysis include isochromosome 7q and trisomy 8, while activating mutations of the JAK/STAT pathway have been reported [4]. Some of the main differential diagnoses to consider when making the diagnosis of HSTCL are aggressive natural killer cell leukemia, gamma/delta-expressing T-cell large granular lymphocytic leukemia (T-LGLL), reactive gamma/delta T-cell proliferations, and more rarely other T-cell lymphomas that may have gamma/delta expression. HSTCL have a dismal prognosis with a mean survival of less than a year and poor response to conventional chemotherapy. New targeted therapies such as pralatrexate, duvelisib, and romidepsin are emerging as potential treatment options as a bridge for allogenic HSCT, which remains the only potential curative treatment modality [5].

2. Case Presentation

A 42-year-old African-American female with a past medical history significant for ductal carcinoma in situ diagnosed five years ago, treated with radiation and lumpectomy, presented with a two months history of progressively worsening left-sided abdominal pain and distension. Lab work showed anemia (hemoglobin of 7.3) and thrombocytopenia (platelets of 126) with leukocytosis (WB of 16.5). Due to concern for hemophagocytic lymphohistiocytosis (HLH), additional labs were drawn; her fibrinogen was 339 mg/dL, triglycerides 217 mg/dL, and ferritin 550 ng/mL, which overall did not support the diagnosis. Imaging studies showed marked splenomegaly and mild hepatomegaly. PET scan showed increased splenic and pharyngeal lymph node uptake (Figure 1).

Her liver biopsy showed infiltration by abnormal lymphocytes (Figures 2 and 3) as did her bone marrow biopsy. The flow cytometry study performed on bone marrow aspirate demonstrated 53% abnormal lymphocytes with a phenotype of CD2+ CD3− CD7+ CD5− CD4− CD8− CD56+ CD57− CD16− TCRa/b− TCRg/d−, which was interpreted as NK cell population. Immunohistochemistery for CD3 performed on live core biopsy confirmed the abnormal lymphocytes are CD3 negative. Notwithstanding these abnormal immunophenotypes, further workup including Epstein–Barr virus (EBV) and T-cell receptor (TCR) gene rearrangement studies demonstrated negative EBV infection and positive monoclonal TCR gene rearrangement, which support the diagnosis of stage IV HSTCL with liver and bone marrow involvement. In order to differentiate between NK and T-cell lymphoma, TCR rearrangement studies are helpful like in this case as they can help finalize the diagnosis as HSTCL. The lack of evidence of any EBV infection in her biopsies or her serum DNA was not supportive of involvement by NK-cell leukemia.

Given her symptoms, she was started on prednisone for 1-2 weeks prior to completing 6 cycles of DA-EPOCH administered at dose level +1 that could not be escalated due to cytopenia. After 4 cycles, her interim PET scan showed diffuse hypermetabolic activity of the axial and appendicular skeleton, attributed to super expansion of the bone marrow secondary to chemotherapy. There was no suspicious lymphadenopathy of the chest, abdomen, and pelvis. She tolerated the cycles fairly well, complicated by one inpatient hospitalization for neutropenic fever with negative workup. The goal was to complete the 6 cycles of DA-EPOCH with positive response to allow for allogeneic HSCT if chemosensitive, ideally in CR1.

Unfortunately, her PET scan 4 weeks after her 6th cycle of DA-EPOCH showed she was primary refractory. Imaging also showed a new splenic infarct with worsening splenomegaly (Figure 4). Her labs at that time were significant for a WBC of 19.8, hemoglobin of 7.5, and platelet count of 77. Her liver function enzymes were within normal limits, except for an LD of 1452. Her main complaint was severe abdominal pain, with physical exam findings of tender splenomegaly occupying the whole left hemiabdomen, extending up to her pelvis. Given her symptoms and cytopenias thought to be worsened by her splenomegaly, she underwent an open splenectomy (~9 lbs), as shown in Figure 5. Her recovery was complicated by small bowel injury and a left-sided pleural effusion.

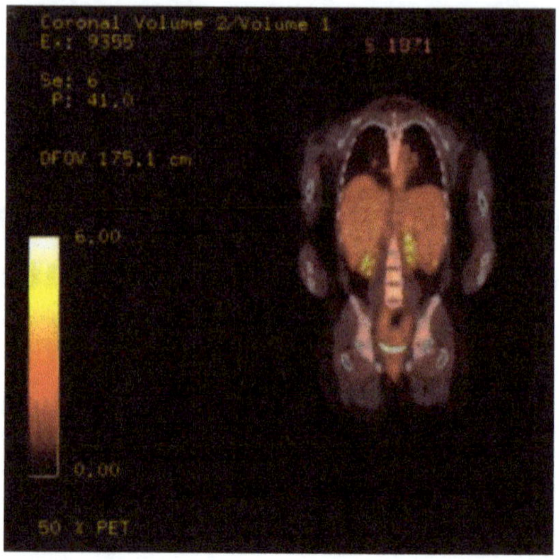

Figure 1: PET scan, initial coronal section at presentation, showing marked splenomegaly. The spleen measured approximately 20 cm in length with relatively focal areas of increased radiotracer uptake in the splenic parenchyma with max SUV 4.4, compared to background max SUV throughout the spleen ranging 2.5–3.0. Background radiotracer uptake throughout the liver was very slightly greater than of the spleen, 2.7–3.2. There was also a focus of asymmetric increased radiotracer uptake in the left parapharyngeal soft tissues with associated soft tissue thickening on CT images and maximum SUV 3.5.

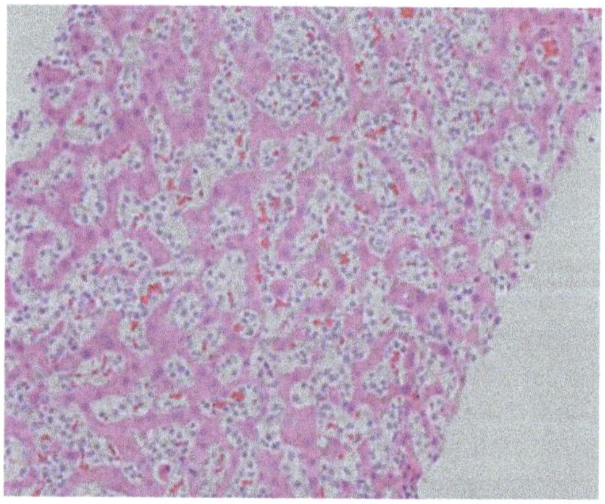

Figure 2: H&E staining of the liver core biopsy shows abnormal diffuse sinusoidal lymphoid infiltration. The lymphocytes are small to intermediate in size with clear cytoplasm and devoid of azurophilic granules, 20x.

The original plan was for salvage therapy with the combination of pralatrexate and romidepsin as a bridge to an allogeneic HSCT from her 10/10 HLA-match sister, but given her counts and performance status, we started her on single agent pralatrexate 10–20–30 mg/m^2, of which she received 4 doses. Repeat PET scan showed disease progression, but given improvement in her performance status and counts, she was started on pralatrexate 25 mg/m^2 and romidepsin 12 mg/m^2·q for 2 weeks (days 1 and 15 of a 28-day treatment cycle).

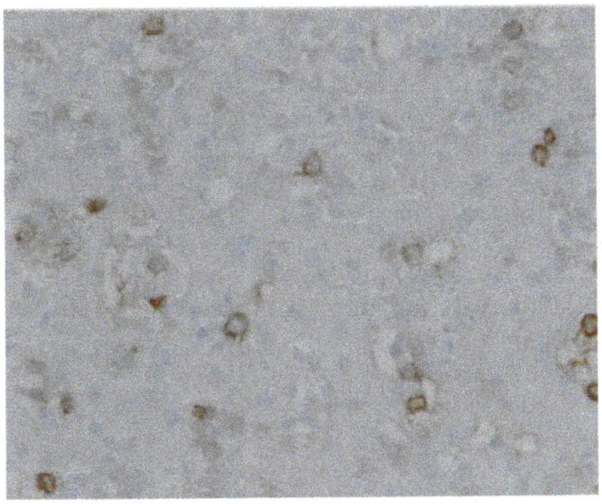

FIGURE 3: Immunohistochemistery for CD3 shows the abnormal lymphocytes are negative for CD3. Rare scattered T-cells are highlighted in the background, 40x.

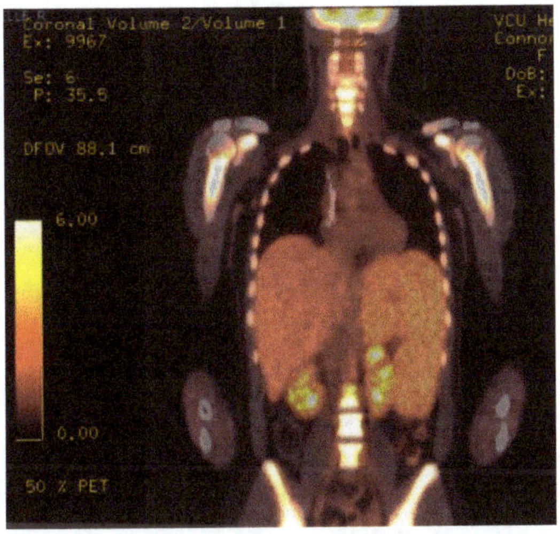

FIGURE 4: Pet scan 4 weeks after 6 cycles of DA-EPOCH showed massive splenomegaly. The spleen measures up to 27.7 cm in length with pronounced hypermetabolic activity throughout the spleen with a maximal SUV of up to 9.8. There are new peripheral wedge-shaped areas of photopenia consistent with infarcts. There is a pronounced mass effect on the stomach and left kidney from the massive splenomegaly. There is ongoing hepatomegaly as well, with the right hepatic lobe measuring 23.1 cm in length compared to 22.0 previously. Hepatic radiotracer uptake is homogenous but decreased from what would normally be expected (the average maximum SUV is approximately 1.9). This diffusely reduced radiotracer uptake could be secondary to a sequestration of radiotracer in the spleen. The previously described area of low-grade uptake in the left parapharyngeal soft tissues now demonstrates a maximal SUV of 2.0, previously 3.5.

Unfortunately, a few months after initiating combination therapy, she was hospitalized with a nosebleed, pancytopenia, and neutropenic fever. This progressed into worsening multiorgan failure of which she expired.

3. Discussion

This case highlights the diagnostic challenges in differentiating CD3 negative HSTCL from NK-cell neoplasm, which is crucial for guiding therapy. While her liver biopsy was suggestive of an NK-cell neoplasm given the presence of NK-cells and CD3 negativity, her clinical presentation was highly suggestive of HSTCL. The characteristic immunophenotype for HSTCL are $CD2^+/CD3^+$, $CD5^-$, and $CD4^-/CD8^-$. Aggressive NK-cell leukemias share a similar immunophenotypic profile with HSTCL, with a negative surface CD3. HSTL is characterized by clonal rearrangement of TCR genes, whereas in aggressive NK-cell leukemia, the genes are typically in germline configuration [6], making TCR arrangement studies an important tool for reaching the correct diagnosis. Furthermore, aggressive NK-cell leukemia is EBV driven, whereas there is no association with EBV and HSTCL. Our patient was negative for EBV infection. It is essential to differentiate between the two entities since the treatment vary significantly. NK-cell lymphomas in the limited stage are usually treated with radiation either preceding or in combination with chemotherapy, which has been shown to improve overall survival. NK-cell lymphomas are generally resistant to CHOP-based chemotherapy regimens but are in many cases sensitive to asparaginase-containing regimens such as SMILE (dexamethasone, methotrexate, ifosfamide, L-asparaginase, and etoposide). Advanced stage NK-cell lymphomas are generally treated with aggressive asparaginase-containing regimens such as SMILE alone [7]. HSTCL cancers on the other hand are usually treated with anthracycline-based aggressive chemotherapy regimens such as DA-EPOCH followed by stem cell transplantation at first remission.

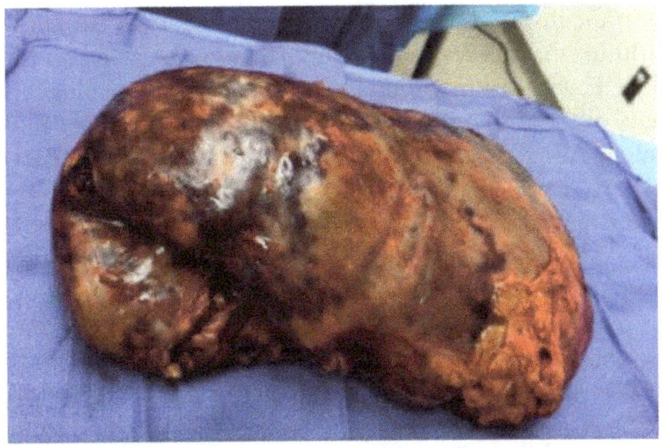

FIGURE 5: Patient underwent open splenectomy. Pathology reported a hepatosplenic T-cell lymphoma diffusedly involving a markedly enlarged spleen, 4025 grams, 29.5 × 22.0 × 10.9 cm. The capsule is tan, remarkable for adhesions and multiple defects ranging in size from 3.7 × 1.0 cm to 16.5 × 11.5 cm. The specimen is remarkable for three possible hilar nodes ranging in size from 1.2 × 0.7 × 0.5 cm to 4.5 × 2.1 × 2.0 cm. Sectioning through the spleen reveals gray-white to yellow hemorrhagic lobular cut surfaces. No definitive grossly unremarkable splenic parenchyma can be identified.

HSTCL is a rare subtype of PTCL, carries a poor prognosis, and has no single standard of care regimen. One of the major challenges for studying this disease is the rarity of the disease itself, which poses challenges in collecting enough data in order to assess efficacy of current therapies and conduct prospective clinical trials. Another challenge is the difficulty in developing risk stratification treatment algorithms that guide therapy. This patient was started on DA-EPOCH with the intention to consolidate with an allogeneic stem cell transplantation given that her sister is a 10/10 match. Allogenic HCT is considered the ultimate curative therapy. In a recent study, 54 patients with HSTCL that underwent allogeneic stem cell transplantation had an improvement in the median overall survival (68 months) compared to historical control (6–11 months) [8, 9]. Given her primary refractory disease, she underwent splenectomy, in order to improve her symptoms and cytopenias, with the hope to increase her count in order to tolerate her salvage therapy with single agent pralatrexate and then in combination with romidepsin [10]. Pralatrexate and romidepsin have shown a broad spectrum of activity across several T-cell histological subtypes, suggesting unique mechanism of actions, and have been increasingly used in all subtypes of peripheral T-cell lymphomas, including HSTCL, at relapse [11]. Case reports already suggest high efficacy with these novel agents in HSTCL. A recent phase 1 study showed that the combination of romidepsin and pralatrexate was well tolerated and resulted in an impressive overall response rate of 71% (10/14 patients) in patients with peripheral T-cell lymphomas including HSTCL [12].

References

[1] L. H. Kapur, Y. Khaled, M. Solh, D. Ward, and C.-C. Chang, "De novo CD3 negative hepatosplenic T-cell lymphoma: diagnostic challenges and pitfalls," *Archives of Pathology & Laboratory Medicine*, vol. 138, no. 7, pp. 969–973, 2014.

[2] A. R. Shustov, W. Hw, A. W. Beaven et al., "Hepatosplenic T-cell lymphoma: clinicopathological features and treatment outcomes: report from the North American peripheral T-cell lymphoma consortium," *Blood*, vol. 122, no. 21, p. 3032, 2013.

[3] M. Montgomery, M. M. van Santen, B. J. Biemond, R. H. Diamond, and S. T. Pals, "Hepatosplenic T-cell lymphoma: a population-based study assessing incidence and association with immune-mediated disease," *Gastroenterology & Hepatology*, vol. 11, no. 3, pp. 160–163, 2015.

[4] M. Travert, Y. Huang, L. de Leval et al., "Molecular features of hepatosplenic T-cell lymphoma unravels potential novel therapeutic targets," *Blood*, vol. 119, no. 24, pp. 5795–5806, 2012.

[5] K. Laribi, M. Alani, C. Truong, and A. Baugier de Materre, "Recent advances in the treatment of peripheral T-cell lymphoma," *Oncologist*, vol. 23, no. 9, pp. 1039–1053, 2018.

[6] Y. Shi and E. Wang, "Hepatosplenic T-cell lymphoma: a clinicopathologic review with an emphasis on diagnostic differentiation from other T-cell/natural killer-cell neoplasms," *Archives of Pathology & Laboratory Medicine*, vol. 139, no. 9, pp. 1173–1180, 2015.

[7] Y. T. Tang, D. Wang, H. Luo et al., "Aggressive NK-cell leukemia: clinical subtypes, molecular features, and treatment outcomes," *Blood Cancer Journal*, vol. 7, no. 12, p. 660, 2017.

[8] A. Rashidi and A. F. Cashen, "Outcomes of allogeneic stem cell transplantation in hepatosplenic T-cell lymphoma," *Blood Cancer Journal*, vol. 5, no. 6, article e318, 2015.

[9] A. W. Chalmers, D. A. Katz, I. J. Miller, and S. A. Gregory, "Successful treatment of hepatosplenic T-cell lymphoma with ESHAP followed by autologous stem cell transplant," *Clinical Advances in Hematology & Oncology*, vol. 11, no. 2, pp. 109–113, 2013.

[10] A. A. Gumbs, J. Zain, O. A. O'Connor, B. MacGregor-Cortelli, M. Patterson, and O. A. O'Connor, "Importance of early splenectomy in patients with hepatosplenic T-cell lymphoma and severe thrombocytopenia," *Annals of Surgical Oncology*, vol. 16, no. 7, pp. 2014–2017, 2009.

[11] A. Shustov, "Hepatosplenic T-cell lymphoma: is cure possible?," *Clinical Advances in Hematology & Oncology*, vol. 11, no. 2, pp. 113–115, 2013.

[12] J. E. Amengual, R. Lichtenstein, J. Lue et al., "A phase 1 study of romidepsin and pralatrexate reveals marked activity in relapsed and refractory T-cell lymphoma," *Blood*, vol. 131, no. 4, pp. 397–407, 2018.

20

A Rare Case of Extramedullary Relapse of Multiple Myeloma Causing Bowel Obstruction

Prarthna V. Bhardwaj,[1] **Shrinkhala Khanna**,[2] **Majd D. Jawad**,[3] **and Syed S. Ali**[4]

[1]*Resident, Department of Internal Medicine, Baystate Medical Center, Springfield, MA, USA*
[2]*Assistant Professor, Department of Hematology/Oncology, UMass Medical Center, Worcester, MA, USA*
[3]*Resident, Department of Pathology, Baystate Medical Center, Springfield, MA, USA*
[4]*Assistant Professor, Department of Hematology Oncology, Baystate Medical Center, Springfield, MA, USA*

Correspondence should be addressed to Prarthna V. Bhardwaj; prarthnabhardwaj@gmail.com

Academic Editor: Marie-Christine Kyrtsonis

Extramedullary myeloma, defined by presence of plasma cells outside the bone marrow, is a rare entity accounting for about 3–9% of all cases. It usually is aggressive with a median survival of <6 months. It is also associated with adverse prognostic factors including 17p deletions and high-risk gene profiles. While common extramedullary sites include bones, there have been several case reports of hematogenous extramedullary myeloma to the liver, lungs, pancreas, breast, skin, and soft tissues. Extramedullary myeloma to the mesentery is a rare entity with only a handful of cases reported. We present a case of 69-year-old man presenting with relapse of multiple myeloma to the mesentery, resulting in bowel obstruction to highlight the various presentations of myeloma.

1. Introduction

Multiple myeloma is characterized by malignant proliferation of plasma cells that usually produce a unique monoclonal immunoglobulin or parts of it. Although it is an incurable disease, there have been several advances in treatment over the past two decades that have greatly improved the overall survival.

The most common presentation of multiple myeloma is clonal expansion in the bone marrow. Roughly 3–9% of patients have pathogenic clonal plasma cell infiltrates that can be found at various anatomical sites, such as the liver, kidney, breasts, testes, skin, lungs, bones, and other tissues which is called extramedullary disease [1, 2].

Clinically, extramedullary disease can be characterized as follows: tumor masses adjacent to bone and extending into soft tissues; soft tissue or visceral tumors that are not connected to the bone; or diffuse infiltration by plasma cells without any obvious focal lesion [2, 3]. Extramedullary disease tends to have an unfavorable prognosis with a significantly shorter overall survival, even in the era of novel agents [4].

Mesenteric myeloma is a very rare condition with about 12 case reports on the same [5–11]. Here, we present a case of extramedullary myeloma relapse, resulting in bowel obstruction which is a very rare entity and highlights its varied presentation.

2. Case Presentation

A 69-year-old Caucasian male was referred to our hospital with 3 weeks of abdominal distension and worsening right lower quadrant pain. He was diagnosed with IgG kappa multiple myeloma four years prior to presentation. He was initially treated with bortezomib/dexamethasone with monthly zolendronic acid with good response initially; however, a year after diagnosis, he was found to have disease progression which manifested as a right radius fracture. His regimen was switched to lenalidomide with dexamethasone with good response and clinically depressed levels of paraproteins. After completion of 9 months of therapy, he underwent autologous stem cell transplant with high-dose melphalan. 7 months after bone marrow transplant, his

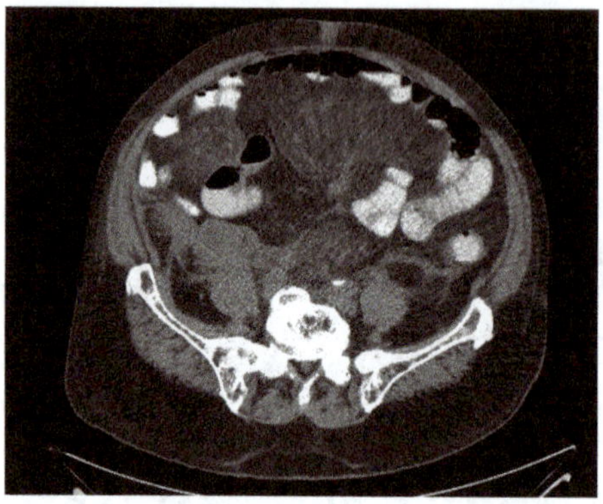

FIGURE 1: CT scan of the abdomen without contrast revealing mesenteric thickening with edema.

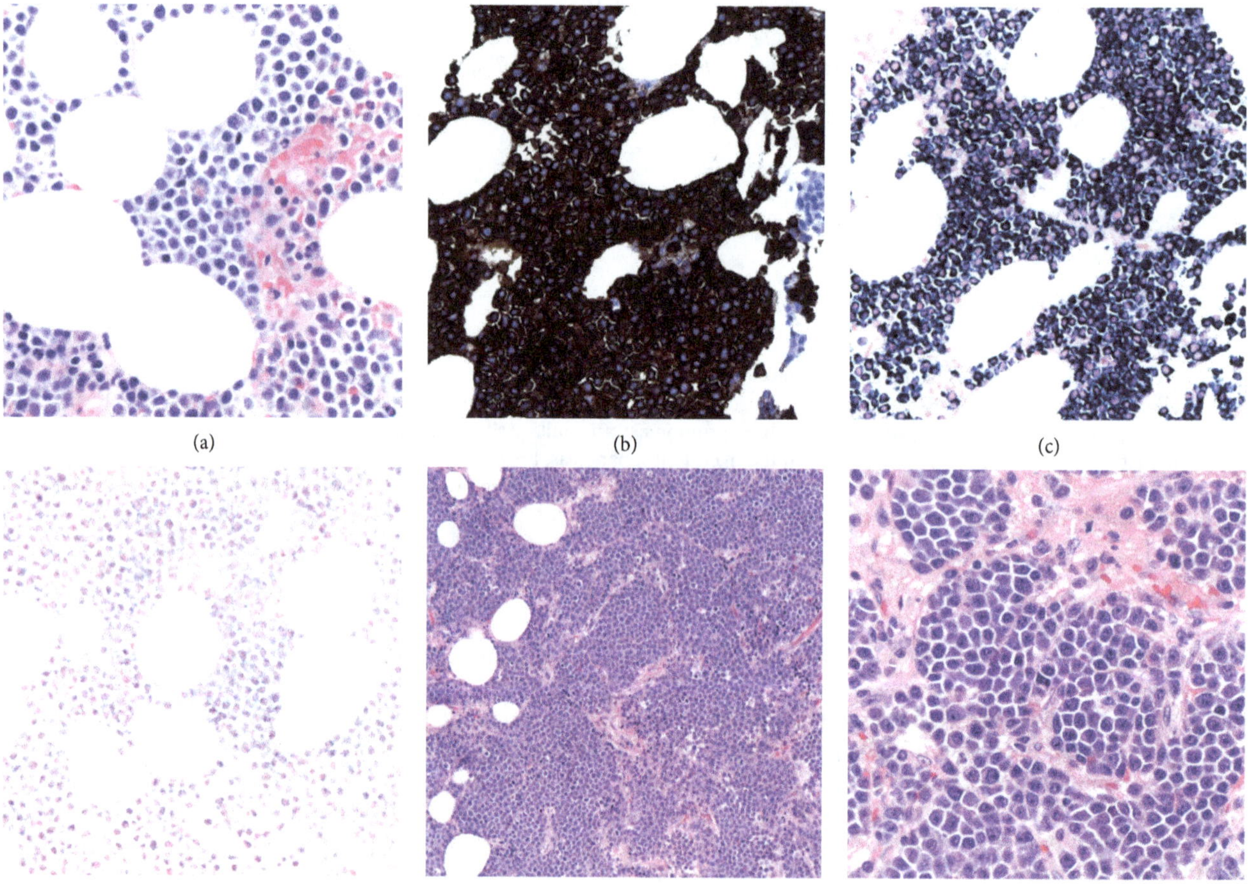

(a) (b) (c)

(d) (e) (f)

FIGURE 2: (a) Bone marrow infiltrated by plasma cells. (b) Bone marrow immunohistochemistry revealing CD138 positive cells. (c) Bone marrow immunohistochemistry positive for kappa light chains. (d) Bone marrow immunohistochemistry negative for lambda light chains. Mesenteric invasion (e) by myeloma cells (10x) and (f) by plasma cells (40x).

disease progressed with involvement of pericardial fluid. Salvage therapy was initiated with pomalidomide, bortezomib, and dexamethasone which was discontinued a year later due to peripheral neuropathy; however, at the end of treatment, there was no evidence of ongoing disease.

When the patient presented to our hospital, he had an acute abdomen. Initial blood work revealed a normocytic anemia with hemoglobin of 8.4 g/dl and elevated ESR of 44. He also had acute kidney injury with creatinine of 3 mg/dl (baseline of 1.9 mg/dl). CT scan of the abdomen and pelvis revealed extensive stranding seen throughout the abdomen within the peritoneal space with edema in the mesentery (Figure 1).

He underwent an exploratory laparotomy which revealed induration of the entire base of the mesentery and retroperitoneum. He had an IgG level of 4407 units with predominantly kappa light chains whose level was 4833 units (kappa to lambda ratio 540). Pathology revealed extensive

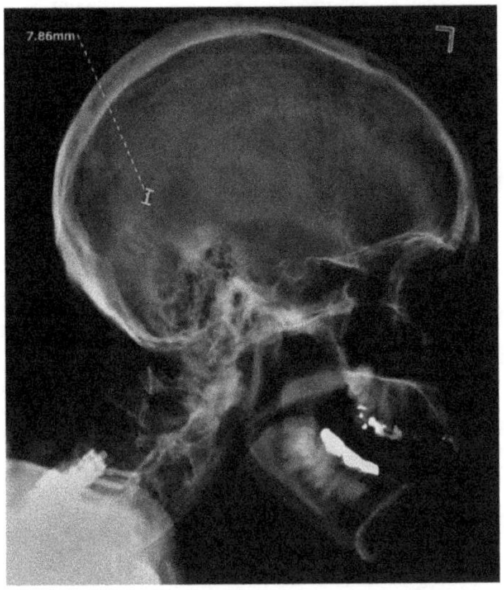

FIGURE 3: Lytic lesions on the skull.

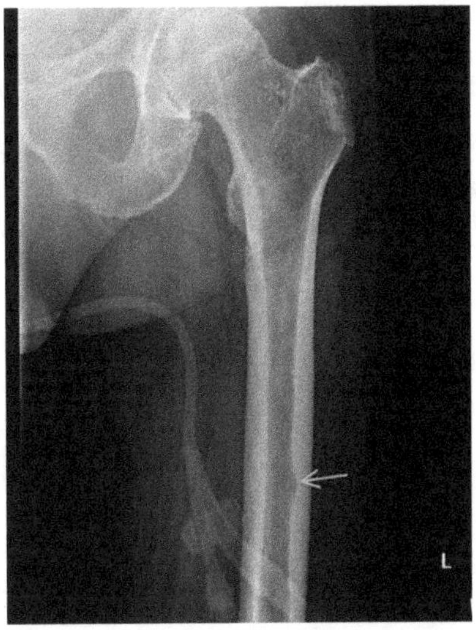

FIGURE 4: Lytic lesions on the L femur.

mesenteric infiltration by kappa restricted plasma cells positive for CD138 on immunohistochemistry, without evidence of amyloidosis. Bone marrow biopsy revealed a 30% involvement by plasma cells (Figures 2(a)–2(f)). Cytogenetics showed 1q22 duplication, trisomy 7 and 15, and gain of 8q24.1. The skeletal survey revealed lytic lesions in the left femur and skull (Figures 3 and 4).

He was started on carfilzomib and dexamethasone therapy for relapsed multiple myeloma. Unfortunately, he died within one day of start of the chemotherapy from surgical complications of bowel obstruction.

3. Discussion

Extramedullary disease is common at the time of relapse in multiple myeloma. At the time of relapse, there is no rationale to favor a specific therapeutic class of drugs. Previous lines of therapy and the duration of response should clearly be considered. We treated with carfilzomib (CFZ), a second-generation proteasome inhibitor. Stewart et al. in their study noted that the progression-free survival (PFS) was significantly improved with CFZ (median, 26.3 months vs. 17.6 months in control group) especially among patients previously treated with bortezomib and lenalidomide and in patients with high-risk cytogenetics (defined by the presence of *t* (4; 14) and *t* (14; 16) or deletion 17p) [12].

Our case is the one of few case reports of a patient presenting with an abdominal catastrophe from relapsed multiple myeloma, causing tethering of the bowel loops due to plasma cell infiltration in the peritoneum.

As patients live longer with myeloma, multiple relapses may occur from different subclones of plasma cells, and this may be the reason for the more frequent occurrence of extramedullary relapse observed today. PET/CT may have role in close follow-up of patients with extramedullary symptoms.

In conclusion, although extramedullary plasmacytomas occur mainly in the upper aerodigestive tract, mesentery may also be involved with very few case reports in the current literature. The sound combination of radiological, laboratory, and histopathological workup leads to the correct diagnosis for a disease with diverse presentations.

References

[1] K. B. Ghimire, S. V. Rajkumar, A. Dispenzieri et al., "Incidence and survival outcomes of extramedullary myeloma," *Blood*, vol. 122, no. 21, p. 3141, 2013.

[2] K. D. Short, S. V. Rajkumar, D. Larson et al., "Incidence of extramedullary disease in patients with multiple myeloma in the era of novel therapy and the activity of pomalidomide on extramedullary myeloma," *Leukemia*, vol. 25, no. 6, pp. 906–908, 2011.

[3] M. Weinstock and I. M. Ghobrial, "Extramedullary multiple myeloma," *Leukemia and Lymphoma*, vol. 54, no. 6, pp. 1135–1141, 2013.

[4] S. Z. Usmani, C. Heuck, A. Mitchell et al., "Extramedullary disease portends poor prognosis in multiple myeloma and is over-represented in high-risk disease even in the era of novel agents," *Haematologica*, vol. 97, no. 11, pp. 1761–1767, 2012.

[5] R. Galhotra, K. Saggar, K. Gupta, and P. Singh, "Primary isolated extramedullary plasmacytoma of the mesentery: a rare case report," *Gastroenterology Research*, vol. 12, pp. 81–84, 2012.

[6] G. Mitropoulou, A. Zizi-Sermpetzoglou, H. Moschouris et al., "Solitary plasmacytoma of the mesentery: a systematic clinician's diagnosis," *Case Reports in Oncological Medicine*, vol. 2017, Article ID 5901503, 4 pages, 2017.

[7] J. Jarry, "Solitary mesenteric plasmacytoma revealed by an acute intestinal obstruction," *Gastroentérologie Clinique et Biologique*, vol. 33, no. 5, pp. 432–434, 2009.

[8] A. Ikeda, N. Takiguchi, Y. Nabeya et al., "Extramedullary plasmacytoma in the mesentery," *The Japanese Journal of Gastroenterological Surgery*, vol. 49, no. 8, pp. 746–753, 2016.

[9] S. Kulkarni, S. Agashe, V. Mane, and M. Ingty, "Solitary extramedullary plasmacytoma of mesentery: a rare presentation," *Medical Journal of Dr. D.Y. Patil University*, vol. 7, no. 6, pp. 798–801, 2014.

[10] T. Rosic, D. Ross, and G. D. Nethathe, "Mesenteric plasmacytoma: an unusual cause of an abdominal mass," *South African Journal of Surgery*, vol. 52, no. 2, pp. 61-62, 2014.

[11] M. T. Sugeeth, H. Vishnu, R. Nandini Devi, and N. Geetha, "Plasmacytoma of the mesentry—a case report," *Scholars Journal of Medical Case Reports*, vol. 4, no. 7, pp. 312–314, 2016.

[12] A. K. Stewart, S. V. Rajkumar, M. A. Dimopoulos et al., "Carfilzomib, lenalidomide, and dexamethasone for relapsed multiple myeloma," *New England Journal of Medicine*, vol. 372, no. 2, pp. 142–152, 2015.

21

Hypercalcemia in Small Lymphocytic Lymphoma with an Elevated Parathyroid Hormone-Related Peptide Associated with Early Richter Transformation

Ashish Bains,[1] Pedro Covas,[2] Olga Timofeeva,[3] and Michael Bromberg[4]

[1]*Department of Pathology and Laboratory Medicine, Lewis Katz School of Medicine at Temple University, Philadelphia, PA, USA*
[2]*Department of Internal Medicine, George Washington University, Washington, DC, USA*
[3]*Department of Pathology, Georgetown University Hospital, Washington, DC, USA*
[4]*Department of Internal Medicine, Section of Hematology, Lewis Katz School of Medicine at Temple University, Philadelphia, PA, USA*

Correspondence should be addressed to Ashish Bains; ashish.bains@tuhs.temple.edu

Academic Editor: Pier Paolo Piccaluga

Hypercalcemia in malignancy is associated with multiple mechanisms and occurs in up to 20–30% of cancer patients. We report a case of small lymphocytic lymphoma/chronic lymphocytic leukemia (SLL/CLL) associated with hypercalcemia and an elevation in parathyroid hormone-related peptide (PTHrP) in the setting of a Richter transformation. Real-time reverse transcriptase PCR on lymph node biopsy specimens obtained before and after transformation showed an 8-fold increase in PTHrP mRNA levels and about 2-fold decrease in the levels of its cognate receptor PTHR1. The findings of this case suggest that parathyroid hormone-related peptide might be useful in monitoring a specific group of patients with SLL/CLL who develop hypercalcemia during the course of their disease and could suggest an autocrine-like mechanism involving PTHrP in Richter transformation.

1. Introduction

Hypercalcemia occurs in up to 20–30% of patients with malignancy [1]. One of the main contributors of hypercalcemia in malignancy is an elevation in parathyroid hormone-related peptide (PTHrP), most commonly seen in squamous cell carcinomas and breast and bladder cancers [1]. Small lymphocytic lymphoma/chronic lymphocytic leukemia (SLL/CLL) is a low-grade, indolent malignancy that usually is not associated with hypercalcemia or an elevated PTHrP. However, SLL/CLL can transform to an aggressive lymphoma, known as a Richter transformation (RT), which occurs about 5% of the time and usually carries a poor prognosis [2, 3]. We investigated the potential association of PTHrP in Richter transformation in a case involving a 70-year-old woman with SLL/CLL who developed hypercalcemia during the course of her disease.

2. Materials and Methods

An IRB approval was obtained to conduct testing on the available biopsy materials. The biopsy material used for RT-PCR was routinely processed, fixed in 10% formalin, and paraffin embedded. Total RNA was extracted from FFPE tissues (2 sections x 5 μm thickness) using Qiagen FFPE RNeasy Kit and deparaffinization solution (Qiagen, Valencia, CA, USA) according to the manual. cDNA synthesis and qRT-PCR were carried out using the Invitrogen SuperScript IV One-Step RT-PCR System (ThermoFisher Scientific, Waltham, MA, USA). PTHR1R and PTHrP levels were quantified using TaqMan assays Hs00896826_g1 and Hs00174969_m1, respectively. The expression levels were normalized using GAPDH expression levels (Hs02786624) (ThermoFisher Scientific, Waltham, MA, USA). The comparative cycle threshold (CT) method was used to analyze the data by generating relative values of the amount of target

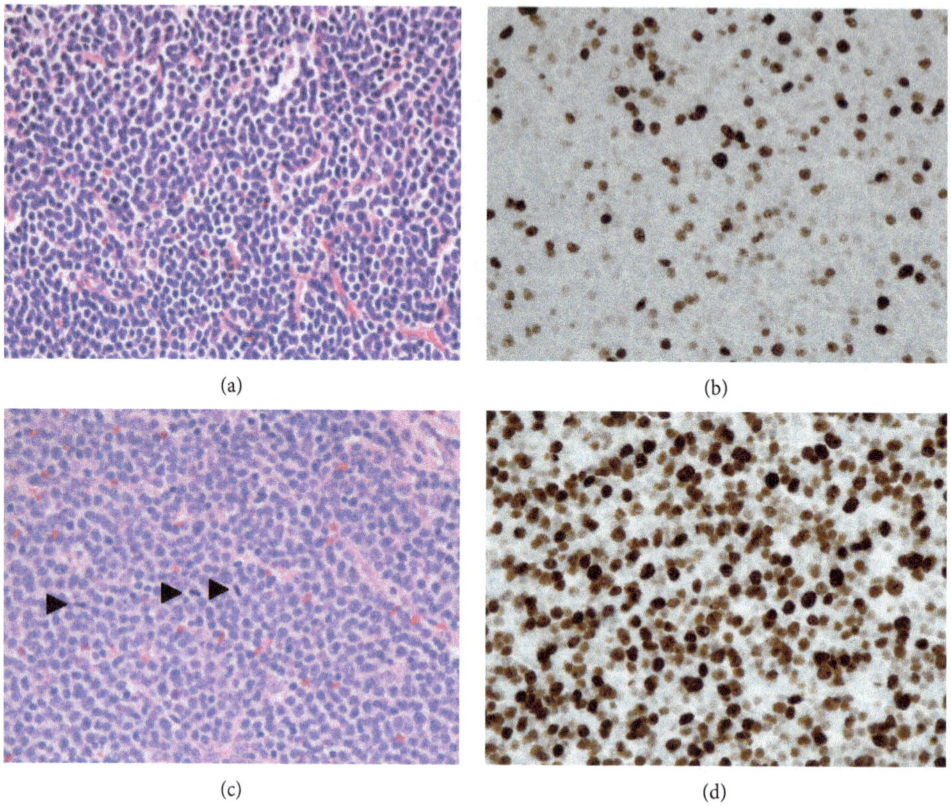

Figure 1: H&E sections of the lymph node excisional biopsy before transformation, demonstrating small round B-lymphocytes with clumped chromatin and rare mitosis (1a); Ki67 showing a low proliferation index (1b). 1c and 1d demonstrate increased cell size with numerous mitotic figures (arrowheads) and a significantly increased proliferation index by Ki67, respectively, at the time of early transformation. All images are taken at 400X magnification.

cDNA (Applied Biosystems) using the following formula: 2–ΔCT, where CT represents the number of cycles for the amplification of target to reach a fixed threshold and correlates with the amount of starting material present; ΔCT = difference between the threshold cycles of the target and an endogenous reference (GAPDH).

3. Results

The patient initially presented in 2010 for evaluation of a left cervical mass in the absence of constitutional symptoms. An excisional biopsy of the left cervical lymph node revealed SLL without evidence of transformation. A metabolic panel at the time of diagnosis was normal and showed a total calcium of 9.2 mg/dL (normal 8.5–10.2 mg/dL), albumin of 4.4 gm/dL (normal 3.5–5.0 gm/dL), BUN 16 mg/dL (normal 8–20 mg/dL), and creatinine 0.94 mg/dL (normal 0.40–1.30 mg/dL). She was observed expectantly and did well until 2013, when the neck mass enlarged. A repeat biopsy of the mass showed SLL with a low proliferation rate (Ki67 approximately 10%) still without evidence of transformation (Figures 1(a) and 1(b)). Her calcium levels at that time and until late 2015 were normal (10.6 mg/dL). She was treated with rituximab and bendamustine for a total of four cycles, which yielded a partial response, and was closely observed until 2016 when she presented with dyspnea and generalized lymphadenopathy. CT scan evaluation revealed diffuse lymphadenopathy above and below the diaphragm. Her total and ionized calcium levels at this time and subsequently were elevated, 12.1 mg/dL and 5.6 mg/dL (normal 4.6–5.3 mg/dL), respectively. She was treated with aggressive intravenous fluid repletion and started on bisphosphonate therapy. PTH and PTHrP levels were 4 pg/mL (normal 10–65 pg/mL) and 151 pmol/L (normal <2 pmol/L), respectively. A follow-up excisional biopsy of a right axillary lymph node demonstrated persistent involvement by CLL/SLL with larger sized neoplastic B-cells, frequent mitotic activity, and a markedly increased proliferation index compared with the prior biopsies, with evidence of early RT (Figures 1(c) and 1(d)). At this time, her peripheral blood was involved by clonal lambda restricted B-cells with an absolute lymphocyte count of 1.6 K/uL and CD45+, CD19+, CD20+ dim, CD23+, and CD5+ immunophenotype by flow cytometry. Peripheral blood cytogenetic analysis demonstrated trisomy 8 and 13q deletion. Immunohistochemical stain on the biopsy material did not provide a definitive staining for PTHrP. However, qRT-PCR showed an 8-fold increase in PTHrP mRNA levels and about 2-fold decrease in the levels of its cognate receptor PTHR1 in 2016 compared with 2013 (Figure 2). These results suggest that the site of PTHrP production was in the lymph node and possibly involved the transformed lymphocytes.

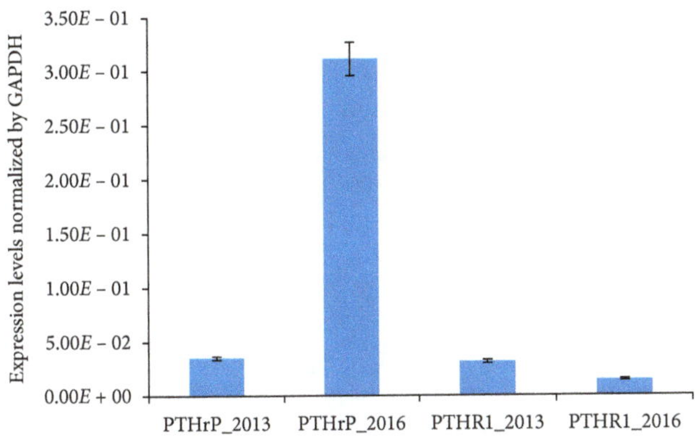

FIGURE 2: The mRNA expression of PTHrP and its receptor PTHR1 in the lymph nodes. The PTHrP levels increased, while PTHR1 levels have decreased in 2016 compared to 2013. The mRNA was extracted from formalin-fixed paraffin-embedded lymph node tissue collected in 2013 and 2016. The expression levels of PTHrT and PTHR1 were normalized using GAPDH expression levels. Each bar represents a mean of three independent experiments for one cell line; bars represent SD.

The patient was treated with five cycles of R-CHOP chemotherapy and achieved a partial response. A follow-up PTHrP level was 46 pmol/L, at least a three-fold decline, with R-CHOP therapy. In 2017, she had a recurrence of her disease with persisting hypercalcemia (ionized calcium elevated up to 6.0 mg/dL) and at this time the total vitamin *D*, 1,25 $(OH)_2$, level was <17 pg/mL (normal range 18–72 pg/mL). She was treated with ibrutinib, but progressed, and electively chose hospice care.

4. Discussion

The etiology for transformation of an indolent small lymphocytic lymphoma into an aggressive variant is not fully known. There are possible risk factors including Epstein–Barr Virus infection and cytogenetic evolution such as trisomy 21 and chromosome 11 abnormalities. [2] Genetic markers such as polymorphisms of CD38, BCL2, and lipoprotein receptor-related protein 4 have also been shown as risk factors to developing a RT. *NOTCH1* mutation has also been noted to increase the risk for a RT. [4, 5].

The symptoms of RT are frequently nonspecific and there is no well-established biomarker to help with diagnosis. FDG/PET imaging can be of ancillary benefit in suspected RT, but FDG avid lymphadenopathy is also nonspecific and ultimately an excisional biopsy is required. [6, 7] Although hypercalcemia is not a common characteristic, it has been regarded in the literature as a precursor to RT. In a review of four case reports of patients with low-grade non-Hodgkin lymphomas, one of the two with CLL/SLL had an elevated PTHrP level nearly two times the upper limit of normal, possibly indicating an association.[8]. Another study described a patient with CLL/SLL with hypercalcemia and 2,500-fold higher peripheral blood PTHrP mRNA level compared to healthy controls at the time of RT.[9]. Other previous studies have also suggested a poorer outcome following the detection of hypercalcemia with higher incidence of histologic transformation and leukemic cell production of PTHrP that may have a pathogenic role in hypercalcemia observed as a rare complication of CLL/SLL [10, 11]. Our data further suggest that the transformed lymphocytes in the lymph node can be the source of PTHrP production. Further studies are needed to establish the correlation between timing of RT and increased PTHrP mRNA levels to determine whether this may be a novel biomarker for early large cell transformation of CLL/SLL.

5. Conclusion

PTHrP might be a novel biomarker to follow in patients with SLL/CLL; although rarely upregulated, in patients who develop hypercalcemia on routinely tested chemistry panels, an increase in PTHrP levels could suggest early RT. This case illustrates that PTHrP can be useful in monitoring a specific group of patients with CLL/SLL who develop hypercalcemia during the course of their disease and might suggest an autocrine-like mechanism involving PTHrP in early large cell transformation.

Authors' Contributions

A Bains and P Covas performed the literature search and drafted the manuscript. M Bromberg and A Bains critically reviewed the manuscript. O Timofeeva performed and analyzed RT-PCR and critically reviewed the manuscript.

References

[1] A. Stewart, "Hypercalcemia associated with cancer," *New England Journal of Medicine*, vol. 352, pp. 373–379, 2005.
[2] A. M. Tsimberidou and M. J. Keating, "Richter syndrome: biology, incidence, and therapeutic strategies," *Cancer*, vol. 103, no. 2, p. 216, 2005.
[3] N. Montgomery and S. Mathews, "Transformation in low grade B-cell neoplasms," *Surgical Pathology Clinics*, vol. 9, no. 1, pp. 79–92, 2016.
[4] D. Rossi and G. Gaidano, "Richter syndrome: pathogenesis and management," *Seminars in Oncology*, pp. 311-319, 2016.
[5] C. Vitale and A. Ferrajoli, "Richter syndrome in chronic lymphocytic leukemia," *Current Hematologic Malignancy Reports*, vol. 11, pp. 43–51, 2016.
[6] L. Falchi and M. Keating, "Correlation between FDG/PET, histology, characteristic, and survival in 332 patients with chronic lymphoid leukemia," *Blood*, vol. 123, no. 18, pp. 2783–2790, 2014.
[7] N. Pemmaraju and P. Jain, "PET-positive lymphadenopathy in CLL-Not always Richter Transformation," *Americal Journal of Hematology*, vol. 92, no. 4, pp. 405-406, 2017.
[8] J. Beaudreuil, "Hypercalcemia may indicate Richter's Syndrome," *Cancer*, vol. 79, pp. 1211–1215, 1997.
[9] N. Watanabe, "Richter's syndrome with hypercalcemia induced by tumor- associated production of parathyroid hormone-related peptide," *Case Reports in Oncology*, vol. 10, pp. 123–126, 2017.

[10] J. F. Seymour, I. F. Khouri, R. E. Champlin, and M. J. Keating, "Refractory chronic lymphocytic leukemia complicated by hypercalcemia treated with allogeneic bone marrow transplantation. Case report and review," *American Journal of Clinical Oncology*, vol. 17, no. 4, pp. 360–368, 1994.

[11] J. F. Seymour and M. J. Keating, "Parathyroid hormone related protein in hypercalcaemia in CLL," *British Journal of Haematology*, vol. 89, no. 3, pp. 685-686, 1995.

22

Pulmonary Lymphangitic Spread of Multiple Myeloma as Early Relapse after Autologous Stem Cell Transplantation

Bicky Thapa,[1] **Gulrayz Ahmed**,[1] **Meera Mohan**,[1] **Volodymyr Shponka**,[2] **and Parameswaran Hari**[1]

[1]*Division of Hematology and Oncology, Department of Medicine, Medical College of Wisconsin, Milwaukee, WI, USA*
[2]*Division of Pathology and Laboratory Medicine, Department of Medicine, Medical College of Wisconsin, Milwaukee, WI, USA*

Correspondence should be addressed to Gulrayz Ahmed; gahmed@mcw.edu

Academic Editor: Pier Paolo Piccaluga

Clinical relapses early after autologous stem cell transplantation portrays an inferior clinical outcome. Early relapse in this setting with extramedullary disease (EMD) of lung involvement in multiple myeloma is rare. To our knowledge, this is the first reported case of lymphangitic spread of myeloma with pulmonary parenchymal and pleural involvement occurring at first relapse.

1. Introduction

Multiple myeloma (MM) is characterized by malignant clonal proliferation of plasma cells and is known for relapsing disease course with a small cure fraction. Extramedullary disease (EMD) in MM exemplifies a clonally evolved population of myeloma cells that can survive independent of the bone marrow (BM) microenvironment and confers treatment resistance and adverse clinical outcome. Herein, we report a rare case of fulminant pulmonary lymphangitic relapse of myeloma with extramedullary pulmonary involvement as the first clinical presentation of relapse occurring within 90 days after an upfront autologous stem cell transplantation (ASCT).

2. Case

A 63-year-old female presented with R-ISS stage II IgG kappa MM after disease progression from monoclonal gammopathy of undetermined significance (MGUS). She had high-risk cytogenetics del17p (unknown clone size) on FISH with complex karyotype. She presented with back pain resulting from a thoracic vertebral paramedullary mass at T12 with no neurological compromise. ^{18}F-FDG PET at diagnosis showed multiple focal lesions with no extramedullary disease. The patient proceeded with 30 Gy local radiation to thoracic spine and induction therapy with KRD for 4 cycles achieving a partial response (IMWG criteria), followed by high dose chemotherapy (HDC) and ASCT. ASCT did not further deepen the response and the patient attained partial response, hence the plan was to proceed with additional KRD consolidation followed by maintenance therapy. However, the patient presented with worsening shortness of breath (SOB) and cough approximately D + 90 after ASCT requiring hospitalization. A computed tomography (CT) at admission showed new bilateral lower lobe infiltrates with consolidation and innumerous pulmonary nodules (Figure 1). She was started on broad-spectrum antibiotics for suspected bacterial pneumonia. Incidentally, she was also found to have worsening pancytopenia with an elevated lactate dehydrogenase 609 unit/L without laboratory evidence of hemolysis. Peripheral smear reported 1% circulating plasma cells by morphology. An extensive infectious workup was unrevealing. Bronchoscopy with bronchoalveolar lavage (BAL) revealed atypical plasma cells with a malignant pleural effusion. A repeat CT scan was performed for persistent hypoxia, which showed further worsening of bilateral lower lobe consolidation along with extensive ground-glass density, interlobular septal thickening, and patchy consolidation throughout the upper lobes as well as superior segments of the lower lobes (Figure 1).

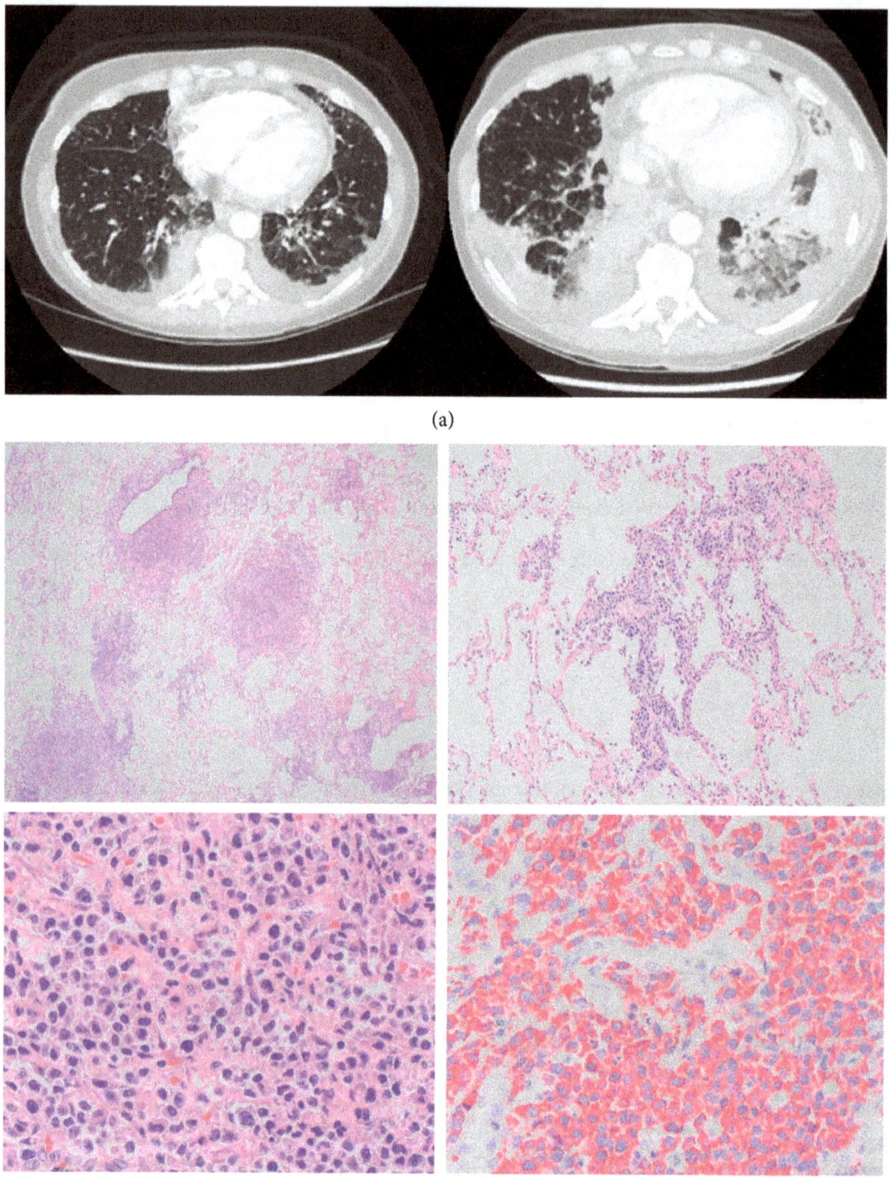

(a)

(b)

Figure 1: (a) Coronal sections of computed tomography showing worsening of bilateral lower lobe consolidation along with extensive ground-glass density, interlobular septal thickening. (b) Pathological specimen showing infiltration of lung parenchyma by kappa light chain restricted atypical plasma cells with a large, round to irregular nuclei, variably prominent nucleoli, and moderate amounts of eosinophilic cytoplasm. Flow cytometry showed 17.9% plasma cells with the following immunophenotypic markers (CD5 (−), CD10 (−), CD19 (−), CD20 (−), CD38 (bright+), CD45 (dim+), CD56 (partial dim+), CD138 (variably+), and CD319 (+)) (Hematoxylin and eosin; 20*x*, 100*x*, 500*x*, and 500*x*, respectively.)

Video-assisted thoracoscopy and lung biopsy showed extensive patchy involvement of lung parenchyma by clonal kappa-restricted plasma cells in perivascular, peribronchial, and periseptal distribution in addition to focally forming variably sized aggregates (Figure 1). Bone marrow (BM) biopsy was 95% cellular, with 88.9% monotypic kappa-restricted plasma cells. FISH studies on the BM aspirate showed deletion of 1p with a gain of 1q, a gain of FGFR3 (4p16), the gain of MYC (8q24), the gain of CCND1 (11q13), monosomy 13, a complex *t* (14; 16) IGH-MAF translocation, TP53 deletion, and gain of MAFb (20q12) observed in 29–96% of plasma-cell-enriched cells analyzed. This is in contrast to the FISH studies at initial diagnosis which showed 1q21 gain, the gain of MYC, *t* (14; 16) in addition to the original TP53 clone. Cytogenetics showed a complex tetraploid karyotype with (del)17P. Taken together, the clinical picture was consistent with a marrow relapse and extramedullary myelomatous lung involvement with lymphangitic spread and malignant pleural effusion. The patient became progressively hypoxic, requiring admission to the intensive care unit. She was started on methylprednisolone 1 gram daily for 3 days followed by bendamustine (90 mg/

Table 1: Summary of case reports with myelomatous lung involvement and their outcomes.

Case reports	Age and gender	Diagnostic modality	Subtype of myeloma	Cytogenetics	EMD involvement of the lung	Treatments	Status
Marmor et al. [13]	65, F	Lung biopsy	IgG kappa	NA	At initial diagnosis of MM	None	Expired
Nitu et al. [14]	60, M	BAL	IgG	NA	At initial diagnosis of MM	None	Unknown
Yuan et al. [15]	58, M	BAL	IgG kappa	*t* (11; 14) (q13; q32) and del 13q14.3	4 years after ASCT	Induction: vincristine, adriamycin, and dexamethasone (VAD) followed by ASCT while hospitalized: thalidomide, dexamethasone, bortezomib, and doxorubicin.	Expired
Kushwaha et al. [18]	60, M	Lung biopsy and BMBx	IgG	NA	At initial diagnosis of MM	None	Expired
Sahin Balcik et al. [18]	62, M	Lung biopsy	IgA kappa	Del(13q), hypodiploidy	At initial diagnosis of MM	Vincristine, adriamycin, dexamethasone (VAD)	Expired
Ravinet et al. [17]	61, M	Lung tissue autopsy	IgG kappa	*t* (4; 14)	6 months after diagnosis of MM; EMD lung within 2 months of ASCT	Induction: bortezomib, thalidomide, and dexamethasone followed by ASCT	Expired
Lok et al. [16]	64, M	Chest wall mass biopsy and BAL	Lambda light chain	NA	5 months after diagnosis of MM	NA	Expired
Rai et al. [19]	55, F	CT guided lung biopsy, BMBx	NR	NA	At initial diagnosis of MM	NA	NR
Abhishek et al. [20]	58, M	Lung biopsy	NR	NA	1 year after diagnosis of MM	Induction therapy: bortezomib, thalidomide, and dexamethasone. Treatment for relapse not reported.	NR
Shah et al. [21]	60, M	CT guided FNAC of lung mass, BMBx	IgG	NA	At initial diagnosis of MM	Melphalan, prednisone	Unknown
Furuncuoglu et al. [22]	42, M	CT guided lung biopsy	Lambda light chain	NA	At initial diagnosis of MM	NA	Unknown

NA, not available; NR, not reported; BAL, bronchoalveolar lavage; BMBx, bone marrow biopsy; ASCT, autologous stem cell transplant; CT, computed tomography; EMD, extramedullary disease.

m^2) × 2 days. Unfortunately, the MM was proved difficult to control, thus we proceeded with salvage KPACE with minimal symptomatic improvement. Given the incurable nature of disease and limited prognosis, the patient opted for hospice care.

3. Discussion

The incidence of EMD in MM had increased from 6.5% in 2005 to 23.7% in 2014 based on a recent registry study, and this is ascribed to the improving survival of MM patients and routine integration of novel imaging techniques such as PET CT and MRI DWIBS in clinical practice [1]. It has been postulated that repeated relapse after exposure to novel agents promote a clonal evolution and establishment of more aggressive clones, which account for an increase in EMD, but this theory had been refuted by more recent studies [2]. As expected, EMD is more frequent in the relapsed refractory setting with distribution showing mostly a predominance of liver involvement in the posttransplant setting compared to more skin and soft tissue at diagnosis [3]. EMD in general portends poor prognosis due to the aggressive nature of the disease and resistance to chemotherapy. While EMD is rare at the initial diagnosis, it confers an inferior 5-year progression free survival (PFS) of 21% overall survival (OS) of 31%[3].

EMD correlates with a high-risk 70-gene expression profiling signature with enrichment of MF molecular subgroup and the PR molecular subgroup [3]. In addition, EMD at the time of diagnosis is a robust predictor of EMD in the relapse setting [4]. It had been postulated that EMD develops because of a "bone marrow escape" of more clonally evolved plasma cells capable of surviving independently of bone marrow microenvironment akin to primary plasma cell leukemia (pCL). Indeed, whole-exome sequencing and gene expression profiling analysis of pCL showed enrichment for high-risk mutations in addition to downregulation of adhesion molecules present in the extracellular matrix supporting their extramedullary survival [5, 6]. TP53 deletions and MYC overexpression by FISH were shown to be presented in a significant proportion of patients presenting with EMD like our patient driving a state of increased proliferation and decreased apoptosis analogous to double-hit lymphoma. Furthermore, discordance in the cytogenetic markers between the bone marrow and EMD has also been observed in keeping with the clonal evolution of these populations [7, 8]. Cytogenetic or FISH analyses were not performed in the lung EMD in our patient, and the genetics is unknown. Concomitant secondary central nervous system involvement has a distinctive association with EMD and spinal fluid examination in our patient was unremarkable.

Our case is unique due to the clinical presentation of early fulminant relapse within 90 days of ASCT with lymphangitic and parenchymal involvement of the lung along with the pleura. The relapse pattern could be due to a hematogenous inoculum of plasma cells in the lung followed by perivascular lymphatic spread into pulmonary parenchyma. In addition, early relapse within the first 24 months of ASCT occurring in 35–38% of newly diagnosed multiple myeloma (NDMM) confers an inferior clinical outcome [9]. More recently, a study reported a unique subset (12.9%) of NDMM relapsing within 12 months of ASCT. Cytogenetics defined high risk and ultra-high risk was significantly greater in this subset of patients with a progression free survival of 18 months and overall survival of 26 months, once again underscoring the dismal outcome in this subset of patients [10, 11].

Our case highlights the very aggressive nature of the disease depicted by the presence of high-risk cytogenetics of (del)17p at initial diagnosis, suboptimal response to induction therapy, early relapse within 3 months of ASCT with additional high-risk cytogenetics including 1q21, and complex tetraploid karyotype with poor response to salvage therapy. Interestingly, in our case, there is a striking discordance in the flow cytometry expression of CD56 or neural cell adhesion molecule (NCAM) with BM being negative and extramedullary lung site positive perhaps suggesting a clonal evolution [12]. Published case reports of EMD with lung involvement demonstrated high mortality with dismal prognosis [13–17] (Table 1). So far, 11 cases have been published in the last 15 years with pulmonary parenchymal EMD. Majority of these described cases presented with lung EMD at the time of diagnosis while only two cases had lung EMD after ASCT (one within 2 months of ASCT and the other 4 years after ASCT). Overall clinical outcome has been dismal (Table 1). Clinical presentation is variable and a high index of suspicion is crucial [13–17, 23]. Besides, our patient was perplexing with COVID-19-related pneumonia high on the differential. Due to rarity and underrepresentation in clinical trials, there is no consensus on the optimal management of these subsets of patients; we opted for salvage multiagent chemotherapy in combination with novel agents. Long-term favorable outcomes have been described following alloSCT [24], which option our patient declined to pursue. Indeed, the expression of CD 38 is preserved in the BM and EMD possibly implying the role of novel CD 38 targeting antibodies, bispecific T-cell engager (BiTE), and chimeric antigen receptor (CAR) T-cell therapy. Extramedullary involvement of lung parenchyma with a lymphangitic spread as the first evidence of an early relapse after an upfront ASCT is extremely rare and associated with poor outcomes.

Abbreviations

KRD: Kyprolis (carfilzomib), Revlimid (lenalidomide), and low-dose dexamethasone
KPACE: Kyprolis (carfilzomib) 20 mg·m^2 D1,2 and 36 mg/m^2 D8, 9, cisplatin 10 mg/m^2 D1-4, adriamycin 10 mg/m^2 D1-4, cyclophosphamide 400 mg/m^2 D1-4, and etoposide 40 mg/m^2 D1-4^{18}F-FDG
PET: ^{18}F-2-Fluoro-2-deoxyglucose positron emission tomography/computed tomography
FISH: Fluorescence in situ hybridization
MRI DWIBS: Diffusion-weighted whole-body imaging with background body signal suppression
IMWG: International myeloma working group.

Authors' Contributions

Bicky Thapa and Gulrayz Ahmed are co-first authors and contributed equally to this article.

References

[1] N. Gagelmann, D.-J. Eikema, S. Iacobelli et al., "Impact of extramedullary disease in patients with newly diagnosed multiple myeloma undergoing autologous stem cell transplantation: a study from the chronic malignancies working party of the EBMT," *Haematologica*, vol. 103, no. 5, pp. 890–897, 2018.
[2] C. Varga, W. Xie, J. Laubach et al., "Development of extramedullary myeloma in the era of novel agents: no evidence of increased risk with lenalidomide-bortezomib combinations," *British Journal of Haematology*, vol. 169, no. 6, 2015.
[3] S. Z. Usmani, C. Heuck, A. Mitchell et al., "Extramedullary disease portends poor prognosis in multiple myeloma and is over-represented in high-risk disease even in the era of novel agents," *Haematologica*, vol. 97, no. 11, pp. 1761–1767, 2012.
[4] C. Varga, W. Xie, J. Laubach et al., "Development of extramedullary myeloma in the era of novel agents: no evidence of increased risk with lenalidomide-bortezomib combinations," *British Journal of Haematology*, vol. 169, no. 6, pp. 843–850, 2015.
[5] C. Schinke, E. M. Boyle, C. Ashby et al., "Genomic analysis of primary plasma cell leukemia reveals complex structural alterations and high-risk mutational patterns," *Blood Cancer Journal*, vol. 10, no. 6, pp. 1–9, 2020.

[6] C. J. Neuse, O. C. Lomas, C. Schliemann et al., "Genome instability in multiple myeloma," *Leukemia*, vol. 34, no. 11, p. 2887, 2020.

[7] L. Billecke, E. M. Murga Penas, A. M. May et al., "Cytogenetics of extramedullary manifestations in multiple myeloma," *British Journal of Haematology*, vol. 161, no. 1, pp. 87–94, 2013.

[8] L. Rasche, C. Bernard, M. S. Topp et al., "Features of extramedullary myeloma relapse: high proliferation, minimal marrow involvement, adverse cytogenetics: a retrospective single-center study of 24 cases," *Annals of Hematology*, vol. 91, no. 7, pp. 1031–1037, 2012.

[9] S. K. Kumar, A. Dispenzieri, R. Fraser et al., "Early relapse after autologous hematopoietic cell transplantation remains a poor prognostic factor in multiple myeloma but outcomes have improved over time," *Leukemia*, vol. 32, no. 4, pp. 986–995, 2018.

[10] C. Bygrave, C. Pawlyn, F. Davies et al., "Early relapse after high-dose melphalan autologous stem cell transplant predicts inferior survival and is associated with high disease burden and genetically high-risk disease in multiple myeloma," *British Journal of Haematology*, 2020.

[11] B. A. Walker, K. Mavrommatis, C. P. Wardell et al., "A high-risk, double-hit, group of newly diagnosed myeloma identified by genomic analysis," *Leukemia*, vol. 33, no. 1, pp. 159–170, 2019.

[12] A. M. Harrington, P. Hari, and S. H. Kroft, "Utility of CD56 immunohistochemical studies in follow-up of plasma cell myeloma," *American Journal of Clinical Pathology*, vol. 132, no. 1, pp. 60–66, 2009.

[13] D. B. Marmor, J. L. Farber, and J. E. Gottlieb, "Acute respiratory distress syndrome due to pulmonary involvement by neoplastic plasma cells in multiple myeloma," *Thorax*, vol. 61, no. 5, pp. 455-456, 2006.

[14] M. Niţu, E. Crişan, M. Olteanu, C. Călăraşu, M. Olteanu, and M. R. Popescu, "Lung involvement in multiple myeloma-case study," *Current Health Sciences Journal*, vol. 40, no. 4, pp. 274–276, 2014.

[15] Y. Yuan, R. Wieczorek, D. L. Green, P. Cook, H. Ballard, and D. J. Araten, "Multiple myeloma involving skin and pulmonary parenchyma after autologous stem cell transplantation," *Journal of Hematology & Oncology*, vol. 2, no. 1, p. 48, 2009.

[16] R. Lok, D. Golovyan, and J. Smith, "Multiple myeloma causing interstitial pulmonary infiltrates and soft-tissue plasmacytoma," *Respiratory Medicine Case Reports*, vol. 24, pp. 155–157, 2018.

[17] A. Ravinet, S. Perbet, R. Guièze et al., "Lung postmortem autopsy revealing extramedullary involvement in multiple myeloma causing acute respiratory distress syndrome," *Case Reports in Hematology*, vol. 2014, Article ID 635237, 2014.

[18] O. Sahin Balcik, M. Albayrak, S. Dagdas et al., "A rare extramedullary involvement in myeloma: lung parenchyma and association with unfavorable chromosomal abnormalities," *Turkish Journal of Hematology*, vol. 27, no. 2, pp. 109–112, 2010.

[19] S. Rai, H. B. Sridevi, V. Acharya, F. Lobo, and J. Kini, "Pulmonary plasmacytoma in multiple myeloma: a rare case of extramedullary spread," *Egyptian Journal of Bronchology*, vol. 9, no. 3, p. 293, 2015.

[20] K. Abhishek, M. Ejazi, Z. Hashim, R. Chaudhary, and K. Niharika, "Multiple myeloma with different thoracic manifestations: case series," *Indian Journal of Respiratory Care*, vol. 7, no. 2, p. 108, 2018.

[21] K. Saha, N. K. Sit, A. Maji, and D. Jash, "A case of multiple myeloma with lung involvement," *Middle East Journal of Cancer*, vol. 3, no. 2-3, pp. 75–78, 2012.

[22] Y. Furuncuoglu, "Multiple myeloma mimicking metastatic lung cancer," *Turkish Journal of Oncology*, vol. 30, no. 3, 2015.

[23] R. S. Kushwaha, S. Kumar, S. Mehra, and R. Prasad, "Pulmonary and nodal multiple myeloma with a pleural effusion mimicking bronchogenic carcinoma," *Journal of Cancer Research and Therapeutics*, vol. 5, no. 4, pp. 297–299, 2009.

[24] M. C. Minnema, N. W. C. J. Van De Donk, S. Zweegman et al., "Extramedullary relapses after allogeneic non-myeloablative stem cell transplantation in multiple myeloma patients do not negatively affect treatment outcome," *Bone Marrow Transplantation*, vol. 41, no. 9, pp. 779–784, 2008.

23

Case of Stroke from Cerebral Vasculitis following Carfilzomib, Lenalidomide and Dexamethasone Therapy in a Patient with Relapsing Multiple Myeloma

Deborah Osafehinti and Kaveh Zivari

Department of Internal Medicine, Maimonides Medical Center, Brooklyn, NY, USA

Correspondence should be addressed to Deborah Osafehinti; dosafehinti@maimonidesmed.org

Academic Editor: Sergio Storti

Lenalidomide, a synthetic derivation of thalidomide, in recent years, has been the backbone of multiple myeloma treatment leading to improved survival. Common adverse effects from lenalidomide-based regimens include hypertension, heart disease, and venous thromboembolism. Hence, thromboprophylaxis is recommended to reduce the risk of stroke. We report a case of stroke from cerebral vasculitis in a patient receiving carfilzomib, lenalidomide, and dexamethasone for relapsing multiple myeloma, not previously published. Medical oncologists should be aware of other causes of stroke among multiple myeloma patients receiving a lenalidomide-based regimen to prevent its occurrence.

1. Introduction

Multiple myeloma (MM) is a hematological malignancy characterized by the neoplastic proliferation of plasma cells leading to monoclonal immunoglobulin production [1–3]. It accounts for 10 to 15% of all hematological malignancies [2, 4], and in the United States, there are more than 20,000 new cases of multiple myeloma every year [4]. Treatment choice is mainly dependent on the functional status of the patient and the aggressiveness of the disease. These include autologous stem cell transplant (for those who are transplant eligible) and chemotherapy [3, 4]. The overall survival rates and treatment response have improved over the past decade following the introduction of novel targeted therapies such as the immunomodulatory agents (IMiD), thalidomide, and proteasome inhibitors (PI), bortezomib [5, 6]. However, MM remains an incurable disease, and many patients will relapse despite receiving appropriate treatment.

The US FDA recently approved the combination of carfilzomib (Kyprolis), a proteasome inhibitor, lenalidomide (Revlimid), a synthetic derivative of thalidomide [7], and dexamethasone for patients with relapsed/refractory multiple myeloma after reports showed better survival outcomes compared to earlier regimens [8, 9]. In the ASPIRE trial, patients treated with the carfilzomib (Kyprolis), lenalidomide (Revlimid), and dexamethasone regimen (i.e., KRd regimen) resulted in a progression-free survival median of 26.3 months compared to 17.6 months in patients treated with lenalidomide and dexamethasone (Rd) regimen [9]. However, grade≥3 adverse effects and serious effects were higher in the KRd arm than the Rd arm, some of which include hypertension, ischemic heart disease, heart failure, and venous thromboembolism [9, 10]. Specifically, by substituting an amino group in the phthaloyl ring, lenalidomide has less adverse side effects compared to thalidomide [11]. The same change in the phthaloyl ring of lenalidomide results in a complex immune modulation effect that is responsible for its activity. However, this complex can lead to lenalidomide toxicity. Most cases of lenalidomide toxicity include skin lesions [11–14], urticaria [15], but rarely vasculitis [13]. We report a case of a patient on the KRd regimen who presented with stroke caused by cerebral vasculitis.

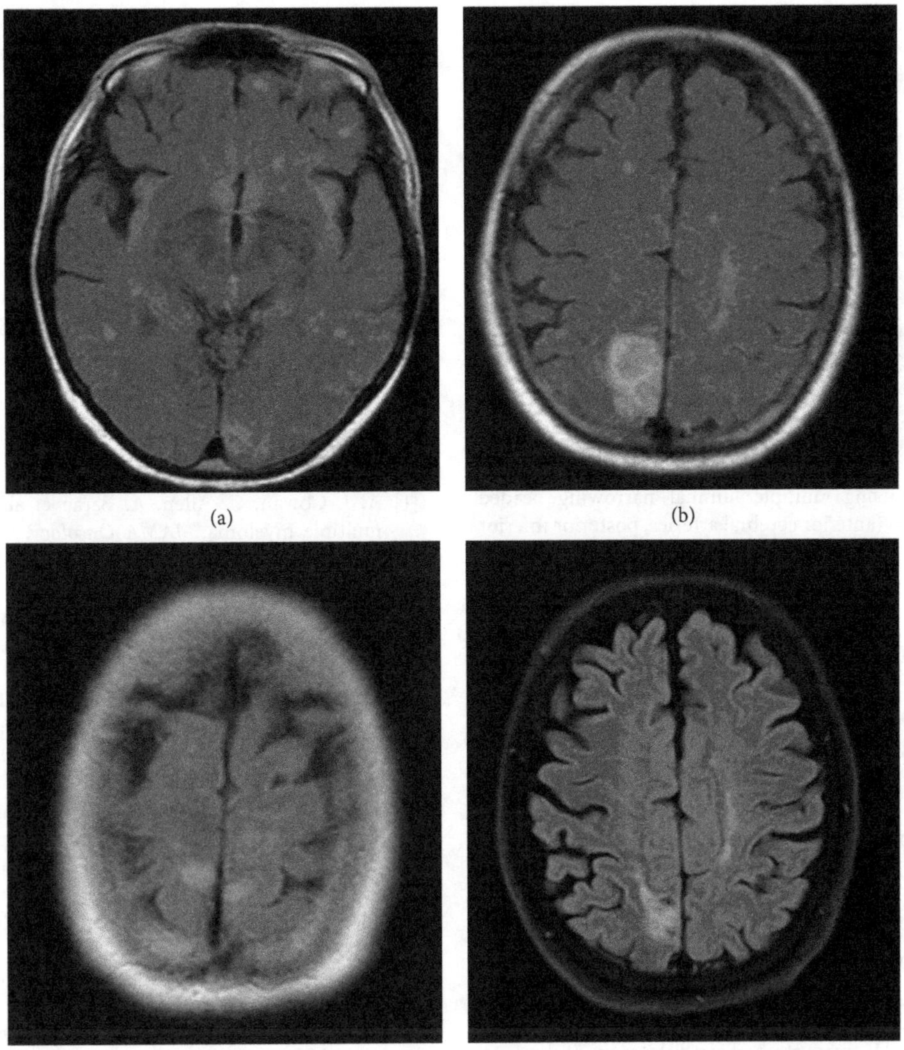

FIGURE 1: MRI brain showing acute ischemic regions. (a-b) Acute infarcts in the posterior circulation involving bilateral cerebellar hemispheres, medial bilateral occipital and parietal lobes, and the posterior watershed region at the vertex with small amount of hemorrhagic conversion within the right parietal parasagittal lesion. (c-d) MRI image of infarct in the medial occipital lobe and parietal lobes bilaterally.

2. Case

We present a 59-year-old female with a history of multiple myeloma diagnosis in 2015. Laboratory results at the time of diagnosis had shown hemoglobin of 6.4 g/dl, platelet of 43,000/Ul, and creatinine of 1.2 mg/dl increased from her baseline of 0.7 mg/dl. Serum protein electrophoresis showed an immunoglobulin A level of 9680 mg/dl with low immunoglobulin G and M levels. She had induction chemotherapy with cyclophosphamide, bortezomib, and dexamethasone (CyBorD) regimen, received autologous bone marrow transplantation in 2016, and subsequently went into remission. Unfortunately, she relapsed in 2017 and then started a salvage regimen with carfilzomib, lenalidomide, and dexamethasone every two weeks to 1 month as well as daily low-dose aspirin.

In February 2019, she was admitted to our hospital with complaints of increased lethargy, multiple falls, and worsening headaches for 4 to 5 days. Physical examination showed mild left facial droop. Aside from being a current everyday smoker (about five cigarette sticks per day) with COPD and a former heroin abuser on a methadone maintenance program, she had no history of diabetes, hypertension, or previous strokes. CT of the head revealed a mass-like structure in the right precentral region measuring approximately 1.5 cm by 0.9 cm surrounded by a large area of vasogenic edema without midline shift and a small age-indeterminate infarct in the left posterior paramedian parietal lobe. MRI of the brain (Figure 1) revealed non-enhancing acute infarcts in the posterior circulation involving bilateral cerebellar hemispheres, medial bilateral occipital and parietal lobes, and the posterior watershed region at the vertex with small amount of hemorrhagic

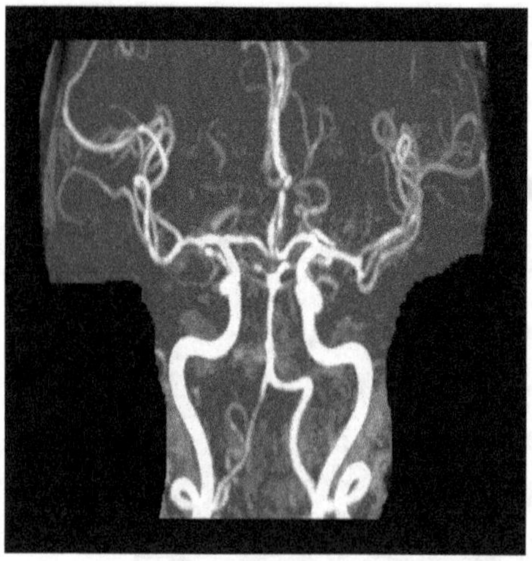

Figure 2: MRA showing multiple luminal narrowing beaded pattern in most vessels (anterior cerebral arteries, posterior inferior M2 division of the right middle cerebral artery, and posterior cerebral arteries).

conversion within the right parietal parasagittal lesion. MRA of the brain (Figure 2) without contrast further revealed multiple long and short segments of luminal narrowing with a beaded pattern in the anterior cerebral arteries, posterior inferior M2 division of the right middle cerebral artery, and posterior cerebral arteries indicating vasculitis as the etiology. CRP was more than 40 mg/dl. dsDNA and ANCA testing were both negative. A thromboembolic phenomenon was ruled-out as transthoracic echocardiography showed no evidence of valvular disease, vegetation, patent foramen ovale, or thrombosis. Also, carotid Doppler showed no significant carotid stenosis.

We withheld further chemotherapy, and a short course of dexamethasone IV was started and later switched to prednisone PO before discharge. She also received anticoagulation with apixaban. After outpatient follow-up, she resumed carfilzomib, cyclophosphamide, and dexamethasone regimen, which responded briefly as M spike returned to near baseline but later developed myelomatous meningitis. As a result, she received intrathecal methotrexate and cytarabine and commenced salvage therapy with DCEP (dexamethasone, cyclophosphamide, etoposide, and cisplatin). Three weeks after receiving the first cycle, she was admitted for severe pancytopenia, septic shock with *Klebsiella* bacteremia, acute respiratory distress syndrome (ARDS), and gastrointestinal bleeding secondary to thrombocytopenia and apixaban use. Unfortunately, she died from multiorgan failure.

3. Discussion

There have been no prior reports of stroke in a patient with relapsed multiple myeloma treated with carfilzomib, lenalidomide, and dexamethasone regimen [8, 9]. However, the lenalidomide and dexamethasone regimen approved for patients with newly diagnosed multiple myeloma has an increased risk for arterial thromboembolism, including stroke and myocardial infarction [16, 17]. Lenalidomide carries a black box warning for thromboembolic risks, and thromboprophylaxis with either low-molecular-weight heparin, warfarin, or low-dose aspirin is recommended for patients treated with a lenalidomide-based regimen [18–20]. Our patient, however, had a stroke with cerebral vasculitis being the underlying etiology.

Although the KRd regimen may have a promising safety profile from previous clinical trials, we expect that market surveillance will offer more data about rare or idiosyncratic adverse effects. We hope that such knowledge will identify patients who are at high risk and provide preventive measures to improve their quality of life.

References

[1] A. J. Cowan, C. Allen, A. Barac et al., "Global burden of multiple myeloma," *JAMA Oncology*, vol. 4, no. 9, p. 1221, 2018.

[2] C. Gerecke, S. Fuhrmann, S. Strifler, M. Schmidt-Hieber, H. Einsele, and S. Knop, "The diagnosis and treatment of multiple myeloma," *Deutsches Äerzteblatt International*, vol. 113, no. 27-28, pp. 470–476, 2016.

[3] S. Jewell, Z. Xiang, A. Kunthur, and P. Mehta, "Multiple myeloma: updates on diagnosis and management," *Federal Practitioner*, vol. 32, no. Suppl 7, pp. 49S–56S, 2015.

[4] S. V. Rajkumar, "Multiple myeloma: 2014 update on diagnosis, risk-stratification, and management," *American Journal of Hematology*, vol. 89, no. 10, pp. 998–1009, 2014.

[5] O. Landgren and K. Iskander, "Modern multiple myeloma therapy: deep, sustained treatment response and good clinical outcomes," *Journal of Internal Medicine*, vol. 281, no. 4, pp. 365–382, 2017.

[6] S. Lonial and K. C. Anderson, "Association of response endpoints with survival outcomes in multiple myeloma," *Leukemia*, vol. 28, no. 2, pp. 258–268, 2014.

[7] U. Vitolo, A. Chiappella, S. Franceschetti et al., "Lenalidomide plus R-CHOP21 in elderly patients with untreated diffuse large B-cell lymphoma: results of the REAL07 open-label, multicentre, phase 2 trial," *The Lancet Oncology*, vol. 15, no. 7, pp. 730–737, 2014.

[8] D. S. Siegel, M. A. Dimopoulos, H. Ludwig et al., "Improvement in overall survival with carfilzomib, lenalidomide, and dexamethasone in patients with relapsed or refractory multiple myeloma," *Journal of Clinical Oncology*, vol. 36, no. 8, pp. 728–734, 2018.

[9] A. K. Stewart, S. V. Rajkumar, M. A. Dimopoulos et al., "Carfilzomib, lenalidomide, and dexamethasone for relapsed multiple myeloma," *New England Journal of Medicine*, vol. 372, no. 2, pp. 142–152, 2015.

[10] W. Li, R. F. Cornell, D. Lenihan et al., "Cardiovascular complications of novel multiple myeloma treatments," *Circulation*, vol. 133, no. 9, pp. 908–912, 2016.

[11] V. Kotla, S. Goel, S. Nischal et al., "Mechanism of action of lenalidomide in hematological malignancies," *Journal of Hematology & Oncology*, vol. 2, no. 1, p. 36, 2009.

[12] M. A. Dimopoulos, A. Palumbo, M. Attal et al., "Optimizing the use of lenalidomide in relapsed or refractory multiple myeloma: consensus statement," *Leukemia*, vol. 25, no. 5, pp. 749–760, 2011.

[13] M. Breccia, L. Cannella, R. Latagliata et al., "Unexpected erythroid and cytogenetic responses after discontinuation of a short course of lenalidomide as a result of severe skin rash in a

patient with 5q syndrome," *Journal of Clinical Oncology*, vol. 29, no. 14, pp. e402–e403, 2011.

[14] N. W. van de Donk, G. Görgün, R. W. Groen et al., "Lenalidomide for the treatment of relapsed and refractory multiple myeloma," *Cancer Management and Research*, vol. 4, pp. 253–268, 2012.

[15] H. P. Sviggum, M. D. P. Davis, S. V. Rajkumar, and A. Dispenzieri, "Dermatologic adverse effects of lenalidomide therapy for amyloidosis and multiple myeloma," *Archives of Dermatology*, vol. 142, no. 10, pp. 1298–1302, 2006.

[16] P. Shridhar, R. Khalil, D. Lasorda, and Y. Chun, "Lenalidomide induced stroke in multiple myeloma," *Journal of Integrative Cardiology*, vol. 2, no. 6, 2016.

[17] A. Hinduja, K. Limaye, R. Ravilla et al., "Spectrum of cerebrovascular disease in patients with multiple myeloma undergoing chemotherapy-results of a case control study," in *PLoS One*, J. Hendrikse, Ed., vol. 11, no. 11, Article ID e0166627, 2016.

[18] S. P. Menon, S. V. Rajkumar, M. Lacy, P. Falco, and A. Palumbo, "Thromboembolic events with lenalidomide-based therapy for multiple myeloma," *Cancer*, vol. 112, no. 7, pp. 1522–1528, 2008.

[19] E. Zamagni, A. Brioli, P. Tacchetti, B. Zannetti, L. Pantani, and M. Cavo, "Multiple myeloma, venous thromboembolism, and treatment-related risk of thrombosis," *Seminars in Thrombosis and Hemostasis*, vol. 37, no. 3, pp. 209–219, 2011.

[20] M. P. Cruz, "Lenalidomide (revlimid): a thalidomide analogue in combination with dexamethasone for the treatment of all patients with multiple myeloma," *P & T*, vol. 41, no. 5, pp. 308–313, 2016.

24

Prolonged Pediatric Extracorporeal Membrane Oxygenation Support with Cardiopulmonary Failure in Juvenile Myelomonocytic Leukemia

Maris Bartkevics,[1] Bert Hennig,[2] Tayfun Gungor,[3] Roland Ammann,[2] and Alexander Kadner[1]

[1]*Center for Congenital Heart Disease, Department of Cardiovascular Surgery, Inselspital University Hospital, Bern University, Bern, Switzerland*
[2]*Department of Pediatrics, University Children's Hospital, Bern University, Bern, Switzerland*
[3]*Department of Stem Cell Transplantation, University Children's Hospital Zurich, University Zurich, Zürich, Switzerland*

Correspondence should be addressed to Alexander Kadner; alexander.kadner@insel.ch

Academic Editor: Sergio Storti

We report a case of a child survival after extracorporeal membrane oxygenation (ECMO) support of 25 days for cardiopulmonary failure and septic shock in the context of juvenile myelomonocytic leukemia (JMML). ECMO support is still a matter of debate for the management of septic patients with malignancy. However, these patients are at increased risk for early death secondary to pulmonary complications due to leukostasis, direct pulmonary infiltration with WBC, and systemic inflammatory response syndrome following malignant cell lysis. Despite the high risk of complications, ECMO support must be discussed as part of management, providing better outcome in this group of patients.

1. Introduction

Extracorporeal membrane oxygenation (ECMO) support is still a matter of debate for the management of septic patients with malignancy. However, these patients are at increased risk for early death secondary to pulmonary complications due to leukostasis, direct pulmonary infiltration with WBC, and systemic inflammatory response syndrome following malignant cell lysis [1].

We report a case of successful management of a child with juvenile myelomonocytic leukemia (JMML), who required prolonged ECMO support secondary to cardiopulmonary failure following initiation of chemotherapy.

2. Patients' Medical Report

A 4-year-old boy presented with an intermittent fever for two weeks, cold symptoms, and loss of appetite. On physical examination, the child was found moderately dehydrated, tachycardic, and tachypneic and demonstrated a hepatosplenomegaly. His peripheral blood tests showed 10% myeloid blasts with WBC (16.2×10^9/L), severe anemia (Hb 2.8 g/dL), and thrombocytopenia (platelets 6×10^9/L), as well as a monocyte count of 4.61×10^9/l. A bone marrow aspiration was performed and revealed 10% of myeloid blast cells. The patient was started on an induction regimen with cytarabine and rasburicase. Less than 24 hours after initiation of therapy, he developed fever and progressive respiratory failure. A chest X-ray showed a bilateral pulmonary infiltration. In the context of suspected sepsis, the broad-spectrum antibiotic treatment was started. Echocardiography showed signs of severe pulmonary hypertension (PHT). Despite inotropic support, mechanical ventilation, and early antibiotics, the patient deteriorated and was referred to our tertiary pediatric intensive care unit.

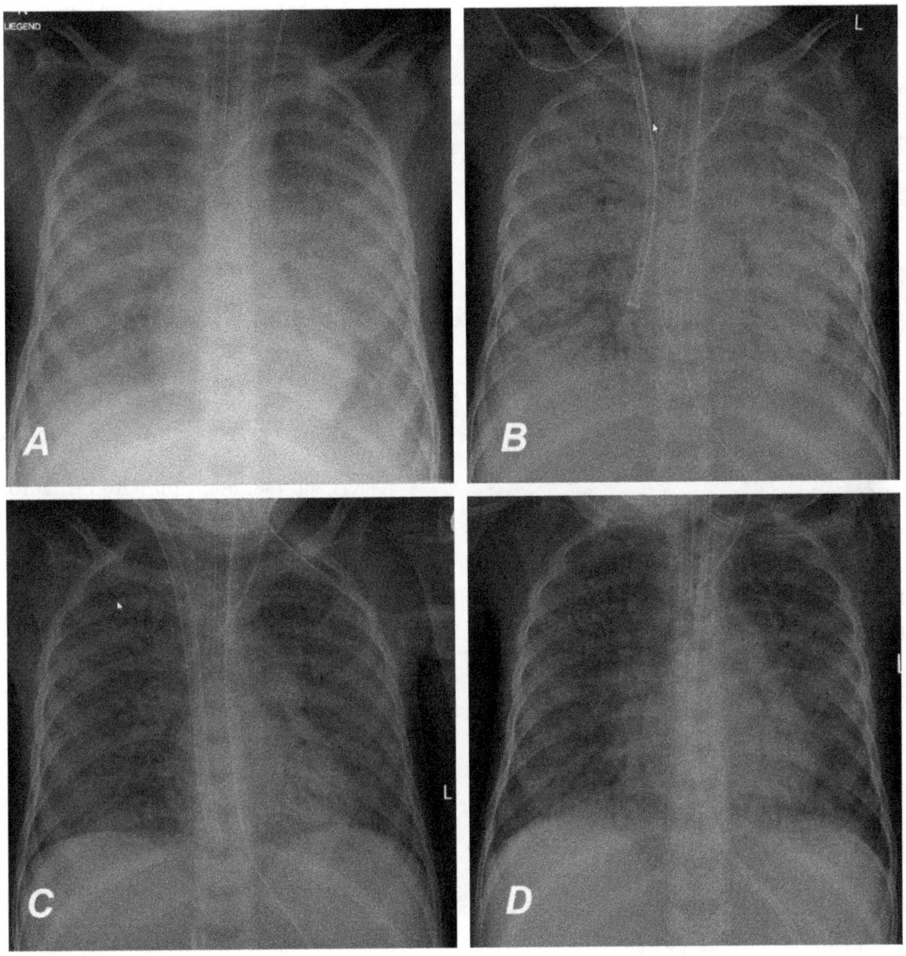

FIGURE 1: (a) Chest X-ray on admission. (b) Chest X-ray after ECMO cannulation via neck vessels. (c) Chest X-ray after conversion to veno-venous ECMO by using single venous neck cannula. (d) Chest X-ray after ECMO weaning.

At arrival, his general condition was critical with signs of multiorgan failure and severe lactic acidosis. The neurological status appeared to be normal. His acute respiratory distress syndrome necessitated high-pressure ventilation (Figure 1(a)). Despite optimized conventional therapy, he rapidly developed cardiogenic shock. A veno-arterial (VA) ECMO was initiated via neck vessel cannulation, and immediate improvement in oxygenation was achieved (Figure 1(b)). ECMO flow was stable between 1.2 - 1.7 L/min during the whole support period. ACT was kept at 180 seconds. No major bleeding complications occurred. Mechanical ventilation was continued, and PHT therapy was initiated with sodium nitroprusside and nitrous oxide. First improvements in ventilation were observed on day 12 on ECMO support. On day 18, VA ECMO could be converted to a veno-venous (VV) ECMO by using a dual lumen Avalon ELITE cannula (MAQUET Cardiopulmonary AG, Germany) (Figure 1(c)). After seven days of VV ECMO support, the patient was successfully weaned on day 25 (Figure 1(d)). The neurologic assessment of the patient was limited during ECMO support due to pharmacological sedation. Following further hemodynamic improvement and weaning of sedation, the patient demonstrated a quadriplegia, global aphasia, and conjugate eye deviation. Subsequent MRI diagnostic revealed a central pontine myelinolysis. Certainly, it was caused by dyselectrolaemia with severe hypernatremia. Despite severe neurological impairment, his respiratory condition improved further, and 2 days later (day 30), he was extubated (Figure 2). Following extubation, a bilateral vocal cord paralysis of probably central origin was noticed.

Given the fast improvement of the patient, the initially paused chemotherapy with cytarabine was restarted early, thus allowing a cytogenetic remission on day 21 of ECMO support.

On day 34 of hospitalization, the patient was referred for evaluation for allogeneic hematopoietic stem cell transplantation to the transplantation center. A genetic testing revealed a KRAS and SETBP1 mutation. Given the severe neurological impairment, the decision was taken to proceed with bridging chemotherapy until improvement of the neurological status could be observed.

Five weeks later, the patient's clinical condition was normal with a remarkably improved neurological status and normalized vocal chord function. The patient could walk, even drive a 3-wheel bike, while his cognitive function was still impaired with a stammer requiring further speech and language therapy.

Six months later, he underwent allogeneic hematopoietic stem cell transplantation with a 10/10 HLA-matched

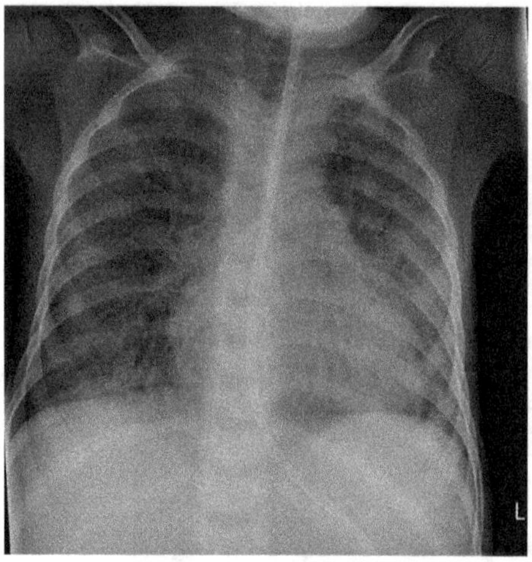

Figure 2: Chest X-ray after extubation.

unrelated donor donating bone marrow. The conditioning comprised fludarabine, targeted busulfan, and melphalan including rabbit ATG. He engrafted at day +26 and +23 with neutrophils and platelets of donor origin. The child was discharged home with minor cognitive impairment.

3. Discussion

To our knowledge, this is the first report of survival after prolonged ECMO support (25 days) in a child with JMML and cardio-respiratory failure secondary to tumor lysis syndrome. Meister et al. published a case report of an infant with JMML, who was on ECMO support for 5 days and died because of pulmonary failure [2]. JMML is a rare, aggressive, clonal hematopoietic disorder of childhood characterized by overproduction of monocytic and granulocytic cells with organ infiltration, such as spleen, liver, and lungs [3]. A life-threatening complication is the occurrence of a TLS arising most commonly after initiation of chemotherapy. Mortality is reported between 21–66% [4]. Generally, the main principles of management include early recognition of metabolic and renal complications and the prompt administration of inotropic and respiratory support. However, there are no data and recommendations on the application of ECMO therapy in those cases. Considering that in JMML hemorrhagic and thrombotic complications are frequent and survival for refractory shock in pediatric patients with or without sepsis is limited, the initiation of ECMO therapy is debatable and might be withheld from those patients. The reported case demonstrates that successful management of cardiorespiratory failure in the setting of TLS in JMML can be achieved. Early administration of ECMO should be considered and allows for immediate stabilization of cardiorespiratory function in this context. Despite the high risk of hemorrhagic and thromboembolic complications in patients with JMML, prolonged ECMO support should be attempted.

Abbreviations

ECMO: Extracorporeal membrane oxygenation
JMML: Juvenile myelomonocytic leukemia
PHT: Pulmonary hypertension
VA: Veno-arterial
VV: Veno-venous
WBC: White blood cells.

References

[1] M. Huang, E. Owen, S. Myers, and A. Raj, "Cardiopulmonary failure requiring ECMO bypass resulting from leukemia cell lysis in a patient with childhood acute myelomonocytic leukemia," *Case Reports in Hematology*, vol. 2015, Article ID 640528, 3 pages, 2015.

[2] B. Meister, B. Zelger, G. Kropshofer et al., "Extracorporeal membrane oxygenation as a rescue therapy for leukaemic children with pulmonary failure," *British Journal of Haematology*, vol. 148, no. 1, pp. 126–131, 2010.

[3] J. L. Y. Cheong and M. H. Moorkamp, "Respiratory failure, juvenile myelomonocytic leukemia, and neonatal Noonan syndrome," *Journal of Pediatric Hematology/Oncology*, vol. 29, no. 4, pp. 262–264, 2007.

[4] F. P. Wilson and J. S. Berns, "Tumor lysis syndrome: new challenges and recent advances," *Advances in Chronic Kidney Disease*, vol. 21, no. 1, pp. 18–26, 2014.

25

An Unusual Presentation of Extracavitary Primary Effusion Lymphoma: Internal Jugular Vein Occlusion, Intractable Symptoms of Intracranial Hypertension, and Prolonged Remission after Highly Active Antiretroviral Therapy

Anindita Ghosh,[1] **Rodrick Chitaurirwa Zvavanjanja**,[2] **and Joshua Baalwa**[1]

[1]*Departments of Pathology, Laboratory Medicine, McGovern Medical School, University of Texas Health Sciences Center at Houston, Houston, Texas, USA*
[2]*Diagnostic and Interventional Imaging, McGovern Medical School, University of Texas Health Sciences Center at Houston, Houston, Texas, USA*

Correspondence should be addressed to Joshua Baalwa; joshua.baalwa@uth.tmc.edu

Academic Editor: Pier Paolo Piccaluga

Primary involvement of the skeletal muscle by extracavitary primary effusion lymphoma (PEL) is an extremely rare phenomenon. We report an unusual case of PEL involving the jugulodigastric skeletal muscle without serous cavity involvement which resulted in complete occlusion of the ipsilateral proximal internal jugular vein, causing the patient to present with clinical features of intractable throbbing headache, photophobia, acute confusion state, sporadic syncopal attacks, and dyspnea without obvious palpable neck swellings. This led to an initial clinical suspicion, dedicated diagnostic workup, and empiric therapy for acute meningoencephalitis, severe atypical pneumonia, and acute pulmonary embolism. Owing to his refractory symptoms, exploratory CT imaging eventually revealed a heterogenous jugulodigastric mass, and finally, a pathologic diagnosis of extracavitary PEL was identified as the cause of his intracranial hypertension. The patient remains in remission 22 months after commencing a dolutegravir-based HAART regimen without any chemotherapeutic intervention.

1. Introduction

Primary effusion lymphoma (PEL) commonly presents as malignant effusions in the serous cavity. Extracavitary PEL without serous cavity involvement is rare and usually involves the lymph nodes, spleen, visceral organs, and bone marrow among other locations [1]. Similar to other non-Hodgkin lymphomas, primary soft tissue involvement is rare and is usually seen in advanced stages of nodal lymphoma as secondary involvement [2].

The jugulodigastric region is located below the posterior belly of the digastric and anterior to the proximal portion of the sternocleidomastoid muscle and provides space for major neck vessels coursing in and out of the cranium. Of the major neck vasculature, the internal jugular vein courses most closely to the proximal portion of the sternocleidomastoid muscle where it is susceptible to occlusion by jugulodigastric mass lesions. Occlusion of the internal jugular vein has been reported to cause significant morbidity including fatal intracranial hypertension [3].

The mechanism of pathogenesis of human herpesvirus type-8 (HHV8)-related PEL is multifaceted. HHV8 preferentially infects postgerminal center B cells and plasma cells and, upon integrating into their genome, produces multiple oncogenic viral transcripts which promote viral latency (latent-associated nuclear antigen), host cell proliferation (latent-associated nuclear antigen and viral cyclin), and resistance to apoptosis (viral FLICE inhibitory protein) [1]. It is therefore not surprising that antiviral therapy improves outcomes of patients with HHV8-associated primary effusion lymphoma.

Here, we report the first case of extracavitary PEL primarily involving the jugulodigastric skeletal muscle and causing symptoms consistent with intracranial hypertension. The patient remains in remission 22 months after commencing a dolutegravir-based HAART regimen without any chemotherapeutic intervention.

2. Case Report

A 31-year-old male presented with worsening dyspnea, excruciating throbbing headache, photophobia, and spotting in his vision for three days in November 2019. He reports that his symptoms were insidious during onset beginning approximately in July 2019. The dyspnea eventually became associated with a nonproductive cough and frequent episodes of fevers and chills, and in October of the same year, the symptoms became intolerable resulting in one week's hospitalization and empiric treatment for pneumocystis jiroveci pneumonia (PJP). He was discharged after feeling better on HAART and Bactrim regimens, for which he was poorly compliant. Three weeks later, he was again hospitalized with further worsening of dyspnea and throbbing headache, nausea, vomiting, diarrhea, and a syncopal episode. He did not require intubation but did require supplemental oxygen. After a week in hospital, he was discharged but at this time, he was off HAART. This recovery was short lived, and within three weeks from discharge, he presented again with rapid worsening of the same symptoms, as alluded to above in November 2019. His other past medical history included living with HIV/AIDS for 10 years, neurosyphilis, and hypertension. He is reported to have been compliant with HAART for only the first three years following HIV/AIDS diagnosis.

On examination, he was found to be tachypneic, mildly hypoxic, tachycardic, and hypotensive and his neck was supple with no obvious cervical lymphadenopathy. He had elevated serum lactate, but his LDH was within normal limits. His absolute CD4 count was 267 cells/μL, and the HIV RNA viral load was 5.27 logs. Direct fluorescent antibody (DFA) studies on a bronchial alveolar lavage sample revealed neither *Pneumocystis jirovecii* organisms nor influenza A and B, parainfluenza 1, 2, and 3, adenovirus, nor respiratory syncytial viruses. Workup on sputum samples detected no acid-fast bacilli by Ziehl–Neelsen staining or culture. A QuantiFERON Gold test was ordered but was not performed by the reference laboratory due to sampling issues. EBV peripheral blood serology tests were ordered but not performed due to sample lipemia. A buffy coat smear exam for white blood cell intracellular microorganisms and urine histoplasma antigen were negative. Anerobic and aerobic blood cultures were negative. A chest X-ray showed retrocardiac atelectasis but no other definitive evidence of pneumonia or pulmonary edema. A chest CT for the pulmonary embolism protocol was also emergently performed and showed neither evidence of pulmonary embolism nor right heart strain but showed increased soft tissue density in the right lower neck with surrounding subcutaneous edema, noting that these findings are nonspecific and may represent contusion, represent neoplasm, or be related to a lymphoproliferative disorder or HIV. Nuclear medicine imaging also showed low probability of pulmonary embolism.

In view of his throbbing headache and photophobia, an urgent CT head followed by MRI head was performed to assess for space-occupying lesions and meningoencephalitis; however, both showed no acute abnormalities. A lumbar puncture was performed, and cerebrospinal fluid (CSF) analysis revealed a clear sample with a normal protein level and no pleocytosis. Additional CSF studies were negative for cryptococcal antigen, VDRL and treponemal antigen, aspergillus/blastomyces/histoplasma (both yeast phase/mycelial phase) antibodies, and herpes simplex virus and varicella zoster virus DNA by polymerase chain reaction. Due to findings of right neck edema and a dense lesion on the prior chest CT PE protocol, CT of the neck soft tissue was performed four days later due to further deterioration in presenting symptoms, and it revealed an enlarged and heterogenous right sternocleidomastoid muscle and a heterogenous right jugulodigastric confluent mass measuring approximately 7.4 cm in the greatest craniocaudal dimension. Transient compression upon the right internal jugular vein and complete occlusion of the proximal internal jugular vein by the heterogenous mass were also noted (Figure 1). An abdominal ultrasound scan was performed at the same time due to right upper quadrant discomfort, and it revealed no significant findings except for mild hepatosplenomegaly. CT abdomen was not performed.

Consequently, ultrasound-guided fine core needle biopsies of the 7 cm heterogenous mass stained by hematoxylin and eosin revealed tissue cores of the skeletal muscle infiltrated by sheets of large atypical plasmacytoid cells with predominantly vesicular chromatin, high nuclear to cytoplasmic ratio, variably conspicuous nucleoli, and scant to moderate cytoplasm (Figure 2). On immunohistochemical staining, the neoplastic cells were strongly and diffusely positive for MUM-1, EMA, and HHV8 and weakly for CD45, while in situ hybridization staining also revealed diffuse and strong staining for EBV-encoded RNA and strong lambda light chain restriction (Figure 3). They were negative for CD20, PAX5, CD79a, CD138, CD30, CD15, ALK-1, CD10, BCL6, and BCL2. Flow cytometric analysis of the same tissue biopsy revealed an abnormal B-cell population positive for CD45 (dim), CD38, CD138 (occasional cells), and cytoplasmic lambda light chain and negative for CD19, CD20, CD56, and cytoplasmic kappa light chain. In addition, fluorescent in situ hybridization studies on the core biopsies utilizing target DNA and control probes for MYC oncogene on the long arm of chromosome 8 (8q) revealed MYC amplification in 20 of 100 nuclei analyzed, further providing clonal support for a lymphoid neoplasm. Therefore, based on these morphological, immunophenotypical, and genetic findings, a final diagnosis of extracavitary PEL was made.

He was treated with oxygen therapy by nasal canula, intravenous fluids, broad-spectrum antibiotics, and prednisone empirically for PJP pneumonia, and his acute symptoms subsided. His HAART regimen was also changed from Genvoya (elvitegravir, cobicistat, emtricitabine, and tenofovir alafenamide) to dolutegravir and Descovy (emtricitabine and tenofovir alafenamide). Surprisingly, during the course of his HAART treatment, his right neck mass steadily resolved with eventual complete restoration of the right internal jugular vein patency as seen on consecutive staging PET scans (Figures 4 and 5). Additionally, both initial staging and

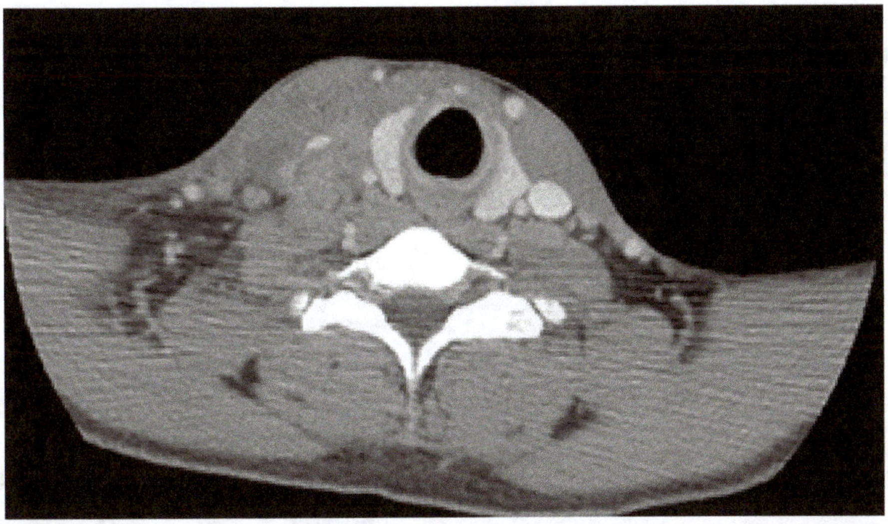

FIGURE 1: Pretreatment computed tomography of neck soft tissue with contrast, axial image shows right internal jugular vein compressed to a slit by a large heterogenous jugulo-digastric mass.

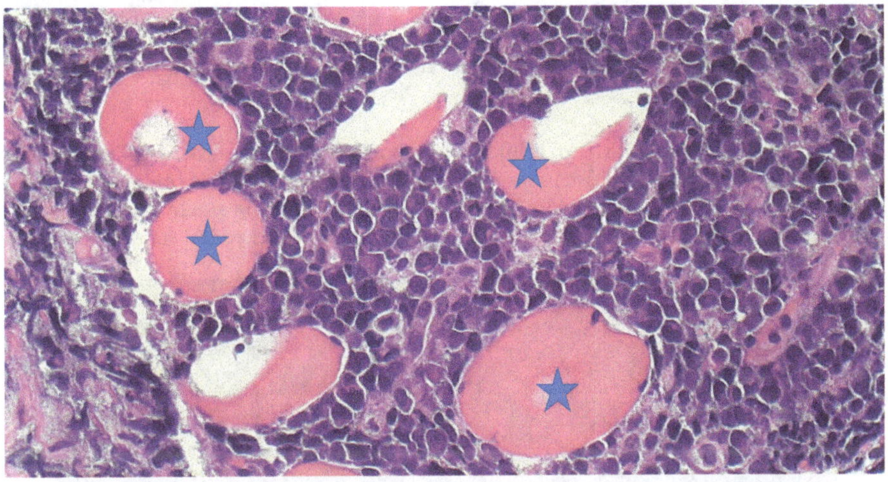

FIGURE 2: Primary effusion lymphoma involving skeletal muscle. Hematoxylin and Eosin stain shows skeletal muscle (blue asterixes) infiltrated and replaced by large neoplastic plasmacytoid cells. All images at 400X magnification.

restaging PET scans, approximately 7 and 42 weeks after diagnosis, revealed no FDG abnormal activity within the spleen nor within his abdomen or pelvic lymph nodes. After nearly two years of follow-up, the patient continues to experience sustained remission of his PEL without ever having received any chemotherapeutic intervention.

3. Discussion

The extracavitary variant of PEL is very rare and has unusual clinical presentations leading to significant diagnostic challenges. Its morphological and immunohistochemical findings are similar to classic PEL, although extracavitary varieties have a slightly better prognosis. Multiple previous case reports have shown the extracavitary form presenting as visceral, cutaneous, and intravascular tumors [4–7]. However, data on primary soft tissue involvement are sparse, yet their involvement could compromise function of adjacent vital neurovascular structures. This report thus adds information to the known possible protean de novo presentations of the extracavitary variant of PEL.

We found our case diagnostically challenging because it took multiple hospitalizations over at least four months before arriving at an unexpected diagnosis of hematological malignancy involving the nuchal skeletal muscle. Although our patient repeatedly presented with the same symptoms, progressively localizable to the head, a cause for symptoms remained an enigma after routine microbiological, biochemical, and imaging studies. Factors likely contributing to the diagnostic challenge for our case were masking of neck symptoms by excruciating headaches and the lack of obvious palpable neck lesions. In addition, heterogenous involvement of the jugulodigastric muscles by lymphoma, together with their deep location in the neck, likely precluded easy visibility of neck masses. Our diagnostic challenges were therefore not entirely unexpected and were further compounded by the fact that early diagnosis of nuchal lymphomas can be notoriously difficult [8].

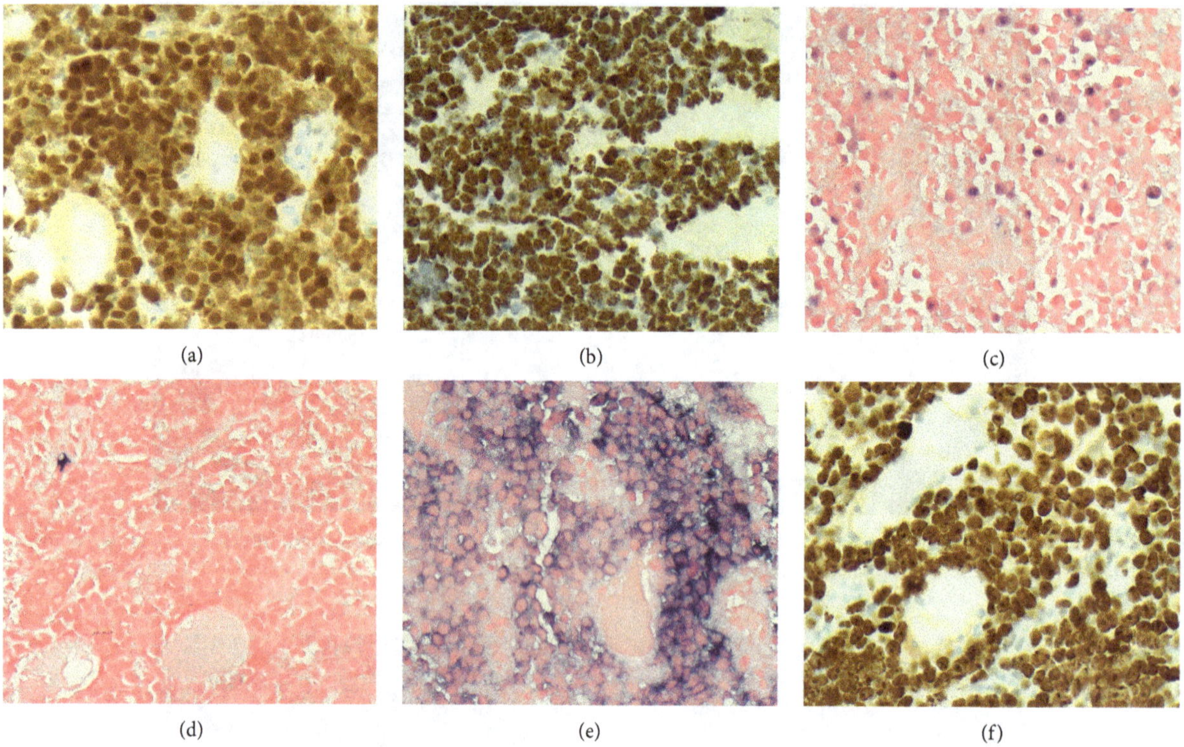

Figure 3: (a) Neoplastic cells diffusely positive for MUM-1. (b) HHV8 immunohistochemical stain is diffusely positive in neoplastic cells, while (c) a subset of neoplastic cells are positive for Epstein Barr virus encoded RNA by in situ hybridization staining. (d, e) The neoplastic cells show strong lambda light chain restriction (e) compared to kappa (d) light chain by in situ hybridization staining. (f) The neoplastic cells demonstrate a high proliferation index (<90%) as measured by Ki67 immunohistochemical stain. All images at 400X magnification.

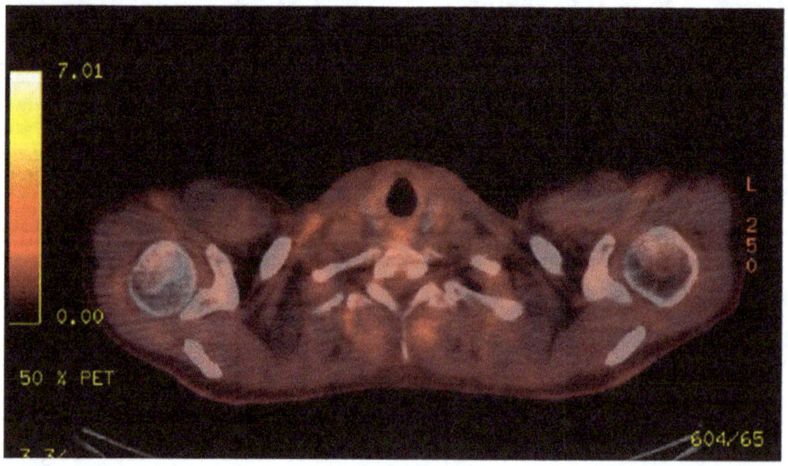

Figure 4: Immediate post treatment fused PET/CT. Seven weeks post initial head and neck CT. Approximate similar level demonstrating total resolution of the previous right heterogenous mass and right internal jugular compression. No fluorodeoxyglucose (FDG) avid lymph nodes seen.

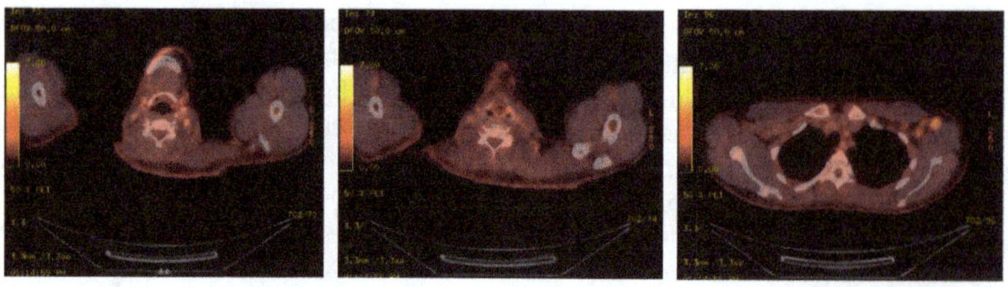

Figure 5: Second post treatment fused PET/CT demonstrating some FDG avidity in bilateral level 2 nodes and left axillary nodes which are reactive. The treated right jugulo-digastric mass not active or enlarged as demonstrated in Figure 1.

Nuchal extraluminal vascular occlusion by lymphoma as a cause of cerebrovenous insufficiency including intracranial hypertension is very rare. In one study of 128 individuals, the commonest cause of cerebrovenous insufficiency due to extraluminal internal jugular vein compression was osseous bone lesions, with neck swollen lymph nodes accounting for only 1% [9]. Our patient manifested symptoms of intracranial hypertension secondary to extraluminal internal jugular vein compression as outlined in the modified Dandy criteria, with the exception that an increase in cerebrospinal fluid opening pressure was not measured. These symptoms included intractable headaches associated with photophobia and lack of a demonstrable CNS lesion on imaging. Due to these symptoms, our patient was worked up and empirically treated for meningoencephalitis, albeit with no sustained improvement.

Achieving prolonged remission of HIV-associated PEL with a HAART regimen alone without concurrent chemotherapy is extremely rare with less than ten published reports in the literature [10–13]. In these rare case reports, the benefit from HAART treatment is thought to be due to HHV8 viral burden control by antiretroviral-induced immune reconstitution and/or direct antiviral action of some antiretroviral medications on HHV8 [14]. The control of HHV8 infection results in elimination of viral-derived oncogenes and therefore tumor remission. Therefore, considering the rarity of primary effusion lymphoma and its overall poor treatment outcomes, we feel that continued reporting of rare clinical scenarios of treatment successes on a case-by-case basis is warranted to inform novel treatment strategies.

Notably, our patient developed primary effusion lymphoma while on an integrase inhibitor-based HAART regimen, Genvoya^R. Following diagnosis of primary effusion lymphoma, his antiretroviral treatment was changed from Genvoya^R to a dolutegravir-based HAART regimen, and within four weeks, his neck mass resolved. This rapid remission coincided with a drop in the HIV viral load from 184,000 copies/mL to 7370 copies/mL although, paradoxically, his CD4 count instead dropped from 267 to 105 cells/microliter. He has remained in clinical remission without requiring chemotherapy for at least 22 months after switching to a dolutegravir-based HAART regimen, also an integrase inhibitor-based HAART regimen. Whether there might be differences in antitumoral efficacy among various integrase inhibitor-based HAART regimens against HHV8-associated PEL is still unknown and may be worthy exploring in larger case series. Differences in antitumoral efficacy have been reported for HHV8-associated Kaposi's sarcoma where protease inhibitors were shown to have better antitumoral efficacy compared to integrase and nonnucleoside reverse transcriptase inhibitors [15, 16]. Of note, Genvoya^R contains a boosted second-generation integrase inhibitor, while dolutegravir is a nonboosted third-generation integrase inhibitor. To our knowledge, our case is the second to report prolonged tumor remission on a dolutegravir-based HAART regimen [13].

4. Conclusion

In patients with unexplained symptoms of intracranial hypertension, it is worthwhile pursuing a differential diagnosis of nuchal lymphoma such as PEL as a possible cause.

References

[1] K. Shimada, F. Hayakawa, and H. Kiyoi, "Biology and management of primary effusion lymphoma," *Blood*, vol. 132, no. 18, pp. 1879–1888, 2018.

[2] B. D. Cheson, R. I. Fisher, S. F. Barrington et al., "Recommendations for initial evaluation, staging, and response assessment of Hodgkin and non-Hodgkin lymphoma: the Lugano classification," *Journal of Clinical Oncology*, vol. 32, no. 27, pp. 3059–3067, 2014.

[3] W. Schummer, C. Schummer, and W.-D. Niesen, "Unrecognized internal jugular vein obstruction: cause of fatal intracranial hypertension after tracheostomy?" *Journal of Neurosurgical Anesthesiology*, vol. 14, no. 4, pp. 313–315, 2002.

[4] G. M. Crane, R. R. Xian, K. H. Burns, M. J. Borowitz, A. S. Duffield, and J. M. Taube, "Primary effusion lymphoma presenting as a cutaneous intravascular lymphoma," *Journal of Cutaneous Pathology*, vol. 41, no. 12, pp. 928–935, 2014.

[5] G. Liao, J. Cai, C. Yue, and X. Qing, "Extracavitary/solid variant of primary effusion lymphoma presenting as a gastric mass," *Experimental and Molecular Pathology*, vol. 99, no. 3, pp. 445–448, 2015.

[6] Y. Kim, V. Leventaki, F. Bhaijee, C. C. Jackson, L. J. Medeiros, and F. Vega, "Extracavitary/solid variant of," *Annals of Diagnostic Pathology*, vol. 16, no. 6, pp. 441–446, 2012.

[7] U. Pielasinski, C. Santonja, S. M. Rodríguez-Pinilla, and L. Requena, "Extracavitary primary effusion lymphoma presenting as a cutaneous tumor: a case report and literature review," *Journal of Cutaneous Pathology*, vol. 41, no. 9, pp. 745–753, 2014.

[8] K. Storck, M. Brandstetter, U. Keller, M. Brandstetter, U. Keller, and A. Knopf, "Clinical presentation and characteristics of lymphoma in the head and neck region Head Face," *Med*, vol. 15, p. 1, 2019.

[9] D. Zhou, J.-Y. Ding, Y. Jing-Yuan et al., "Understanding jugular venous outflow disturbance," *CNS Neuroscience and Therapeutics*, vol. 24, no. 6, pp. 473–482, 2018.

[10] E. Oksenhendler, J. P. Clauvel, S. Jouveshomme, F. Davi, and G. Mansour, "Complete remission of a primary effusion lymphoma with antiretroviral therapy," *American Journal of Hematology*, vol. 57, no. 3, pp. 266–363, 1998.

[11] L. Hocqueloux, F. Agbalika, E. Oksenhendler, and J. M. Molina, "Long-term remission of an AIDS-related primary effusion lymphoma with an-tiviral therapy," *AIDS*, vol. 15, no. 2, pp. 280–282, 2001.

[12] D. Ripamonti, B. Marini, A. Rambaldi, and F. Suter, "Treatment of primary effusion lymphoma with highly active antiviral therapy in the setting of HIV infection," *AIDS*, vol. 22, no. 10, pp. 1236-1237, 2008.

[13] L. Campogiani, C. Cerva, G. Maffongelli et al., "Remission of an HHV8-related extracavitary in an HIV-positive patient during antiretroviral treatment containing dolutegravir," *AIDS Research and Therapy*, vol. 16, 2019.

[14] M. Narkhede, S. Arora, and C. Ujjani, "Primary effusion lymphoma: current perspectives," *OncoTargets and Therapy*, vol. 11, pp. 3747–3754, 2018.

[15] F. R. Simonetti, D. Ricaboni, D. Cattaneo, V. Micheli, S. Rusconi, and C. Gervasoni, "Relapse of Kaposi's sarcoma and HHV-8 viremia in an HIV-infected patient switching from protease inhibitor to integrase inhibitor-based antiretroviral therapy," *Journal of Clinical Virology*, vol. 74, pp. 75–77, 2016.
[16] F. Bani-Sadr, S. Fournier, and J. M. Molina, "Relapse of Kaposi's sarcoma in HIV-infected patients switching from a protease inhibitor to a non-nucleoside reverse transcriptase inhibitor-based highly active antiretroviral therapy regimen," *Journal of AIDS*, vol. 17, no. 10, pp. 1580-1581, 2003.

26

Bortezomib use for a Critically Ill Patient with Angioimmunoblastic T-Cell Lymphoma

Motoharu Shibusawa

IMS Group, Shinmatsudo Central General Hospital, Department of Hematology, Chiba, Japan

Correspondence should be addressed to Motoharu Shibusawa; m_sibusawa@hotmail.com

Academic Editor: Kostas Konstantopoulos

Angioimmunoblastic T-cell lymphoma (AITL) accounts for 18.5% of all peripheral T-cell lymphomas. There is still no gold standard chemotherapy for treating newly diagnosed AITL. This case describes the use of bortezomib in newly diagnosed AITL. A 53-year-old man with no previous illness presented with erythema and swelling in the left neck. A diagnosis of AITL was made based on the results of lymph node biopsies. AITL progression led the patient to a severely deteriorated general condition. Bortezomib was thus administered, which resulted in a reduction in lymphadenopathies, the disappearance of tumor fever, and a decrease in serum lactate dehydrogenase levels. Subsequently, the patient's general condition gradually improved. Despite the patient's poor condition, bortezomib was well tolerated. After bortezomib administration, the patient did not require chemotherapy for approximately 10 months. The present case indicates that bortezomib is a possible treatment option for patients with AITL.

1. Background

Angioimmunoblastic T-cell lymphoma (AITL) accounts for 18.5% of all peripheral T-cell lymphomas, and it occurs frequently in Europe, Asia, and North America [1]. AITL is a neoplasm comprising mature *T* follicular helper cells. *T* follicular helper cells release various factors, including C-X-C motif chemokine ligand 13, interleukin (IL)-21, IL-10, IL-6, transforming growth factor-β, vascular endothelial growth factor (VEGF), and angiopoietin. A complex network of interactions exists between tumor cells and various cellular components in the reactive microenvironment [2]. The clinical presentations of AITL include lymphadenopathies, bone marrow involvement, skin rash, and laboratory test abnormalities (anemia, positive result on direct antiglobulin test, thrombocytopenia, hypergammaglobulinemia, and hypereosinophilia) [3]. Patients with AITL may also present with plasmacytosis [4–6].

To date, there is no gold standard chemotherapy for treating newly diagnosed AITL. AITL is usually treated with the CHOP regimen, which includes cyclophosphamide, doxorubicin, vincristine, and prednisone; CHOEP, which includes etoposide in addition to CHOP; and ACVBP, which includes doxorubicin, cyclophosphamide, vindesine, bleomycin, and prednisone. [3].

Bortezomib is an anticancer drug that inhibits the proteasome, inducing the accumulation of unfolded and misfolded proteins, which in turn leads to apoptosis and cell death. In addition, bortezomib inhibits the production of cytokines such as IL-6, insulin-like growth factor-1, and VEGF in bone marrow stromal cells. [7] Bortezomib is also an effective agent for the treatment of B-cell neoplasms, such as multiple myeloma, mantle cell lymphoma, and lymphoplasmacytic lymphoma. [7,8] Moreover, several previous studies have reported the efficacy of bortezomib for the treatment of T-cell neoplasms. [9–11].

This case report describes the successful use of bortezomib in a critically ill patient with AITL.

2. Case Presentation

A 53-year-old man with no previous illness presented with erythema throughout the body 4 weeks before and with

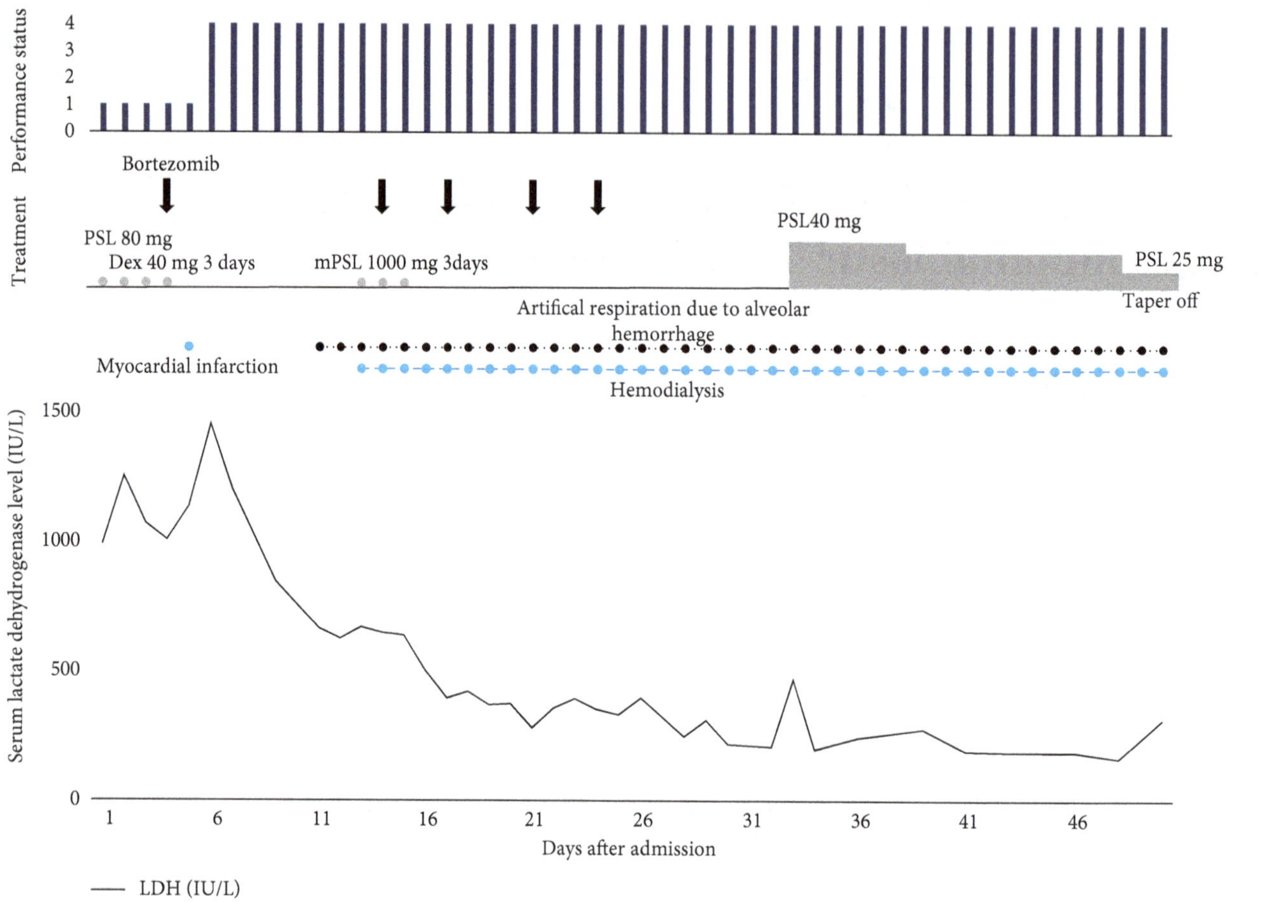

FIGURE 1: Clinical course after admission to our hospital. After bortezomib administration, the serum lactate dehydrogenase level decreased. LDH; lactate dehydrogenase. PSL; prednisolone, Dex:dexamethasone, and mPSL; methylprednisolone.

swelling in the left neck 6 weeks before admission to our hospital. The patient was admitted to another hospital 18 days before admission to our hospital. A whole-body computed tomography (CT) revealed lymphadenopathies and a ground-glass appearance in the lung. His soluble IL-2 receptor level was 5,445 U/mL. Prednisolone (PSL) administration was started at a dose of 30 mg daily. A left axilla lymph node biopsy was performed on the fourth day after another hospital admission. Then, the patient was transferred to our hospital. The clinical course after admission to our hospital is summarized in Figure 1. On the first hospital day, his consciousness was clear. His vital signs were as follows: body temperature, 38.3°C; blood pressure, 162/97 mmHg; pulse rate, 122 beats/min; and oxygen saturation, 91% in ambient air. Moreover, his Eastern Cooperative Oncology Group (ECOG) performance status was 1, and his Karnofsky scale score [12] was 80 points. Erythema in the face, arms, and trunk and palpable lymphadenopathies in the bilateral cervical and left axilla areas were noted. Regarding B symptoms, the patient had a fever of >38°C but no drenching night sweats or unintentional weight loss. Laboratory tests on admission revealed leukocytosis (white blood cell count, 28,800/μL) with an increase in the level of eosinophils (17.0%) and plasma cells (11.0%); anemia (hemoglobin level, 10.0 g/dL); decreased percentage of reticulocytes (2.0%); elevated serum levels of lactate dehydrogenase (LDH) (991 IU/L), creatinine (1.56 mg/dL), and C-reactive protein (4.75 mg/dL); and polyclonal gammaglobulinemia (immunoglobulin (Ig) G, IgA, and IgM levels were 5,366 mg/dL, 378 mg/dL, and, 660 mg/dL, respectively). Serum and urinary protein electrophoresis did not reveal a localized band. A clonally rearranged Ig heavy chain JH gene was not detected. Whole-body CT showed lymphadenopathies in the bilateral cervical, subclavian, axillary, mediastinal, para-abdominal aortic, and bilateral inguinal regions; splenomegaly; and a ground-glass pattern in both lungs. A bone marrow examination was performed and it revealed no evidence of malignant cell invasion. However, flow cytometry analysis revealed an increase in the level of plasma cells (accounting for 25.8% of all nucleated cells) with no restriction of light chains. The dosage of PSL was up to 80 mg on the first hospital day, but the treatment was switched to dexamethasone at a dose of 40 mg daily for 3 days on the second hospital day because PSL failed to improve the lymphadenopathies. Biopsy of the left axillary lymph nodes was performed again on the fourth hospital day. A diagnosis of AITL accompanied by reactive plasmacytosis was made based on the results of the two lymph node biopsies and other aforementioned tests. The Ann Arbor stage was IIIB. The international prognostic index was

TABLE 1: Previous case reports of bortezomib use in angioimmunoblastic T-cell lymphoma.

	Age/Sex	Treatment	Response	Duration of effectiveness	Reference
case1	63/ Female	Bortezomib and dexamethasone	Lymphadenopathies reduced in size	4 months	14
case2	76/ Female	Bortezomib, mitoxantrone, and dexamethasone	Disappearance of lymphadenopathy	18 months	15

high-intermediate risk. Treatment with subcutaneous administration of bortezomib at a dose of 1.3 mg/m^2 was started on the fourth hospital day, but the patient experienced chest discomfort on the fifth hospital day. Electrocardiography showed an elevated ST segment elevation in aVf and V2–V4. The patient's serum creatine phosphokinase-MB level was increased to 115 IU/L. These findings led to a diagnosis of acute myocardial infarction (AMI). The patient was admitted to the intensive care unit. Percutaneous coronary angioplasty was performed, and antiplatelet therapy with aspirin at a dose of 200 mg and prasugrel at a dose of 20 mg daily and anticoagulant therapy with intravenous administration of heparin were started. An intra-aortic balloon pump was introduced. Chemotherapy with bortezomib was temporarily discontinued. Chest radiography showed shadows in both lungs, which were extended on the seventh hospital day. On the 11th hospital day, the patient experienced respiratory failure, resulting in the need for artificial respiration followed by prone positioning. Bronchoscopy was performed, which revealed that there were no mucosal abnormalities, lesions, or obstructions in the airways. Serial bronchoalveolar lavage was performed with the sequential administration of normal saline. The return was erythematous effluent. Based on the bronchoscopy and chest radiography findings, a diagnosis of respiratory failure due to alveolar hemorrhage was made. Subsequently, antiplatelet therapy was discontinued, but heparin administration was continued because the coronary artery thrombus remained. An artificial cardiac pacemaker was inserted because of the onset of atrioventricular block. On the 14th hospital day, the patient's consciousness level dropped to Glasgow coma scale $E_4M_4M_5$. A fever of 39.2 °C developed and his ECOG performance status increased to 4. His Karnofsky scale score decreased to 10 points. The patient required noradrenaline administration for hypotension and hemodialysis for acute renal failure secondary to hypotension. The patient received steroid pulse therapy with methylprednisolone at a dose of 1,000 mg for 3 days for alveolar hemorrhage, followed by PSL administration. However, the patient's general condition severely deteriorated, and he required chemotherapy because the developing fever was considered tumor fever secondary to AITL recurrence. Therefore, five doses of bortezomib were administered, following which the tumor fever disappeared and his serum LDH level decreased. On the 20th hospital day, the patient no longer required artificial respiration only hemodialysis. Compared with the CT scans of the 13th hospital day, those of the 30th hospital day showed a reduction in lymphadenopathies (<50% reduction), and the size of the splenomegaly remained the same. The patient's general condition gradually improved. On the 135th hospital day, the patient was discharged and followed up as an outpatient thereafter. After discharge from the hospital, approximately 1 month later, positron-emission tomography revealed ^{18}F-fluorodeoxyglucose uptake in the lymph nodes as follows: bilateral cervical region (maximum standardized uptake value [SUV max], 7.5), around the stomach on the lesser curvature side (SUV max, 6.02), and para-abdominal aortic region (SUV max, 8.76). Thus, there were lymphadenopathies with ^{18}F-fluorodeoxyglucose uptake as revealed via positron-emission tomography, but they had not progressed. Therefore, the patient did not require chemotherapy for approximately 10 months. However, lymphadenopathies progressed thereafter. The patient had received cytotoxic chemotherapy and died of AITL progression approximately 10 months after starting cytotoxic chemotherapy.

3. Discussion

Bortezomib is known to be effective for the treatment of B-cell neoplasms. [7, 8] Moreover, several clinical and in vitro studies have demonstrated the efficacy of bortezomib in the treatment of T-cell neoplasms, as described below.

Regarding the safety of using bortezomib for AITL treatment, a previous phase 2 study reported the outcomes of CHOP therapy plus bortezomib use for the treatment of peripheral T-cell lymphoma. [13] The study was conducted in 46 previously untreated patients with peripheral T-cell lymphomas, including 8 patients with AITL. Twenty-nine patients completed the planned treatment schedule (median number of cycles: 6), and the response was assessed in 44 patients because 2 patients dropped out early as they developed grade 4 hepatic dysfunction and pneumonia. Grade 3–4 leucopenia (common terminology criteria for adverse events (CTCAE) ver 3.0) was the most frequent adverse event, whereas neurotoxicity was tolerable (grade 1–2 peripheral neuropathy). The findings pertaining to the present case suggest the safety of using bortezomib for the treatment of T-cell lymphomas, where the only adverse effect was leukopenia grade 1 (CTCAE ver 5.0). The patient developed AMI the day after bortezomib administration, but it is speculated that AMI was caused by hypercoagulation associated with the administration of a high dose of dexamethasone. Furthermore, the most noteworthy aspect was that chemotherapy with bortezomib was well tolerated despite the patient's severely deteriorated condition.

There are two case reports of bortezomib use in patients with AITL (Table 1). [14, 15] In Case 1, similar to that in our case, bortezomib was used in combination with steroids, which resulted in a reduction in lymphadenopathies. The clinical effectiveness of bortezomib was indicated. In Case 2, because bortezomib was used in combination with other anticancer drugs, it is not clear whether bortezomib was effective for AITL. In our case, the patient did not require chemotherapy for 10 months. This clinical course indicates that bortezomib is a possible treatment option for patients with AITL.

4. Conclusion

The present case indicates that bortezomib is a possible treatment option for patients with AITL. Furthermore, it may be well tolerated, even if the patient's general condition deteriorates.

References

[1] M. Federico, T. Rudiger, M. Bellei et al., "Clinicopathologic characteristics of angioimmunoblastic T-cell lymphoma: analysis of the international peripheral T-cell lymphoma project," *Journal of Clinical Oncology*, vol. 31, no. 2, pp. 240–246, 2013.

[2] A. Dogan, P. Gaulard, E. S. Jaffe, H. K. Müller-Hermelik, and L. d. Leval, "Angioimmunoblastic T-cell lymphoma and other nodal lymphomas of T follicular helper cell origin," *WHO Classification of Tumours of Haematopoietic and Lymphoid Tissues*, vol. 129, pp. 407–410, 2017.

[3] M. A. Lunning and J. M. Vose, "Angioimmunoblastic T-cell lymphoma: the many-faced lymphoma," *Blood*, vol. 129, no. 9, 2017.

[4] H. Sakai, H. Tanaka, T. Katsurada, Y. Yoshida, E. Okamoto, and H. Ohno, "Angioimmunoblastic T-cell lymphoma initially presenting with replacement of bone marrow and peripheral plasmacytosis," *Internal Medicine*, vol. 46, no. 7, pp. 419–424, 2007.

[5] A. N. Ahsanuddin, R. K. Brynes, and S. Li, "Peripheral blood polyclonal plasmacytosis mimicking plasma cell leukemia in patients with angioimmunoblastic T-cell lymphoma: report of 3 cases and review of the literature," *International Journal of Clinical and Experimental Pathology*, vol. 4, no. 4, pp. 416–420, 2011.

[6] H. Nagoshi, J. Kuroda, T. Kobayashi et al., "Clinical manifestation of angioimmunoblastic T-cell lymphoma with exuberant plasmacytosis," *International Journal of Hematology*, vol. 98, no. 3, pp. 366–374, 2013.

[7] S. Ito, "Proteasome inhibitors for the treatment of multiple myeloma," *Cancers*, vol. 12, no. 2, p. 265, 2020.

[8] J. P. Leonard, R. R. Furman, and M. Coleman, "Proteasome inhibition with bortezomib: a new therapeutic strategy for non-Hodgkin's lymphoma," *International Journal of Cancer*, vol. 119, no. 5, pp. 971–979, 2006.

[9] Z. X. Yan, L. L. Wu, K. Xue et al., "MicroRNA187 overexpression is related to tumor progression and determines sensitivity to bortezomib in peripheral T-cell lymphoma," *Leukemia*, vol. 28, no. 4, pp. 880–887, 2014.

[10] S. Iwata, S. Yano, Y. Ito et al., "Bortezomib induces apoptosis in T lymphoma cells and natural killer lymphoma cells independent of Epstein-Barr virus infection," *International Journal of Cancer*, vol. 129, no. 9, 2011.

[11] M. Ri, S. Iida, T. Ishida et al., "Bortezomib-induced apoptosis in mature T-cell lymphoma cells partially depends on upregulation of Noxa and functional repression of Mcl-1," *Cancer Science*, vol. 100, no. 2, pp. 341–348, 2009.

[12] H. J. West and J. O. Jin, "Performance status in patients with cancer," *JAMA Oncology*, vol. 1, no. 7, p. 998, 2015.

[13] S. J. Kim, D. H. Yoon, H. J. Kang et al., "Bortezomib in combination with CHOP as first-line treatment for patients with stage III/IV peripheral T-cell lymphomas: a multicentre, single-arm, phase 2 trial," *European Journal of Cancer*, vol. 48, no. 17, 2012.

[14] H. P. Du, Q. Q. Yang, and Y. E. Zhang, "Bortezomib-based chemotherapy to treat refractory angioimmunoblastic T-cell lymphoma: a case report and review of the literature," *Oncology Letters*, vol. 11, no. 3, 2016.

[15] S. Liu, Z. Yuan, C. Zhang, W. Fu, and J. Hou, "Bortezomib-based treatment for relapsed and refractory angioimmunoblastic T-cell lymphoma: case report and literature review," *Oncology Letters*, vol. 4, no. 2, pp. 262–264, 2012.

27

Successful Treatment of Myeloid Sarcoma in an Elderly Patient with Myelodysplastic Syndrome with Reduced-Dose Azacitidine

Kazuya Sato[1] **Nodoka Tsukada**[1] **Junki Inamura,**[1] **Shigetsuna Komatsu,**[2] **Keisuke Sato,**[3] **Masayo Yamamoto**[4] **Motohiro Shindo**[4] **Kentaro Moriichi**[4] **Yusuke Mizukami**[4] **Mikihiro Fujiya**[4] **Yoshihiro Torimoto,**[4] **and Toshikatsu Okumura**[4]

[1]*Department of Hematology/Oncology, Asahikawa Kosei General Hospital, 1-24, Asahikawa 078-8211, Japan*
[2]*Department of Dermatology, Asahikawa Kosei General Hospital, 1-24, Asahikawa 078-8211, Japan*
[3]*Department of Clinical Laboratory, Asahikawa Kosei General Hospital, 1-24, Asahikawa 078-8211, Japan*
[4]*Division of Gastroenterology and Hematology/Oncology, Department of Medicine, Asahikawa Medical University, Asahikawa, Hokkaido, Japan*

Correspondence should be addressed to Kazuya Sato; satofam@wine.plala.or.jp

Academic Editor: Sudhir Tauro

Myeloid sarcoma (MS), which involves extramedullary lesions, is classified as a unique subtype of acute myeloid leukemia (AML). At present, no standard treatments for MS have been established. The patient was an 89-year-old man with myelodysplastic syndrome-excess blast-2 (MDS-EB-2) with a 2-year history of intermittent treatment with azacitidine (AZA) during a 4-year history of MDS. He developed painful cutaneous tumors 8 months after the second discontinuation of AZA. They were refractory for antibiotics and topical tacrolimus hydrate. A tumor biopsy was performed, and the histological findings of the tumor lesion showed a proliferation of tumor cells that were positive for myeloperoxidase and CD68 and negative for CD4 and CD123. The patient was diagnosed with MDS-associated MS. MDS-EB-2 quickly progressed to AML with the appearance of peripheral blood blasts and 25% bone marrow blasts. Monotherapy with reduced-dose AZA (37.5 mg/m^2 for 7 days, every 4–6 weeks) was restarted, and the MS quickly disappeared. The patient's MS was successfully treated with 16 cycles of AZA treatment over a 22-month period. There have been 10 reported cases in which MS was successfully treated with AZA. Among the 10 cases, the patient in the present case was the oldest. Treatment with reduced-dose AZA should be considered as a therapeutic option for MS in elderly patients with MDS, especially patients who are ineligible for intensive chemotherapy.

1. Introduction

Myeloid sarcoma (MS), which involves extramedullary lesions at sites such as the skin, lymph nodes, gastrointestinal tract, bone, soft tissue, and testis, is classified as a unique subtype of acute myeloid leukemia (AML) [1–3]. MS may precede or coincide with AML or represent acute blastic transformation of myelodysplastic syndrome (MDS), myeloproliferative neoplasms, or chronic myelogenous leukemia [1, 2, 4]. No standard treatment for MS has been established; thus, intensive chemotherapy consisting of anthracycline and cytarabine is generally selected as the initial therapy, according to chemotherapy for AML. In addition, allogeneic hematopoietic stem-cell transplantation (allo-HSCT) or radiation therapy may also be considered [2, 4]. However, elderly patients are generally not eligible for intensive chemotherapy and allo-HSCT; thus, further strategies are required, especially for elderly patients with MS.

A hypomethylating agent, azacitidine (AZA), which improved overall survival in comparison to conventional care treatment in higher-risk MDS patients who were not eligible for allo-HSCT [5], is widely used in clinical practice for the treatment of patients with MDS, as well as a proportion of patients with AML [6, 7]. However, there are few reports of patients with MS who were successfully treated with AZA [8–13].

We herein report a case of MS in an elderly patient with MDS, which was successfully treated with 16 cycles of AZA treatment over a 22-month period. This is a rare case of MS that was successfully treated with AZA monotherapy.

2. Case Presentation

An 85-year-old man with pancytopenia was diagnosed with MDS with multilineage dysplasia (MDS-MLD) based on bone marrow aspiration (BMA), which revealed 2.6% myeloblasts with trilineage dysplasia and normal karyotype. Based on these findings, the case was categorized as intermediate-1 or low risk according to the International Prognostic Scoring System (IPSS) [14] or Revised IPSS (IPSS-R) [15], respectively. At this point, the patient had been treated with vitamin K2 (menatetrenone) and active vitamin D3 (calcitriol) because combination therapy of these two drugs was reported to be effective against low-risk MDS [16]. At 87 years of age, the patient undertook BMA again because his pancytopenia had progressed, and he was diagnosed with MDS with excess blasts-2 (MDS-EB-2) based on the BMA findings, which revealed 11% myeloblasts and multilineage dysplastic changes of bone marrow cells (Figures 1(a)–1(d)), with a normal karyotype. The disease status was categorized as intermediate-2 risk according to the IPSS and high risk according to the IPSS-R; thus, AZA treatment was initiated on hospitalization at the standard dose of 75 mg/m^2/day, subcutaneously, for 7 days every month. The patient achieved a hematological improvement (HI) with manageable adverse events (AEs), including constipation and general malaise after the first cycle of AZA. The second cycle was therefore administered in an outpatient setting. However, the treatment was discontinued due to septic shock after the second cycle of AZA. The patient became dependent on red blood cell (RBC) transfusions due to a clinical progression of MDS because one year after the discontinuation of AZA (at 88 years of age), we did not perform any histological examinations, such as BMA. Therefore, additional 3 cycles of AZA were administered in an outpatient setting with a reduced dose of 37.5 mg/m^2 (50% dose reduction) daily. The dose of AZA was decided according to the prescribing information for AZA [17] based on the nadir absolute neutrophil count $<0.5 \times 10^9$/L in the preceding (second) cycle. Treatment with AZA was discontinued again because the patient refused to continue the treatment due to the AEs, which included constipation and general malaise, as well as the inconvenience of going to the hospital.

At eight months after the second discontinuation of AZA (at 89 years of age), a painful cutaneous tumor, the top of which showed yellow-colored necrosis (Figure 2(a)), developed at the left groin lesion. Laboratory tests revealed the following: white blood cell count, 2,900/μL, with 63.6% neutrophils, 32.6% lymphocytes, 3.5% monocytes, 0.3% eosinophils, and no blast cells; hemoglobin, 6.6 g/dL; platelet count, 8.7×10^4/μL; and C-reactive protein, 0.57 mg/dL. No treatments, including oral and topical antibiotics, topical tacrolimus hydrate, and analgesics, had any effect on the tumor. A biopsy of the tumor was performed one month after its development. Histological examination revealed the proliferation of tumor cells with a high nuclear/cytoplasmic ratio (Figure 3(a)). Immunohistochemically, the neoplastic cells were positive for myeloperoxidase (Figure 3(b)), partially positive for cluster of differentiation (CD) 68 (Figure 3(c)) and CD33, but negative for CD3, CD4 (Figure 3(d)), CD20, CD34, CD56, CD117, and CD123 (Figure 3(e)). A diagnosis of MDS-associated MS was made. One month after the development of the first cutaneous lesion, another cutaneous tumor appeared on the left cheek (Figure 2(b)). BMA revealed a hypercellular marrow with 25% myeloblasts, which were positive for CD13, CD33, CD34, and HLA-DR; a G-band analysis revealed a normal karyotype. A diagnosis of AML secondary to MDS was made.

Considering the patient's age, clinical conditions, and the previously experienced AEs, treatment with AZA was started again at a dose of 37.5 mg/m^2/day, subcutaneously, for 7 days every 4–6 weeks (in total, this was the 6th cycle of AZA treatment) during short-term hospitalization, which consisted of 9 days of inpatient treatment per cycle, in order to manage the acute-phase AEs caused by AZA. The cutaneous MS lesion located on the left groin (Figures 4(a)–4(c)) and that on the left cheek (Figures 4(d)–4(f)) promptly disappeared after the 6th and 7th cycles of AZA treatment. Although myeloblasts had appeared in peripheral blood after several cycles of retreatment with AZA, the treatment was continued because of persistence of the response on MS, and the pain caused by his lesions remained relieved, with tolerable AEs, by AZA. The patient had received 16 cycles (over a 22-month period) of AZA treatment with the same dose on repeated short-term hospitalization until he died of progression of AML. He eventually received 21 cycles of AZA treatment in total. No exacerbation of cutaneous MS had been confirmed during AZA treatment.

3. Discussion

We experienced a case of MS in an elderly man with MDS, which was successfully treated with AZA over a 22-month period. Although cytarabine-based intensive chemotherapy is generally selected as the initial therapy for MS (based on its efficacy) [2, 3], the patient in the present case was 89 years of age, and there were concerns about AEs. Radiation therapy may be a therapeutic option for MS; however, the patient had already developed multiple MS lesions; thus, it was not selected. For these reasons, reduced-dose AZA monotherapy was restarted again, and AZA-associated AEs were managed by short-term hospitalization. While the present patient was expected to have an approximately 2-year survival after starting AZA treatment, based on the result of the AZA-001 phase III trial for higher-risk MDS (median overall survival of 24.5 months) [5], he received 21 cycles of AZA treatment in total and eventually survived for 49 months despite developing MS.

To our knowledge, there are 10 reported cases in which MS including leukemia cutis (LC), a phenotype of

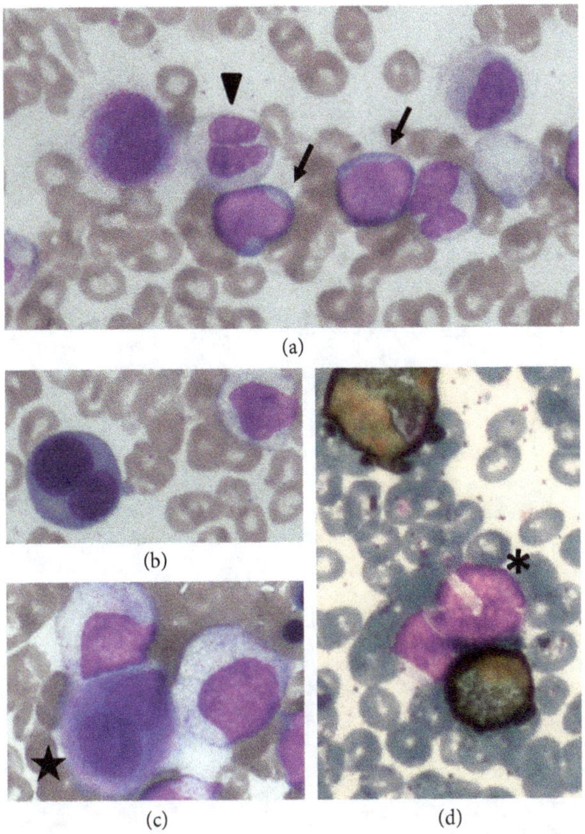

FIGURE 1: Microscopic findings of the bone marrow smears. Bone marrow aspirate smears (May–Giemsa staining; magnification: ×400) showed (a) myeloblasts (arrows) and a hyposegmented mature neutrophil (arrowhead), (b) a binucleated erythroblast, and (c) a micromegakaryocyte (indicated with a star). (d) Myeloperoxidase staining (magnification: ×400) of the bone marrow cells showed a hypogranular neutrophil (indicated with an asterisk).

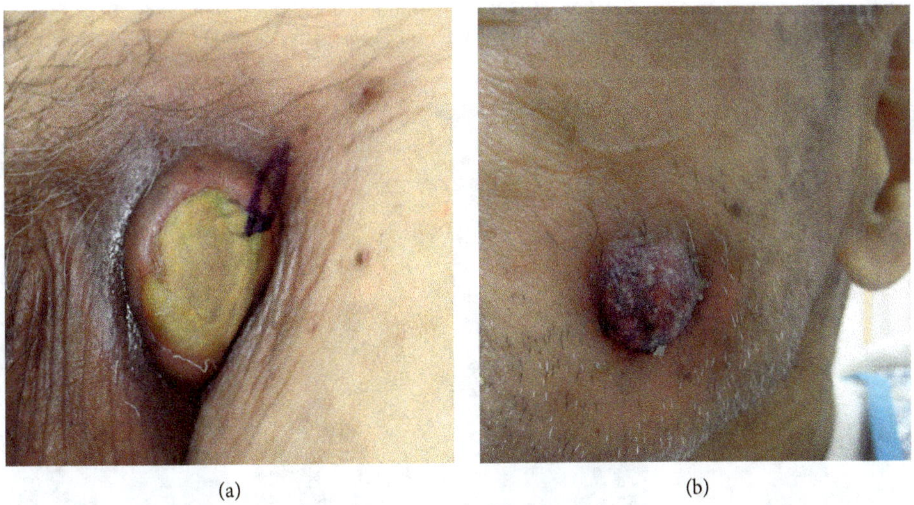

FIGURE 2: Cutaneous tumor lesions. (a) A painful cutaneous tumor, the top of which showed yellow-colored necrosis, which developed at the left groin 8 months after the second discontinuation of azacitidine. (b) Another cutaneous tumor, which appeared on the left cheek one month after the development of the first cutaneous lesion at the left groin.

extramedullary leukemia induced by the infiltration of leukemic cells into the epidermis, the dermis, or the subcutis [18], was successfully treated with AZA [8–13]. The clinical characteristics of the cases are shown in Table 1. Aside from two cases, most were elderly patients; our patient was the oldest. In all of these cases, AZA treatment was performed for MS that developed in a patient with preceding hematological malignancies (MDS, chronic myelomonocytic leukemia

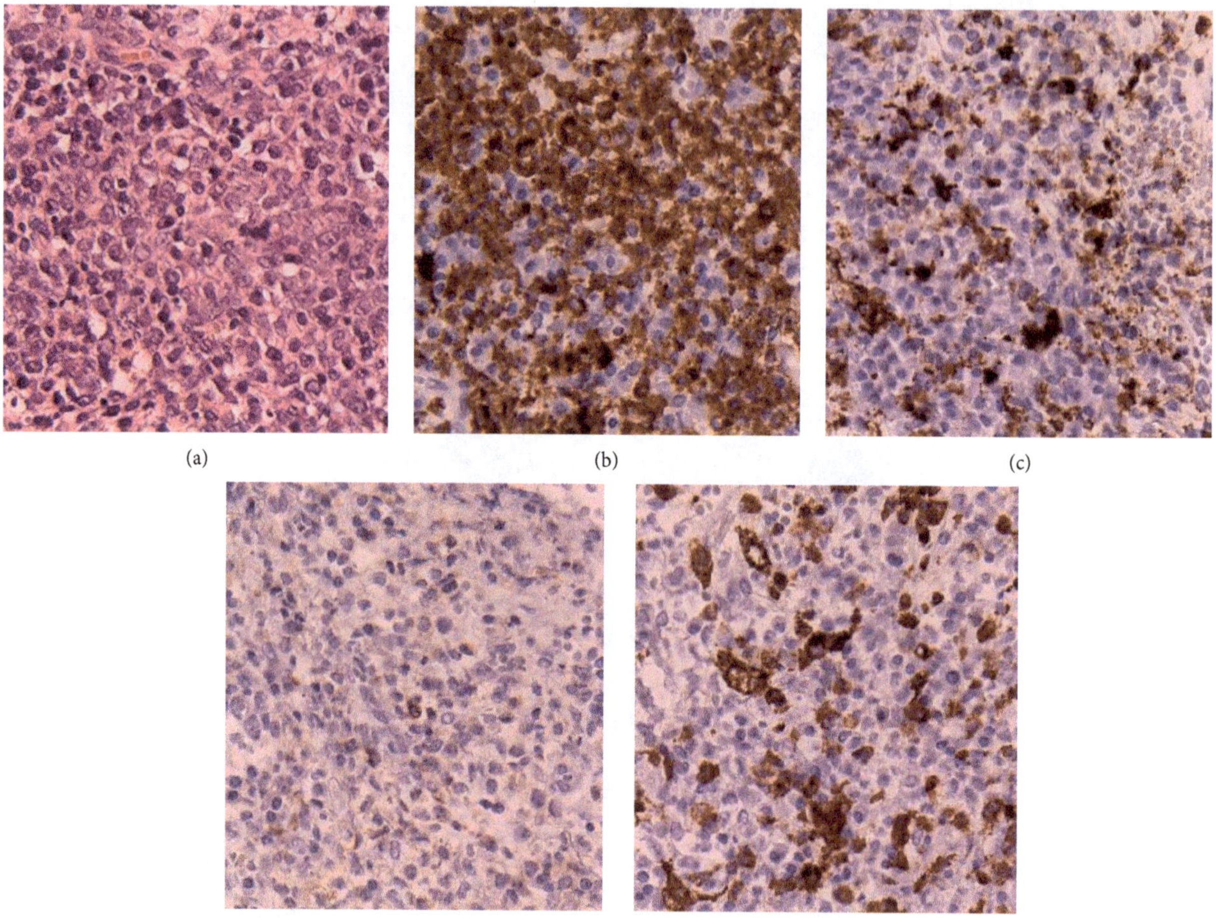

(a) (b) (c) (d) (e)

FIGURE 3: The histological findings of the tumor located in the left groin. A biopsy specimen showed the proliferation of tumor cells with a high nuclear/cytoplasmic ratio on hematoxylin and eosin staining (×20) (a). Immunohistochemical staining (×20) of tumor cells was positive for myeloperoxidase (b), partially positive for cluster of differentiation (CD) 68 (c), negative for CD4 (d), and negative for CD123 (e).

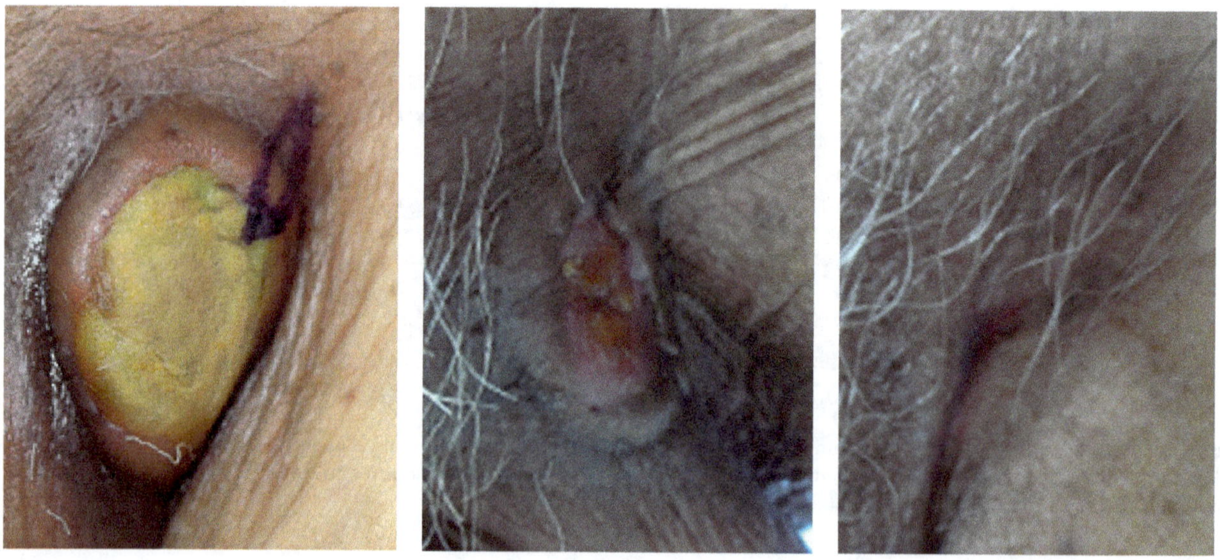

(a) (b) (c)

FIGURE 4: Continued.

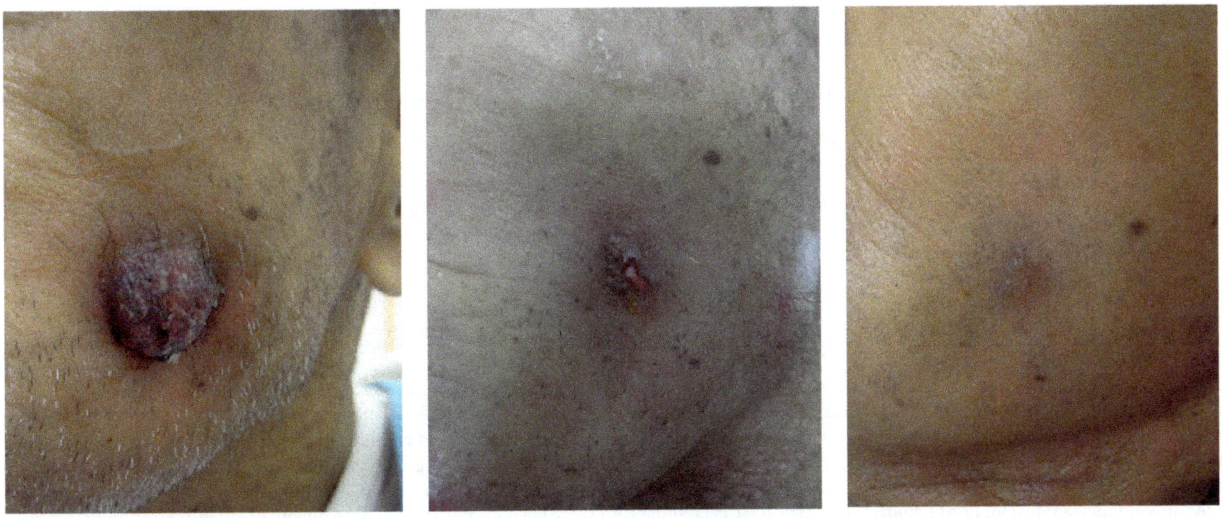

(d) (e) (f)

Figure 4: The response of cutaneous myeloid sarcoma (MS) to treatment with azacitidine. An MS located at the left groin before the first (6th in total) cycle of azacitidine retreatment (a). Before the second (7th in total) cycle (b). After the second cycle (c). An MS on the left cheek before the first cycle (d). Before the second cycle (e). After the second cycle (f).

Table 1: The clinical characteristics of cases of myeloid sarcoma that were successfully treated with azacitidine.

Case/ reported year	Age/ sex	Diagnosis at development of MS	Sites of origin	Treatment for MS	Cycles of AZA for MS	Maximum response of AZA for MS	Outcome (cause of death)	Reference
1 (2013)	62/M	CMML type-2	Right humerus	AZA (75 mg/m^2 × 7 days) + RT (25 Gy)	6*	Decreased in size	Alive	[8]
2 (2013)	34/M	Monoblastic leukemia cutis	Multiple skin nodules, groin mass	IDR + Ara C followed by allo-HSCT ⟶ CLAG followed by DLI and RT ⟶ a cycle of AZA (32 mg/m^2 × 5 days) ⟶ 4 cycles of AZA (75 mg/m^2 × 7 days) ⟶ RT	5	Decreased in size	Died (multiorgan failure)	[9]
3 (2013)	39/F	Relapse of AML-M2 after allo-HSCT	Gingiva	FLAG with GO ⟶ FLAG and DLI ⟶ AZA (75 mg/m^2 × 7 days)	17*	Clinical resolution	Alive	[9]
4 (2015)	72/M	MDS EB-2	Disseminated skin papules (LC)	36 cycles of AZA (75 mg/m^2 × 5 days) for MDS ⟶ 41 cycles of the same dose of AZA after the onset of LC	41*	Pathological resolution	Alive	[10]
5 (2015)	78/M	MDS MLD	Multiple skin lesions (LC)	AZA (75 mg/m^2 × 7 days) ⟶ 6-MP	7	Clinical resolution	Died (N/A)	[10]
6 (2015)	76/M	CMML type-1	Multiple skin lesions (LC)	9 cycles of AZA (75 mg/m^2 × 5 days) for CMML ⟶ 4 cycles of AZA (75 mg/m^2 × 7 days) after the onset of LC	4	Regression of LC	Died (N/A)	[10]
7 (2016)	80/F	MDS ⟶ AML	Left eyelid	CAG ⟶ AZA (75 mg/m^2 × 7 days)	At least 1	Decreased in size	Died (AML progression)	[11]
8 (2017)	71/F	MDS EB-2	Nasopharynx, tonsil, spleen, multiple lymph nodes, skin	DNR + Ara C ⟶ AZA (100 mg/body × 7 days, as maintenance therapy)	20*	Skin: clinical and radiological resolution; others: a marked reduction in the FDG uptake on PET-CT	Alive	[12]

Table 1: Continued.

Case/ reported year	Age/ sex	Diagnosis at development of MS	Sites of origin	Treatment for MS	Cycles of AZA for MS	Maximum response of AZA for MS	Outcome (cause of death)	Reference
9 (2018)	70/F	Therapy-related MDS (MDS-RS-MLD)	Multiple skin lesions (LC)	A cycle of AZA (75 mg/ m^2) ⟶ 6 cycles of biomodulatory therapy: AZA (75 mg/body × 7 days), pioglitazone and ATRA	7	Clinical resolution	Died (AML progression)	[13]
10 (present case)	89/M	MDS EB-2	Skin	AZA (37.5 mg/m^2 × 7 days)	16	Clinical resolution	Died (AML progression)	N/A

F: female; M: male; MS: myeloid sarcoma; CMML: chronic myelomonocytic leukemia; MDS: myelodysplastic syndrome; AML: acute myeloid leukemia; EB: excess blasts; AZA: azacitidine; RT: radiotherapy; Ara C: cytarabine; CAG: cytarabine, aclarubicin, and granulocyte colony-stimulating factor (G-CSF); DNR: daunorubicin; FDG: fluorodeoxyglucose; PET-CT: positron emission tomography-computed tomography; N/A: not available; LC: leukemia cutis; MLD: multilineage dysplasia; IDR: idarubicin; allo-HSCT: allogeneic hematopoietic stem-cell transplantation; CLAG: cladribine, high-dose cytarabine, and G-CSF; DLI: donor lymphocyte infusion; FLAG: fludarabine, high-dose cytarabine, and G-CSF; GO: gemtuzumab ozogamicin; 6-MP: 6-mercaptopurine; MDS-RS: MDS with ring sideroblasts; ATRA: all-trans-retinoic acid. *"Ongoing."

(CMML), monoblastic LC, or AML). AZA treatment was effective for MS originating at various sites; 7 cases (including our case) involved skin lesions. Four cases (cases 1 and 7–9) with MS were successfully treated with AZA in combination with sequential radiotherapy, multidrug chemotherapy, or biomodulatory drugs. One of the 4 cases (case 8) was treated with AZA as a maintenance therapy. Including the present case—in which AZA monotherapy was administered for remission induction and maintenance therapy—six cases (cases 2–6 and 10) with MS were successfully treated with AZA monotherapy, and five of them had skin leukemic lesions. MS resolved clinically, radiologically, or pathologically with AZA treatment in six cases (cases 3–5 and 8–10). One to 41 cycles of AZA therapy were performed for the 10 patients with MS; 6 of the patients eventually died of the progression of AML or other causes. The dose of AZA was reduced in 4 cases (cases 2, 4, 9, and 10) or modified in 1 case (case 8) among the 10 patients, and the present patient received the lowest dose of AZA (37.5 mg/m^2 for 7 days) among the cases with repeated treatment for a long period. From these findings, AZA probably has some benefit for MS in a certain group of patients with myeloid malignancies.

Sporadic case studies [19–23] have reported that decitabine—another hypomethylating agent that is used for the treatment of MDS or for the treatment of elderly patients with AML who are not eligible for standard chemotherapy in Western countries—was effective for treating MS in patients with myeloid malignancies (e.g., AML or CMML). Some of those cases with MS involved the skin [19, 22], similar to our case. As shown in Table 1, successful treatment with AZA in MS patients with involvement of the skin or with LC has also been reported [9, 10, 12, 13]. Thus, hypomethylating agents may have some effects in certain patients with MS, including patients who develop cutaneous lesions.

In this case, the appearance of blasts in peripheral blood was observed after AZA treatment, which eventually led to the progression of leukemia, but the exacerbation of the skin lesions was not observed during the treatment. The first reason for this issue would be that a dose of sufficient intensity for the marrow or peripheral leukemic cells could not be maintained due to the dose reduction and the prolonged treatment interval (>4 weeks). Second, the activation of the immune system by AZA treatment may contribute to the antitumor effect on the skin MS lesions. It has been reported that AZA induces cytotoxic CD8 T cells for some tumor antigens, such as melanoma-associated antigens (MAGE antigens) and Wilm's tumor antigen 1 [24]. In addition, it has been reported that AZA and valproate upregulate MAGE antigens in AML cell lines [25]. Antigen-presenting cells, such as dendritic cells, which are necessary for the activation of antigen-specific cytotoxic T cells, are abundant in the skin. Thus, leukemic cells in the MS lesions on the skin might be controlled by not only the inhibition of DNA synthesis by AZA treatment but also by the antileukemic effect of the activation of cytotoxic T cells against the leukemia-specific antigens. Further accumulation of such cases is required to clarify this issue.

However, a case of LC has been reported in a patient with acute myelomonocytic leukemia on AZA treatment [26]. That case was considered refractory to the AZA treatment. The responsiveness of cutaneous lesions of MDS/AML to AZA treatment might differ by disease status or histology of underlying disease. Physicians should consider the possibility of such a case developing.

We did not have a good treatment plan for this patient other than repeating the treatment with AZA. Venetoclax, which is an inhibitor of the antiapoptotic BCL2 protein, is reported to be clinically beneficial in hypomethylating agent-(HMA-) resistant patients with MDS/AML in combination with an HMA [27]. While venetoclax is not currently available for patients with MDS/AML in our country, combination therapy of venetoclax and AZA will likely be a good treatment option for patients such as the present case.

4. Conclusion

We reported a case of MS that developed in an elderly patient with MDS, which was successfully treated with AZA monotherapy for a 22-month period, despite a reduction in the dose. Although further accumulation of such cases is needed, treatment with AZA should be considered as a potential treatment strategy when MS develops in patients with myeloid malignancies, such as MDS, especially elderly patients who are ineligible for intensive treatment. If an effect on MS is confirmed in such cases, AZA treatment should be continued as much as possible.

Consent

Written informed consent was obtained from the family of the patient for publication of this case report and any accompanying images.

References

[1] S. A. Pileri, S. Ascani, M. C. Cox et al., "Myeloid sarcoma: clinico-pathologic, phenotypic and cytogenetic analysis of 92 adult patients," *Leukemia*, vol. 21, no. 2, pp. 340–350, 2007.

[2] D. A. Arber, A. Orazi, R. Hasserjian et al., "The 2016 revision to the World Health Organization classification of myeloid neoplasms and acute leukemia," *Blood*, vol. 127, no. 20, pp. 2391–2405, 2016.

[3] K. Kant Sahu, A. Adrian Sherif, A. Kumar Mishra et al., "Testicular myeloid sarcoma: a systematic review of the literature," *Clinical Lymphoma, Myeloma & Leukemia*, vol. 19, pp. 603–618, 2019.

[4] R. Bakst, A. Powers, and J. Yahalom, "Diagnostic and therapeutic considerations for extramedullary leukemia," *Current Oncology Reports*, vol. 22, no. 7, p. 75, 2020.

[5] P. Fenaux, G. J. Mufti, V. E. Santini et al., "Efficacy of azacitidine compared with that of conventional care regimens in the treatment of higher-risk myelodysplastic syndromes: a randomised, open-label, phase III study," *The Lancet Oncology*, vol. 10, no. 3, pp. 223–232, 2009.

[6] T. Bernal, P. Martínez-Camblor, P. Martínez-Camblor et al., "Effectiveness of azacitidine in unselected high-risk myelodysplastic syndromes: results from the Spanish registry," *Leukemia*, vol. 29, no. 9, pp. 1875–1881, 2015.

[7] A. Nakaya, S. Fujita, A. Satake et al., "Evaluation of azacitidine in patients with transplant-ineligible myelodysplastic syndromes and acute myeloid leukemia with myelodysplasia-related changes in a Japanese clinical setting," *Oncology Letter*, vol. 19, no. 2, pp. 1317–1321, 2020.

[8] A. Serrao, G. Loglisci, A. Salaroli, I. Zacheo, G. Alimena, and M. Breccia, "Azacitidine followed by radiotherapy as effective treatment for chronic myelomonocytic leukemia with extramedullary localization," *Leukemia & Lymphoma*, vol. 54, no. 2, pp. 411-412, 2013.

[9] A. Antar, Z. K. Otrock, M. Kharfan-Dabaja et al., "Azacitidine in the treatment of extramedullary relapse of AML after allogeneic hematopoietic cell transplantation," *Bone Marrow Transplantation*, vol. 48, no. 7, pp. 994-995, 2013.

[10] I. María Stefania, M. Carolina, C. Heras et al., "Leukemia cutis in myelodysplastic syndrome and chronic myelomonocytic leukemia patients treated with adjusted dose 5-azacitidine," *European Journal of Dermatology*, vol. 25, pp. 622-623, 2015.

[11] H. Kang, Y. Takahashi, E. Takahashi et al., "Myeloid sarcoma in an eyelid that developed during chemotherapy for acute myeloid leukemia," *Case Reports in Ophthalmology*, vol. 7, no. 1, pp. 25–29, 2016.

[12] T. Kakizaki, T. Ushiki, M. Masuko et al., "Successful 5-azacytidine treatment of myeloid sarcoma and leukemia cutis associated with myelodysplastic syndrome A case report and literature review," *Medicine*, vol. 96, no. e7975, p. 36, 2017.

[13] D. Heudobler, S. Klobuch, S. Thomas et al., "Cutaneous leukemic infiltrates successfully treated with biomodulatory therapy in a rare case of therapy-related high risk MDS/AML," *Frontier Pharmacology*, vol. 9, p. 1279, 2018.

[14] P. Greenberg, C. Cox, M. M. LeBeau et al., "International scoring system for evaluating prognosis in myelodysplastic syndromes," *Blood*, vol. 89, no. 6, pp. 2079–2088, 1997.

[15] P. L. Greenberg, H. Tuechler, J. Schanz et al., "Revised International prognostic scoring system for myelodysplastic syndromes," *Blood*, vol. 120, no. 12, pp. 2454–2465, 2012.

[16] N. Akiyama, K. Miyazawa, Y. Kanda et al., "Multicenter phase II trial of vitamin K2 monotherapy and vitamin K2 plus 1α-hydroxyvitamin D3 combination therapy for low-risk myelodysplastic syndromes," *Leukemia Research*, vol. 34, no. 9, pp. 1151–1157, 2010.

[17] D. P. Steensma and R. M. Stone, "Practical recommendations for hypomethylating agent therapy of patients with myelodysplastic syndromes," *Hematology/Oncology Clinics of North America*, vol. 24, no. 2, pp. 389–406, 2010.

[18] R. L. Bakst, M. S. Tallman, D. Douer, and J. Yahalom, "How I treat extramedullary acute myeloid leukemia," *Blood*, vol. 118, no. 14, pp. 3785–3793, 2011.

[19] A. Castelli, M. L. Mosca-Siez, A. Patriarca, D. Liscia, and A. Conconi, "Efficacy and safety of decitabine against cutaneous granuloblastic sarcoma: a case report," *Annals of Hematology*, vol. 97, no. 8, pp. 1485-1486, 2018.

[20] D. Riccomagno, B. M. A. M. Bär, M. Gotthardt, and W. J. F. M. van der Velden, "Activity of decitabine in pericardial myeloid sarcoma," *International Journal of Hematology*, vol. 108, no. 2, pp. 121-122, 2018.

[21] M. Gornicec, A. Wölfler, S. Stanzel, H. Sill, and A. Zebisch, "Evidence for a role of decitabine in the treatment of myeloid sarcoma," *Annals of Hematology*, vol. 96, no. 3, pp. 505-506, 2017.

[22] D. P. Steensma and B. B. Friday, "Monocytic skin nodules in chronic myelomonocytic leukemia: clinical response to decitabine therapy," *Leukemia & Lymphoma*, vol. 48, no. 8, pp. 1628-1629, 2007.

[23] S. N. Singh, Q. Cao, I. Gojo, A. P. Rapoport, and G. Akpek, "Durable complete remission after single agent decitabine in AML relapsing in extramedullary sites after allo-SCT," *Bone Marrow Transplantation*, vol. 47, no. 7, pp. 1008-1009, 2012.

[24] O. C. Goodyear, M. Dennis, N. Y. Jilani et al., "Azacitidine augments expansion of regulatory T cells after allogeneic stem cell transplantation in patients with acute myeloid leukemia (AML)," *Blood*, vol. 119, no. 14, pp. 3361–3369, 2012.

[25] O. Goodyear, A. Agathanggelou, I. Novitzky-Basso et al., "Induction of a CD8+ T-cell response to the MAGE cancer testis antigen by combined treatment with azacitidine and sodium valproate in patients with acute myeloid leukemia and myelodysplasia," *Blood*, vol. 116, no. 11, pp. 1908–1918, 2010.

[26] A. Kara, A. Akın Belli, V. Karakuş, Y. Dere, and E. Kurtoğlu, "A case of leukemia cutis with acute myeloid leukemia on azacitidine therapy," *Turkish Journal of Hematology*, vol. 4, pp. 192-193, 2017.

[27] B. Liu, Y. Guo, L. Deng, Y. Qiao, and J. Jian, "The efficacy and adverse events of venetoclax in combination with hypomethylating agents treatment for patients with acute myeloid leukemia and myelodysplastic syndrome: a systematic review and meta-analysis," *Hematology (Amsterdam, Netherlands)*, vol. 25, no. 1, pp. 414–423, 2020.

28

Aggressive Disease Course of Multiple Myeloma with Concomitant ALK-Negative Anaplastic Large Cell Lymphoma: A Case Report with an Unusual Presentation

Michela Staderini,[1] **Lara Mannelli**,[1,2] **Elisabetta Antonioli**,[1] **Benedetta Puccini**,[1] **Valentina Berti**,[3] **Francesco Mungai**,[4] **Federica Vergoni**,[5] **Valentina Carrai**,[1] **Luigi Rigacci**,[1,6] **and Alberto Bosi**[1]

[1]*Haematology Unit, Careggi University Hospital, Florence, Italy*
[2]*Medical Genetics, University of Siena, Siena, Italy*
[3]*Nuclear Medicine Unit, Department of Biomedical, Experimental and Clinical Sciences, Careggi University Hospital, Florence, Italy*
[4]*Diagnostic Radiology Unit, Careggi University Hospital, Florence, Italy*
[5]*Pathological Anatomy Unit, Careggi University Hospital, Florence, Italy*
[6]*Hematology and Stem Cell Transplant Unit, San Camillo Forlanini Hospital, Rome, Italy*

Correspondence should be addressed to Michela Staderini; michelastaderini@gmail.com

Academic Editor: Yusuke Shiozawa

ALK-negative anaplastic large cell lymphoma is a rare T-cell neoplasm with an aggressive course requiring prompt diagnostic work-up and treatment. Few cases of concomitant multiple myeloma and T-cell neoplasm are described in the literature, mainly regarding primary cutaneous anaplastic large cell lymphoma. We present the case of a 65-year-old man, simultaneously diagnosed with ALK-negative anaplastic large cell lymphoma with extranodal localization in the gastrocnemius muscle (stage 1AE) and IgG lambda multiple myeloma (ISS 2, Durie-Salmon stage 3A). Both diseases required therapeutic intervention due to the high proliferative index of lymphoma and the presence of bone lesions attributable to myeloma. The therapeutic program initially included chemotherapy (cyclophosphamide, doxorubicin, vincristine, etoposide, and prednisone; CHOEP), radiotherapy on the leg, bortezomib, and then consolidation with autologous hematopoietic stem cell transplantation. Despite being on bortezomib treatment and waiting for transplantation, the patient experienced an early myeloma progression that turned out to be refractory to second-line lenalidomide-based treatment. To our knowledge, this is the first case of concurrent diagnosis of extranodal ALK-negative anaplastic large cell lymphoma of the muscle and multiple myeloma. Simultaneous onset can be challenging for clinicians as both diseases may have an aggressive course requiring multiple treatments with increased risk of toxicity and complicated management.

1. Introduction

ALK-negative anaplastic large cell lymphoma (ALK-ALCL) is a rare CD30+ T-cell neoplasm involving both lymph nodes and extranodal sites, often presenting with B symptoms and advanced stage disease [1]. Primary involvement of the skeletal muscles is extremely rare in adults and has been associated with rapid dissemination and poor prognosis [2–4].

On the other side, multiple myeloma (MM) is characterized by clonal plasma cell (PC) infiltration in the bone marrow and, rarely, in extramedullary sites, leading to signs of organ damage typically summarized by the acronym

CRAB (hypercalcemia, renal failure, anaemia, and bone lesions).

Few cases of concomitant diagnosis of multiple myeloma and T-cell neoplasms are described, mainly regarding CD30+ cutaneous anaplastic large cell lymphoma. Often the plasma cell dyscrasia precedes the diagnosis of the T-cell neoplasm [5–7]. Some authors have hypothesized a causal relationship between the two diseases, but the potential pathogenic mechanism has not been fully understood [7]. Currently, only one case of contemporary diagnosis of aggressive ALK-negative ALCL and IgA lambda multiple myeloma is described in the literature [8]; that case was characterized by 15% plasma cell infiltration in the bone marrow (suggestive of smoldering MM), and no information on follow-up or response to treatment was available because the patient died quickly after diagnosis.

To the best of our knowledge, this is the first report of a simultaneous diagnosis of symptomatic extranodal ALK– ALCL and MM, requiring to start a treatment aiming to target both diseases.

2. Case Presentation

In June 2017, a Caucasian 65-year-old man was admitted to the Hematology Unit of Careggi Hospital (Florence, Italy) with swelling and pain in his right leg. At MRI, a large spindle-shaped lesion (size 3 × 2.2 × 8.4 cm) was detected at his right gastrocnemius muscle. The lesion had the same signal intensity of the surrounding normal muscular tissue in the T1-weighted sequence and intermediate signal intensity in the T2-weighted sequence; it was hyperintense in sequences with fat suppression and showed a high contrast-enhancement.

He underwent a core needle biopsy of the lesion with morphologic examination demonstrating a dense infiltrate of large pleomorphic cells with prominent nucleoli, many of which having horseshoe or kidney-shaped eccentric nuclei resembling hallmark cells (Figure 1). Immunohistochemical staining showed expression of CD45 and CD4, strong and uniform expression of CD30, and negativity of CD19, CD20, Pax-5, CD3, CD5, CD8, EMA, Perforin, CD56, CD34, and ALK in the neoplastic cells; TIA1 was only expressed in a minority of cells (−/+); MIB-1 was >90%. These findings were consistent with ALK-negative anaplastic large cell lymphoma (Figure 2).

The patient did not complain about any systemic symptom; his physical exam was normal. He had no previous medical history of cancer or autoimmune diseases. In his medical records, atrial fibrillation and ventricular flutter on treatment with beta-blockers were reported. Blood tests showed normal white blood cell and platelet counts, with mild anaemia (haemoglobin 12.5 g/d); LDH and liver enzymes were normal, creatinine 1.25 mg/dl, calculated GFR 54 ml/min, and beta2 microglobulin 4.5 mg/L. In addition, a serum IgG lambda monoclonal component (1.53 g/dl) was found, with increased lambda light chains (106 mg/L), and the sFLC ratio was lower than 100, albumin 33.7 g/L, and calcium 8.9 mg/dl.

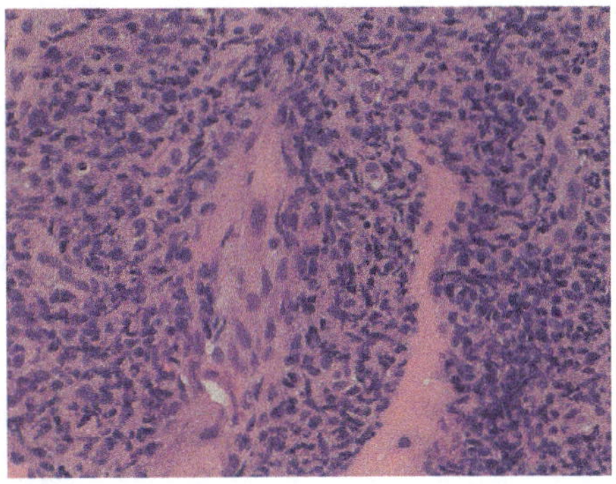

FIGURE 1: Core needle biopsy of the lesion in the right gastrocnemius muscle. H&E stain showing a dense infiltrate of large pleomorphic cells with prominent nucleoli and horseshoe or kidney-shaped nuclei (hallmark cells) consistent with ALCL.

A whole-body computed tomography (CT) scan did not show any other pathologic finding; in particular, no bone lytic lesions were revealed. In order to complete lymphoma staging procedures, a bone marrow biopsy was performed, and a relevant infiltration (roughly 70%) by atypical plasma cells with lambda light-chain restriction was detected (Figure 3).

Multiparameter flow cytometry on the bone marrow sample showed plasma cells, accounting for 45% of cellularity, that were positive for CD138 and CD38 and negative for CD19, CD56, and CD45; CD117 was partially expressed. No signs of bone marrow clonal T-cell infiltration were found. Cytogenetic analysis was not performed because of insufficient bone marrow sample.

An F18-FDG PET/CT confirmed the lesion in the right gastrocnemius muscle, which was intensely hypermetabolic, and revealed three additional vertebral hypermetabolic lesions in D5, L2, and S1, that were ascribed to myeloma (Figure 4(a)).

Based on these findings, the patient was diagnosed with an aggressive CD30+ ALK-negative ALCL (stage 1AE) and a concomitant IgG lambda multiple myeloma (MM, ISS score 2, and Durie-Salmon stage IIIA). Due to one MM-defining event (bone lesions at F18-FDG PET/CT) and one biomarker of malignancy (bone marrow infiltration over 60%), myeloma was defined as symptomatic, thus indicating the need to start an effective treatment.

The concurrence of two aggressive diseases led us to adopt a treatment approach taking into account the high proliferative index of lymphoma and therefore was based on the immediate application of standard ALCL treatment, followed by a consolidation program including autologous stem cell transplantation (ASCT), preceded by a conditioning regimen also active on myeloma.

From August 2017 to November 2017, the patient received 4 courses of polychemotherapy according to the CHOEP regimen (21-day cycles of cyclophosphamide 750 mg/sqm, doxorubicin 50 mg/sqm, and vincristine 1.4 mg/sqm on day 1; etoposide 100 mg/sqm on days 1–3; prednisone 100 mg/sqm on days 1–5).

In January 2018, after chemotherapy, an MRI showed a complete response of the ALCL lesion, and a 18F-FDG PET/

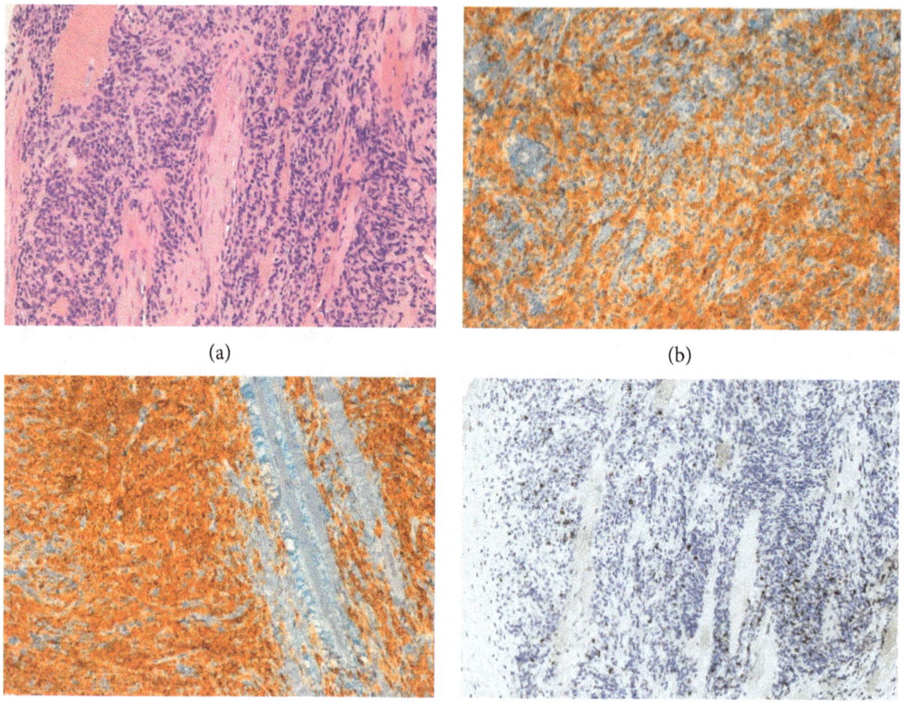

Figure 2: Immunohistochemical features of the lymphoma. (a) Hematoxylin and eosin staining; (b) CD30 and (c) CD4 immunostaining showing a strong and uniform expression in the neoplastic cells; (d) TIA1 immunostaining; this marker was only expressed in a minority of cells (−/+).

CT revealed the complete disappearance of the right gastrocnemius muscle and of D5 and L2 lesions, with persistence of moderate metabolic activity in the left sacral lesion (Deauville score = 3) (Figure 4(b)). Serum M-component decreased (0.4 gr/dl), and a re-evaluation of bone marrow biopsy displayed the reduction of plasma cell infiltration to 10% of marrow cellularity. As such, MM was in partial response. On February 2018, peripheral blood stem cell (PBSC) mobilization was achieved following high-dose cyclophosphamide (2 gr/sqm) and granulocyte-colony stimulating factor (G-CSF), and an amount of CD34+ cells adequate for a single ASCT was collected. Then, in March 2018, the patient received localized radiotherapy on the right gastrocnemius muscle for a total of 36 Gy, without any relevant complication. Waiting to be transplanted, on April 2018, the patient started VD treatment (bortezomib 1.3 mg/smq twice a week, days 1-4-8-11 and oral dexamethasone 40 mg, days 1-2-4-5-8-9-11-12, cycles every 21 days), completing two cycles. On June 2018, during the third course, he was hospitalized because of an *E. coli* infection complicated by sepsis and congestive heart failure; he was discharged one month later. Serum M-protein remained permanently around 0.3 g/dl, and serum lambda light chains were 30 mg/L, confirming a MM partial response.

Unfortunately, on July 2018, few days later, he was hospitalized again due to paraplegia and neurogenic bladder dysfunction. An MRI of the spine showed a spinal cord compression due to neoplastic tissue extending from vertebrae D6 to D10 (size 10 × 5 × 2.5 cm). Considering the severity of the neurologic impairment, a new biopsy of the lesion was not performed, and radiotherapy in association to high-dose dexamethasone was immediately started, obtaining a rapid neurologic improvement.

M-protein kept stable (0.3 g/dl), but lambda sFLC were increased to 860 mg/L. A new bone marrow biopsy showed an increased monoclonal plasma cell infiltration (50% of marrow cellularity) with morphologic atypia and aberrant phenotype. Fluorescent in situ hybridization (FISH) performed on purified bone marrow plasma cells, which was not available at the diagnosis, showed *t*(14;16) in 100% and del17p13 in 64% of the cells analyzed. On August 2018, we started a second line therapy with weekly daratumumab in combination with lenalidomide and dexamethasone (DRd). After one cycle, the patient's conditions deteriorated, and a new MRI of the spine revealed two additional neoplastic lesions that extended from vertebrae D2 to D6 and from vertebrae D12 to L4. In September 2018, the patient was deceased due to disease progression.

3. Discussion

ALK− ALCL usually presents with advanced stage disease (stage III-IV), B symptoms, lymph nodes, and extranodal tissue involvement [1]. The median age at presentation of ALK− ALCL patients is 54–61 years [9].

Our case instead presented with an extranodal noncutaneous ALK− ALCL showing muscular involvement as a unique lesion without systemic symptoms. This clinical onset coincided with a symptomatic IgG lambda MM. According to the last edition of WHO classification, ALK− ALCL is defined as a CD30+ T-cell neoplasm that is not

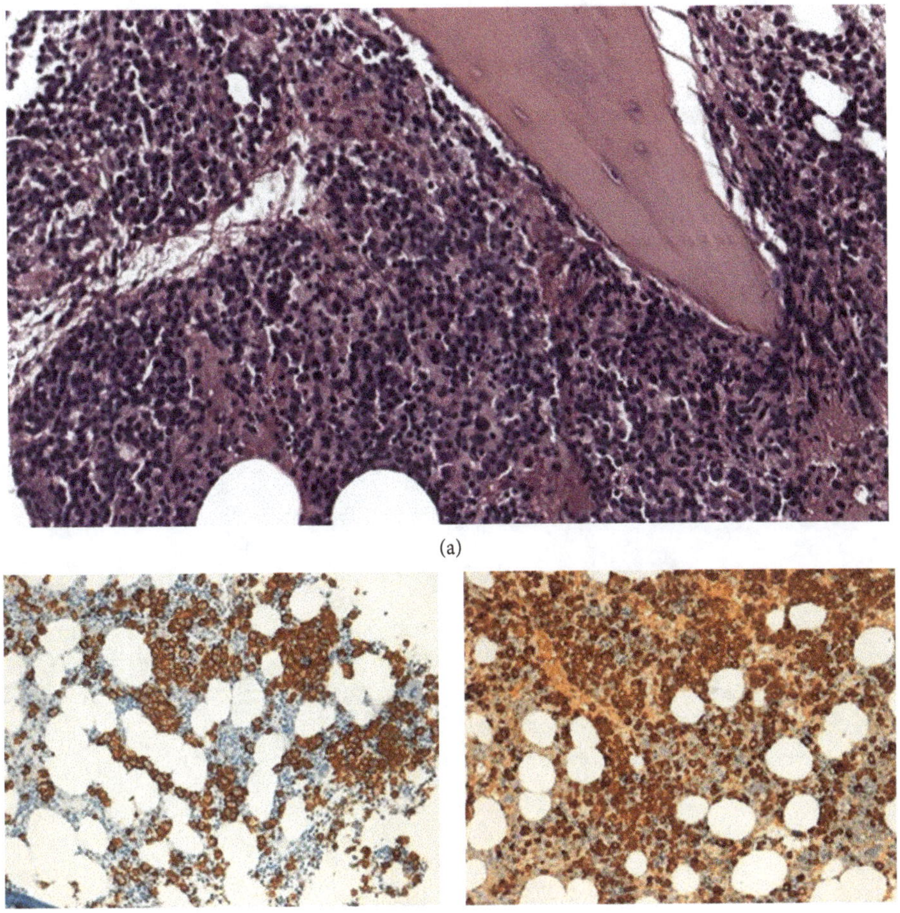

(a) (b) (c)

FIGURE 3: Bone marrow biopsy performed at diagnosis showed plasma cell infiltration with lambda-chain restriction. (a) H&E staining; (b) CD138 staining; (c) lambda staining.

reproducibly distinguishable by morphology from ALK-positive (ALK+) ALCL, but lacks ALK protein expression [1]. T-cell/cytotoxic markers can be lacking in ALCL as well as EMA which is only positive in 43% of the cases [10]. While both Pax-5 negativity and cell morphology helped us to rule out classical Hodgkin lymphoma, distinguishing ALCL from PTCL-NOS can be challenging. The occurrence of hallmark cells together with strong and uniform CD30 expression in the neoplastic proliferation appeared more consistent with ALCL than PTCL-NOS in this case.

Regarding concomitant diagnosis of T-cell lymphoma and MM, in the few other cases described in the literature [5–7], the diagnosis of a T-cell neoplasm occurred later than the diagnosis of MM, leading to surmise a pathogenic role for acquired cellular immunity impairment, on turn caused by PC disorders or previous therapies. In our patient the relationship between the two neoplasms was unclear, and the chronologic sequence of onset could not be proven. Nevertheless, the patient did not have any prior history of MGUS or other plasma cell dyscrasias. Moreover, the incidence of lymphoproliferative disorders is generally increased in immunosuppressed patients, but our patient was not previously treated with any chemo-radiotherapy and blood tests excluded an active viral infection.

The optimal treatment for ALK-negative ALCL is still debated because of the rarity of the disease and the related lack of prospective randomized trials. ALK– ALCL generally responds well to doxorubicin-containing chemotherapy, but frequently relapses [11]. The role of autologous stem cell transplant in first remission in ALCL has been investigated in small trials with 5-year overall survival (OS) rates of up to 80%. However, in many of these studies, ALK expression was not assessed [12, 13]. The prognosis of ALK– ALCL patients is poor, with a 5-year (OS) of 30–49%, versus 70–86% in ALK+ ALCL [14, 15]. On the contrary, multiple myeloma treatment is well standardized and includes upfront autologous stem cell transplantation for younger patients [16]. However, the prognosis can be quite heterogeneous according to cytogenetic and biochemical markers [17]: specifically, the outcome of patients harbouring one of the high-risk chromosomal aberrations, such as *t*(4;14), *t*(14;16), *t*(14;20), and especially del17p, is dismal and not completely overcome by the new drug combinations so far [18].

In our patient, both diseases required therapeutic intervention. Because of the high proliferation index (MIB-1 > 90%), we decided to treat lymphoma first. Afterwards, we observed an aggressive behaviour and a rapid progression of multiple myeloma which led the patient to death, eventually

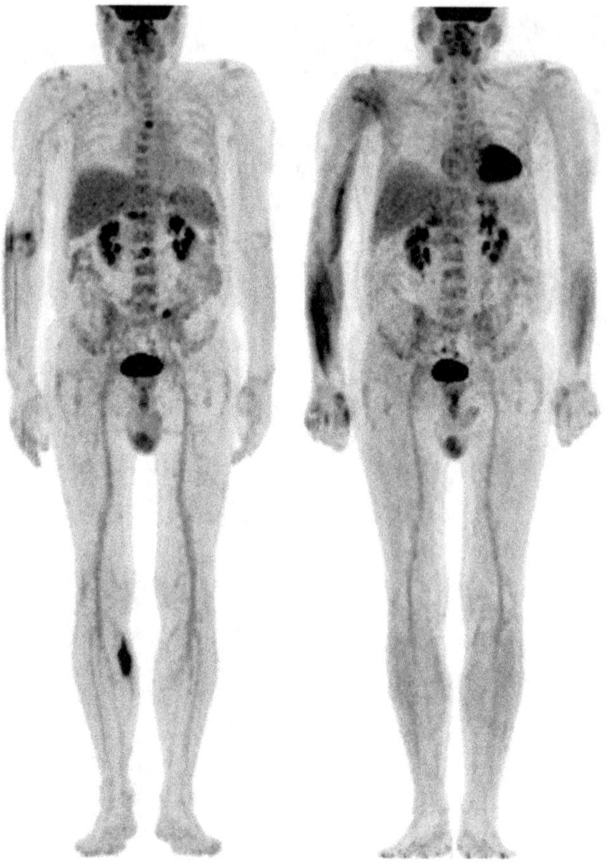

(a) (b)

FIGURE 4: F18-FDG PET/CT performed at staging showed an intensely hypermetabolic lesion in the right leg and revealed three additional vertebral hypermetabolic lesions in D5, L2, and S1 (a). After chemotherapy, the hypermetabolic lesions in the right leg, D5, and L2 had completely disappeared, with persistence of moderate metabolic activity in the left sacral lesion (DS = 3) (b).

explained by the double high-risk cytogenetic alterations identified at relapse.

Unfortunately, no cytogenetic data were available at diagnosis, and we cannot exclude a clonal selection secondary to chemotherapy treatment for lymphoma.

Consent

Written informed consent was obtained from the patient's relatives for publication of this case report and any accompanying images.

Authors' Contributions

Michela Staderini and Lara Mannelli are contributed equally to the manuscript.

References

[1] S. H. Swerdlow, E. Campo, S. A. Pileri et al., "The 2016 revision of the World Health Organization classification of lymphoid neoplasms," *Blood*, vol. 127, no. 20, pp. 2375–2390, 2016.

[2] M. Emori, M. Kaya, S. Takahata, H. Tobioka, Y. Minaki, and T. Yamashita, "Anaplastic lymphoma kinase-negative anaplastic large cell lymphoma with extranodal involvement of the thigh muscle: a case report," *Journal of Medical Case Reports*, vol. 8, no. 1, p. 9, 2014.

[3] Y. Kubo, J. Aoi, T. Johno et al., "A case of anaplastic large cell lymphoma of skeletal muscle," *The Journal of Dermatology* vol. 41, no. 41, pp. 999–1002, 2014.

[4] Y. Zongyou, L. Yueju, G. Fuqian et al., "Anaplastic large cell lymphoma with primary involvement of the skeletal muscle: a case report," *Oncology Letters*, vol. 9, no. 6, pp. 2815–2818, 2015.

[5] R. C. Romano, D. N. Cohen, M. T. Howard, and C. N. Wieland, "A primary cutaneous CD30-positive T-cell lymphoproliferative disorder arising in a patient with multiple myeloma and cutaneous amyloidosis," *The American Journal of Dermatopathology*, vol. 38, no. 5, pp. 388–392, 2016.

[6] M. Nassiri, G. E. Byrne, C. C. Whitcomb, and J. J. Byrnes, "Synchronous null-cell anaplastic large cell lymphoma and multiple myeloma," *Annals of Hematology*, vol. 88, no. 9, pp. 923–925, 2009.

[7] M. Tangour, I. Chelly, S. Haouet, M. Zitouna, and N. Kchir, "Multiple myeloma and cutaneous anaplastic large T-cell lymphoma in the same patient: is there a causal relation?," *Journal of Cutaneous Pathology*, vol. 38, no. 3, pp. 298–300, 2011.

[8] S. Nassif, N. El-Majzoub, O. Abbas, S. Temraz, and Z. Chakhachiro, "Simultaneous occurrence of a CD30 positive/ALK-negative high grade T-cell lymphoma and plasma cell myeloma: report of a case," *Hematology/Oncology and Stem Cell Therapy*, vol. 8, no. 1, pp. 40–42, 2015.

[9] C. Querfeld, I. Khan, B. Mahon, B. P. Nelson, S. T. Rosen, and A. M. Evens, "Primary cutaneous and systemic anaplastic large cell lymphoma: clinicopathologic aspects and therapeutic options," *Oncology (Williston Park)*, vol. 24, no. 7, pp. 574–587, 2010.

[10] K. J. Savage, N. L. Harris, J. M. Vose et al., "ALK− anaplastic large-cell lymphoma is clinically and immunophenotypically different from both ALK+ ALCL and peripheral T-cell lymphoma, not otherwise specified: report from the International Peripheral T-Cell Lymphoma Project," *Blood*, vol. 111, no. 12, pp. 5496–5504, 2008.

[11] A. J. M. Ferreri, S. Govi, S. A. Pileri, and K. J. Savage, "Anaplastic large cell lymphoma, ALK-negative," *Critical Reviews in Oncology/Hematology*, vol. 85, no. 2, pp. 206–215, 2013.

[12] R. Fanin, F. Silvestri, A. Geromin et al., "Primary systemic CD30 (Ki-1)-positive anaplastic large cell lymphoma of the adult: sequential intensive treatment with the F-MACHOP regimen (+/− radiotherapy) and autologous bone marrow transplantation," *Blood*, vol. 87, no. 4, pp. 1243–1248, 1996.

[13] R. Fanin, A. Sperotto, F. Silvestri et al., "The therapy of primary adult systemic CD30-positive anaplastic large cell lymphoma: results of 40 cases treated in a single center," *Leukemia & Lymphoma*, vol. 35, no. 1-2, pp. 159–169, 1999.

[14] K. J. Savage, "Prognosis and primary therapy in peripheral T-cell lymphomas," *Hematology*, vol. 2008, no. 1, pp. 280–288, 2008.

[15] H. Stein, H. D. Foss, H. Dürkop et al., "CD30(+) anaplastic large cell lymphoma: a review of its histopathologic, genetic, and clinical features," *Blood*, vol. 96, no. 12, pp. 3681–3695, 2000.

[16] F. Gay, M. Engelhardt, E. Terpos et al., "From transplant to novel cellular therapies in multiple myeloma: European Myeloma Network guidelines and future perspectives," *Haematologica*, vol. 103, no. 2, pp. 197–211, 2018.

[17] A. Palumbo, H. Avet-Loiseau, S. Oliva et al., "Revised International Staging System for multiple myeloma: a report from International Myeloma Working Group," *Journal of Clinical Oncology*, vol. 33, no. 26, pp. 2863–2869, 2015.

[18] P. Sonneveld, H. Avet-Loiseau, S. Lonial et al., "Treatment of multiple myeloma with high-risk cytogenetics: a consensus of the International Myeloma Working Group," *Blood*, vol. 127, no. 24, pp. 2955–2962, 2016.

29

Venetoclax Combined with Hypomethylating Agents for Treatment-Naïve B/Myeloid Mixed Phenotype Acute Leukemia

Di Wu, Wenlan Chen, Zhichao Chen, and Qiubai Li

Institute of Hematology, Union Hospital, Tongji Medical College, Huazhong University of Science and Technology, Wuhan 430022, Hubei, China

Correspondence should be addressed to Qiubai Li; qiubaili@hust.edu.cn

Academic Editor: Yusuke Shiozawa

Mixed phenotype acute leukemia (MPAL) is a rare hematological malignancy that lacks consensus on optimal management. We report for the first time two cases of treatment-naïve B/myeloid MPAL patients treated with a novel chemo-free regimen using venetoclax combined with hypomethylating agents, which successfully induced complete remission with tolerable toxicities.

1. Introduction

Mixed phenotype acute leukemia (MPAL) is a heterogeneous group of rare acute leukemias defined as those with coexpression of myeloid and lymphoid antigens on the same blasts or those that have two separate populations of cells expressing distinct lineage characteristics, accounting for no more than 5% of all acute leukemias [1]. Due to the rarity of MPAL and the limited understanding of its pathophysiology, there is no consensus regarding optimal management. Its prognosis remains dismal, with the risk of death increased by 59% and 26% compared to that of acute lymphoblastic leukemia (ALL) and acute myeloid leukemia (AML), respectively [1].

Here, we present the first two cases of treatment-naïve B/myeloid MPAL successfully treated with a chemo-free regimen of venetoclax, a potent and selective small-molecule B-cell lymphoma/leukemia (BCL)-2 inhibitor, combined with a hypomethylating agent (HMA).

2. Case Report

2.1. Case #1. A 23-year-old female was admitted with one-week history of low fever and petechiae on her left lower extremity. Peripheral blood results showed hyperleukocytosis (112.73×10^9/L), anemia (6.9 g/dL), and thrombocytopenia (51×10^9/L). Physical examination revealed no hepatomegaly, lymphadenopathy, or splenomegaly. The Eastern Cooperative Oncology Group Performance Status (ECOG PS) was 1. Bone marrow evaluation showed myeloid blasts (27.5%) and primitive lymphocyte (59.5%) by cytomorphology analysis, with about 4% of the tumor cells positive for myeloperoxidase (MPO) staining. Immunophenotyping by flow cytometry revealed expression of B-cell antigens and myeloid antigens on two distinct populations of blast cells. To be specific, one population (61.64%) was phenotypically abnormal B-lineage blasts expressing CD19, CD34, cCD79a part, CD38 part, CD22, HLA-DR, CD33, and CD13, and the other (29.44%) was aberrant myeloid cells expressing CD33, CD15, CD64, CD11b part, CD11c dim, CD13 part, CD38, and CD45 dim. Chromosomal karyotyping revealed a 46, XX karyotype. First- and next-generation sequencing found no mutations of BCL-2, BRAF, KRAS, PHF6, and FBXW7. Detection for MLL-AF4, E2A-HLF, E2A-PBX1, SIL-TAL1, TEL-AML1, HOX11, HOX11L2, CAML-AF10, and BCR-ABL genes showed negative results. The patient was subsequently diagnosed as B/myeloid MPAL. BH3 profiling was not performed due to unavailability of this technique in our hospital.

After leukapheresis sessions, her white blood cell count reduced to 11.52×10^9/L. For induction therapy, she received decitabine (DAC) (50 mg, intravenous infusion for 7 consecutive days) and venetoclax (100 mg p.o. day 1, 200 mg day 2, and 400 mg days 3–28). Complete remission with incomplete blood count recovery (CRi) was achieved after the first cycle, with 2.56% abnormal B-cell blasts (expressing CD19, CD34, TdT part, CD22, CD38 dim, HLA-DR, CD33, and cCD79a) detected in minimal residual disease (MRD) test by flow cytometry. We repeated this regimen for consolidation. However, her disease relapsed after this consolidation cycle, with primitive cells (42.0%) found in cytomorphology, with abnormal immunophenotyping of B-cell blasts (expressing CD19, CD34 part, CD33 part, HLA-DR, CD13 dim, CD10 part, CD22, CD38, and cCD79a part). Then, ALL-based therapy (idarubicin 12 mg/m^2 days 1-3; vindesine 4 mg days 1, 8, 15, and 22; dexamethasone 15 mg days 1–28) was applied intravenously for one cycle, after which second CR was achieved with residual abnormal B-cell blasts (0.03%; expressing CD19, CD34, TdT dim, CD22, CD38, CD33, and CD79a part). After that, DAC (50 mg, days 1–7), venetoclax (100 mg day 1, 200 mg day 2, 400 mg days 3–28), dexamethasone (10 mg days 1–16, 5 mg days 17–20, and 2.5 mg days 21-22), and vindesine (4 mg days 1, 8, 15, and 22) were subsequently coadministered for the consolidation therapy, after which she remained CR, with 0.48% abnormal B-cell blasts (expressing CD19, CD22, CD38 dim, HLA-DR, CD33, CD34, and cCD79a) detected in the MRD test by flow cytometry. Treatment-related toxicities during the 4 cycles according to the National Cancer Institute Common Terminology Criteria for Adverse Events Version 5.0 [2] are summarized (Table 1). The patient has completed allogeneic peripheral blood stem cell transplantation (allo-PBSCT) in August 2019 and remains CR.

2.2. Case #2. A 24-year-old male patient was admitted with high fevers for 5 days, with a white blood cell count of 0.60×10^9/L, hemoglobin of 8.3 g/dL, and platelets at 26×10^9/L. There were no obvious abnormalities in his physical examination, and ECOG PS was 1. A subsequent morphology analysis of bone marrow cells revealed myeloid blasts (56.5%) and primitive lymphocyte (17%) with about 8% of the tumor cells positive for MPO staining, and flow cytometry analysis showed aberrant myeloid blasts (64.31%; expressing CD34, CD117, CD7, CD33 part, CD22 dim, CD38, CD13, CD64 part, and HLA-DR) and B-lymphoid blasts coupling with myeloid expression (3.39%; CD34, CD19, CD117 part, cCD79a, CD7, CD13, CD22, CD20, and CD38). Next-generation sequencing detected a mutation of PTPN11 gene (36.41%), and BCL-2 gene was negative. Analysis of chromosomal karyotyping, fused gene detection, fluorescence in situ hybridization, and IGH/TCR test showed negative results. Thus, a diagnosis of B/myeloid MPAL coupling with PTPN11 mutation was established. BH3 profiling was not performed either.

Antibiotics and supportive care were used to treat the severe pneumonia before the coming induction chemotherapy. However, the infection was hard to control and infectious shock occurred on the 28th day of hospitalization. Thus, to lower the infection-related risk, chemo-free induction therapy was initiated using venetoclax (100 mg day 1, 200 mg day 2, and 400 mg days 3–28) combined with azacitidine (AZA) (100 mg, subcutaneous injection for 7 consecutive days). When completed, there were no abnormal myeloid or lymphoid blasts in bone marrow morphology, and immunophenotyping revealed MRD negative status. Besides, the mutant PTPN11 gene became negative. He successfully received one more cycle of consolidation chemotherapy using IA regimen (idarubicin 20 mg days 1-3 and cytarabine 200 mg days 1–7) intravenously, after which allo-PBSCT was performed in December 2019 on patient request, and he remains CR now. Treatment-related toxicities during the 2 cycles are summarized (Table 1).

TABLE 1: Summary of treatment response and related toxicities.

	Case 1				Case 2	
Cycle	1	2	3	4	1	2
Treatment	DAC[a] +VEN[b]	DAC +VEN	IVP[c]	DAC +VEN +VP[d]	AZA[e] +VEN	IA[f]
Response	CRi[g]	Relapse	CR[h]	CR	CR	CR
Anemia†	3-4	2–4	2–4	2-3	3-4	2-3
Thrombocytopenia†	1–4	1–4	1–4	1–4	1–4	1–4
Neutropenia†	1–4	1–4	3-4	4	1–4	1–4
Gastrointestinal toxicities†	1-2	1-2	1-2	1-2	1-2	1-2

[a]DAC, decitabine; [b]VEN, venetoclax; [c]IVP, idarubicin, vindesine, and dexamethasone; [d]VP, vindesine and dexamethasone; [e]AZA, azacitidine; [f]IA, idarubicin and cytarabine; [g]CRi, complete remission with incomplete blood count recovery; [h]CR, complete remission. †CTCAE V5.0: National Cancer Institute Common Terminology Criteria for Adverse Events, version 5.0. [2].

3. Discussion

Three mainstream regimens exist for MPAL patients: ALL-based, AML-based, and "hybrid" therapy (ALL plus AML). Based on retrospective data, experts recommend ALL-based rather than AML-based chemotherapy for its superiority in remission rates [3, 4], whereas there still exist contradictory research results. One study presented that overall responses of MPAL did not differ significantly to AML-type and ALL-type induction (84% vs 91%, $P = 0.999$) [5]. Another study analyzed 27 patients with MPAL and concluded that the CR rate of those treated with genome-wide methylation matched therapy (AML-directed therapy for AML-like MPAL and ALL-directed therapy for ALL-like MPAL) was significantly higher than those treated with unmatched regimen (72% vs 22%, $P = 0.037$). They highlighted that their data's consistency of ALL-based regimen's preponderance in response and survival rates with previous studies may be attributed to higher incidence of ALL-like MPAL, raising the question of ALL-like therapy's applicability in methylation-defined AML-like MPAL [6]. However, all these different research results have not been verified in multicenter, prospective clinical trials. In addition, complications of conventional chemotherapy, like fatal infections and hemorrhage, remain a threat to MPAL patients' survival [7].

Members of the BCL-2 protein family play a crucial role in maintaining cancer cells' survival through antagonizing proapoptotic proteins. Venetoclax, a potent and selective BCL-2 inhibitor, has shown clinical activity in hematological malignancies, including B-ALL, T-ALL, and AML, but venetoclax monotherapy is modest and explorations on combinational therapy become the mainstream choice [8, 9].

Aberrant DNA methylation contributes to the pathogenesis of both myeloid and lymphoid malignancies and is also discovered to possibly participate in aberrant transformation of hematopoietic stem cells in MPAL [10]. Decitabine (DAC) and AZA both act as HMA, and their performance in convincing response, outstanding survival benefit, and well-tolerated safety profile has enabled them to become first-line treatment options in elderly AML patients [11]. Several clinical researches also suggest their promising feasibility in B-ALL and T-ALL, especially decitabine in relapsed/refractory ALL, whereas data of this area are still limited [12–16]. An 81-year-old female MPAL, T/myeloid patient was treated by 4 cycles of DAC monotherapy to induce CR, first showing the efficacy and tolerability of HMA in MPAL [17].

When venetoclax and HMA were coadministered, the synergistic effect achieved an outstanding CR rate of 67% with manageable adverse events. The adverse events were mainly hematological and gastrointestinal toxicities in elderly AML patients unfit for standard chemotherapy [18]. In ALL, two reported cases of T-ALL who relapsed after HSCT were treated with venetoclax and decitabine and achieved second CR [19, 20]. Two cases of relapsed or refractory T/myeloid MPAL were reported to receive venetoclax combined with azacitidine or decitabine, both induced CR [21, 22]. In our female patient, whose lymphoid-linage blasts dominated, this combinational regimen did show efficacy at cycle 1 induction therapy, particularly for myeloid-linage aberrant cells, whereas the lymphoid blasts relapsed after the consolidation cycle. Subsequently, ALL-based re-induction was effective for those lymphoid blasts, and the later coadministration of DAC, venetoclax, dexamethasone, and vindesine for consolidation therapy was successful to prepare her for allo-PBSCT. As for our male patient who was frail to receive conventional intensive chemotherapy and whose myeloid-linage blasts accounted for a larger part, this regimen successfully achieved leukemia-free state and abnormal gene mutation was also cleared. Hematological and gastrointestinal toxicities were tolerable (Table 1).

In conclusion, BCL-2 inhibitor combined with HMA could be a potential option to treat MPAL, especially for those that are not suitable to receive standard chemotherapy, which needs to be further verified in future clinical trials.

Authors' Contributions

Di Wu and Wenlan Chen contributed equally to this study.

Acknowledgments

This work was supported by the National Natural Science Foundation of China (NSFC) (nos. 81974009 and 81974221).

References

[1] R. Shi and R. Munker, "Survival of patients with mixed phenotype acute leukemias: a large population-based study," *Leukemia Research*, vol. 39, no. 6, pp. 606–616, 2015.

[2] National CI, "National cancer institute common terminology criteria for adverse events (CTCAE) v5.0," https://ctep.cancer.gov/protocolDevelopment/electronic_applications/ctc.htm#ctc_50.

[3] O. Wolach and R. M. Stone, "Optimal therapeutic strategies for mixed phenotype acute leukemia," *Current Opinion in Hematology*, vol. 27, no. 2, pp. 95–102, 2020.

[4] M. Maruffi, R. Sposto, M. J. Oberley, L. Kysh, and E. Orgel, "Therapy for children and adults with mixed phenotype acute leukemia: a systematic review and meta-analysis," *Leukemia*, vol. 32, no. 7, pp. 1515–1528, 2018.

[5] B. M. Getta, M. Roshal, J. Zheng et al., "Allogeneic hematopoietic stem cell transplantation with myeloablative conditioning is associated with favorable outcomes in mixed phenotype acute leukemia," *Biology of Blood and Marrow Transplantation*, vol. 23, no. 11, pp. 1879–1886, 2017.

[6] K. Takahashi, F. Wang, K. Morita et al., "Integrative genomic analysis of adult mixed phenotype acute leukemia delineates lineage associated molecular subtypes," *Nature Communications*, vol. 9, no. 1, p. 2670, 2018.

[7] X.-Q. Xu, J.-M. Wang, S.-Q. Lu et al., "Clinical and biological characteristics of adult biphenotypic acute leukemia in comparison with that of acute myeloid leukemia and acute lymphoblastic leukemia: a case series of a Chinese population," *Haematologica*, vol. 94, no. 7, pp. 919–927, 2009.

[8] R. Valentin, S. Grabow, and M. S. Davids, "The rise of apoptosis: targeting apoptosis in hematologic malignancies," *Blood*, vol. 132, no. 12, pp. 1248–1264, 2018.

[9] A. Hantel, J. Wynne, N. Lacayo et al., "Safety and efficacy of the BCL inhibitors venetoclax and navitoclax in combination with chemotherapy in patients with relapsed/refractory acute lymphoblastic leukemia and lymphoblastic lymphoma," *Clinical Lymphoma Myeloma and Leukemia*, vol. 18, pp. S184–S185, 2018.

[10] O. S. Eckstein, L. Wang, J. N. Punia et al., "Mixed phenotype acute leukemia (MPAL) has a high frequency of mutations in epigenetic regulatory genes: results from whole exome sequencing," *Blood*, vol. 124, no. 21, p. 3560, 2014.

[11] M. S. Tallman, E. S. Wang, J. K Altman et al., "Acute myeloid leukemia, version 3.2019, NCCN clinical practice guidelines in Oncology," *Journal of the National Comprehensive Cancer Network*, vol. 17, no. 6, pp. 721–749, 2019.

[12] K. Paulson, R. Kumar, A. Ahsanuddin, and M. D. Seftel, "Azacytidine as a novel agent in the treatment of acute lymphoblastic leukemia," *Leukemia & Lymphoma*, vol. 52, no. 1, pp. 134–136, 2011.

[13] J.-k. Cui, Y. Xiao, Y. You et al., "Decitabine for relapsed acute lymphoblastic leukemia after allogeneic hematopoietic stem cell transplantation," *Current Medical Science*, vol. 37, no. 5, pp. 693–698, 2017.

[14] M. J. Burke, J. K. Lamba, S. Pounds et al., "A therapeutic trial of decitabine and vorinostat in combination with chemotherapy for relapsed/refractory acute lymphoblastic leukemia," *American Journal of Hematology*, vol. 89, no. 9, pp. 889–895, 2014.

[15] C. B. Benton, D. A. Thomas, H. Yang et al., "Safety and clinical activity of 5-aza-2′-deoxycytidine (decitabine) with or with-

out Hyper-CVAD in relapsed/refractory acute lymphocytic leukaemia," *British Journal of Haematology*, vol. 167, no. 3, pp. 356–365, 2014.

[16] G. Garcia-Manero, D. A. Thomas, M. E. Rytting et al., "Final report of a phase I trial of decitabine with or without hyperCVAD in relapsed acute lymphocytic leukemia (ALL)," *Blood*, vol. 116, no. 21, p. 379, 2010.

[17] J.-Y. Lee, S.-m. Lee, J.-Y. Lee, K.-H. Kim, M.-Y. Choi, and W.-S. Lee, "Mixed-phenotype acute leukemia treated with decitabine," *The Korean Journal of Internal Medicine*, vol. 31, no. 2, pp. 406–408, 2016.

[18] C. D. DiNardo, K. Pratz, V. Pullarkat et al., "Venetoclax combined with decitabine or azacitidine in treatment-naive, elderly patients with acute myeloid leukemia," *Blood*, vol. 133, no. 1, pp. 7–17, 2019.

[19] L. T. Rahmat, A. Nguyen, H. Abdulhaq, S. Prakash, A. C. Logan, and G. N. Mannis, "Venetoclax in combination with decitabine for relapsed T-cell acute lymphoblastic leukemia after allogeneic hematopoietic cell transplant," *Case Reports in Hematology*, vol. 2018, Article ID 6092646, 4 pages, 2018.

[20] N. Farhadfar, Y. Li, W. S. May, and C. B. Adams, "Venetoclax and decitabine for treatment of relapsed T-cell acute lymphoblastic leukemia: a case report and review of literature," *Hematology/Oncology and Stem Cell Therapy*, 2020.

[21] X. Wu, J. Zhang, Q. Chen et al., "Efficacy of venetoclax in combination with azacitidine followed by haploidentical transplantation in refractory acute myeloid leukaemia and mixed phenotype acute leukaemia," *British Journal of Haematology*, vol. 189, no. 5, pp. e200–e204, 2020.

[22] H. Klocke, Z. M. Dong, C. O'Brien et al., "Venetoclax and decitabine for T/myeloid mixed-phenotype Acute leukemia not otherwise specified (MPAL NOS)," *Case Reports in Hematology*, vol. 2020, Article ID 8811673, 4 pages, 2020.

Immunogenicity of Pfizer mRNA COVID-19 Vaccination Followed by J&J Adenovirus COVID-19 Vaccination in Two Patients with Chronic Lymphocytic Leukemia

Zoe L. Lyski,[1] Myung Sun Kim,[2] David Xthona Lee,[1] David Sampson,[2] Hans-Peter Raué,[3] Vikram Raghunathan,[2] Debbie Ryan,[2] Amanda E. Brunton,[4] Mark K. Slifka,[3] William B. Messer,[1,3,5] and Stephen E. Spurgeon[2]

[1]*Department of Molecular Microbiology & Immunology, Oregon Health & Science University (OHSU), Portland, OR 97239, USA*
[2]*Knight Cancer Institute, Oregon Health & Science University (OHSU), Portland, OR 97239, USA*
[3]*Division of Neuroscience, Oregon National Primate Research Center, Oregon Health & Science University, Beaverton, OR 97239, USA*
[4]*OHSU-PSU School of Public Health, Portland, OR 97239, USA*
[5]*Department of Medicine, Division of Infectious Diseases, Oregon Health & Science University (OHSU), Portland, OR 97239, USA*

Correspondence should be addressed to Stephen E. Spurgeon; spurgeos@ohsu.edu

Academic Editor: Pier Paolo Piccaluga

Individuals with chronic lymphocytic leukemia (CLL) have significant immune disfunction, often further disrupted by treatment. While currently available COVID-19 vaccinations are highly effective in immunocompetent individuals, they are often poorly immunogenic in CLL patients. It is important to understand the role a heterologous boost would have in patients who did not respond to the initial two-dose mRNA vaccine series. SARS-CoV-2 specific immune responses, including antibodies and memory B-cells, CD4 and CD8 T-cells were assessed prior to vaccination, as well as postinitial vaccination series and post-third dose in two subjects. One subject seroconverted, had RBD-specific memory B-cells and spike-specific CD4 T-cells while the other did not. Both subjects had a spike-specific CD8 T-cell response after the original mRNA vaccination series that was further boosted after the third dose or remained stable. The results of this study, however small, are especially promising to CLL individuals who did not seroconvert following the initial mRNA vaccination series.

1. Introduction

Chronic lymphocytic leukemia (CLL) is characterized by the monoclonal proliferation of dysfunctional B-cells, leading to a broad range of immune defects. CLL patients face significant risk of morbidity and mortality from infections [1], including from SARS-CoV-2, the causative agent of COVID-19 [2]. Vaccines can be instrumental in mitigating the risk of infections in CLL; however, responses to vaccination are highly variable and significantly influenced by CLL disease status, baseline characteristics, types of vaccine, and active CLL therapy [3].

Although current COVID-19 vaccines elicit robust immunity in immunocompetent hosts [4], the antibody response in CLL patients is highly variable [5–7] and particularly poor in patients with low total immunoglobulin levels, those that have had anti-CD20 monoclonal antibodies within the past year, or those that are undergoing active therapy with agents such as Bruton's tyrosine kinase inhibitors (BTKi). The best responses to date have been in CLL patients who are in remission and/or years out from active treatment.

Given decreased vaccine efficacy in CLL, an additional dose of vaccine may be beneficial in CLL patients, especially given the rise of variants of concern (VoCs). Initial data from solid organ transplant recipients on immunosuppression as well as individuals with solid tumors on active therapy showed a role for additional vaccination [8, 9]. This led to the FDA extending the EUA for Pfizer-BioNTech and Moderna mRNA vaccines to include additional doses in immunocompromised patients. However, these results may not be generalizable to CLL, and additional studies are needed to better define vaccine responses in the CLL patient population, including the role of mixing mRNA vaccination with other vaccine formulations, such as the adenovirus vectored vaccine Ad26COV2.s, commonly known as the Johnson and Johnson (J&J) vaccine.

2. Case Report

Here we describe two CLL patients who "self-referred" to outside pharmacies for an additional vaccination with the J&J COVID-19 vaccine following 2 doses of the BNT162b2 vaccine (Pfizer-BioNTech). Both patients had previously been enrolled as study subjects in an IRB-approved observational study (OHSU IRB# 21230) to investigate immune response following COVID-19 vaccination. The additional J&J dose was subsequently self-reported to the study team. On initial enrollment, demographics, CLL disease characteristics, and treatment details were collected (Table 1), and baseline laboratory values were obtained, including semi-quantitative SARS-CoV-2 spike antibody titer, serum IgG, a complete blood count, and multicolor flow cytometry measuring immune cell populations (Table 1). Whole blood was collected for additional serologic and cellular studies.

SARS-CoV-2 spike receptor binding domain (RBD)-specific antibody levels were tested by ELISA and endpoint titers were calculated as previously described [10]. In addition, baseline PBMC samples were functionally tested for the presence of SARS-CoV-2 spike RBD-specific memory B-cells (MBCs) by limiting dilution assay as previously described [11, 12]. Briefly, PBMCs were serially diluted and incubated with a stimulation cocktail in which the MBCs present within PBMCs differentiated and became antibody-secreting cells. The supernatants were collected 7 days later and assayed for antigen specificity by RBD-ELISA. This allows one to functionally test MBC-derived antibodies and back-calculate the frequency of total IgG-secreting MBCs as well as RBD-specific MBCs [11, 12]. In addition, CD4+ and CD8+ T-cells were also functionally assessed for the presence of IFNγ and TNFα secretion following spike protein-derived peptide stimulation. Briefly, PBMCs were stimulated with 2 peptide pools of overlapping (10AA) 17mers representing the SARS-CoV-2 spike protein (BEI Resources). Following stimulation, the cells were stained as previously described [13, 14]. Data was acquired on an LSR Fortessa (Becton Dickenson) and analyzed using FlowJo software. Cytokine expression in medium-alone cultures was subtracted from peptide-stimulated cultures to calculate peptide-specific cytokine expression. Responses to both peptide pools were added together to yield the total frequency of SARS-CoV-2-specific cytokine-producing CD4+ and CD8+ T cells.

Neither subject had prevaccination B-cell responses as measured by RBD-specific antibodies or MBCs. Neither had a virus-specific CD8+ response at baseline. While Subject 2 had spike peptide-reactive CD4+ T-cells at baseline, these cells were unresponsive and did not expand following vaccination. In contrast, CD8+ responses were observed after mRNA vaccination in both subjects (Figure 1). It has previously been reported that SARS-CoV-2 naïve individuals may have preexisting cross-reactivity to SARS-CoV-2 peptides through prior infection by common cold coronaviruses: SARS-CoV-2 specific CD4+ T-cells have been identified in 20–50% of people without SARS-CoV-2 exposure or vaccination [15].

Approximately four weeks after initial vaccination, neither subject had detectable RBD-specific SARS-CoV-2 antibodies or MBCs. Both had measurable vaccine-induced CD8+ T-cell responses following mRNA vaccination, although CD4+ responses did not appear to increase above baseline (Figure 1).

Subject 1 received the J&J vaccine 104 days and Subject 2 received 81 days after completion of the BNT162b2 vaccine series. Following J&J vaccination, additional samples were obtained from Subject 1, 30 days after the third vaccine, and Subject 2, 27 days following the third vaccine. Interestingly, Subject 1 had undetectable RBD-specific antibodies, RBD-specific MBCs, and virus-specific CD4+ T-cells after the initial vaccination series. However, following an additional vaccination, all three measures increased above the limit of detection: RBD-ELISA titer of 625, RBD-specific MBC frequency of 3.6/10^6 B-cells, and 166 spike-specific CD4+ T-cells/10^6, and a spike-specific CD8+ T-cell response that remained stable and did not boost appreciably following the 3rd vaccination (Figure 1). Subject 2 did not seroconvert or have detectable virus-specific MBCs after their primary mRNA vaccination series; however, they had a spike-specific CD8+ T-cell response that was further boosted after a 3rd dose and a virus-specific CD4+ response that did not change following the original vaccine series or the 3rd dose of J&J.

3. Discussion

Other than subject age (60s vs 80s), the most notable difference between the subjects' baseline characteristics (Table 1) is that Subject 1 was treatment naive, while Subject 2 had undergone previous treatment (6 years ago) with obinutuzumab, an anti-CD20 mAb, and is currently on active treatment with ibrutinib since 2017. Both had baseline B-cell frequencies outside of the normal range, with Subject 1 exhibiting a low percentage of naïve B-cells (0.092) and a high percentage of MBCs (59.1), while Subject 2 had a low percentage of naïve B-cells (11.37) and MBCs (0.45). Although Subject 2 had mild hypogammaglobulinemia, neither had a history of recurring infections or a need for IgG supplementation. Levels of baseline CD4+ and CD8+ T-cells (absolute values) were also normal in each subject prior to vaccination (data not shown). Both had very low percentages of naïve B cells which could explain the initial poor response to vaccination. The significance of the increased percentage of MBCs in Subject 1 is unclear, but does suggest some broader preservation of normal B cell maturation and

TABLE 1: Baseline characteristics and demographics for subjects included in the study.

Subject ID	Age	Gender	Date of diagnosis	Current treatment	Prior treatment	IgG mg/dL	Absolute lymphocyte Count (K/mm3)	B-cells (CD19+) %	Naïve B-cells (IgD+CD27−) %	Memory B-cells (IgD−CD27+) %	B1 B-cells (CD5+CD19+) %
						(768–1632)	(1.00–4.80)	(4–17)	(50–80)	(5–21)	(<6)
1	60's	F	17/02/2014	None	None	834	21.09	76	0.092	59.1	76.18
2	80's	F	02/01/2014	Ibrutinib (2017)	Obinutuzumab × 6 cycles (completed 2015)	510	5.93	61	11.37	0.45	59.96

Note. Normal ranges for each of the B-cell subsets are in parenthesis under each B-cell type.

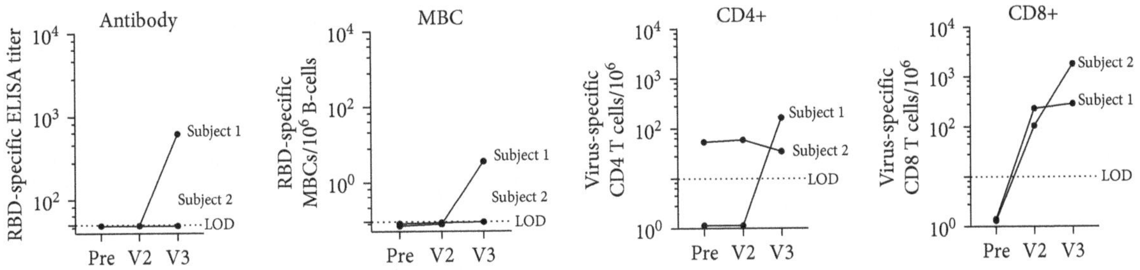

FIGURE 1: Immune response to COVID-19 vaccination in CLL subjects. RBD-specific antibody titer. Subjects without a detectable antibody titer (<1 : 50 serum dilution) were assigned a value of 49. The limit of detection (LOD) is 50. Frequency of RBD-specific MBCs per 10^6 CD19+ B-cells following ex vivo stimulation. Subjects who did not have a detectable response were assigned a value between 0.07 and 0.09. The limit of detection (LOD) is 0.1. SARS-CoV-2 spike peptide-reactive CD4 and CD8 T-cells are defined as double positive for IFNγ and TNFα cytokine secretion. Patients who did not have a detectable T-cell response were assigned an arbitrary number less than 2. The limit of detection (LOD) is 10. Visit 1 (pre) blood draw was taken 21 and 40 days prior to the Pfizer vaccine series (2-doses). Visit 2 (V2) blood draw was taken 33 and 24 days post vaccination, and Visit 3 (V3) was drawn 30 and 27 days after the 3rd vaccination with J&J.

immune function. Although Subject 1 did have an immune response, antibody levels were relatively low as compared to some of the levels observed in immunocompetent postvaccine populations [16] and certain CLL populations [4]. The clinical significance of specific antibody levels remains unknown.

Active treatment with Bruton's tyrosine kinase (BTK) inhibitors like ibrutinib may have a profound impact on B-cell survival, differentiation, and production of antibodies as the absence of intact BTK-dependent B-cell receptor mediated signaling prevents B-cells from differentiating into mature peripheral B-cells. Immune responses following vaccination or natural infection are limited in these patients [17]. Recall to antigens encountered prior to treatment appears to remain largely intact; however, response to novel antigens encountered during treatment seems to be abrogated. Subject 2 has been on ibrutinib for over four years. The impact of prolonged treatment vs. shorter-term BTK inhibition on immune responses is unknown. However, clinical data [18] suggest some improvement in humoral immunity with prolonged (>6 months) treatment. T-cells are also disrupted in individuals with CLL and even further disrupted with BTK treatment [19]. In the cases presented here, both subjects did have an increase in virus-specific CD8+ T-cells; however, the significance is unclear in terms of protection, as neutralizing antibodies are often viewed as the correlate of protection against COVID-19.

4. Conclusion

The results of this study, however small, provide initial evidence that a 3rd vaccination against COVID-19 with the heterotypic vaccine Ad26COV2.s results in an immune response that was not observed following the recommended 2-dose mRNA vaccination series. This is especially promising news to subjects who are treatment naïve, not currently in active treatment, or who may consider vaccination before beginning active treatment.

Disclosure

The funders had no involvement in study design; in the collection, analysis, and interpretation of data; in the writing of the report; or in the decision to submit the article for publication.

Authors' Contributions

Zoe L. Lyski contributed to formal analysis, investigation, and visualization, prepared the original draft, and edited and reviewed the manuscript. Myung Sun Kim was responsible for investigation, project administration, visualization, and resources. David Xthona Lee contributed to investigation and formal analysis. David Sampson was responsible for project administration and resources. Hans P. Raué contributed to formal analysis and investigation and edited and reviewed the manuscript. Vikram Raghunathan was responsible for investigation, project administration, and recourses. Debbie Ryan was responsible for project administration and resources. Amanda E. Brunton performed formal analysis and was responsible for resources. Mark K. Slifka was involved in funding acquisition and supervision and reviewed and edited the manuscript. William B. Messer was responsible for conceptualization, funding acquisition and supervision and reviewed and edited the manuscript. Stephen E. Spurgeon was responsible for conceptualization, funding acquisition, project administration, and supervision, prepared the original draft and reviewed and edited the manuscript.

Acknowledgments

The authors would like to thank the subjects for participating in this research study. This work was funded in part by the National Institute of Allergy and Infectious Diseases NIAID 1R01AI145835 (WBM), US National Institute of Health grant P51 OD011092 (MKS), and endowed funds from the Knight Cancer Institute's Scholar Award for Leukemia and Lymphoma Research (SES).

References

[1] P. Wadhwa and V. Morrison, "Infectious complications of chronic lymphocytic leukemia," *Seminars in Oncology*, vol. 33, no. 2, pp. 240–249, 2006.

[2] L. Scarfò, T. Chatzikonstantinou, G. M. Rigolin et al., "COVID-19 severity and mortality in patients with chronic lymphocytic leukemia: a joint study by ERIC, the European Research Initiative on CLL, and CLL Campus," *Leukemia*, vol. 34, no. 9, pp. 2354–2363, 2020.

[3] J. A. Whitaker, S. A. Parikh, T. D. Shanafelt et al., "The humoral immune response to high-dose influenza vaccine in persons with monoclonal B-cell lymphocytosis (MBL) and chronic lymphocytic leukemia (CLL)," *Vaccine*, vol. 39, no. 7, pp. 1122–1130, 2021.

[4] F. P. Polack, S. J. Thomas, N. Kitchin et al., "Safety and efficacy of the BNT162b2 mRNA covid-19 vaccine," *New England Journal of Medicine*, vol. 383, no. 27, pp. 2603–2615, 2020.

[5] Y. Herishanu, I. Avivi, A. Aharon et al., "Efficacy of the BNT162b2 mRNA COVID-19 vaccine in patients with chronic lymphocytic leukemia," *Blood*, vol. 137, no. 23, pp. 3165–3173, 2021.

[6] L. E. Roeker, D. A. Knorr, M. C. Thompson et al., "COVID-19 vaccine efficacy in patients with chronic lymphocytic leukemia," *Leukemia*, vol. 35, no. 9, pp. 2703–2705, 2021.

[7] Z. Lyski, M. S. Kim, D. Xthona Lee et al., "Cellular and humoral Immune response to mRNA COVID-19 vaccination in subjects with chronic lymphocytic leukemia," *medRxiv*, 2021.

[8] N. Kamar, F. Abravanel, O. Marion, C. Couat, J. Izopet, and A. Del Bello, "Three doses of an mRNA covid-19 vaccine in solid-organ transplant recipients," *New England Journal of Medicine*, vol. 385, no. 7, pp. 661-662, 2021.

[9] R. T. Shroff, P. Chalasani, R. Wei et al., "Immune responses to two and three doses of the BNT162b2 mRNA vaccine in adults with solid tumors," *Nature Medicine*, vol. 27, no. 11, pp. 2002–2011, 2021.

[10] A. Thomas, W. B. Messer, D. E. Hansel et al., "Establishment of monoclonal antibody standards for quantitative serological diagnosis of SARS-CoV-2 in low-incidence settings," *Open Forum Infectious Diseases*, vol. 8, no. 3, p. ofab061, 2021.

[11] Z. L. Lyski, A. E. Brunton, M. I. Strnad et al., "SARS-CoV-2 specific memory B-cells from individuals with diverse disease severities recognize SARS-CoV-2 variants of concern," *The Journal of Infectious Diseases*, 2021.

[12] I. J. Amanna and M. K. Slifka, "Quantitation of rare memory B cell populations by two independent and complementary approaches," *Journal of Immunological Methods*, vol. 317, no. 1-2, pp. 175–185, 2006.

[13] H. P. Raué and M. K. Slifka, "Pivotal advance: CTLA-4+ T cells exhibit normal antiviral functions during acute viral infection," *Journal of Leukocyte Biology*, vol. 81, no. 5, pp. 1165–1175, 2007.

[14] H. P. Raué and M. K. Slifka, "CD8+ T cell immunodominance shifts during the early stages of acute LCMV infection independently from functional avidity maturation," *Virology*, vol. 390, no. 2, pp. 197–204, 2009.

[15] J. Mateus, A. Grifoni, A. Tarke et al., "Selective and cross-reactive SARS-CoV-2 T cell epitopes in unexposed humans," *Science*, vol. 370, no. 6512, pp. 89–94, 2020.

[16] T. A. Bates, H. C. Leier, Z. L. Lyski et al., "Age-dependent neutralization of SARS-CoV-2 and P.1 variant by vaccine immune serum samples," *JAMA*, vol. 326, 2021.

[17] C. Pleyer, M. A. Ali, J. I. Cohen et al., "Effect of Bruton tyrosine kinase inhibitor on efficacy of adjuvanted recombinant hepatitis B and zoster vaccines," *Blood*, vol. 137, no. 2, pp. 185–189, 2021.

[18] C. Sun, X. Tian, Y. S. Lee et al., "Partial reconstitution of humoral immunity and fewer infections in patients with chronic lymphocytic leukemia treated with ibrutinib," *Blood*, vol. 126, no. 19, pp. 2213–2219, 2015.

[19] P. M. Roessner and M. Seiffert, "T-cells in chronic lymphocytic leukemia: guardians or drivers of disease?" *Leukemia*, vol. 34, no. 8, pp. 2012–2024, 2020.

31

Coexisting *BRAF*-Mutated Langerhans Cell Histiocytosis and Primary Myelofibrosis with Shared *JAK2* Mutation

Johanne Marie Holst,[1,2] Marie Beck Enemark,[1,2] Trine Lindhardt Plesner,[3] Martin Bjerregaard Pedersen,[1] Maja Ludvigsen,[1,2] and Francesco d'Amore[1,2]

[1]*Department of Hematology, Aarhus University Hospital, Palle Juul-Jensens Boulevard 35, Aarhus N 8200, Denmark*
[2]*Department of Clinical Medicine, Aarhus University, Palle Juul-Jensens Boulevard 82, Aarhus N 8200, Denmark*
[3]*Department of Pathology, Copenhagen University Hospital, Blegdamsvej 3B, København N 2200, Denmark*

Correspondence should be addressed to Johanne Marie Holst; johahols@rm.dk

Academic Editor: Stephen E. Langabeer

Langerhans cell histiocytosis (LCH) is an infrequent disease, characterized by oligoclonal proliferation of immature myeloid-derived cells. However, the exact pathogenesis remains unknown. In rare cases, LCH is present in patients with concomitant myeloid proliferative neoplasms. Here, we describe a 69-year-old male, who presented with a maculopapular rash covering truncus, face, and scalp. A cutaneous ulcerating lesion on the right cheek led to a biopsy showing LCH. Lesional cells were $BRAF^{V600E}$ and $JAK2^{V617F}$ mutated. A bone marrow aspirate showed no infiltration of Langerhans cells, but alterations consistent with primary myelofibrosis (PMF) and a polymerase chain reaction test were positive for $JAK2^{V617F}$. Our case highlights an uncommon condition of two hematological malignancies present in the same patient. The identification of the $BRAF^{V600E}$ mutation supports previous findings of this mutation in LCH. Interestingly, a $JAK2^{V617F}$ mutation was found in both LCH and PMF cells, indicating a possible clonal relationship between the two malignancies.

1. Introduction

Langerhans cell histiocytosis (LCH) is a clonal neoplastic proliferation of immature myeloid-derived cells similar to Langerhans cells [1–3]. The disease is rare and affects adults at a rate of approximately 1-2 cases per million [3, 4]. It may present as localized to a single site or occur as more disseminated disease with multiorgan involvement. The clinical course is highly related to disease stage and type of organ involvement with high survival rates in unifocal disease as opposed to multisystem disease, particularly if resistant to therapy [1]. The pathogenesis of LCH is poorly understood, but the neoplastic cells are believed to originate from immature myeloid-derived dendritic cells, similar to epidermal Langerhans cells [1, 3]. Approximately 50% of LCH cases harbor $BRAF^{V600E}$ mutations in LCH cells resulting in constitutive Ras/Raf/MEK/ERK signaling and increased mitogen-activated protein kinase (MAPK) activity [4–7]. LCH has previously been reported associated with other hematological disorders, including cases of myeloid proliferative neoplasia (MPN) [8, 9]. Here, we present a rare case presentation of $BRAF^{V600E}$-mutated LCH and coexisting primary myelofibrosis (PMF) both sharing a Janus kinase 2 $(JAK2)^{V617F}$ mutation.

2. Case Presentation

A 69-year-old man was admitted to our department after skin biopsies from the ear and right cheek (Figure 1(a)) had revealed a histopathological picture morphologically and immunohistochemically consistent with LCH (Figure 2). Due to a painless, nonitching maculo-papular rash on face, scalp, and truncus (Figure 1(b)), he was treated with phototherapy (i.e., UVB) and topical steroids by a local dermatologist for approximately one year. During the last three months prior to admission, a 2.5 cm × 2.5 cm ulcerative

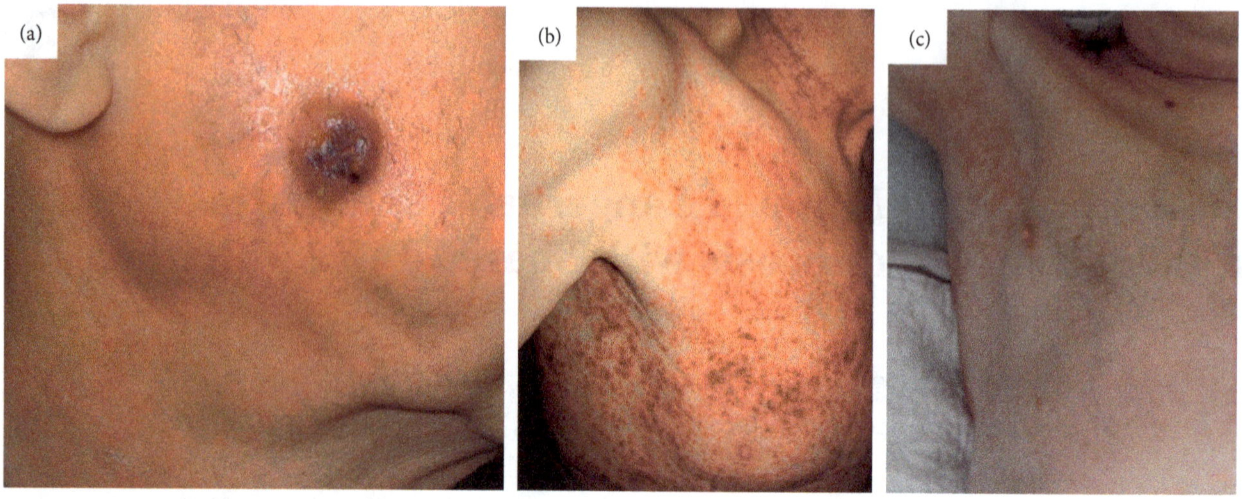

FIGURE 1: (a) Tumor localized to the cheek of the patient. (b) Painless, nonitching maculopapular rash on the patient's truncus. (c) Normalization of the skin after BRAF-inhibitor treatment.

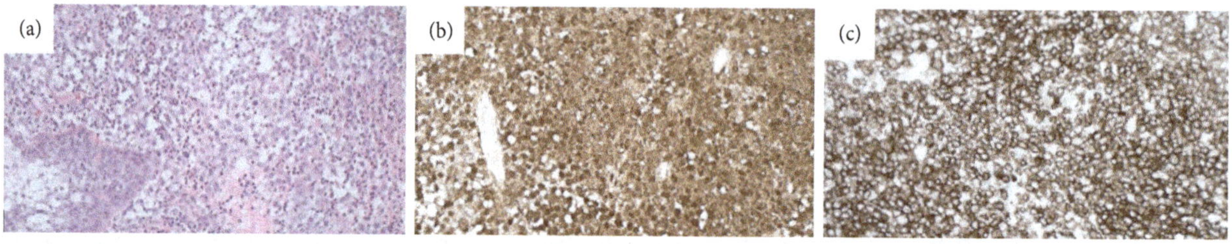

FIGURE 2: Skin sample at the time of diagnosis showing histopathological and immunohistochemical features consistent with Langerhans cell histiocytosis. (a) Haematoxylin and eosin staining (100x), and immunohistochemical staining for (b) S100 (100x) and (c) CD1a (100x).

cutaneous lesion had developed on his cheek. He had symptomatic generalized pruritus and fatigue but no night sweats, weight loss, or bone pain. Neither peripheral lymph adenopathy nor hepatosplenomegaly were found. Blood counts showed mild anemia with hemoglobin of 12.9 g/dL, a total leucocyte count of 14.5×10^9/L, and platelets of 451×10^9/L. During the following year, the patient continued to have anemia, sustained leukocytosis, and a varying level of thrombocytes. At diagnosis, serum-bilirubin, serum-aminotransferase, serum-lactate dehydrogenase, and serum-creatinine levels were normal.

Immunohistochemically, a biopsy from the skin and ear showed a tumor cell population with a strong expression of S100 and CD1a (CD207) and moderate expression of CD68 (Figures 2(b) and 2(c)). The proliferation rate of the neoplastic cells was 40% (Ki-67). Both *BRAF*^{V600E} mutation and *JAK2*^{V617F} mutation (variant allele frequency (VAF) 0.08%) were detected in the sample using a quantitative polymerase chain reaction (qPCR) assay with a sensitivity of 1% and 0.01%, respectively.

A trephine biopsy showed no evidence of LCH in the bone marrow, but the histomorphology was consistent with a chronic myeloproliferative neoplasia of PMF type (Figure 3). The bone marrow was hypercellular with an elevated number of clustered atypic megakaryocytes (large hyperlobulated in varying shapes and with large hyperchromatic nuclei). Increased reticulin and early-stage collagen fibrosis

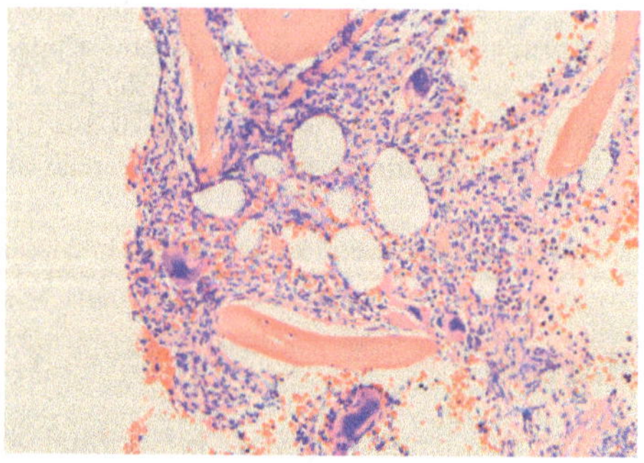

FIGURE 3: Giemsa staining of the bone marrow sample showing histopathological features consistent with primary myelofibrosis (200x).

were seen. A *JAK2*^{V617F} mutation (VAF 0.2%) was identified, while other common MPN-associated mutations in genes such as *CALR* or *MPL* were not found. No *BRAF* mutation was identified in the bone marrow.

In order to determine the extent of disease dissemination, a combined positron emission tomography-computed tomography (PET/CT) scan was performed. It revealed increased focal ^{18}F-FDG uptake localized to the right cheek lesion, a cutaneous lesion in the occipital area, a cervical lymph node, the soft tissue anterior to the pubic bone (Figure 4(a)), and several foci in pelvic bones (Figure 4(b)). Thus, the patient suffered from multifocal LCH. The CT scan

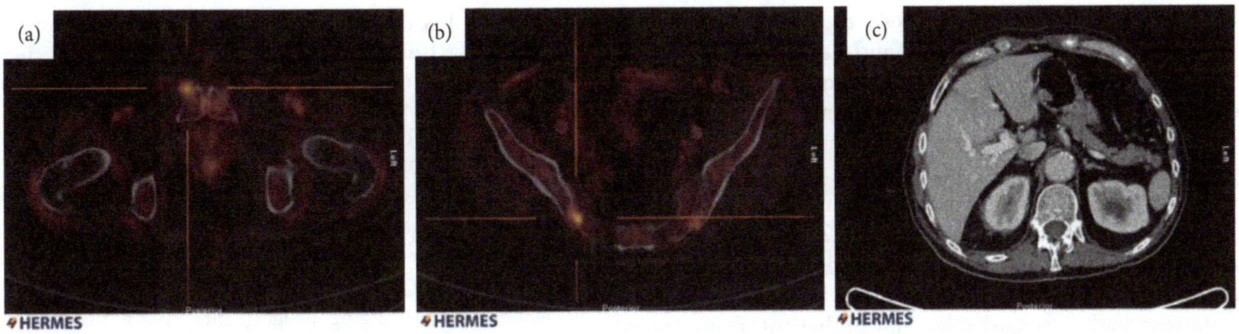

FIGURE 4: Elevated ^{18}F-FDG uptake localized corresponding to (a) the right cheek, cutaneous portion of the back head (occipital) and in one lymph node at the neck and (b) several foci in the pelvic bones, and a soft tissue process ahead of right os pubis showing increased ^{18}F-FDG activities. (c) The CT scan showing pathological edematous appearance of the kidney surrounded by adipose tissue.

revealed an edematous appearance of both kidneys surrounded by adipose tissue similar to the appearance described in patients with Erdheim–Chester disease (Figure 3(c)). However, a kidney biopsy showed no infiltration of LCH.

The patient had a medical history of multiple cardiovascular events on an atherosclerotic background including coronary bypass grafting, bypass surgery of the leg, and a cerebral insult with moderate cognitive sequelae. His medication consisted of tamsulosin, clopidogrel, and simvastatin. He was a nonsmoker and had no history of alcohol abuse.

His family history included several cases of cancer, including a brother with chronic lymphoid leukemia and a niece treated for acute lymphocytic leukemia.

The patient was treated with IV cytarabine (100 mg/m^2), which had to be prematurely discontinued due to infectious complications. The patient was mainly affected by the LCH skin alterations, and as the disease progressed, subsequently, the patient was treated with the oral BRAF-inhibitor vemurafenib for three months. This considerably improved his skin alterations (Figure 1(c)). Nine treatments of topical application of mechlorethamine were performed in the same period. Following a planned lower-extremity thrombectomy, the patient developed an acute coronary infarction. Sadly, he died of infectious complications one year after the initial diagnosis of LCH and PMF.

3. Discussion

Here, we describe the clinical, histopathological, and molecular findings in a patient who was diagnosed with two rare coexisting cancers of hematopoietic origin, i.e., LCH and PMF. While a *BRAF* mutation seemed limited to the LCH-associated lesions, a *JAK2*^{V617F} mutation was found in both the cutaneous LCH lesion and in the LCH-void, but PMF involved bone marrow. The latter observation may suggest a possible pathogenetic relationship between the two malignant conditions in this patient. To our knowledge, the occurrence of coexisting LCH and PMF has only been described once before [10]. In that report, LCH and PMF were demonstrated to share the *JAK2*^{V617F} mutation by performing a molecular genetic analysis on laser microdissected single LCH and PMF cells, suggesting a possible clonal relationship between the two cell populations.

LCH is characterized by proliferating clonal neoplastic cells with surface markers similar to those of normal Langerhans cells found in the skin [1–3]. However, the origin of the malignant cell population in LCH has been questioned [11], and a comparison of global gene and protein expression patterns between LCH cells and epidermal Langerhans cells shows surprisingly low overall correlation [12]. Furthermore, numerous of the overexpressed genes in LCH cells are known to be associated with myeloid-derived dendritic cells. Some previous reports have found LCH associated with other hematopoietic disorders, including myelo- and lymphoproliferative malignancies [8, 9, 13, 14]. It has therefore been hypothesized that mutations in common hematopoietic precursor cells may explain the development of occasional co-occurrence of two hematological diseases [8, 15]. Interestingly, Milne et al. found *BRAF*^{V600E} mutations present both in myeloid progenitors and CD34$^+$ cells from LCH patients [16]. Our finding of a shared *JAK2* mutation in the LCH and PMF lesions of our patient supports the hypothesis of common pathogenetic steps, possibly at the hematopoietic progenitor cell level, leading to the development of both diseases. Both *BRAF* and *JAK2* are genes whose regulatory impact lies upstream of the MAPK and Pi3K pathways [5, 17]. Hence, the occurrence of a shared *JAK2* mutation may suggest a concurrent development of LCH and PMF from clonally related hematopoietic progenitor cell populations.

The qPCR was performed on DNA extracted from bone marrow and skin biopsies with a substantial contribution from nonneoplastic cells. This may in part explain the low allelic frequencies of *JAK2* mutations identified in the samples. Presence of blood cells in the LCH skin biopsy resulting in identification of the same *JAK2* mutation in the LCH skin biopsy may therefore also represent a possible pitfall.

Both LCH and PMF are associated with chronic inflammation, and this may contribute to the pathophysiology in both diseases [1, 18–20]. With this case, we show interesting possible insight into the pathogenesis of LCH with the association of both the MAPK and JAK-STAT pathways, which are both involved in various immunologic and inflammatory responses. Furthermore, the identification of *BRAF*^{V600E} and constitutive MAPK and Ras/Raf/MEK/ERK signaling has contributed to the establishment of LCH as a malignant process [4, 21]. BRAF signaling is involved in various cellular functions, such as proliferation, apoptosis, angiogenesis, and survival. Accordingly, *BRAF* mutations have been associated with various cancers, e.g., hairy cell leukemia and metastatic melanoma [4, 22, 23]. The *BRAF* enzyme inhibitor vemurafenib represents an attractive novel treatment option in *BRAF*^{V600E}-mutated cancers [24]. Also, our patient had a remarkable clinical benefit from the treatment with vemurafenib leading to considerable improvement of the original facial skin alterations. The short observation period on vemurafenib treatment due to the patient's death following complications after a planned vascular surgery procedure does not allow us to evaluate whether vemurafenib also was beneficial on PMF.

4. Conclusion

In conclusion, here we describe a patient with coexisting *BRAF*^{V600E}-mutated LCH and PMF sharing a *JAK2*^{V617F} mutation. Whether a possible molecular relationship between LCH and MPN exists—and if the diseases, in some cases, share common pathologic driving events—will require further investigations on a larger number of cases, and, if possible, investigated with careful single-cell analysis.

Consent

Written consent was obtained from the patient.

Authors' Contributions

Johanne Marie Holst and Marie Beck Enemark contributed equally and share first authorship.

Acknowledgments

This work was supported by grants from Aarhus University, iLymph, SEB pension, the Danish Lymphoma Group, and the Ølufgaard P. N. Kristensen Foundation.

References

[1] B. H. Durham, "Molecular characterization of the histiocytoses: neoplasia of dendritic cells and macrophages," *Seminars in Cell & Developmental Biology*, vol. 86, pp. 62–76, 2019.

[2] C. E. Allen, M. Merad, and K. L. McClain, "Langerhans-cell histiocytosis," *New England Journal of Medicine*, vol. 379, no. 9, pp. 856–868, 2018.

[3] J.-F. Emile, O. Abla, S. Fraitag et al., "Revised classification of histiocytoses and neoplasms of the macrophage-dendritic cell lineages," *Blood*, vol. 127, no. 22, pp. 2672–2681, 2016.

[4] M. Papo, F. Cohen-Aubart, L. Trefond et al., "Systemic histiocytosis (Langerhans cell histiocytosis, erdheim-chester disease, destombes-rosai-dorfman disease): from oncogenic mutations to inflammatory disorders," *Current Oncology Reports*, vol. 21, no. 7, p. 62, 2019.

[5] G. Tran, T. N. Huynh, and A. S. Paller, "Langerhans cell histiocytosis: a neoplastic disorder driven by Ras-ERK pathway mutations," *Journal of the American Academy of Dermatology*, vol. 78, no. 3, pp. 579–590, 2018.

[6] D. J. Zinn, R. Chakraborty, and C. E. Allen, "Langerhans cell histiocytosis: emerging insights and clinical implications," *Oncology (Williston Park, N. Y.)*, vol. 30, no. 2, pp. 122–139, 2016.

[7] M. Kobayashi and A. Tojo, "Langerhans cell histiocytosis in adults: advances in pathophysiology and treatment," *Cancer Science*, vol. 109, no. 12, pp. 3707–3713, 2018.

[8] K. Kiavash and J. C. Malone, "Langerhans cell histiocytosis associated with underlying hematolymphoid disorders in adults: report of 2 cases and review of the literature," *The American Journal of Dermatopathology*, vol. 40, no. 8, pp. 588–593, 2018.

[9] T. Iwasaki, I. Takahashi, T. Nagashima et al., "Cutaneous Langerhans cell histiocytosis in elderly with chronic myelomonocytic leukemia," *The Journal of Dermatology*, vol. 41, no. 3, pp. 262–265, 2014.

[10] A. Bonometti, F. Bagnoli, D. Fanoni et al., "*JAK2*-mutated Langerhans cell histiocytosis associated with primary myelofibrosis treated with ruxolitinib," *Human Pathology*, vol. 73, pp. 171–175, 2018.

[11] M. Merad, F. Ginhoux, and M. Collin, "Origin, homeostasis and function of Langerhans cells and other langerin-expressing dendritic cells," *Nature Reviews Immunology*, vol. 8, no. 12, pp. 935–947, 2008.

[12] C. E. Allen, L. Li, T. L. Peters et al., "Cell-specific gene expression in Langerhans cell histiocytosis lesions reveals a distinct profile compared with epidermal Langerhans cells," *The Journal of Immunology*, vol. 184, no. 8, pp. 4557–4567, 2010.

[13] A. L. Feldman, F. Berthold, R. J. Arceci et al., "Clonal relationship between precursor T-lymphoblastic leukaemia/lymphoma and Langerhans-cell histiocytosis," *The Lancet Oncology*, vol. 6, no. 6, pp. 435–437, 2005.

[14] J. R. Edelbroek, M. H. Vermeer, P. M. Jansen et al., "Langerhans cell histiocytosis first presenting in the skin in adults: frequent association with a second haematological malignancy," *British Journal of Dermatology*, vol. 167, no. 6, pp. 1287–1294, 2012.

[15] S. L. Yohe, C. B. Chenault, E. E. Torlakovic, S. L. Asplund, and R. W. McKenna, "Langerhans cell histiocytosis in acute leukemias of ambiguous or myeloid lineage in adult patients: support for a possible clonal relationship," *Modern Pathology*, vol. 27, no. 5, pp. 651–656, 2014.

[16] P. Milne, V. Bigley, C. M. Bacon et al., "Hematopoietic origin of Langerhans cell histiocytosis and Erdheim-Chester disease in adults," *Blood*, vol. 130, no. 2, pp. 167–175, 2017.

[17] F. Perner, C. Perner, T. Ernst, and F. H. Heidel, "Roles of *JAK2* in aging, inflammation, hematopoiesis and malignant transformation," *Cells*, vol. 8, no. 8, 2019.

[18] F. Halbritter, M. Farlik, R. Schwentner et al., "Epigenomics and single-cell sequencing define a developmental hierarchy in Langerhans cell histiocytosis," *Cancer Discovery*, vol. 9, no. 10, pp. 1406–1421, 2019.

[19] S. Ruberti, E. Bianchi, E. Bianchi et al., "Involvement of MAF/SPP1 axis in the development of bone marrow fibrosis in PMF patients," *Leukemia*, vol. 32, no. 2, pp. 438–449, 2018.
[20] S. Koschmieder, T. I. Mughal, H. C. Hasselbalch et al., "Myeloproliferative neoplasms and inflammation: whether to target the malignant clone or the inflammatory process or both," *Leukemia*, vol. 30, no. 5, pp. 1018–1024, 2016.
[21] G. Badalian-Very, J.-A. Vergilio, B. A. Degar et al., "Recurrent *BRAF* mutations in Langerhans cell histiocytosis," *Blood*, vol. 116, no. 11, pp. 1919–1923, 2010.
[22] H. Davies, G. R. Bignell, C. Cox et al., "Mutations of the *BRAF* gene in human cancer," *Nature*, vol. 417, no. 6892, pp. 949–954, 2002.
[23] E. Tiacci, V. Trifonov, G. Schiavoni et al., "*BRAF*Mutations in hairy-cell leukemia," *New England Journal of Medicine*, vol. 364, no. 24, pp. 2305–2315, 2011.
[24] J. Haroche, F. Cohen-Aubart, J.-F. Emile et al., "Reproducible and sustained efficacy of targeted therapy with vemurafenib in patients with brafv600e-mutated erdheim-chester disease," *Journal of Clinical Oncology*, vol. 33, no. 5, pp. 411–418, 2015.

32

Bone Marrow Aspirate Clot: A Useful Technique in Diagnosis and Follow-Up of Hematological Disorders

Lucas Oliveira Cantadori,[1] **Rafael Dezen Gaiolla**,[1] **Ligia Niero-Melo**,[1] **and Cristiano Claudino Oliveira**[2,3]

[1]*São Paulo State University (UNESP), Medical School of Botucatu, Department of Internal Medicine, Botucatu, SP, Brazil*
[2]*São Paulo State University (UNESP), Medical School of Botucatu, Department of Pathology, Botucatu, SP, Brazil*
[3]*São Luiz/D'or Hospital, Department of Pathology, São Paulo, SP, Brazil*

Correspondence should be addressed to Lucas Oliveira Cantadori; lucascantadori@gmail.com

Academic Editor: Shaji Kumar

Bone marrow biopsy is a diagnostic tool largely used in the evaluation of a broad number of disorders that could affect the hematopoietic system. Differently, bone marrow aspirate clot technique is rarely performed even though it has been described in literature. Here, we highlight the utility of the bone marrow aspirate clot, exemplifying through the discussion of three clinical cases in which this technique was used for diagnosis and follow-up purposes: megaloblastic hemopathy, multiple myeloma, and chronic lymphocytic leukemia. Bone marrow clot analysis increases sensitivity to diagnose hemopathies and offers the possibility of morphological evaluation and anatomopathological study, with the advantage of not needing decalcification processes, hence improving antigenic expression in immunohistochemical and FISH techniques. It is an easy-to-perform technique, offering a quick, reliable, and more comfortable procedure for patients.

1. Introduction

Bone marrow (BM) evaluation is essential for the diagnosis of primary hemopathies, neoplastic or not, and other diseases that may occur with hematological repercussion. Moreover, this analysis is mandatory for lymphoma staging and can also provide material for analysis of potential prognostic and predictive factors that could drive treatment in specific diseases. BM evaluation is important, for example, for the setting of cytogenetic and molecular profile in acute leukemia or multiple myeloma and the continuous assessment of these pathologies [1, 2].

The procedure usually results in an aspirate sample and a bone fragment sample (trephine biopsy). A smear (myelogram) is obtained from the aspirate for a qualitative and quantitative cytological assessment of BM cells. This material can also be used for flow cytometry, conventional and molecular cytogenetics, and microbiological exam when infections are suspected. The bone fragment is technically processed for histopathologic and immunophenotypic analysis by immunohistochemistry (IHC) allowing not only the morphological assessment but also an analysis of BM architecture, based mainly on the relationships established between the hematopoietic tissue and bone trabeculae and central sinusoids and the grade of extracellular matrix deposition. [2, 3].

It is important to point out that, in Brazil, the analysis of the myelogram is restricted to hematologists, whereas the analysis of the trephine biopsy (bone fragment) is a pathologist's responsibility.

After performing the myelogram, the resulting clot from this procedure is commonly discarded although it may also be utilized for histopathological evaluation with IHC and molecular research studies, for example, *in situ* hybridization technique [4, 5], which allows, therefore, the histological evaluation to supplement the cytological analysis and broadens exam sensitivity.

BM aspirate clot (BMC) technique is not frequently utilized in medical practice. Even though it has been described in the literature, few studies evaluated its applicability in the diagnosis and follow-up of several hematological diseases.

In this article, the technique to make BMC will be described and its practical applicability will be shown through the description of three clinical cases.

2. Materials and Methods

2.1. Trephine Biopsy and Bone Marrow Aspirate Technique. Bone marrow biopsy is done in the posterior iliac crest while the patient is in right or left lateral decubitus position. In this procedure, sedation is optional. After asepsis and antisepsis, local anesthesia with xylocaine 1% without a vasoconstrictor is applied. The most used needle is an 11-*gauge* Jamshidi needle which is inserted perpendicularly to the bone surface from the posterior iliac crest and directed to the anterior iliac crest, avoiding the needle penetration in the sacroiliac component. The aim is to collect a bone fragment that is approximately 1.5 cm long, which is firstly stored in a flask with buffer formaldehyde at 10% and then processed with a decalcification period which is a critical step to guarantee materials with conditions for evaluation and utilization of complementary techniques [1].

Bone marrow aspirate for myelogram and aspirate clot is done preferably in the sternum manubrium (in adults) with the patient in dorsal decubitus position. However, caution should be taken in cases of multiple myeloma due to the higher risk of sternum perforation. In these cases, the aspiration is preferably done in the posterior iliac crest, right before the bone marrow biopsy. Sedation is usually not needed. After asepsis and antisepsis, local anesthesia with xylocaine 1% without a vasoconstrictor is applied. There are several needles available in the market, all disposable ones. The currently utilized model in our service is an 18-*gauge* needle by 90 millimeters (18G × 90 mm). The needle is inserted perpendicularly to the medium point of the sternum manubrium, 1 cm above the angle of Louis. After needle fixation, the spindle is removed to couple a 5-ml syringe and aspirate the maximum amount from 1 to 2 ml of bone marrow, avoiding sample hemodilution. Next, the smear is prepared for a total of 6 slides, and the rest of the exceeding material is separated on an extra slide until coagulation. If extra material is needed for other exams (BM karyotype, for instance), a new syringe is coupled to the needle and aspiration is done without new punctures.

2.2. Bone Marrow Aspirate Clot Processing Technique. After a bone marrow aspirate, the material left on the extra slide must be placed, after coagulation, in a flask with buffer formaldehyde at 10% or Bouin liquid similarly to the procedures in other biopsy handlings (Figure 1). The technique is quite similar to the cell-block procedure after fine-needle aspiration.

Once the material is fixed, the same procedure for a common biopsy is followed. Briefly, it is measured in macroscopy, placed in a cassette and submitted to five alcohol baths, followed by five xylol baths and, finally, impregnated with paraffin. The whole procedure is done overnight. Afterwards, the sample is removed from the cassette and immersed in liquid paraffin at 60°C, forming a paraffin block. Slides are made from 3- to 4-millimicron cuts of this block.

The cuts are stained according to the standard staining of our service which is hematoxylin and eosin (H&E), Perls (or prussian blue stain), and reticulin. It is noteworthy to point out that reticulin staining, even without the presence of bone support, results in excellent-quality slides for visualization and quantification. Specific immunohistochemical staining is carried out accordingly when indicated.

2.3. Clinical Cases. In order to exemplify the clinical applicability of the described technique, samples of bone marrow clot at the time of the diagnosis of three different patients attended in the Hematology Service of the Clinical Hospital of Botucatu Medical School, UNESP, in Brazil, will be presented.

In all three patients, both the diagnosis and follow-up assessment were based only on bone marrow aspirate clot technique.

3. Results

3.1. Case 1. A 78-year-old woman was referred from the internal medicine due to symptoms of progressive fatigue, tiredness at small efforts, and intermittent claudication. During physical exam, she presented paleness and atrophic glossitis. Hemogram with pancytopenia and macrocytosis and high lactate dehydrogenase (LDH) (Figure 2).

3.2. Case 2. An 87-year-old man was checked in the emergency room presenting symptoms of mental confusion, tiredness at small efforts, and intense lumbar pain. During physical exam, he was clumsy and dehydrated. Lab exams showed he had anemia, hypercalcemia, and renal insufficiency. X-rays showed multiple lytic lesions in the axial skeleton (Figure 3).

3.3. Case 3. This is the case of a 65-year-old man, undergoing clinical follow-up due to lymphocytosis and thrombocytopenia in routine exams, and is asymptomatic (Figure 4).

4. Discussion

Conventional trephine bone marrow biopsies have bone trabeculae, requiring material decalcification before histological processing. Decalcification process is the removal of mineral from the bone tissue with the utilization of chemical agents in order to submit the tissue to histotechnical chelation in microtome.

The mineralization level of tissue bone directly influences decalcification protocols. It takes longer to decalcify bones with high mineral density. Time and the utilized chemical agent can damage the tissue either a lot or less, leading to quality loss in the cell analysis of different staining, immunohistochemistry, and/or molecular techniques.

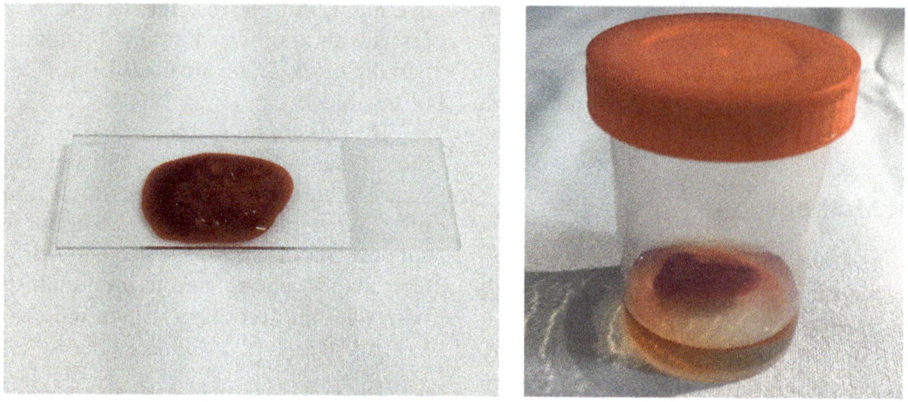

(a) (b)

FIGURE 1: Sample of bone marrow clot after bone marrow aspirate harvest. (a) Material after harvest placed on a slide. (b) After clot formation, the material is fixed in buffer formaldehyde at 10% and processed conventionally with the advantage of dismissing decalcification.

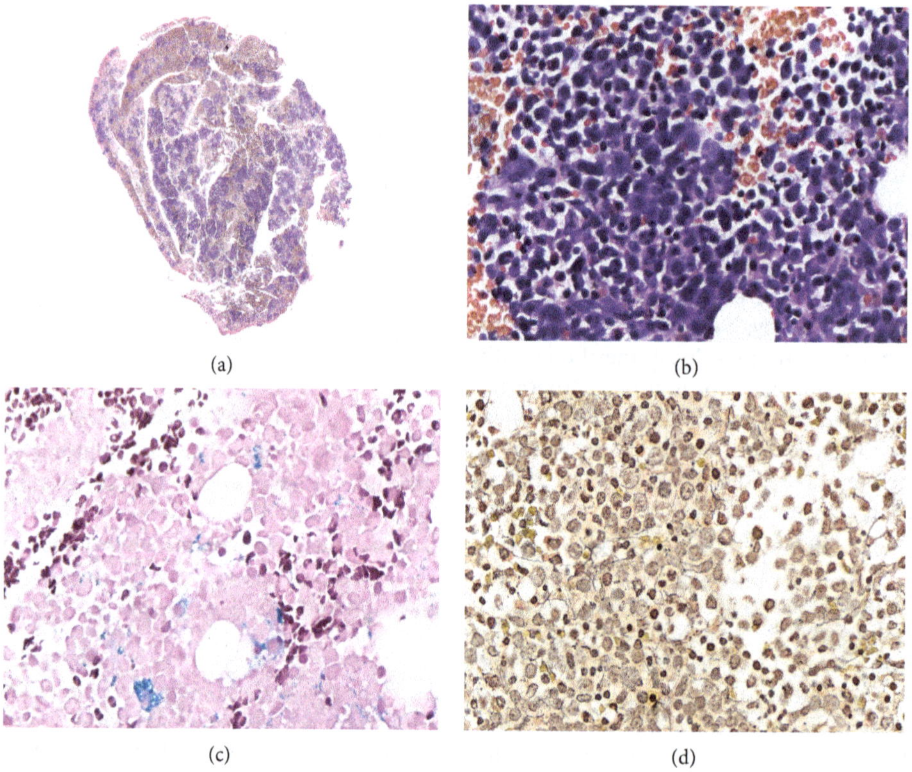

FIGURE 2: Case 1. The patient with final diagnosis of megaloblastic hemopathy (pernicious anemia). (a) Microscopic panoramic image to show the general aspect of BMC (H&E, 10x). Each grouping of hematopoietic material is called spicule. Five spicules are necessary to consider a material representative for analysis. The utilized criteria to render MC are the same used to interpret BMB. (b) Erythroid hyperplasia with numerous megaloblasts (H&E, 400x). (c) Demonstration of histochemical staining application on MC (Perls, 400x). In the image, hemosiderin deposits are stained blue. (d) Application of reticulin histochemical staining on MC (reticulin, 400x). Reticulin fibers are stained black. It is possible to evaluate this network with this technique similarly to BMB.

In bone marrow biopsy, the fragment is delicate with trabeculae that are little thickened and in which the hematopoietic, adipose, and bone tissues are closely related and have different distribution patterns. In normal hematopoiesis or in disease setting, the bone marrow analysis depends on the evaluation of these components individually or together.

The biological nature of these elements is very different among themselves and, although in bone marrow biopsy the main aim is to analyze the hematopoietic tissue, its architectural relationship with the bone component takes an important place as well. Thus, the decalcification of this material is quite challenging since it is necessary to apply a technique that allows to cut bone

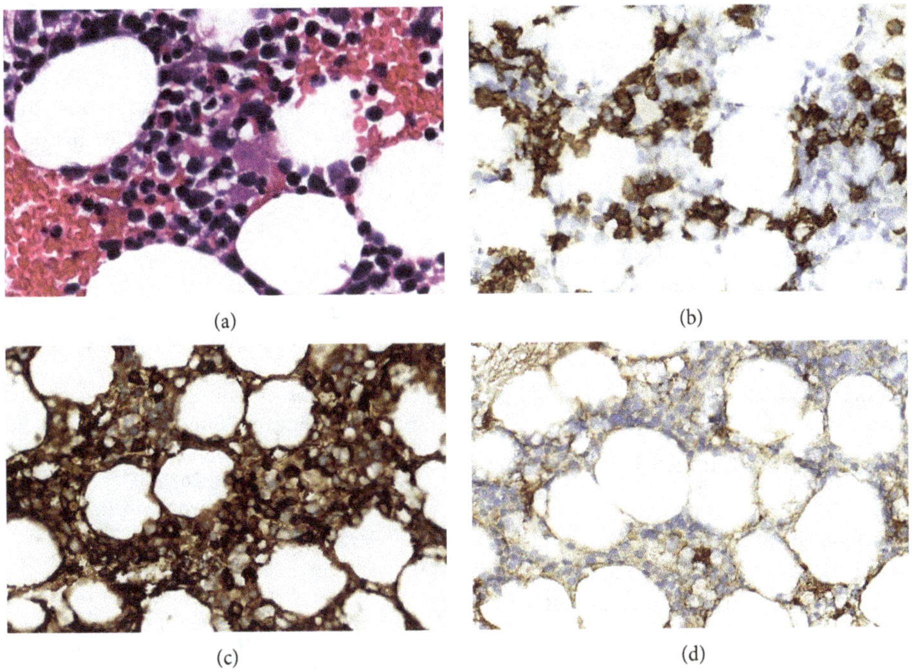

FIGURE 3: Case 2. The patient with final diagnosis of multiple myeloma. (a) Histological section showing a small grouping of plasmocytes in the middle (H&E, 400x). (b) Utilization of IHC to detect, confirm, and quantify plasmocytes (IHQ, CD138, 400x). Resource applied for diagnosis and posttreatment reevaluations. IHC evaluation confirming that plasmocytes present restriction of immunoglobulin light kappa chain, indicating the diagnosis of multiple myeloma: (c) (kappa, 400x) and (d) (lambda, 400x).

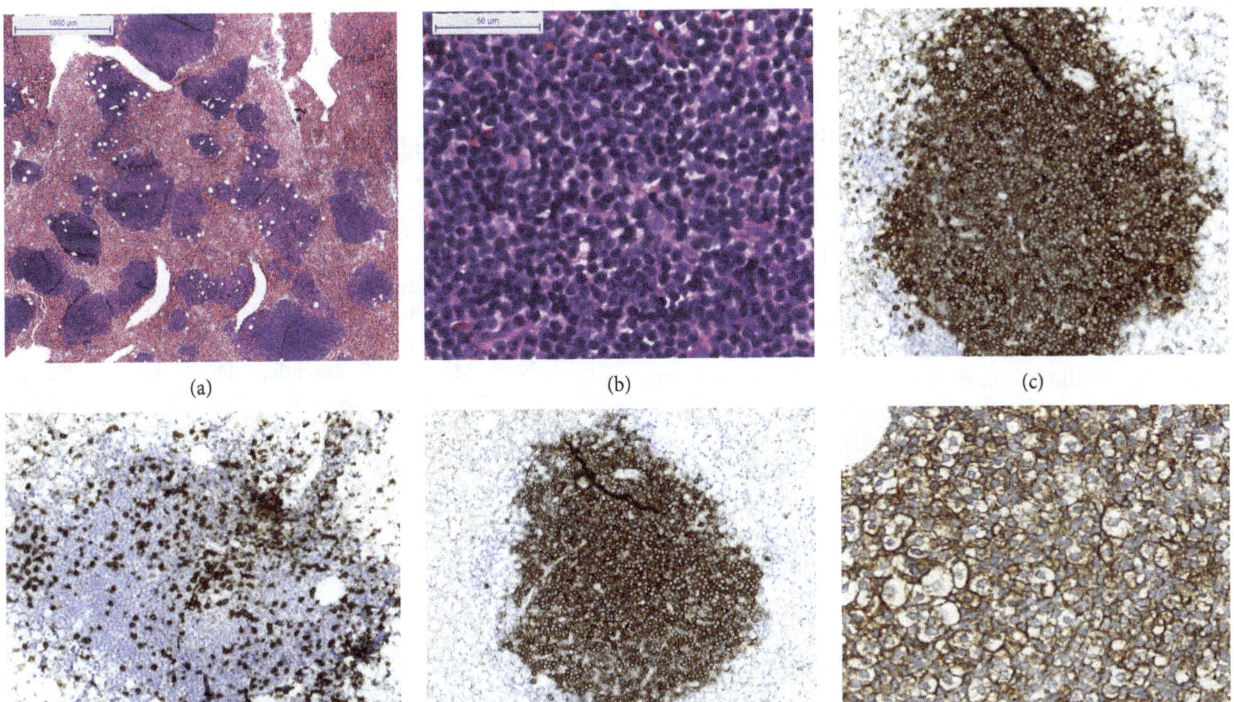

FIGURE 4: Case 3. The patient with final diagnosis of chronic lymphocytic leukemia (CLL). (a) BMC, in small magnification, showing intense hypercellularity of bone marrow with lymphoid accumulation (H&E, 40x). (b) Cell details, characterizing lymphocytes as small and typical of this neoplasia with hyperchromatic nuclei and regular membrane (H&E, 400x). (c) Immunopositivity for CD20, confirming B-cell origin of the neoplasia (IHC, CD20, 200x). (d) Contrast in lymphoid accumulation, showing a small percentage of T lymphocytes (IHC, CD3, 200x). (e) Immunopositivity overlapping for CD5 in neoplastic B cells (IHC, CD5, 200x). (f) Immunopositivity for CD23 allows diagnosis of CLL (IHQ, CD23, 200x). Note the quality of immunostaining in the images. In BMB samples, due to calcification, color irregularities can compromise analysis and make precise diagnostics sometimes difficult.

trabeculae without influencing negatively the morphological, immunophenotypical, and molecular evaluations of the hematopoietic tissue.

There are different options available to perform this decalcification. The main examples are

(a) nitric oxide (NO_3 10%)

(b) formic acid 25% with sodium citrate

(c) hydrochloric acid (HCl 10%) associated with EDTA (ethylene diamine tetra acetic acid) and potassium sodium tartrate

(d) HCl 3.5%

(e) HCl 3.5% associated with EDTA and potassium sodium tartrate

(f) EDTA 10% in pH 8.0 and adjusted with sodium hydroxide

The targeted histological cut in the microtome is 3.0-millimicron thick. In general, the most successful decalcification protocols with the smallest cell damage for complementary exams are those that apply EDTA with hydrochloric acid.

Bone marrow aspirate clot (BMC) is an alternative to this methodology because it does not need decalcification. The clot allows the same kind of histological evaluation as bone marrow biopsy, except for the analysis of architectural relationship between parenchyma/bone. The hematopoietic tissue is enriched in the clot exam, allowing adequate cuts, utilization of several histochemical staining, and/or immunophenotypical evaluation and/or molecular analysis [5, 6]

When compared to BMB, BMC presents better antigenic expression in IHC techniques, mainly because it does not need decalcification procedure. Moreover, in situ hybridization techniques showed better results in BMC [5].

Although occasionally BMC isolated analysis is not enough to diagnose architectural alterations of bone marrow, its use results in complementary data to myelogram and BMB and may substitute the latter in cases of immediate unavailability of the exam, technical difficulty in accessing the bone, or regarding the patient's comfort if multiple evaluations are necessary for the follow-up of hematological diseases [3, 7]. Therefore, it is advantageous with histological characterization from a single anesthesia event and single bone marrow puncture.

Due to its complementarity with BMB, BMC increases sensitivity to diagnose hemopathies because it provides an additional site for anatomopathological analysis, which is especially useful for lymphoma staging [8]. Moreover, BMC allows histological evaluation and pathologist's opinion in clinical contexts in which BMB is not routinely done, such as in megaloblastic hemopathies and immune-mediated thrombocytopenic purpura [9]. Our service experience for more than 4 decades using BMC confirms the validity of this procedure for diagnosis, many times fortunate ones, which would be seen only in BMB (e.g., granulomas, lymphoid aggregates, necrosis focus, edema, and megakaryocyte clustering) [9].

Therefore, BMC represents a simpler technique without the need of additional analgesia but local anesthesia, in which a quick bone marrow aspirate offers the possibility of not only morphological evaluation but also anatomopathological analysis equivalent to BMB, speeding up the diagnosis and improving the patient's comfort.

References

[1] R. S. Riley, D. Williams, M. Ross et al., "Bone marrow aspirate and biopsy: a pathologist's perspective. II. interpretation of the bone marrow aspirate and biopsy," *Journal of Clinical Laboratory Analysis*, vol. 23, no. 5, pp. 259–307, 2009.

[2] J. D. Cotelingam, "Bone marrow biopsy: interpretive guidelines for the surgical pathologist," *Advances in Anatomic Pathology*, vol. 10, no. 1, pp. 8–26, 2003.

[3] B. J. Bain, "Bone marrow aspiration," *Journal of Clinical Pathology*, vol. 54, no. 9, pp. 657–663, 2001.

[4] K. Matsue, Y. Matsue, K. Kumata et al., "Quantification of bone marrow plasma cell infiltration in multiple myeloma: usefulness of bone marrow aspirate clot with CD138 immunohistochemistry," *Hematological Oncology*, vol. 35, no. 3, pp. 323–328, 2017.

[5] R. N. Miranda, H. F. L. Mark, and L. J. Medeiros, "Fluorescent in situ hybridization in routinely processed bone marrow aspirate clot and core," *Biopsy Sections*, vol. 145, no. 6, pp. 1309–1314, 1994.

[6] M. G. Ong, M. Lowery-Nordberg, S. Pillarisetti, D. Veillon, and J. Cotelingam, "Maximizing the diagnostic yield from bone marrow aspirate material using the cell block technique on clot sections," *Laboratory Medicine*, vol. 46, no. 1, pp. e24–e27, 2015.

[7] E. E. Torlakovic, R. K. Brynes, E. Hyjek et al., "ICSH guidelines for the standardization of bone marrow immunohistochemistry," *International Journal of Laboratory Hematology*, vol. 37, no. 4, pp. 431–449, 2015.

[8] J. W. Dee, M. Valdivieso, and B. Drewinko, "Comparison of the efficacies of closed trephine needle biopsy, aspirated paraffin-embedded clot section, and smear preparation in the diagnosis of bone-marrow involvement by lymphoma," *American Journal of Clinical Pathology*, vol. 65, no. 2, pp. 183–194, 1976.

[9] L. Niero-Melo, L. S. R. Resende, R. D. Gaiolla et al., "Guidelines for morphological diagnosis of myelodysplastic syndromes," *Revista Brasileira de Hematologia e Hemoterapia*, vol. 28, no. 3, pp. 167–174, 2006.

33

Systemic Relapse in a Young Adult Patient with Primary CNS Diffuse Large B-Cell Lymphoma

Adam Khorasanchi,[1] Zachary Benson,[1] Misty Hall,[2] Nelya Ebadirad,[3] Mohammad H. Gharavi,[3] Patrick Willard,[1] Miranda Chimzar,[4] John McKay,[1] Gary Simmons,[1,5] and Victor Yazbeck[1,5]

[1]*Department of Internal Medicine, Virginia Commonwealth University, Richmond, VA, USA*
[2]*Department of Pathology, Virginia Commonwealth University, Richmond, VA, USA*
[3]*Department of Radiology, Virginia Commonwealth University, Richmond, VA, USA*
[4]*School of Medicine, Virginia Commonwealth University, Richmond, VA, USA*
[5]*Massey Cancer Center, Virginia Commonwealth University, Richmond, VA, USA*

Correspondence should be addressed to Victor Yazbeck; vyyazbeck@vcu.edu

Academic Editor: Kostas Konstantopoulos

Primary central nervous system diffuse large B-cell lymphoma (PCNS-DLBCL) is a rare form of non-Hodgkin's lymphoma, characterized by an aggressive disease course. While CNS relapse is common, systemic relapse is rare with no consensus on optimal treatment. This paper presents an unusual case of advanced PCNS-DLBCL with systemic relapse, including adrenal gland involvement. A review of the existing literature and a discussion on the management of systemic relapse in PCNS-DLBCL is also provided.

1. Introduction

Primary central nervous system lymphoma (PCNSL) is a rare and aggressive form of non-Hodgkin's lymphoma (NHL) confined to the brain, eyes, spinal cord, leptomeninges, or cranial nerves. [1] 90% to 95% are classified histologically as diffuse large B-cell lymphoma (PCNS-DLBCL) [2]. High-dose methotrexate (HD-MTX) based induction chemotherapy is the preferred first-line treatment. Despite high response rates to initial treatment, up to 60% of patients eventually relapse, with no standardized salvage regimen [3]. Patients with relapsed disease have an extremely poor prognosis with a median survival of 2 months without additional treatment [4].

While CNS relapse is common, systemic relapse is rare, occurring in 7–10% of patients and also represents a major therapeutic challenge [5]. Novel insights into the pathophysiology of PCNSL have identified the B-cell receptor (BCR) pathway as a key mechanism in the pathogenesis of PCNS-DLBCL. The use of targeted agents, such as ibrutinib and immunomodulatory drugs, has demonstrated promising clinical activity and offers additional therapeutic options in patients with relapsed/refractory disease [4].

This paper reports an unusual case of advanced PCNS-DLBCL with systemic relapse, including adrenal gland involvement. A review of the existing literature and a discussion on the management of systemic relapse in PCNS-DLBCL is also provided.

2. Case Report

A 23-year-old African-American male presented to our clinic following a diagnosis of relapsed CNS lymphoma (Figures 1 and 2). The patient's initial workup showed no evidence of systemic lymphoma. The patient had a history of Wolff–Parkinson White syndrome (WPW) and PCNS-DLBCL (nongerminal center B-cell-like (non-GCB) subtype, Figure 3), and had previously been treated with

HD-MTX-based induction chemotherapy and an autologous stem cell transplant (ASCT). The patient maintained a complete response (CR) for 12 months prior to the diagnosis of CNS relapse. The patient was treated according to the radiation therapy oncology group (RTOG) 0227 protocol of preirradiation chemotherapy with HD-MTX, rituximab, and temozolomide for 6 cycles, followed by low-dose whole-brain radiation (WBRT) and postirradiation temozolomide. Posttreatment magnetic resonance imaging (MRI) showed no evidence of CNS disease. One year following therapy, the patient presented to the hospital with complaints of right upper quadrant abdominal pain and emesis. Imaging showed new bilateral adrenal masses. The biopsy demonstrated diffuse lymphoid infiltrate with extensive necrosis on hematoxylin and eosin (H&E) staining. Immunohistochemistry (IHC) detected PAX5+ and CD20+ cells (Figure 4), consistent with systemic relapse from his initial CNS lymphoma. Positron emission and computed tomography (PET-CT) showed increased tracer uptake of bilateral adrenal glands with a small mass inferior to the right adrenal gland (Figure 5). Given the non-GCB subtype, the patient was started on ibrutinib 560 mg daily as a bridge to chimeric antigen receptor T-cell therapy (CAR-T). The lymphodepleting regimen, fludarabine 30 mg/m^2/d and cyclophosphamide 300 mg/m^2/d, was administered for 3 days followed by an infusion of 3.6×10^8 CAR-T cells/kg tisagenlecleucel (Kymriah). The patient's hospital course was complicated by supraventricular tachycardia associated with WPW and grade 1 cytokine release syndrome on day +6, requiring supportive treatment [6]. The patient achieved a complete metabolic response (CMR) on day +60 by PET-CT and MRI with a Deauville score of 3 (Figure 5). Unfortunately, on day +90 the patient was hospitalized with right hip pain and relapsed again with a right psoas mass biopsy proven DLBCL. The patient was treated with radiotherapy (total 36 Gy) to the psoas mass, but this was discontinued due to interval enlargement of the mass and the development of new confluent celiac lymphadenopathy. Next, the patient was started on salvage chemo-immunotherapy with rituximab-ifosfamide, carboplatin and etoposide (R-ICE), as a bridge to an allogeneic stem cell transplant. Following four cycles of R-ICE, the patient achieved near complete resolution of the psoas mass on PET-CT but developed worsening dizziness with a new right cerebellar mass on MRI. This was treated with radiotherapy (total 36 Gy) and one cycle of HD-MTX. Unfortunately, posttreatment MRI showed multiple new lesions in the hypothalamus, lateral ventricles, and enlargement of a known right subcortical parietal mass. The patient died from disease progression on day +310, nearly four years following the initial diagnosis.

3. Discussion

PCNS-DLBCL is characterized by an aggressive disease course and overall long-term survival rates that range from 20% to 40% [5]. Age, performance status, lactate dehydrogenase levels, and elevated cerebrospinal fluid protein are variables used in prognostic models [7]. Risk factors include immunodeficiency states, such as HIV infection. Mutations in the B-cell receptor and Toll-like signaling receptor pathways promote tumor development [7]. Histopathologic examination typically reveals perivascular cuffing of neoplastic cells with an almost constant expression of pan-B-cell markers (CD19, CD20, CD22, and CD79a) on IHC [1]. B-cell lymphoma 6 (BCL6) positivity is seen in 60% of tumors and has been associated with a worse prognosis. Interferon regulatory factor 4/multiple myeloma oncogene 1 and BCL2 are positive in 95% of tumors. Increased MYC expression is also common [7]. Two distinct molecular subtypes of PCNS-DLBCL exist: GCB and non-GCB, with the non-GCB subtype (>85%) being more common and associated with poor overall survival (OS) [8, 9].

Commonly reported symptoms in patients with PCNS-DLBCL include focal neurologic deficits, neuropsychiatric symptoms, and signs of elevated intracranial pressure such as headache, nausea, and vomiting [3]. The classic "B" symptoms are rarely seen [4]. Lesions on contrast-enhanced MRI are often periventricular and involve the deep white matter, basal ganglia, or corpus callosum [3]. A definitive diagnosis of PCNS-DLBCL requires a brain biopsy. An ophthalmic exam, lumbar puncture, whole body PET/CT, and bone marrow examination are recommended to rule out systemic disease [4, 7].

Management of frontline PCNS-DLBCL involves a multimodal approach including chemotherapy, stem cell transplantation, and/or radiotherapy [10]. The role of surgery is limited to diagnostic purposes due to the diffuse and infiltrative disease nature [3]. While PCNS-DLBCL is extremely sensitive to radiotherapy, this modality alone is no longer recommended for initial treatment, given the lack of durable responses and increased risk of neurotoxicity [10]. However, WBRT remains a reasonable alternative in the frontline setting for: (1) patients who are not candidates for HD-MTX-based induction; (2) in the consolidation setting; or (3) as salvage therapy in patients who have not responded adequately to induction chemotherapy [10].

The first step in the management of PCNS-DLBCL is induction chemotherapy with the goal of achieving a complete radiographic response [11]. A HD-MTX-based regimen is the preferred first-line induction therapy for newly diagnosed cases. Following induction therapy, most patients require consolidation treatment to eliminate residual disease and prolong overall survival (OS) [11]. If CR is achieved, consolidation options include: (1) high-dose chemotherapy with ASCT (in younger patients and patients with adequate organ function), (2) high-dose cytarabine with etoposide, (3) low-dose WBRT, or (4) continuous monthly HD-MTX after induction therapy. If residual disease is present, WBRT is recommended [12]. Ongoing trials that randomly assign patients to different consolidation treatments will hopefully shed more light on the optimal consolidation regimen. In addition, age and response to induction therapy should be used to guide the choice of consolidation [2].

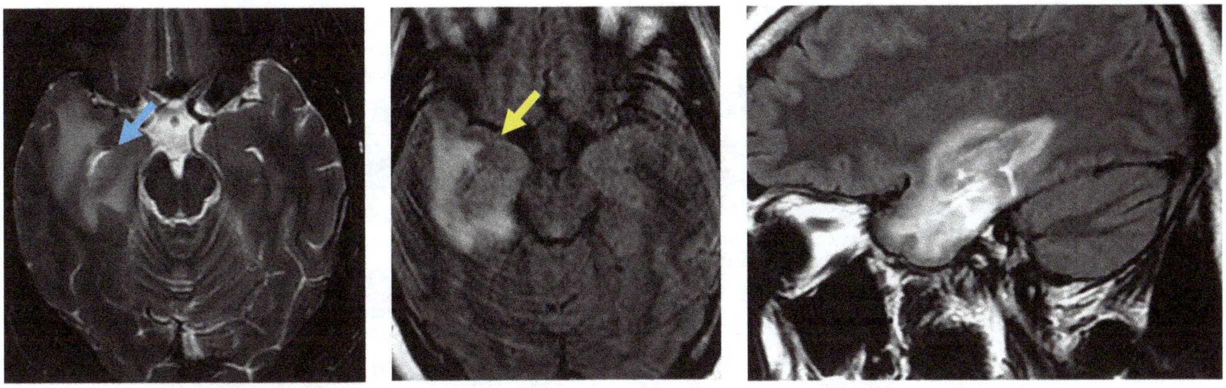

(a) (b) (c)

FIGURE 1: Axial T2-weighted (a), axial FLAIR (b), and sagittal FLAIR (c) views of MRI brain showing CNS relapse. Images show T2 isointense-hypointense signal in right inferior temporal lobe with peripheral edema causing expansion of the uncus (yellow arrow) without mass effect on temporal horn of right lateral ventricle (blue arrow).

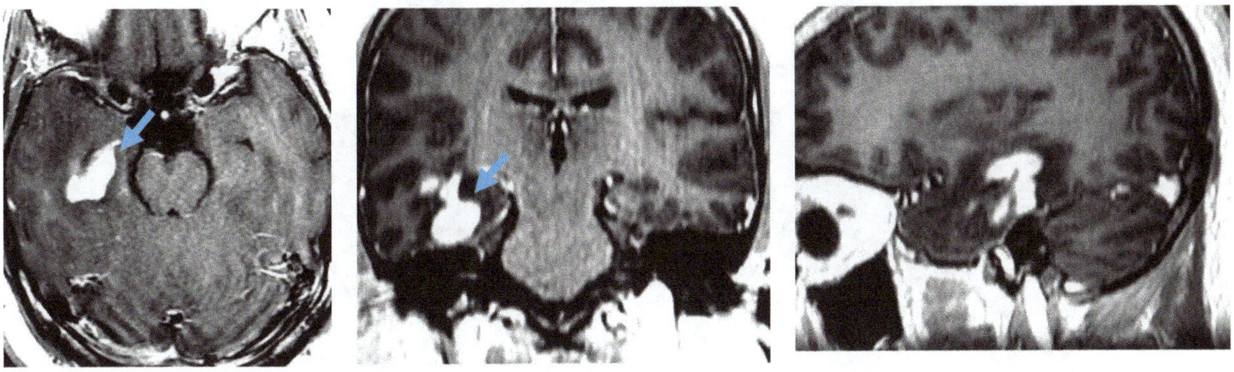

(a) (b) (c)

FIGURE 2: Contrast-enhanced axial (a), coronal (b), and sagittal (c) views of MRI brain showing CNS relapse. Images reveal homogenous enhancement (blue arrows) in periventricular tissues of right temporal lobe.

Despite such therapy, nearly 50% of patients relapse with a median time to relapse of 10–18 months [4]. There is no consensus on optimal treatment following relapse. The choice of salvage treatment depends on age, previous treatment and response, performance status, relapse site (CNS vs. systemic), and comorbidities. Salvage treatment for CNS relapse may include chemotherapy, radiotherapy, stem cell transplantation, or immunotherapy [10]. For MTX-sensitive disease, retreatment with HD-MTX-based regimens should be considered, especially if relapse occurred more than one year after a HD-MTX-based regimen [3]. In a retrospective analysis, rechallenge with HD-MTX led to a significant overall response rate (ORR) of 85–91%, with a median OS of 41–62 months [13, 14]. High-dose cytarabine, either alone or used in combination, has been associated with CR rates of 40–70% [15–19]. Modest activity has also been observed with single-agent bendamustine in a study of 12 patients with relapsed PCNSL with half of the patients responding [20]. Our patient's initial CNS relapse was treated as per the RTOG 0227 protocol. Results from this study for previously untreated PCNSL demonstrated a two year OS rate of 80.8% and a 51% CR with minimal rates of neurotoxicity [21].

While most patients experience CNS relapse, systemic relapse is rarely observed, as seen in our patient with adrenal and psoas involvement [22]. Additional sites of systemic relapse reported in the literature include musculoskeletal, testicular, kidney, and liver involvement [23]. Interestingly, there are few published cases of adrenal relapse. Ma et al. described a patient found to have bilateral adrenal involvement of their PCNS-DLBCL following MTX-based chemotherapy and WBRT, who was started on rituximab-hyper CVAD and then transitioned to R-CHOP [5]. In patients found to have bilateral adrenal involvement, primary adrenal lymphoma (PAL) with secondary CNS involvement should also be considered in the differential [5]. In fact, adrenal involvement has been found to be highly associated with CNS relapse risk and is one of the criteria used in the CNS international prognostic index for DLBCL [24]. Our patient's adrenal biopsy results showed non-GCB subtype which was consistent with his prior PCNSL, and therefore confirmed secondary rather than primary adrenal involvement.

Management of systemic relapse in PCNS-DLBCL is challenging given its rarity and lack of effective treatment options. Patients with systemic relapse in PCNSL-DLBCL

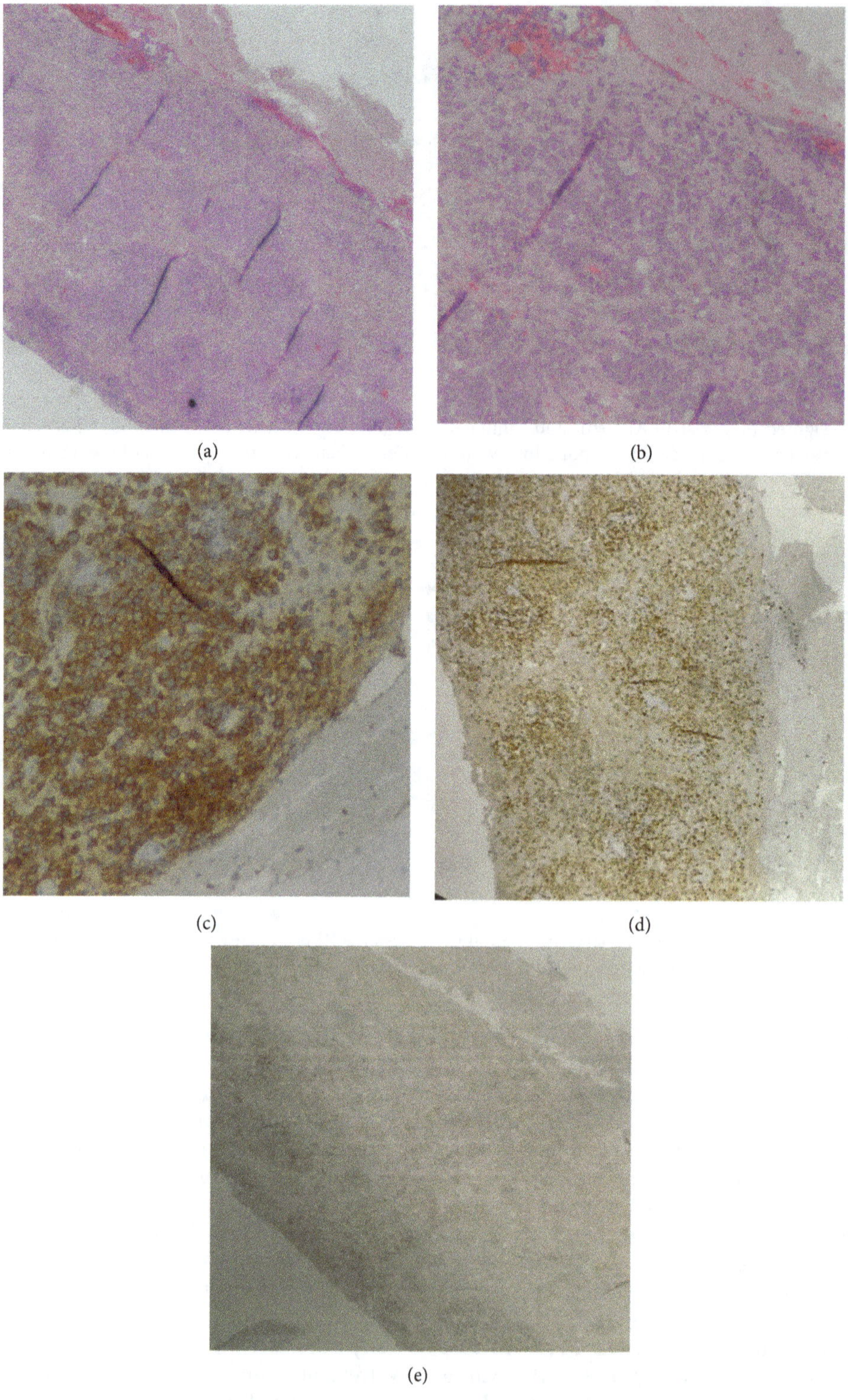

FIGURE 3: Parietal core brain biopsy of initial PCNSL mass. *H* and *E* stain showing neural tissue with infiltration of large round blue cells at 40x (a) and 100x (b). Positive CD20 stain highlighting the infiltration of large round blue cells at 100x (c). Positive MUM1 (d) and negative CD10 stains (e) supporting non-GCB subtype.

are treated similarly to those with relapsed systemic DLBCL [23]. Myeloablative chemotherapy and ASCT are considered important components in first-line and later therapy [25]. Allogeneic stem cell transplant may also be curative and remains an option for patients who relapse following ASCT [25]. An emerging new treatment option for systemic relapse is CAR-T-cell therapy. Studies of anti-CD19 CAR-T cells in relapsed systemic DLBCL have shown up to 50% CR and durable remission [26–28]. Due to safety concerns with immune effector cell associated neurotoxicity and unclear

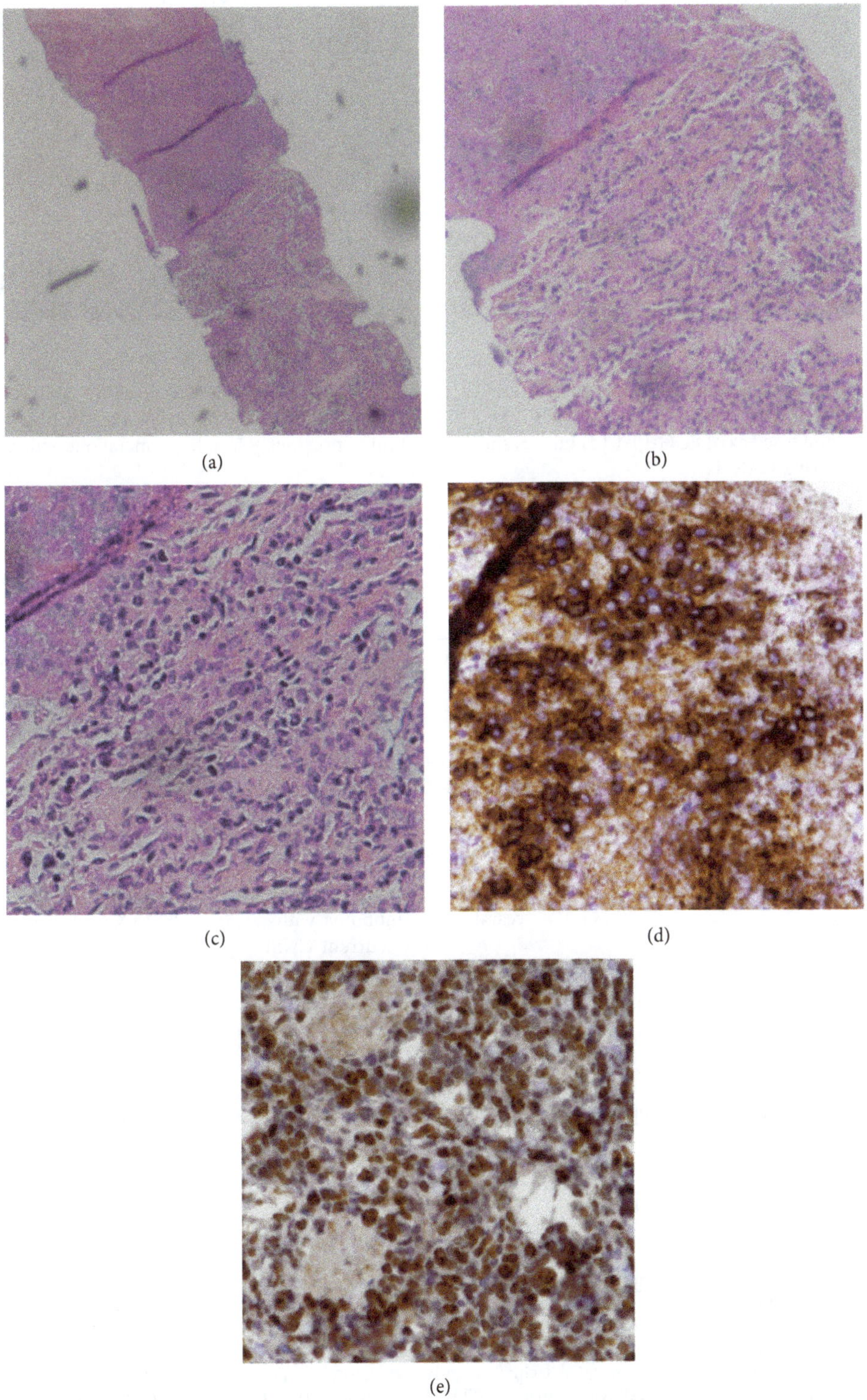

FIGURE 4: FNA and core biopsy of adrenal gland mass. *H* and *E* stain showing infiltration of large round blue cells and necrosis at 40x (a), 100x (b), 400x (c). CD20 stain highlight the infiltration of large round blue cells at 100x (d). Ki-67 stain showing a proliferation rate of >90% of the infiltration of large round blue cells at 100x (e).

efficacy in patients with a history of advanced CNS disease, this cohort of patients has largely been excluded from CAR-T clinical trials [29]. However, subsequent work has demonstrated the safe and efficacious use of CAR-T in patients with CNS malignancies with appropriate management [30]. In an ongoing single center phase 1 trial, investigating the use of CAR-T in seven patients with a history of primary or secondary CNS lymphoma (SCNSL), an ORR of 57% was

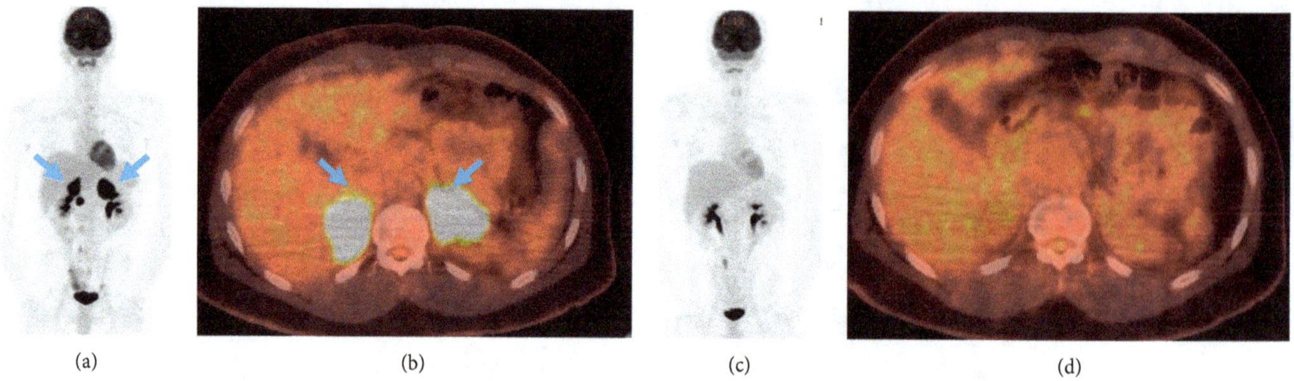

Figure 5: Pretreatment coronal maximum-intensity-projection (a) and axial fused FDG-PET (b) images show enlarged and hypermetabolic bilateral adrenal glands (blue arrows) with SUV max of 17.1 and 14.1 on the right and left respectively. Posttreatment coronal maximum-intensity-projection (c) and fused axial FDG-PET (d) images show resolution of previously seen hypermetabolic activity of bilateral adrenal glands two months following CAR-T.

Table 1: Current CAR-T clinical trials in R/R PCNSL.

Sponsor	Study chair	Study design	Population	Conditions	Interventions	NCT
University College London	Claire Roddie	Phase I	Adults (>16 years)	(i) R/R PCNSL	Anti-CD19 CAR-T cells	NCT04443829
Massachusetts General Hospital	Matthew J. Frigault	Phase I	Adults (>18 years)	(i) R/R PCNSL	Tisagenlecleucel (anti-CD19 CAR-T cells)	NCT04134117
Dana-Farber Cancer Institute	Caron A. Jacobson	Phase I	Adults (>18 years)	(i) R/R CNSL (ii) systemic lymphoma with concurrent CNSL	Axicabtagene ciloleucel (anti-CD19 CAR-T cells)	NCT04608487
Memorial Sloan Kettering Cancer Center	Jae Park	Phase I	Adults (>18 years)	(i) R/R CNSL (ii) systemic lymphoma with concurrent CNSL	Anti-CD19 19 (T2) 28z1XX CAR-T cells	NCT04464200
Celgene	Claudia Schuster-bauer	Phase II	Adults (>18 years)	(i) R/R CNSL (ii) systemic lymphoma with concurrent CNSL	Lisocabtagene maraleucel (anti-CAR-T cells)	NCT03484702
Zhejiang University	He Huang	Phase I	(i) Children (>3 years) (ii) Adults (18–75 years)	(i) ALL with CNS involvement (ii) NHL with CNS involvement	Anti-CD19 CAR-T cells	NCT04532203
UNC Lineberger Comprehensive Cancer Center	Natalie Grover	Phase I	Adults (>18 years)	(i) R/R BCL (ii) R/R PCNSL (iii) R/R CLL/SLL	iC9-anti-CD19 CAR-T cells	NCT03696784
Shenzhen Genoimmune Medical Institute	Lung-Ji Chang	Phase I/II	(i) Children (>6 months) (ii) Adults (18–75 years)	(i) R/R BCL	4SCAR19 and 4scar20/22/70/PSMA/13/79b/GD2	NCT04429438

R/R: relapsed-refractory; PCNSL, primary CNS lymphoma; CAR-chimeric antigen receptor; NCT, national clinical trial identifier; ALL, acute lymphoblastic leukemia; NHL, non-Hodgkin lymphoma; BCL: B-cell lymphoma; CLL/SLL, chronic lymphocytic leukemia/small lymphocytic lymphoma; iC9: inducible caspase 9.

observed with no cases of grade ≥3 neurotoxicity [31]. Another study described 8 SCNSL patients who received CAR-T, none of whom experienced > grade 1 neurotoxicity. Two patients were noted to have CR at day +90 and day +180 respectively, while two patients died within 30 days secondary to disease progression [30]. Several ongoing clinical trials [32, 33] are exploring the use of CAR-T in PCNSL (Table 1).

Despite how promising CAR-T appears to be, 21–35% of patients still experience relapse, as seen with our patient [29]. Unfortunately, in those with multiple disease relapses, treatment outcomes remain poor [34]. Novel targeted therapies, which have demonstrated efficacy both within the CNS and systemically for relapsed-refractory (R/R) PCNSL, should be considered. These agents have been investigated in prospective clinical trials [29, 35–56], and

Table 2: Agents with activity in R/R PCNSL.

Author	Agents	Study type	# of patients	ORR (PR + CR)	Median PFS, mo	Median OS, mo
Fischer et al. [35]	Topotecan	Prospective	27	9/27 (33%)	2	8.4
Voloschin et al. [36]	Topotecan	Prospective	15	6/15 (40%)	2 (60 d)	32.7
Reni et al. [37]	Temozolomide	Prospective	36	11/36 (31%)	2.8	3.9
Soussain et al. [38]	CYVE + SCT	Prospective	43	20/40 (50%)	11.6	18.3
Batchelor et al. [39]	Ritux	Prospective	11	4/11 (36%)	1.9 (57 d)	20.9
Raizer et al. [40]	Pemetrexed	Prospective	11	6/11 (55%)	5.7	10.1
Dietrich et al. [41]	Pemetrexed	Prospective	14	8/14 (57%)	4.2	44.5+
Rubenstein et al. [42]	IT Ritux + IT MTX	Prospective	14 (6 PCNSL)	6/14 (43%)	1.2	NR
Nayak et al. [43]	Ritux + temozolomide+pred	Prospective	16	5/14 (36%)	1.6 (7 wk)	NR
Korfel et al. [44]	Temsirolimus	Prospective	37	20/37 (54%)	2.1	3.7
Grommes et al. [45]	Ibrutinib	Prospective	20 (13 PCNSL)	10/13 (77%)	4.6	15 (PCNSL)
Grommes et al. [46]	Ibrutinib + HD-MTX + Ritux	Prospective	15	12/14 (80%)	9.2	NR
Roschewski et al. [47]	TEDDi-R: ibrutinib + anthracycline	Prospective	18	9/13 (69%)	15.2	NR
Rubenstein et al. [48]	Lenalidomide	Prospective	14	9/14 (64%)	6	NR
Ghesquieres et al. [49]	Revri : Lenalidomide + Ritux	Prospective	50	16/50 (32%)	7.5	14.7
Tun et al. [50]	Pomalidomide + dexamethasone	Prospective	29	12/25 (48%)	5.3	NR
Fox et al. [51]	Tier : Thiotepa + ifos + eto + Ritux	Prospective	27	14/27 (52%)	3	5
Kasenda et al. [52]	HDAra-C + Thiotepa + Ritux + SCT	Prospective	39	28/39 (72%)	12.4	NR
Gavrilenko et al. [53]	Nivolumab	Prospective	9 (8 PCNSL)	7/9 (78%)	12	12
Siddiqi et al. [54]	CD19 CAR-T-cell therapy	Prospective	7 (3 PCNSL)	4/7 (57%)	NR	NR
Li et al. [55]	CD19/CD22 CAR-T-cell therapy	Prospective	5 (1 PCNSL)	5/5 (100%)	3	NR
Tu et al. [29]	CD19/CD70 CAR-T-cell therapy	Case study	1	1/1 (100%)	>17	>17
Siddiqi et al. [56]	CD19 CAR-T-cell therapy	Case series	5	3/5 (60%)	NR	NR

ORR, overall response rate; CR, complete response; PR, partial response; PFS, progression free survival; OS, overall survival; NR, not reported; IT, intrathecal; pred, prednisone; HDAra-C, high-dose cytarabine; CYVE, cytarabine + etoposide; SCT, stem cell transplant; HD-MTX, high-dose methotrexate; Ritux, rituximab; ifos, ifosfamide; eto, etoposide; CAR, chimeric antigen receptor.

are summarized below (Table 2). Single-agent temsirolimus, an mTOR inhibitor, demonstrated an ORR of 54% in a study of 37 patients with refractory PCNSL [44]. Ibrutinib, a Bruton's tyrosine kinase inhibitor, demonstrated excellent single-agent activity with an ORR of 77% in 13 PCNSL patients [45]. Additionally, ibrutinib was added to HD-MTX and rituximab in 15 patients with PCNSL and SCNSL. In PCNSL, 8 patients responded, including 6 patients achieving CR [46]. However, the durability of response to this regimen is unknown since responding patients were allowed treatment with ASCT consolidation [57]. Immunomodulatory drugs (IMiDs), which inhibit NF-Kβ activity, include lenalidomide and pomalidomide [57]. In a multicenter phase 2 study, 50 patients with relapsed PCNSL received lenalidomide and rituximab for eight cycles, followed by maintenance lenalidomide for responders. The observed ORR was 32%, including 13 achieving CR [49]. Pomalidomide and its combination with dexamethasone demonstrated significantly improved survival compared with IMiDs alone [50]. Finally, the use of immune checkpoint inhibitors (ICI) may represent another promising treatment approach in PCNSL [58]. In an immunocompetent preclinical model, anti-PD1 monoclonal antibodies had significant therapeutic activity against CNS lymphoma [59]. Moreover, Nayak et al. reported long-term responses in a small retrospective study of 4 patients with PCNSL [60].

4. Conclusion

This paper describes a rarely reported case of a 23-year-old man with advanced PCNS-DLBCL and systemic relapse, including adrenal gland involvement. Despite achieving near complete resolution of adrenal disease following CAR-T, the patient experienced multiple disease relapses and ultimately died from disease progression. Typically associated with a poor prognosis, this case highlights the challenges associated with management of systemic relapse in PCNS-DLBCL, and the necessity of well-designed clinical trials testing novel treatment options for this rare and often deadly disease.

References

[1] A. J. M. Ferreri, "How i treat primary CNS lymphoma," *Blood*, vol. 118, no. 3, pp. 510–522, 2011.

[2] C. Grommes and L. M. DeAngelis, "Primary CNS lymphoma," *Journal of Clinical Oncology*, vol. 35, no. 21, pp. 2410–2418, 2017.

[3] Q. Cai, Y. Fang, and K. H. Young, "Primary central nervous system lymphoma: molecular pathogenesis and advances in treatment," *Translational Oncology*, vol. 12, no. 3, pp. 523–538, 2019.

[4] Y. S. Choi, "Recent advances in the management of primary central nervous system lymphoma," *Blood Research*, vol. 55, no. S1, pp. S58–S62, 2020.

[5] S. Ma, S. S. Sen, R. Jug et al., "Adrenal relapse of primary central nervous system diffuse large B-cell lymphoma," *Medicine*, vol. 97, no. 38, Article ID e12482, 2018.

[6] D. W. Lee, B. D. Santomasso, F. L. Locke et al., "ASTCT consensus grading for cytokine release syndrome and neurologic toxicity associated with immune effector cells," *Biology of Blood and Marrow Transplantation*, vol. 25, no. 4, pp. 625–638, 2019.

[7] J. Glass, "Current management of primary central nervous system lymphoma," *Chinese Clinical Oncology*, vol. 6, no. 4, p. 38, 2017.

[8] S. Camilleri-Broët, E. Crinière, P. Broët et al., "A uniform activated B-cell-like immunophenotype might explain the poor prognosis of primary central nervous system lymphoma: analysis of 83 cases," *Blood*, vol. 107, pp. 190–196, 2006.

[9] S. Bhagavathi, A. Sharathkumar, S. Hunter et al., "Activated B-cell immunophenotype might be associated with poor prognosis of primary central nervous system lymphomas," *Clinical Neuropathology*, vol. 27, no. 1, pp. 13–20, 2008.

[10] S. Löw, C. H. Han, and T. T. Batchelor, "Primary central nervous system lymphoma," *Therapeutic Advances in Neurological Disorders*, vol. 11, Article ID 1756286418793562, 2018.

[11] K.-W. Song and T. Batchelor, "Treatment of primary CNS lymphoma: maximizing clinical benefit, minimizing neurotoxicity," *Current Oncology Reports*, vol. 23, no. 11, p. 132, 2021.

[12] National Comprehensive Cancer Network, "Central nervous system cancers," 2021, https://www.nccn.org/professionals/physician_gls/pdf/cns.pdf.

[13] S. R. Plotkin, R. A. Betensky, F. H. Hochberg et al., "Treatment of relapsed central nervous system lymphoma with high-dose methotrexate," *Clinical Cancer Research*, vol. 10, no. 17, pp. 5643–5646, 2004.

[14] E. Pentsova, L. M. Deangelis, and A. Omuro, "Methotrexate re-challenge for recurrent primary central nervous system lymphoma," *Journal of Neuro-Oncology*, vol. 117, no. 1, pp. 161–165, 2014.

[15] L. E. Abrey, L. M. DeAngelis, and J. Yahalom, "Long-term survival in primary CNS lymphoma," *Journal of Clinical Oncology*, vol. 16, no. 3, pp. 859–863, 1998.

[16] M. Sierra Del Rio, D. Ricard, C. Houillier et al., "Prophylactic intrathecal chemotherapy in primary CNS lymphoma," *Journal of Neuro-Oncology*, vol. 106, no. 1, pp. 143–146, 2012.

[17] L. M. DeAngelis, "Primary central nervous system lymphoma," *Molecular Neuro-Oncology and Its Impact on the Clinical Management of Brain Tumors*, vol. 135, pp. 155–169, 1994.

[18] L. M. DeAngelis, "Primary CNS lymphoma: treatment with combined chemotherapy and radiotherapy," *Journal of Neurobiology*, vol. 43, pp. 249–257, 1999.

[19] E. Arellano-Rodrigo, A. López-Guillermo, E. M. Bessell, B. Nomdedeu, E. Montserrat, and F. Graus, "Salvage treatment with etoposide (VP-16), ifosfamide and cytarabine (ara-C) for patients with recurrent primary central nervous system lymphoma," *European Journal of Haematology*, vol. 70, no. 4, pp. 219–224, 2003.

[20] M. C. Chamberlain, "Salvage therapy with bendamustine for methotrexate refractory recurrent primary CNS lymphoma: a retrospective case series," *Journal of Neuro-Oncology*, vol. 118, no. 1, pp. 155–162, 2014.

[21] J. Glass, M. Won, C. J. Schultz et al., "Phase I and II study of induction chemotherapy with methotrexate, rituximab, and temozolomide, followed by whole-brain radiotherapy and postirradiation temozolomide for primary CNS lymphoma: NRG oncology RTOG 0227," *Journal of Clinical Oncology*, vol. 34, no. 14, pp. 1620–1625, 2016.

[22] K. Jahnke, E. Thiel, P. Martus et al., "Relapse of primary central nervous system lymphoma: clinical features, outcome and prognostic factors," *Journal of Neuro-Oncology*, vol. 80, no. 2, pp. 159–165, 2006.

[23] M. Igala, "Unusual relapse of primary central nervous system lymphoma," *SpringerPlus*, vol. 5, no. 1, p. 301, 2016.

[24] N. Schmitz, S. Zeynalova, M. Nickelsen et al., "CNS international prognostic index: a risk model for CNS relapse in patients with diffuse large B-cell lymphoma treated with R-CHOP," *Journal of Clinical Oncology*, vol. 34, no. 26, pp. 3150–3156, 2016.

[25] T. Mika, S. Ladigan, A. Baraniskin et al., "Allogeneic hematopoietic stem cell transplantation for primary central nervous system lymphoma," *Haematologica*, vol. 105, pp. e160–e163, 2020.

[26] F. L. Locke, A. Ghobadi, C. A. Jacobson et al., "Long-term safety and activity of axicabtagene ciloleucel in refractory large B-cell lymphoma (ZUMA-1): a single-arm, multicentre, phase 1-2 trial," *The Lancet Oncology*, vol. 20, no. 1, pp. 31–42, 2019.

[27] S. J. Schuster, M. R. Bishop, C. S. Tam et al., "Tisagenlecleucel in adult relapsed or refractory diffuse large b-cell lymphoma," *New England Journal of Medicine*, vol. 380, no. 1, pp. 45–56, 2019.

[28] S. S. Neelapu, F. L. Locke, N. L. Bartlett et al., "Axicabtagene ciloleucel CAR T-cell therapy in refractory large B-cell lymphoma," *New England Journal of Medicine*, vol. 377, no. 26, pp. 2531–2544, 2017.

[29] S. Tu, X. Zhou, Z. Guo et al., "CD19 and CD70 dual-target chimeric antigen receptor T-cell therapy for the treatment of relapsed and refractory primary central nervous system diffuse large B-cell lymphoma," *Frontiers in Oncology*, vol. 9, p. 1350, 2019.

[30] M. J. Frigault, J. Dietrich, M. Martinez-Lage et al., "Tisagenlecleucel CAR T-cell therapy in secondary CNS lymphoma," *Blood*, vol. 134, no. 11, pp. 860–866, 2019.

[31] C. W. Freyer and D. L. Porter, "Advances in CAR T therapy for hematologic malignancies," *Pharmacotherapy: The Journal of Human Pharmacology and Drug Therapy*, vol. 40, no. 8, pp. 741–755, 2020.

[32] ClinicalTrials.gov [Internet], "National library of medicine (US)," 2000, https://clinicaltrials.gov/ct2/results?term=central+nervous+system+lymphoma+CAR-T&draw=2&rank=7#rowId6.

[33] P. Karschnia, J. Blobner, N. Teske et al., "CAR T-cells for CNS lymphoma: driving into new terrain?" *Cancers*, vol. 13, no. 10, p. 2503, 2021.

[34] P.-O. Thuresson, N. Vander Velde, P. Gupta, and J. Talbot, "A systematic review of the clinical efficacy of treatments in relapsed or refractory diffuse large B cell lymphoma," *Advances in Therapy*, vol. 37, no. 12, pp. 4877–4893, 2020.

[35] L. Fischer, E. Thiel, H.-A. Klasen et al., "Prospective trial on topotecan salvage therapy in primary CNS lymphoma," *Annals of Oncology*, vol. 17, no. 7, pp. 1141–1145, 2006.

[36] A. D. Voloschin, R. Betensky, P. Y. Wen, F. Hochberg, and T. Batchelor, "Topotecan as salvage therapy for relapsed or refractory primary central nervous system lymphoma," *Journal of Neuro-Oncology*, vol. 86, no. 2, pp. 211–215, 2008.

[37] M. Reni, F. Zaja, W. Mason et al., "Temozolomide as salvage treatment in primary brain lymphomas," *British Journal of Cancer*, vol. 96, no. 6, pp. 864–867, 2007.

[38] C. Soussain, K. Hoang-Xuan, L. Taillandier et al., "Intensive chemotherapy followed by hematopoietic stem-cell rescue for refractory and recurrent primary CNS and intraocular lymphoma: société française de Greffe de Moëlle osseuse-thérapie cellulaire," *Journal of Clinical Oncology*, vol. 26, no. 15, pp. 2512–2518, 2008.

[39] T. T. Batchelor, S. A. Grossman, T. Mikkelsen, X. Ye, S. Desideri, and G. J. Lesser, "Rituximab monotherapy for patients with recurrent primary CNS lymphoma," *Neurology*, vol. 76, no. 10, pp. 929-930, 2011.

[40] J. J. Raizer, A. Rademaker, A. M. Evens et al., "Pemetrexed in the treatment of relapsed/refractory primary central nervous system lymphoma," *Cancer*, vol. 118, no. 15, pp. 3743–3748, 2012.

[41] J. Dietrich, L. Versmee, J. Drappatz et al., "Pemetrexed in recurrent or progressive central nervous system lymphoma: a phase I multicenter clinical trial," *The Oncologist*, vol. 25, no. 9, pp. 747–e1273, 2020.

[42] J. L. Rubenstein, J. Li, L. Chen et al., "Multicenter phase 1 trial of intraventricular immunochemotherapy in recurrent CNS lymphoma," *Blood*, vol. 121, no. 5, pp. 745–751, 2013.

[43] L. Nayak, L. E. Abrey, J. Drappatz et al., "Multicenter phase II study of rituximab and temozolomide in recurrent primary central nervous system lymphoma," *Leukemia and Lymphoma*, vol. 54, no. 1, pp. 58–61, 2013.

[44] A. Korfel, U. Schlegel, U. Herrlinger et al., "Phase II trial of temsirolimus for relapsed/refractory primary CNS lymphoma," *Journal of Clinical Oncology*, vol. 34, no. 15, pp. 1757–1763, 2016.

[45] C. Grommes, A. Pastore, N. Palaskas et al., "Ibrutinib unmasks critical role of Bruton tyrosine kinase in primary CNS lymphoma," *Cancer Discovery*, vol. 7, no. 9, pp. 1018–1029, 2017.

[46] C. Grommes, S. S. Tang, J. Wolfe et al., "Phase 1b trial of an ibrutinib-based combination therapy in recurrent/refractory CNS lymphoma," *Blood*, vol. 133, no. 5, pp. 436–445, 2019.

[47] M. Roschewski, M. S. Lionakis, C. Melani, J. A. Butman, S. Pittaluga, and A. N. Lucas, "Dose-adjusted teddi-R induces durable complete remissions in relapsed and refractory primary CNS lymphoma," *Blood*, vol. 132, no. Supplement 1, p. 4195, 2018.

[48] J. L. Rubenstein, H. Geng, E. J. Fraser et al., "Phase 1 investigation of lenalidomide/rituximab plus outcomes of lenalidomide maintenance in relapsed CNS lymphoma," *Blood Advances*, vol. 2, no. 13, pp. 1595–1607, 2018.

[49] H. Ghesquieres, M. Chevrier, M. Laadhari et al., "Lenalidomide in combination with intravenous rituximab (REVRI) in relapsed/refractory primary CNS lymphoma or primary intraocular lymphoma: a multicenter prospective "proof of concept" phase II study of the French Oculo-cerebral lymphoma (LOC) network and the lymphoma study association (LYSA)," *Annals of Oncology*, vol. 30, no. 4, pp. 621–628, 2019.

[50] H. W. Tun, P. B. Johnston, L. M. DeAngelis et al., "Phase 1 study of pomalidomide and dexamethasone for relapsed/refractory primary CNS or vitreoretinal lymphoma," *Blood*, vol. 132, no. 21, pp. 2240–2248, 2018.

[51] C. P. Fox, A. S. Ali, G. McIlroy et al., "A phase 1/2 study of thiotepa-based immunochemotherapy in relapsed/refractory primary CNS lymphoma: the TIER trial," *Blood Advances*, vol. 5, no. 20, pp. 4073–4082, 2021.

[52] B. Kasenda, G. Ihorst, R. Schroers et al., "High-dose chemotherapy with autologous haematopoietic stem cell support for relapsed or refractory primary CNS lymphoma: a prospective multicentre trial by the German cooperative PCNSL study group," *Leukemia*, vol. 31, no. 12, pp. 2623–2629, 2017.

[53] A. N. Gavrilenko, N. P. Volkov, D. I. Shmidt et al., "Nivolumab in primary CNS lymphoma and primary testicular lymphoma with CNS involvement: single center experience," *Blood*, vol. 136, no. Supplement 1, p. 4, 2020.

[54] T. Siddiqi, X. Wang, J. Palmer et al., "CD19-targeting CAR-T cell therapy in CNS lymphoma," *Blood*, vol. 134, no. Supplement_1, p. 4075, 2019.

[55] T. Li, L. Zhao, Y. Zhang et al., "CAR T-cell therapy is effective but not long-lasting in B-cell lymphoma of the brain," *Frontiers in Oncology*, vol. 10, p. 1306, 2020.

[56] T. Siddiqi, X. Wang, M. S. Blanchard et al., "CD19-directed CAR T-cell therapy for treatment of primary CNS lymphoma," *Blood Advances*, vol. 5, no. 20, pp. 4059–4063, 2021.

[57] M. Holdhoff, N. Wagner-Johnston, and M. Roschewski, "Systemic approach to recurrent primary CNS lymphoma: perspective on current and emerging treatment strategies," *OncoTargets and Therapy*, vol. 13, pp. 8323–8335, 2020.

[58] C. Grommes, L. Nayak, H. W. Tun, and T. T. Batchelor, "Introduction of novel agents in the treatment of primary CNS lymphoma," *Neuro-Oncology*, vol. 21, no. 3, pp. 306–313, 2019.

[59] Y. Qiu, Z. Li, F. Pouzoulet et al., "Immune checkpoint inhibition by anti-PDCD1 (anti-PD1) monoclonal antibody has significant therapeutic activity against central nervous system lymphoma in an immunocompetent preclinical model," *British Journal of Haematology*, vol. 183, no. 4, pp. 674–678, 2018.

[60] L. Nayak, F. M. Iwamoto, A. LaCasce et al., "PD-1 blockade with nivolumab in relapsed/refractory primary central nervous system and testicular lymphoma," *Blood*, vol. 129, no. 23, pp. 3071–3073, 2017.

Gemtuzumab-Ozogamicin-Related Impaired Hemoglobin-Haptoglobin Scavenging as On-Target/Off-Tumor Toxicity of Anti-CD33 AML Therapy: A Report of Two Cases

Hanna L. M. Rajala,[1] **Veli-Jukka Anttila**,[2] **Mikko Haapio**,[3] **Mikko A. I. Keränen**,[1] **Ulla Wartiovaara-Kautto**,[1,4] **and Riikka Räty**[1]

[1]*Department of Hematology, Helsinki University Hospital Comprehensive Cancer Center and University of Helsinki, Helsinki, Finland*
[2]*Division of Infectious Diseases, Inflammation Center, Helsinki University Hospital and University of Helsinki, Helsinki, Finland*
[3]*Nephrology, Helsinki University Hospital and University of Helsinki, Helsinki, Finland*
[4]*Applied Tumor Genomics Research Program, Faculty of Medicine, University of Helsinki, Helsinki, Finland*

Correspondence should be addressed to Riikka Räty; riikka.raty@hus.fi

Academic Editor: Tatsuharu Ohno

Gemtuzumab-ozogamicin (GO) is a humanized anti-CD33 antibody, which is conjugated to a cytotoxic calicheamicin. It is used to treat acute myeloid leukemia (AML) in combination with chemotherapy. We describe here two GO-treated acute myeloid leukemia (AML) cases: both patients suffered from a toxic syndrome, which manifested as impaired hemoglobin-haptoglobin scavenging and accumulation of hemolysis-related products. Our observations and earlier reports indicated that the reaction was caused by GO-targeted destruction of CD33 + CD163+ monocytes/macrophages, which are responsible for the clearance of hemoglobin-haptoglobin complexes. The rise of plasma lactate dehydrogenase was an early sign of the reaction, and both patients had high levels of free plasma hemoglobin, but plasma haptoglobin and bilirubin levels were paradoxically normal. Symptoms included septic fever and abnormalities in cardiac tests and in the case of the first patient, severe neurological symptoms which required intensive care unit admittance. Therapeutic plasma exchanges supported the patients until the recovery of normal hematopoiesis. The symptoms may be easily confounded with infectious complications-related organ damage. Regarding the increasing use of gemtuzumab-ozogamicin and other emerging CD33-targeted cell therapies, we want to highlight this mostly unknown and probably underdiagnosed toxicity.

1. Introduction

Gemtuzumab-ozogamicin (GO) is a humanized anti-CD33 monoclonal antibody, which is linked to a very potent cytotoxic agent and N-acetyl gamma calicheamicin. CD33 is expressed on the surface of most acute myeloid leukemia (AML) blasts and on immature myeloid cells. [1] Adverse events related to GO, such as cytopenias and liver toxicity, led to its withdrawal from the market in 2010 due to failure to demonstrate survival benefit because of increased toxicity-related mortality. [2] In 2017, GO regained its approval from the FDA and EMA, as studies on lower-dose fractionated GO showed a better safety profile and beneficial results overall, especially in AML patients with favorable cytogenetics [3–6].

In this report, we present two patients who suffered from life-threatening GO-related impaired hemoglobin-haptoglobin scavenging, which manifested as an atypical intravascular hemolytic reaction. Earlier anecdotal reports have suggested that GO-targeted destruction of CD33 + CD163 + monocytes/macrophages leads to abrogated clearance of hemolysis-related products [7, 8]. Regarding the increasing use of GO and other emerging CD33-targeted cell therapies, we want to highlight this unknown and poorly defined on-target/off-tumor toxicity and share our experience of successful salvage with therapeutic plasma exchanges (TPEs). Both patients consented to the publication of the clinical data.

2. Case Presentation

Patient 1: A 21-year-old otherwise healthy female was diagnosed with core-binding factor (CBF)-AML (t (8; 12) (q21.3; q22)), corresponding RUNX1/RUNX1T1 transcript. After the first-line therapies (Table 1), minimal residual disease (MRD) positivity of 0.02% was still detected in the bone marrow (BM). The patient then moved to Finland. At the first visit to our center, a florid BM-relapse was detected only 14 weeks after the start of the last consolidation cycle. We initiated a course of 7 + 3 combined with fractionated GO (Table 1). Along with stomatitis and cytarabine-related cutaneous reaction, from day 13 onwards, the patient suffered from high fever, malaise, *Clostridium difficile* colitis, and oral HSV infection. Moreover, *Enterococcus faecium* septicemia persisted from day 21, though no deep foci of infection or endocarditis were detected. Human herpes virus 6 nucleic acid test (HHV6-NAT) was positive on day 25 (Figure 1). As a first sign of a toxic reaction, plasma lactate dehydrogenase (P-LD) started to rise from day 11. The reaction escalated quickly from day 19, when blood samples became macroscopically hemolytic. Free plasma hemoglobin (P-Hb) rose markedly, but P-haptoglobin (P-Haptog) and P-Bilirubin (P-Bil) were paradoxically normal, unlike in typical intravascular hemolysis (Figure 1, Table 2). Kidney and liver tests remained normal, but plasma troponin I level was elevated and the patient was hypertensive.

To lower the amount of toxic P-Hb and other potentially harmful substances related to the hemolysis-like reaction and to prevent further organ damage, therapeutic plasma exchanges (TPEs) were performed on days 23–25, 36–38, 43–45, and 50–52. In each TPE, one volume of plasma (about 5% of the patient's weight) was exchanged and replaced with 4–5% albumin and Octaplas-LG® plasma via dialysis catheter. We used citrate and the low-molecular weight heparin, enoxaparin, as anticoagulants.

Despite wide-spectrum antibiotics and repeated TPEs, septic fever did not respond to therapy. On day 35, the patient was admitted to the intensive care unit (ICU) for four days after a seizure. MRI scan showed cerebral microhemorrhages. Cerebrospinal fluid (CSF) HHV6-NAT was positive.

High levels of P-Hb and P-LD persisted until the first signs of recovering hematopoiesis on day 45 (Figure 1, Table 2). However, fever continued and new viral pneumonia-like changes were seen in the CT scan with subacute cardiac tamponade requiring percutaneous pericardial drainage. Immunological pericarditis and pneumonitis were suspected and prednisolone 1 mg/kg was started on day 63 with a clinical response. The patient could finally be discharged on day 81.

During follow-up, cardiac function has recovered and pulmonary function improved partially. The patient remained in MRD-negative complete remission (CR) and underwent allogeneic stem cell transplantation.

Patient 2: a 24-year-old female was diagnosed with CBF-AML (inv16, corresponding *CBFB-MYH11* fusion gene). Pulmonary tuberculosis had been cured with nine months of four-drug therapy one and a half years ago, but otherwise her medical history was unremarkable. We initiated a course of 7 + 3 combined with a single dose of GO (Table 1). Widespread cytarabine-related cutaneous reaction and mucositis and high fever were observed from day 4 onwards. Blood cultures and virus samples remained negative. Because of suspected hyperinflammation (P-ferritin >16500 μg/L, P-IL2R 5509 kU/L), we administered corticosteroid from day 16: fever responded but P-LD was rapidly increasing. P-Hb rose (410 mg/L at highest), and the color of patient's plasma slightly darkened while P-Haptog and P-Bil stayed normal. Hypertension and bradycardia were observed. We did not see any other sign of target-organ damage caused by the toxic reaction. We conducted preemptive TPEs daily on days 20–22. No more TPEs were needed, as P-LD and P-Hb declined after day 22 together with recovering hematopoiesis. CR with low MRD-positivity (*CBFB-MYH11* 0.02%) was detected in the BM on day 29.

3. Discussion

We describe here a rare but life-threatening GO-related on-target/off-tumor toxicity, from which the patients were salvaged with TPEs until hematopoietic recovery. Based on earlier publications, we suspected a hemolysis-like reaction and accumulation of hemolysis-related products caused by impaired hemoglobin-haptoglobin scavenging [7, 8]. Previous reports describe patients who experienced septic high fever and overall malaise, hypertension, neurological symptoms, and abdominal pain. None survived, either due to the persistent reaction or progressive disease (Table 1).

In intravascular hemolysis, plasma haptoglobin is depleted as it binds excess free hemoglobin to prevent its toxicity and infiltration by the kidneys. CD33+ mature tissue macrophages internalize the complexes via the CD163 scavenger receptor [9]. Maniecki et al. speculated that anti-CD33-mediated destruction of CD33 + CD163+ macrophages and subsequently impaired CD163-mediated hemoglobin-haptoglobin scavenging leads to the paradoxical accumulation of both plasma hemoglobin and haptoglobin [7]. Our two patients did not have eminent intravascular hemolysis, as they did not require red blood cell transfusions at the beginning of the reaction. The origin of excess P-Hb is not known, but we suspect that it might be partly related to anti-CD33-mediated destruction of red pulp macrophages in the spleen: these cells are responsible for maintaining hemoglobin-haptoglobin scavenging, and their destruction might release free hemoglobin into plasma. [10].

TPE is used to remove antibodies and immune complexes from circulation [11]. It is the standard of care in thrombotic thrombocytopenic purpura, in which it removes ADAMTS13-blocking antibodies [12]. However, TPE is not

Table 1: Summary of the five patients who had impaired hemoglobin-haptoglobin scavenging reaction after gemtuzumab-ozogamicin therapy. The first two cases are described in detail in this paper, and the last three patients are summarized from two previous publications. In addition, Maniecki et al. [7] mentioned one adult patient, from whom clinical details were not reported.

Patient	Diagnosis	Frontline therapy	Therapy of relapse	Time from last GO to hemolysis	Infections	Symptoms during hemolysis	Outcome	Publication
Patient 1: 21-year-old female (index patient)	Relapsed CBF-AML (BM-blasts 65%) *t* (8; 12), corresponding *RUNX1/RUNX1T1*-fusion gene. Additional mutations in *PHF6*, *EZH2*, and *KDM6A*. No extramedullary disease.	7 + 3 (cytarabine + daunorubicin), 3 x HD-AraC. Relapse after 2 mo.	7 + 3 (cytarabine and idarubicin) and **GO (3 mg/m^2, days 1, 4, 7)**	19 days	*Enterococcus faecium* sepsis, *Clostridium difficile* colitis, HHV6 viremia, HSV stomatitis	Fever, convulsions, confusion, mild diastolic hypertension	Recovered after repeated TPEs. Response to therapy: CRi, MRD-neg	Current
Patient 2: 24-year-old female	Primary CBF-AML (BM-blasts 69%) Inv16, corresponding *CBFB-MYH11*-fusion gene. Axillary and inguinal lymphadenopathy.	7 + 3 (cytarabine and idarubicin) and **GO (3 mg/m2 on day 4)**	—	14 days	Suspected infection, blood cultures negative and virus samples negative. No deep foci of infection detected.	Fever, hypertension, bradycardia	Recovered after 3 TPEs. Response to therapy: CR, MRD 0.02%	Current
2-year-old boy	Relapsed AML M4/M5	NOPHO-AML93 + MUD-SCT. Relapse 18 mo after SCT.	FLAG and **2 doses of GO (7.5 mg/m2) at a 2-week interval**	3 weeks	*Staphylococcal* sepsis	Abdominal pain, hypertension, persistent high fever, malaise	Recovery, but died later from PD	Maniecki et al. Blood 2000 [7]
1-year-old girl	Relapsed AML M5	NOPHO-AML 2004 with 2 doses of GO (5 mg/m^2, 2-week interval). Relapse after 3 mo.	FLAG-DaunoXome, **2 doses of GO (6 mg/m^2, 2-week interval)** and NOPHO-AML 2004 induction	5 weeks	Suspected infection, blood cultures negative	Hypertension, confusion, convulsions	Did not recover from hemolytic episode and died from PD 72 days from the first GO	Maniecki et al. Blood 2000 [7]
12-year-old boy	Refractory AML	Relapse after two salvage chemotherapies	**GO on days 1 and 15**, dose not reported	Hemolytic samples from day 5 of GO cycle	Vancomycin-resistant *Enterococcus faecium* and *Trichosporon asahii* infections	Hypertension, multiorgan failure and need for renal replacement therapy	Did not recover from hemolysis and died 40 days after the first GO	Tesfazghi et al. Clin Chem 2018 [8]

Abbreviations. AML: acute myeloid leukemia; BM, bone marrow; CBF, core-binding factor; CR, complete remission; CRi, CR with incomplete recovery of blood counts; FLAG, fludarabine-HD-AraC-granulocyte stimulating factor; GO, gemtuzumab-ozogamicin; HD-AraC, high-dose cytarabine; HHV6, human herpes virus 6; HSV, herpes simplex virus; mo, months; MRD, minimal residual disease; MUD, matched unrelated donor; NA, not accessible; PD, progressive disease; SCT, stem cell transplant; and TPE, therapeutic plasma exchange.

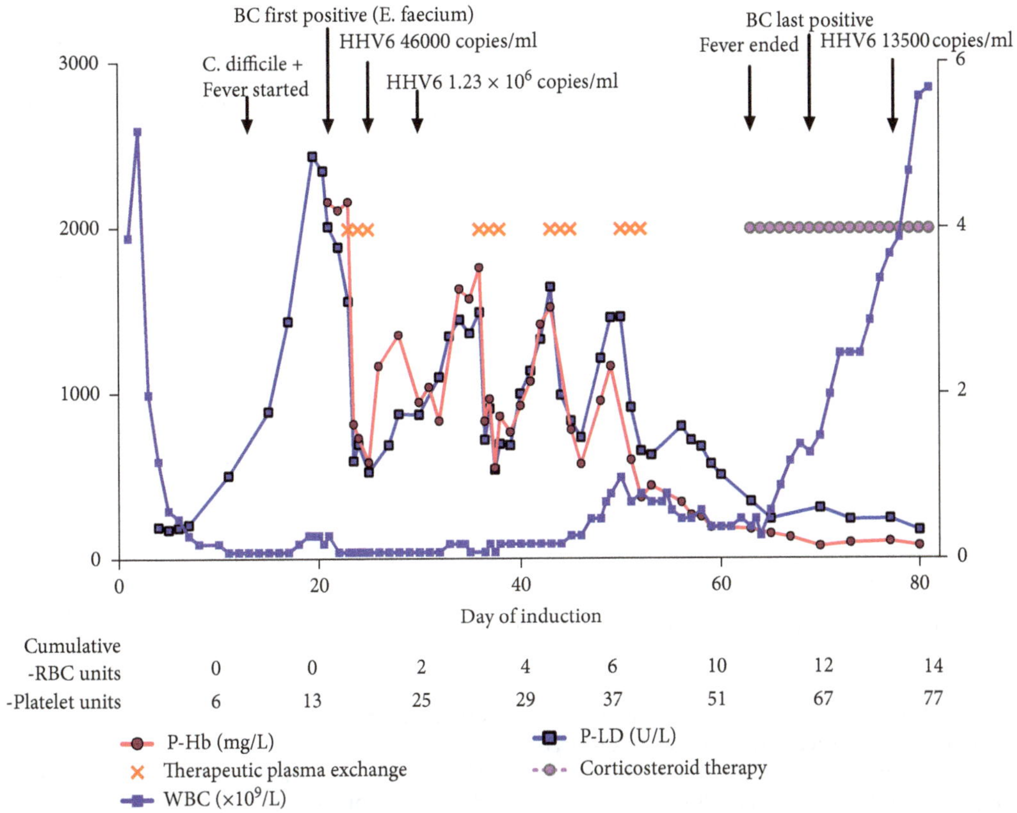

FIGURE 1: The clinical course of patient 1 (index case). Free plasma hemoglobin (P-Hb) and plasma lactate dehydrogenase (P-LD) are shown on the left y-axis, and white blood cell count (WBC) on the right *y*-axis. We used metronidazole and fidaxomicin to treat colitis caused by *Clostridium difficile* and valaciclovir for oral herpes simplex virus (HSV) infection. On day 21, blood culture (BC) was positive as the patient had *Enterococcus faecium* septicemia which continued the following weeks despite repeated removals and replacements of catheters and use of in vitro-effective antibiotics (tigecycline, linezolid, gentamicin, and daptomycin, which were selected because the patient was allergic to vancomycin). The patient tested positive for human herpes virus 6 nucleic acid test (HHV6-NAT) on day 25 and foscarnet was administered from day 31. Therapeutic plasma exchanges started on day 23 with transient responses to P-Hb and P-LD levels. The first signs of granulopoiesis were seen in bone marrow (BM) aspirate on day 46, and we were able to withhold TPEs after day 52, as the reaction subsided along with recovering hematopoiesis. Cumulative number of blood products transfused is shown below: there was no sign of hemolysis-related increased red blood cell (RBC) consumption, as we transfused the first RBC unit on day 25.

TABLE 2: Patient 1: laboratory findings and cumulative number of transfused blood products at different timepoints.

Test unit (normal range)	Day 1 of induction	Day 11 (P-LD rising)	Day 23 (before 1st plasma exchange)	Day 52 (last plasma exchange)	Day 63 (cardiac tamponade)	Day 81 (discharge)	Day 98 (the last BM sample)
B-Hb g/dL (11.7–15.5)	11.9	12.1	NAA	7.4	7.5	9.3	9.9
B-WBC x10^9/L (3.4–8.2)	3.9	0.1	0.1	0.8	0.4	5.7	6.0
B-PLTs x10^9/L (150–360)	83	44	122	14	18	67	29
B-neutrophils x10^9/L (1.5–6.7)	0.39	<0.05	<0.05	0.43	0.14	4.73	4.31
P-CRP mg/L (<4)	<4	28	411	216	266	57	33
P-Hb mg/L (<50)			2167	376	186	87	77
P-LD U/L (115–235)	201	513	1566	660	353	181	175
P-Haptog g/L (0.29–2.0)			4.53	1.46	0.61		

Table 2: Continued.

Test unit (normal range)	Day 1 of induction	Day 11 (P-LD rising)	Day 23 (before 1st plasma exchange)	Day 52 (last plasma exchange)	Day 63 (cardiac tamponade)	Day 81 (discharge)	Day 98 (the last BM sample)
P-Ferritin μg/L (15–125)	11		>16500	1609	1016	1918	2303
P-creatinine μmol/L (50–90)	45	40	49	21	22	29	36
P-ALT U/L (<35)	<9	20	52	42	13	58	31
P-bilirubin μmol/L (<20)	7	5	5	7	29	14	11
P-TnI mg/L (<45)	10		68	136	99	45	18
Cumulative number of RBC units	0	0	0	7	12	14	14
Cumulative number of PLT units	0	7	17	39	57	71	77

Abbreviations: ALT, alanine transferase; B, blood; BM, bone marrow; CRP, C-reactive protein; Hb, hemoglobin; LD, lactate dehydrogenase; NAA, not able to analyze; P, plasma; PLTs, platelets; RBC, red blood cell; TnI, troponine I; WBC, white blood cell.

usually effective in autoimmune hemolytic anemia [13]. In our patients, we used TPE to prevent toxicity related to free plasma hemoglobin, heme, and other potentially toxic molecules related to an inflammatory condition.

The incidence of impaired hemoglobin-haptoglobin scavenging related to GO is probably higher than reported, and the clinical presentation may vary from asymptomatic to life-threatening. Infectious complications and related organ damage during AML therapy may confound or delay the detection of the reaction. The currently recommended lower dose of GO seems to be better tolerated, but the reaction is probably dose-independent. Other CD33-targeting therapies, such as CD33-directed chimeric antigen receptor (CAR) T cells, are under investigation [14]. Similar toxicity seems possible during CD33 CAR T cell therapy, and one might speculate that the reaction could even be prolonged due to the persistence of CAR T cells and enhanced by cytokine release syndrome.

The trigger responsible for tilting the scales towards P-Hb accumulation is not known. Patient 1 had severe infectious problems and patient 2 suffered from widespread cytarabine-related skin toxicity, which might have contributed to the hyperinflammatory status. We did not detect germline mutations linked to immune deficiencies or increased susceptibility to toxicity (skin biopsies and gene panel sequencing).

According to our experiences, P-LD seems to be an early biomarker for this severe adverse event. We suggest that P-LD is followed in GO-treated patients, and if it rises, especially 1–2 weeks after GO administration (outside the time frame for tumor lysis), P-Hb should be analyzed as well. Our first patient survived this toxicity with repeated TPEs, and a similar reaction was suspected in the case of the second patient. Based on our experience, the initiation of TPEs might support patients through bone marrow hypoplasia, until the recovery of normal hemoglobin-haptoglobin scavenging.

Disclosure

All authors are employees of Helsinki University Hospital, Helsinki, Finland.

References

[1] M. L. Linenberger, "CD33-directed therapy with gemtuzumab ozogamicin in acute myeloid leukemia: progress in understanding cytotoxicity and potential mechanisms of drug resistance," *Leukemia*, vol. 19, no. 2, pp. 176–182, 2005.

[2] S. H. Petersdorf, K. J. Kopecky, M. Slovak et al., "A phase 3 study of gemtuzumab ozogamicin during induction and postconsolidation therapy in younger patients with acute myeloid leukemia," *Blood*, vol. 121, no. 24, pp. 4854–4860, 2013.

[3] K. J. Norsworthy, C. W. Ko, J. E. Lee et al., "FDA approval summary: mylotarg for treatment of patients with relapsed or refractory CD33-positive acute myeloid leukemia," *The Oncologist*, vol. 23, no. 9, pp. 1103–1108, 2018.

[4] J. Lambert, C. Pautas, C. Terré et al., "Gemtuzumab ozogamicin for de novo acute myeloid leukemia: final efficacy and safety updates from the open-label, phase III ALFA-0701 trial," *Haematologica*, vol. 104, no. 1, pp. 113–119, 2019.

[5] R. K. Hills, S. Castaigne, F. R. Appelbaum et al., "Addition of gemtuzumab ozogamicin to induction chemotherapy in adult patients with acute myeloid leukaemia: a meta-analysis of individual patient data from randomised controlled trials," *The Lancet Oncology*, vol. 15, no. 9, pp. 986–996, 2014.

[6] S. Ali, H. M. Dunmore, D. Karres et al., "The EMA review of mylotarg (gemtuzumab ozogamicin) for the treatment of acute myeloid leukemia," *The Oncologist*, vol. 24, no. 5, pp. e171–e179, 2019.

[7] M. B. Maniecki, H. Hasle, L. Friis-Hansen et al., "Impaired CD163-mediated hemoglobin-scavenging and severe toxic symptoms in patients treated with gemtuzumab ozogamicin," *Blood*, vol. 112, no. 4, pp. 1510–1514, 2008.

[8] M. T. Tesfazghi, C. W. Farnsworth, S. M. Roper, A. M. Gronowski, and D. J. Dietzen, "Confounding case of hemolysis in a patient with acute leukemia," *Clinical Chemistry*, vol. 64, no. 12, pp. 1690–1694, 2018.

[9] M. J. Nielsen, H. J. Møller, and S. K. Moestrup, "Hemoglobin and heme scavenger receptors," *Antioxidants & Redox Signaling*, vol. 12, no. 2, pp. 261–273, 2010.

[10] T. R. Klei, S. M. Meinderts, T. K. Van Den Berg, and R. van Bruggen, "From the cradle to the grave: the role of macrophages in erythropoiesis and erythrophagocytosis," *Front Immunol*, vol. 8, p. 73, 2017.

[11] E. Zanatta, M. Cozzi, P. Marson, and F. Cozzi, "The role of plasma exchange in the management of autoimmune disorders," *British Journal of Haematology*, vol. 186, no. 2, pp. 207–219, 2019.

[12] A. Picod, F. Provôt, and P. Coppo, "Therapeutic plasma exchange in thrombotic thrombocytopenic purpura," *La Presse Médicale*, vol. 48, no. 11, pp. 319–327, 2019.

[13] M. Ruivard, O. Tournilhac, S. Montel et al., "Plasma exchanges do not increase red blood cell transfusion efficiency in severe autoimmune hemolytic anemia: a retrospective case-control study," *Journal of Clinical Apheresis*, vol. 21, no. 3, pp. 202–206, 2006.

[14] S. K. Tasian, "Acute myeloid leukemia chimeric antigen receptor T-cell immunotherapy: how far up the road have we traveled?" *Therapeutic Advances in Hematology*, vol. 9, no. 6, pp. 135–148, 2018.

35

Double-Expressor Appendiceal Burkitt's Lymphoma: A Case Report and Literature Review

Osama N. Dukmak,[1] **Hamzeh M. I. Abugharbieh**,[1] **Mohammad Farid Emar**,[2] **Iman Khamayseh**,[1] **Salem M. Tos**,[1] **and Rafiq Salhab**[2]

[1]*Al-Quds University, Faculty of Medicine, Jerusalem, State of Palestine*
[2]*Al-Ahli Hospital, Hebron, State of Palestine*

Correspondence should be addressed to Osama N. Dukmak; osama.dukmak112@hotmail.com

Academic Editor: Gergely Feher

Background. Appendiceal lymphoma is a very rare entity accounting for 0.015% of all gastrointestinal lymphoma cases. Acute appendicitis is the most common presentation of primary appendix neoplasms. Burkitt's lymphoma presenting as an acute appendicitis is a rare entity with around 21% of the cases presenting as a lower iliac fossa mass. *Case Presentation.* A 23-year-old male was admitted to the surgical ward as a case of acute appendicitis with localized tenderness in the right iliac fossa, positive rebound tenderness, a positive Rovsing's sign, and ultrasound findings of suspected complicated appendicitis. Appendectomy was performed. Histopathological examination of the appendectomy specimen revealed a double-expressor non-Hodgkin diffuse large cell lymphoma with Burkitt's-like morphology. He was sent for chemotherapy treatment. *Conclusion.* Only 34 cases of Burkitt's lymphoma have been reported to present as acute appendicitis. Histological examination following appendectomy for an apparent appendicitis is essential. Furthermore, complete blood count and a computed tomography scan aid the diagnosis of lymphoma. Double-expressor lymphoma has been shown to have poor outcomes. Therefore, prompt and aggressive treatment is vital.

1. Introduction

Neoplasms of the appendix are rare and account for only 0.5 to 1 percent of intestinal neoplasms [1] and found in ~0.5–1.0% of appendectomy specimens at pathologic evaluation [2]. Appendiceal lymphomas are exceedingly rare and constitute around 0.015% of all gastrointestinal lymphoma cases [2].

Burkitt's lymphoma (BL) is a highly aggressive B-cell non-Hodgkin lymphoma characterized by the translocation and deregulation of the Myc gene on chromosome 8. A case series of 116 patients with appendiceal lymphomas showed that BL was the second most prevalent pathology, diagnosed in 25.9% of patients [2].

This rapidly growing tumor can cause symptoms due to mass effect or direct involvement of the bowel [3] which may manifest as bowel obstruction, intussusception, or appendicitis [4].

Acute appendicitis is the most common presentation of primary appendix neoplasms [5]. Therefore, histological examination following appendectomy for an apparent appendicitis is essential and can provide the diagnosis of BL, which leads to the specific disease management. Herein, we present a 23-year-old male patient who presented with acute appendicitis and was found to have BL.

2. Case Presentation

A 23-year-old male presented to our center complaining of right lower quadrant (RLQ) abdominal pain of 12-hour duration.

The pain started in the periumbilical region and then became more localized to the right iliac fossa where the pain was colicky in nature and was increasing in severity. Moreover, the pain was not related to food or movement.

Furthermore, the patient had nausea and vomiting. However, the patient denied any change in bowel habits or any history of dysuria or change of urine color.

On physical examination, the patient had normal vital signs. The abdomen was normal in shape with a normal inverted umbilicus. There were no visible scars or dilated veins. Moreover, the abdomen was soft with localized tenderness in the right iliac fossa and positive rebound tenderness. Rovsing's sign was also positive. However, there were no features of generalized peritonitis and no masses or organomegaly.

The patient had a sore throat with enlarged cervical lymph nodes 1 week ago and was managed as acute tonsillitis.

Abdominal ultrasound revealed complicated appendicitis.

Urinalysis was normal and laboratory investigations were as follows: hemoglobin level was 16.25 gm/dl (N: 13.5 to 17.5 gm/dl for men); RBC count was 5.663 mCL (N: 4.6–6.2 mCL); WBC was 14.07×10^3 (N: $4–11 \times 10^3$ uL); neutrophils were 70.4% (N: 45–65%); platelets count was 99.39×10^9 L (N: $150–400 \times 10^9$ L); lymphocyte was 3.76% (N: 25–45%); monocyte was 19.3% (N: 0–6%); basophil was 6.51% (N: 0–1%).

The patient was found to have positive Epstein-Barr virus (EBV) IgG antibodies but negative EBV IgM antibodies. Cytomegalovirus antibodies (CMV-IgG and CMV-IgM) were also negative.

We performed an appendectomy through a McBurney's abdominal incision and found a perforated huge appendiceal mass with mild to moderate fluid (Figure 1); the base of the appendix was normal. Free abdominal fluid was not aspirated. The remainder of the intra-abdominal organs appeared unremarkable.

Postoperatively, the patient was sent to the surgical ward and was kept NPO with IV fluids and IV antibiotics. The patient was afebrile and had stable vital signs. Hospital stay was three days with no postoperative complications.

Whole-body CT scan postoperatively showed a soft tissue lesion in the left axilla consistent with lymph node involvement (Figure 2). CT scan also showed liver enlargement (about 20 cm) but no focal lesions. However, there was no mesenteric lymphadenopathy.

Histopathological examination of the appendectomy specimen revealed a non-Hodgkin diffuse large cell lymphoma with Burkitt's-like morphology. Specifically, the hematoxylin and eosin slide demonstrated sheets of highly neoplastic lymphoblasts with high nucleus-to-cytoplasmic (N : C) ratio, hyperchromasia, and apoptotic bodies giving focally starry sky appearance. Zones of necrosis and brisk mitosis were also identified (Figures 3(a)–3(c)).

Immunohistochemistry testing demonstrated the cells being positive for CD20, CD79a, CD10, CD3, Bcl-2, Bcl-6, C-Myc (>40%), and Ki-67 (expressed in >95% of lymphoma cells) and negative for CD30 and CD43.

Genetic testing and FISH were not done unfortunately because they are unavailable at our hospital.

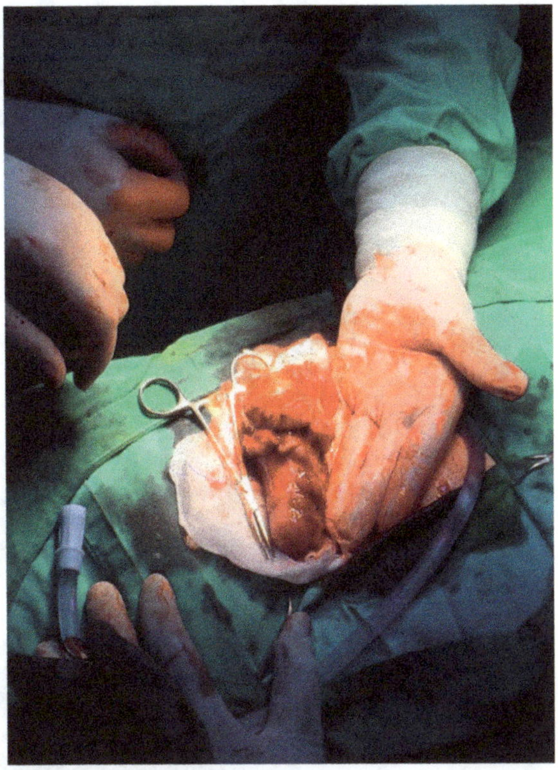

FIGURE 1: The appendiceal mass found intraoperatively.

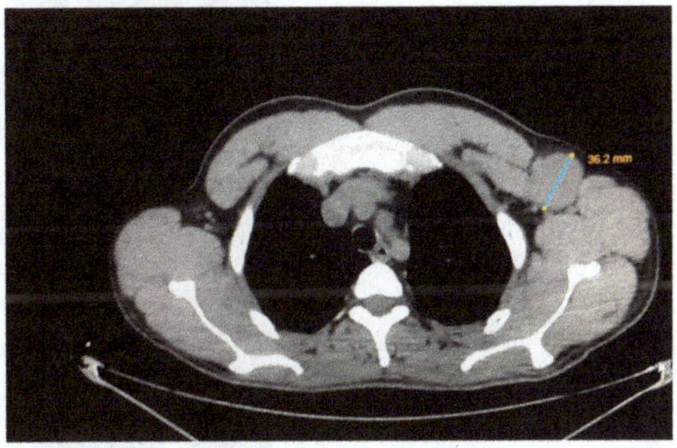

FIGURE 2: CT scan postoperatively showing a soft tissue lesion measuring 36.2 mm in the left axilla consistent of lymph node involvement.

The patient was diagnosed with double-expressor lymphoma according to the immunohistochemistry testing (co-expression of Myc and Bcl2 proteins).

Histology for specimens taken from the bone marrow and cerebrospinal fluid (CSF) showed no evidence of tissue involvement with lymphoma.

The patient thereafter was started on chemotherapy with four cycles of R-IVAC (rituximab, ifosfamide, etoposide, cytarabine), mesna, neupogen, cytarabine, methotrexate, and folic acid. His chemotherapy treatment was complicated with mild anemia, mild thrombocytopenia, nausea, and vomiting.

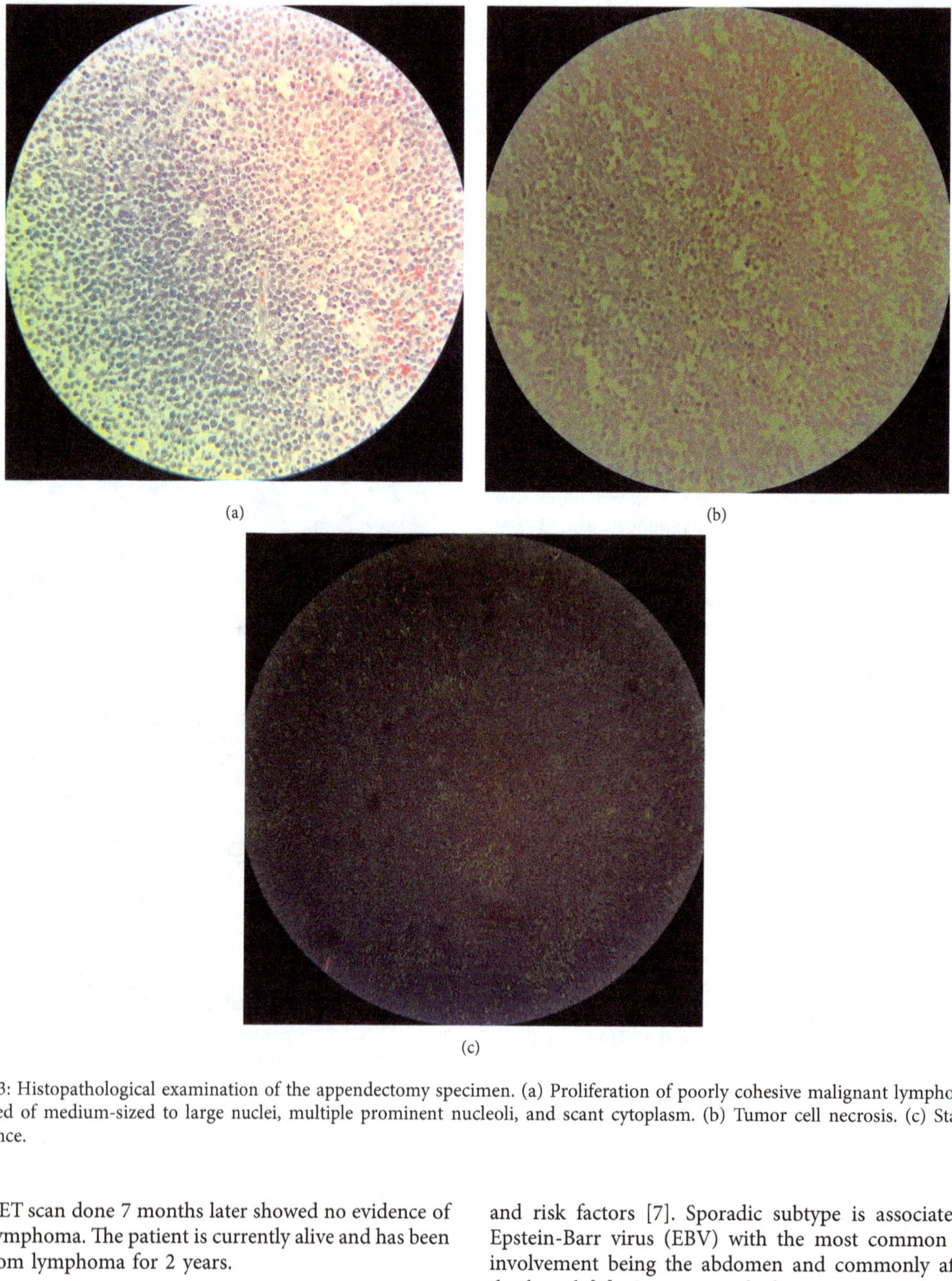

Figure 3: Histopathological examination of the appendectomy specimen. (a) Proliferation of poorly cohesive malignant lymphoid cells, composed of medium-sized to large nuclei, multiple prominent nucleoli, and scant cytoplasm. (b) Tumor cell necrosis. (c) Starry sky appearance.

A PET scan done 7 months later showed no evidence of active lymphoma. The patient is currently alive and has been clear from lymphoma for 2 years.

3. Discussion

Acute appendicitis (AA) is traditionally a clinical diagnosis, but the diagnosis is further supported by laboratory and radiological investigations, such as ultrasound and CT scans [6]. Burkitt's lymphoma is further subdivided into three subtypes (endemic, sporadic, and immunodeficiency-associated) which vary in epidemiology, clinical presentation, and risk factors [7]. Sporadic subtype is associated with Epstein-Barr virus (EBV) with the most common site of involvement being the abdomen and commonly affecting the bowel [7]. Our patient had a positive EBV IgG and appendiceal tumor making the sporadic subtype of Burkitt's lymphoma more likely.

A diagnosis of Burkitt's lymphoma is dependent on a combination of histologic (diffuse lymphoid infiltration with scattered macrophages), immunophenotypic (CD20, CD10, Bcl6 positive, and Ki-67 near 100%), and genetic features (c-Myc translocation) [8]. All of these features were identified in the present case. Although the most common finding on flow

Table 1: Characteristics of Burkett's lymphomas mimicking appendicitis as reported in the literature.

Publication year	Sex	Age	Ethnicity	Presentation	WBC (count/mm^3)	Lymph node involvement	Surgical procedure	Chemo-therapy	Follow-up
2022	M	23	NA	Right lower quadrant (RLQ) pain	14070	Left axillary	Appendectomy	Yes	24 months in remission
2021 [23]	M	18	Not available	Pelvic pain	17400	Not available (NA)	Appendectomy	Yes	30 months in remission
2021 [24]	M	15	NA	RLQ pain	NA	Para-aortic	Appendectomy	Yes	NA
2020 [25]	M	22	NA	RLQ pain	15500	Para-aortic	Appendectomy	Yes	7 months in remission
2020 [9]	F	6	NA	Right iliac fossa (RIF) pain	44600	No	Cecectomy	Yes	NA
2019 [26]	F	40	NA	RIF pain	12400	NA	Appendectomy	Yes	NA
2018 [27]	F	13	NA	Diffuse abdominal pain	15100	NA	Appendectomy and salpingo-oophorectomy	Yes	NA
2018 [28]	M	36	NA	RLQ pain	13200	NA	appendectomy	Yes	NA
2017 [9]	M	16	NA	NA	NA	NA	Appendectomy	NA	NA
2017 [29]	M	20	Middle-Eastern	NA	NA	NA	Appendectomy	NA	NA
2016 [30]	M	53	NA	Diffuse abdominal pain and left flank pain	NA	No	Appendectomy	Yes	NA
2016 [31]	F	27	NA	RLQ pian	NA	Peri-ileal and pericaecal	Right hemi-colectomy	NA	NA
2015 [32]	M	17	NA	RLQ pain	7300	Mesentric	Laparoscopic exploration without appendectomy	Yes	After 2 months, a significant reduction in tumor masses
2015 [33]	16	F	NA	NA	NA	No	Right hemi-colectomy and end-lateral ileotransversostomy	Yes	NA
2014 [34]	10	M	NA	Fatigue and RLQ pain	12800	No	Appendectomy	Yes	14 months in remission
2014 [34]	23	M	NA	Abdominal pain, vomiting, and diarrhea	11800	No	Appendectomy	Yes	17 months in remission
2014 [34]	24	F	NA	RLQ pain	NA	No	Appendectomy	Yes	18 months in remission
2014 [4]	13	F	NA	RIF pain	NA	Ileal	Appendectomy	Yes	96 months in remission
2014 [4]	18	F	NA	Cecal fistula	NA	Ileocecal	Ileocecal resection and end-to-end anastomosis of the ileum and ascending colon	Yes	104 months in remission
2013 [35]	4	M	NA	Abdominal pain	12700	Perirectal and mesenteric	Incision and drainage of abscess	Yes	24 months in remission
2012 [36]	14	M	Caucasian	Periumbilical pain	11500	No	Appendectomy	Yes	12 months in remission
2010 [37]	10	M	NA	Periumbilical pain	15800	No	Appendectomy	Yes	Recurrence after 7 months + died after 8 months
2010 [38]	14	M	Caucasian	RIF pain	15100	No	Right hemi-colectomy	Yes	NA
2010 [5]	49	M	NA	Gross haematuria and RLQ pain	10800	Mesenteric	Right hemi-colectomy	Yes	1 month in remission
2006 [9]	14	M	NA	NA	NA	NA	Right hemi-colectomy	NA	NA
2006 [39]	60	M	Caucasian	RLQ pain	NA	No	Appendectomy	Yes	NA

Table 1: Continued.

Publication year	Sex	Age	Ethnicity	Presentation	WBC (count/ mm^3)	Lymph node involvement	Surgical procedure	Chemo-therapy	Follow-up
2002 [9] [40]	12	M	European	RLQ pain	NA	NA	Right hemi-colectomy	NA	NA
1996 [9]	22	M	NA	NA	NA	NA	NA	NA	NA
1993 [41]	17	M	NA	RLQ pain	NA	No	Cecectomy	Yes	NA
1990 [42]	3	F	Caucasian	RLQ pain	17100	No	Appendectomy	Yes	5.5 months in remission
1984 [43]	22	M	Malay	Right sided abdominal pain	15800	Serosal	Appendectomy	Yes	2 months in remission
1983 [44]	22	M	NA	Epigastric and periumbilical pain	18200	No	Appendectomy	NA	NA
1980 [45]	8	M	Caucasian	Diffuse abdominal pain	10300	No	Appendectomy	Yes	36 months in remission
1980 [45]	10	M	White	Lower abdominal pain	19800	Mesenteric	Appendectomy	Yes	NA

cytometry is an expression of IgM immunoglobulin on the surface of biopsied tissue, mature B-cell markers such as CD19, CD20, CD22, CD79a, and CD10 can be found. However, CD5, CD23, CD34, and tdT are usually negative [9].

Patients with Burkitt's lymphoma who have an abdominal mass may present with nausea, vomiting, loss of appetite, gastrointestinal bleeding, signs and symptoms of acute abdomen, intestinal perforation, or renal failure [9].

Although preoperative CT scans can be used in confirming the presence of appendicitis with high sensitivity [6], they are not great at identifying if the cause is neoplastic [10]. A cohort study was published in 2020 which concluded that even if CT scans cannot identify neoplastic causes, they cannot exclude them either [10]. On the other hand, if the tumor has lymph node involvement, distant metastasis, or features that suggest an underlying malignancy, a preoperative CT scan could give us some hints on the underlying etiology [11]. Our patient did not have any abdominal lymph node involvement or metastasis. However, the patient's liver was enlarged which could indicate a malignancy. Therefore, an abdominal CT scan would give us a suspension but not a conformation. Our management would not have changed except for a more rapid histopathology report and aspirating free fluid in the abdomen in order to test for the presence of malignant cells.

In 2016, the WHO included a new category of lymphoma called high-grade B-cell lymphoma with translocations involving Myc gene and Bcl-6 or Bcl-2 genes. The lymphoma is termed a double hit if two rearrangements are present and triple hit if three rearrangements are present [12]. On the other hand, if the immunohistochemistry exhibits an expression of both Bcl2 and Myc proteins and not related to chromosomal rearrangement, then it is called double-expressor lymphoma [13].

Our patient has positive Myc and Bcl2 making the diagnosis of double-expression diffuse large B-cell lymphoma most likely.

Double-expressor lymphoma has worse outcomes than non-double-expresser lymphoma [14]. Double-expressor lymphoma is standardly treated by R-CHOP chemotherapy which includes rituximab, cyclophosphamide, doxorubicin, vincristine, and prednisone.

Even though there are several induction regimens for diffuse large B-cell lymphoma, patients who received R-HyperCVAD/MA (rituximab, cyclophosphamide, doxorubicin, vincristine, cytarabine, dexamethasone/methotrexate) and DA EPOCH-R (rituximab, cyclophosphamide, methotrexate/ifosfamide, doxorubicin, vincristine, etoposide, cytarabine) had higher rates of complete remission compared to R-CHOP [15].

In 2018, a retrospective study by Ichiro Kawashima and Yoshihiro Inamoto revealed that poor outcomes were noticed after allogeneic transplantation for double-expressor lymphoma [16].

The prognosis of lymphoma is dependent on many factors, such as the primary site of the lymphoma [17]. It has been shown that the 5-year survival rate of lymphomas in the ileocecal region was found to be 64.3% which is higher than that in large intestine (48.8%) and small intestine (32.5%) [17]. Primary central nervous system lymphoma on the other hand showed a low 5-year survival rate of 18% [18]. That being said, appendicular lymphomas have a good prognosis as it was shown that low-grade tumors including lymphomas have a 5-year survival rate of 67%–97% [19].

Another factor that plays a vital role in the prognosis of lymphoma is the histological type [20]. It was found that the 5-year survival rate of double-expressor lymphomas is 33%, which is 5–13 times higher than that of non-double-expressor ones [20]. Similar to double-hit lymphomas, triple-hit lymphomas have worse outcomes than normal ones [21].

Different systems of staging have been used to stage Burkitt's lymphoma, and we would like to emphasize on Murphy's staging system which has emphasis on extranodal disease which also distinguishes CNS disease and bone marrow disease [22].

Including this case, 34 cases of Burkitt's lymphoma have been reported in the literature to present as an acute appendicitis (see Table 1).[5].

A cohort study by Alexander H. Mimery revealed that most of the patients with appendiceal lymphoma were predominantly males accounting for 66.7% of the cases and the average age of onset was around 20 years. A palpable right iliac fossa mass was only identified in around 21% of the cases. However, an appendectomy was done in 65% of the cases (22 out of 34 cases), while 8 of the cases ended up in right hemi-colectomy.

4. Conclusion

Burkitt's lymphoma, although rare, may present as an acute appendicitis. Complete blood count and a computed tomography scan aid the diagnosis of lymphoma. Moreover, immunohistochemistry testing helps in detecting double/triple-hit Burkitt's lymphoma which has worse prognosis.

Only 34 cases of Burkitt's lymphoma have been reported to present as an acute appendicitis.

Acknowledgments

The authors are thankful for Dr. Motaz Abdelrahim Alnatsheh for his help in the data collection and histopathological interpretation. The authors thank Dr. Sadi Abu Khalaf for his help in this case. The authors also thank the patient and his family.

References

[1] K. T. Hesketh, "The management of primary adenocarcinoma of the vermiform appendix," *Gut*, vol. 4, no. 2, pp. 158–168, 1963.

[2] A. Ayub, N. Santana-Rodríguez, W. Raad, and F. Y. Bhora, "Primary appendiceal lymphoma: clinical characteristics and outcomes of 116 patients," *Journal of Surgical Research*, vol. 207, pp. 174–180, 2017.

[3] M. Khanna and S. R. Buddhavarapu, "Primary Burkitt's lymphoma of the appendix presenting as acute abdomen: a case report," *Gastrointestinal Radiology*, vol. 2, pp. 9–14, 2008.

[4] E. P. Weledji, M. N. Ngowe, and J. S. Abba, "Burkitt's lymphoma masquerading as appendicitis—two case reports and review of the literature," *World Journal of Surgical Oncology*, vol. 12, no. 1, 187 pages, 2014.

[5] M. F. Abdalla and H. M. El-Hennawy, "Unusual presentation for primary appendiceal lymphoma: a case report," *Indian Journal of Surgery*, vol. 72, no. S1, pp. 289–292, 2010.

[6] D. J. Humes and J. Simpson, "Acute appendicitis," *BMJ*, vol. 333, no. 7567, pp. 530–534, 2006.

[7] K. Kalisz, F. Alessandrino, R. Beck et al., "An update on Burkitt lymphoma: a review of pathogenesis and multimodality imaging assessment of disease presentation, treatment response, and recurrence," *Insights into imaging*, vol. 10, no. 1, 56 pages, 2019.

[8] J. A. Ferry, "Burkitt's ;lymphoma: clinicopathologic features and differential diagnosis," *The Oncologist*, vol. 11, no. 4, pp. 375–383, 2006.

[9] A. H. Mimery, J. Jabbour, B. Sykes, E. MacDermid, M. Al-Askari, and S. De Clercq, "Burkitt leukemia presenting as acute appendicitis: a case report and literature review," *American Journal of Case Reports*, vol. 21, Article ID e921568, 2020.

[10] H. Kangaspunta, K. Tahkola, E.-V. Wirta, S. Kotaluoto, J. Laukkarinen, and M. Ukkonen, "Preoperative computed tomography is poor in detecting tumors of the appendix among patients with acute appendicitis: a cohort study of 5,224 appendectomies," *Journal of Trauma and Acute Care Surgery*, vol. 88, no. 3, pp. 396–401, 2020.

[11] L. Naar, D. D. Yeh, and H. Kaafarani, "Reply: incorporating preoperative computed tomography (CT) scan and colonoscopy in the practice of acute appendicitis patients at high risk for malignancy," *Surgery*, vol. 169, no. 5, 1260 pages, 2021.

[12] J. W. Friedberg, "Double-hit diffuse large B-cell lymphoma," *Journal of Clinical Oncology*, vol. 30, no. 28, pp. 3439–3443, 2012.

[13] P. A. Riedell and S. M. Smith, "Double hit and double expressors in lymphoma: definition and treatment," *Cancer*, vol. 124, no. 24, pp. 4622–4632, 2018.

[14] A. Dodero, A. Guidetti, A. Tucci et al., "Dose-adjusted EP-OCH plus rituximab improves the clinical outcome of young patients affected by double expressor diffuse large B-cell lymphoma," *Leukemia*, vol. 33, no. 4, pp. 1047–1051, 2019.

[15] P. M. Reagan and A. Davies, "Current treatment of double hit and double expressor lymphoma," *Hematology*, vol. 2017, no. 1, pp. 295–297, 2017.

[16] I. Kawashima, Y. Inamoto, A. M. Maeshima et al., "Double-expressor lymphoma is associated with poor outcomes after allogeneic hematopoietic cell transplantation," *Biology of Blood and Marrow Transplantation*, vol. 24, no. 2, pp. 294–300, 2018.

[17] R. R. Cha, D. H. Baek, G. W. Lee et al., "Clinical features and prognosis of patients with primary intestinal B-cell lymphoma treated with chemotherapy with or without surgery," *Korean Journal of Gastroenterology*, vol. 78, no. 6, pp. 320–327, 2021.

[18] C. Lv, J. Wang, M. Zhou, J.-Y. Xu, B. Chen, and Y. Wan, "Primary central nervous system lymphoma in the United States, 1975-2017," *Therapeutic Advances in Hematology*, vol. 13, Article ID 204062072110661, 2022.

[19] Appendiceal Cancer–National Cancer Institute, 2022.

[20] S. Hatzl, F. Posch, A. Deutsch et al., "Immunohistochemistry for c-myc and bcl-2 overexpression improves risk stratification in primary central nervous system lymphoma," *Hematological Oncology*, vol. 38, no. 3, pp. 277–283, 2020.

[21] N. M. J. Edelstyn, S. J. Ellis, P. Jenkinson, and A. Sawyer, "Contribution of the left dorsomedial thalamus to recognition memory: a neuropsychological case study," *Neurocase*, vol. 8, no. 6, pp. 442–452, 2002.

[22] Y. Y. Li, D. Z. Hu, Y. F. Wang et al., "[Clinical characteristics of 219 patients with primary gastrointestinal non-Hodgkin's lymphoma]," *Zhongguo Shi Yan Xue Ye Xue Za Zhi*, vol. 28, no. 3, pp. 849–854, 2020.

[23] D. Shahmanyan, B. Saway, H. Palmerton et al., "Burkitt-type lymphoma incidentally found as the cause of acute appendicitis: a case report and review of literature," *Surgical Case Reports*, vol. 7, no. 1, 2021.

[24] T. Shaw, H. Cockrell, R. Panchal, A. Abraham, and D. Sawaya, "Burkitt lymphoma presenting as perforated appendicitis," *The American Surgeon*, vol. 88, no. 3, pp. 547-548, 2021.

[25] A. El Bakouri, A. Ballati, M. Bouali, K. Elhattabi, F. Bensardi, and A. Fadil, "Primary appendiceal Burkitt's lymphoma presenting as acute appendicitis: an extremely rare case report and review of the literatture," *Annals of Medicine and Surgery*, vol. 61, pp. 16–18, 2021.

[26] J. A. Villalobos-López, J. C. Gracia-Norzagaray, H. Flores-Nájera, J. G. Valle Leal, and C. D. García Torres, "Primary lymphoma of the appendix: a case report and review of the literature," *Revista de Gastroenterología de México*, vol. 84, no. 2, pp. 254–257, 2019.
[27] D. Hui, J. Rewerska, and B. J. Slater, "Appendiceal and ovarian Burkitt's lymphoma presenting as acute appendicitis," *Journal of Pediatric Surgery Case Reports*, vol. 32, pp. 17–20, 2018.
[28] S. D. de Morais, B. M. Mikhael, S. I. A. Németh, I. M. L. Paulo, É. O. H. de Barros, and O. A. T. Lima, "Burkitt's lymphoma presenting as acute appendicitis: a case report," *Journal of Surgical Case Reports*, vol. 2018, no. 6, 2018.
[29] J. Loh and L. Santos, "Burkitt's lymphoma presenting as acute appendicitis—a case report and review of the literature," *Pathology*, vol. 49, p. S77, 2017.
[30] C. Padma, M. Dovid, and B. Bhavik, "Gastrointestinal Burkitt's lymphoma initially presenting as nephrolithiasis and appendicitis," *American Journal of Gastroenterology*, vol. 111, 2016.
[31] M. M. B. Sangma, S. D. Dasiah, and A. J. Ashok, "Ileo-colic Burkitt lymphoma in a young adult female-a case report," *Journal of Clinical and Diagnostic Research*, vol. 10, no. 4, pp. PD11–PD12, 2016.
[32] I. Van Damme and G. d'Ydewalle, "Elaborative processing in the Korsakoff syndrome: context versus habit," *Brain and Cognition*, vol. 67, no. 2, pp. 212–224, 2008.
[33] V. Alp, N. Ay, N. Söğütçü, R. Duymuş, and Ş. Kaya, "Burkitt lymphoma of appendix not presenting with acute abdomen: case report," *Turkiye Klinikleri Journal of Case Reports*, vol. 23, no. 4, pp. 461–464, 2015.
[34] K. Ziari, K. Alizadeh, O. Rahmani, and M.-R. Kazemi, "Primary lymphoma of appendix: report of three cases and review of literature," *Iranian Journal of Pathology*, vol. 9, no. 2, pp. 160–168, 2014.
[35] D. P. Ryan, A. M. Friedmann, M. D. Schmitz, and R. J. H. Ryan, "Case record of the Massachusetts General Hospital Case 11-2013," *New England Journal of Medicine*, vol. 368, no. 15, pp. 1435–1444, 2013.
[36] J. Gonçalves, A. Cerqueira, H. Antunes, I. Maia, and S. Carvalho, "Ileocecal Burkitt's lymphoma presenting as acute appendicitis: a case report," *Citeseer*, vol. 3, no. 11, 2012.
[37] S.-M. Wang, F.-C. Huang, C.-H. Wu, S.-F. Ko, S.-Y. Lee, and C.-C. Hsiao, "Ileocecal Burkitt's lymphoma presenting as ileocolic intussusception with appendiceal invagination and acute appendicitis," *Journal of the Formosan Medical Association*, vol. 109, no. 6, pp. 476–479, 2010.
[38] S. Bains, G. Ortonowski, P. Murphy, and N. Bhardwaj, "A case of Burkitt's lymphoma presenting as suspected acute appendicitis," *African Journal of Paediatric Surgery*, vol. 7, no. 3, p. 214, 2010.
[39] S. Jaganmohan, B. Chauvin, and G. Burton, "Primary Burkitt's lymphoma of the appendix presenting as acute appendicitis," *The American Journal of Gastroenterology*, vol. 101, pp. 146-147, 2006.
[40] L. Bissen, R. Brasseur, J. S. Azagra, and P. Deirée, "[Burkitt's lymphoma of the appendix]," *JBR-BTR*, vol. 85, no. 5, pp. 257–259, 2002.
[41] K. F. Carstensen and E. Hoffmann, "Primary malignant lymphoma in the appendix vermiformis," *Ugeskr Laeger*, vol. 155, no. 32, pp. 2477-2478, 1993.
[42] Y. Caine, N. Peylan-Ramu, A. Livoff, and M. Schiller, "Primary Burkitt's lymphoma of the appendix," *European Journal of Pediatric Surgery*, vol. 45, no. 4, pp. 251-252, 1990.
[43] S. A. Ghani, N. Syed, and P. E. Tan, "A rare cause of acute appendicitis: Burkitt's lymphoma of the appendix," *Medical Journal of Malaysia*, vol. 39, no. 4, pp. 311–313, 1984.
[44] A. A. Nanji and F. H. Anderson, "Burkitt's lymphoma with acute appendicitis," *Archives of Surgery*, vol. 118, no. 11, 1352 pages, 1983.
[45] I. C. Sin, E.-T. Ling, and R. S. A. Prentice, "Burkitt's lymphoma of the appendix: report of two cases," *Human Pathology*, vol. 11, no. 5, pp. 465–470, 1980.

36

A Case of Aggressive Multiple Myeloma with Extramedullary Involvement of the Female Reproductive System, Thyroid and Breasts

Abdul Moiz Khan,[1] **Ibrahim Azar**,[1] **Saleh Najjar**,[2] **Travis Bevington**,[3] **and Syed Mehdi**[4]

[1]*Department of Internal Medicine, Albany Medical College, Albany, NY, USA*
[2]*Department of Pathology, Albany Medical College, Albany, NY, USA*
[3]*Department of Radiology, Albany Medical College, Albany, NY, USA*
[4]*Section of Hematology/Oncology, Stratton VA Medical Center, Albany, NY, USA*

Correspondence should be addressed to Abdul Moiz Khan; khana13@amc.edu

Academic Editor: Takashi Sonoki

Extramedullary disease at the time of diagnosis of multiple myeloma is a rare finding that portends poor prognosis and necessitates aggressive treatment strategies. We present a case of multiple myeloma with extramedullary plasmacytomas of the female reproductive system, thyroid and breasts. The patient was treated with lenalidomide, bortezomib, cyclophosphamide, and dexamethasone. Follow-up PET-CT scans confirmed clinical complete response, and the patient underwent autologous stem cell transplantation. The patient will be continued on lenalidomide and bortezomib maintenance therapy. To the best of our knowledge, simultaneous involvement of these sites has never been reported. The case highlights that there are no established guidelines on the treatment of multiple myeloma with extramedullary disease leading to great variability based on clinician preference. We will also discuss the treatment options and prognosis of multiple myeloma with extramedullary disease.

1. Introduction

Multiple myeloma (MM) is a disorder of clonal proliferation of plasma cells. MM is defined as clonal bone marrow plasma cells ≥10% or biopsy-proven bony or extramedullary plasmacytoma, and one or more myeloma-defining features (hypercalcemia, renal failure, anemia, lytic bone lesions, ≥60% clonal bone marrow plasma cells, and serum-free light chain ratio ≥100) [1]. It constitutes 10–13% of all hematologic malignancies [2, 3] with an age-adjusted incidence rate of about 4–6 per 100,000 persons per year [2, 4]. Extramedullary disease (EMD) at the time of diagnosis of MM is rare (0.4% to 2%) [5, 6], but during the course of the disease, as many as 13% to 30% of the patients may exhibit extramedullary involvement [7, 8]. The most common extramedullary sites of plasmacytosis are the upper respiratory tract and sinonasal region [9]. However, on reviewing the literature, it is evident that virtually any organ can be affected [7, 10]. Involvement of multiple organs with EMD at the same time is extremely unusual. Of note, plasma cell disorders involving the female reproductive system, thyroid and breasts, are exceptionally uncommon.

Here, we present a case of multiple myeloma with extramedullary plasmacytomas of the female reproductive system, thyroid gland and breasts.

2. Case

A 41-year-old female presented with pelvic pain, profuse menorrhagia, and severe symptomatic anemia (near syncope and shortness of breath). She underwent total abdominal hysterectomy with bilateral salpingo-oophorectomy (TAH/BSO) as the continuous bleeding was not responding to conservative measures and the patient had no further desire of fertility. Biopsy showed an infiltrate in the endomyometrium, fallopian tubes, and cervix of mature-appearing plasma cells that stained positive for CD56, CD38, CD79A, and MUM1 with lambda light chain restriction, consistent with plasmacytosis. Bone marrow (BM) biopsy demonstrated a hypercellular marrow and atypical plasmacytosis (25%) with lambda restriction. BM flow cytometry was positive for CD38, CD138, and CD19 and negative for CD56, CD20, and CD45 consistent with plasma cell neoplasm. FISH showed 46, [XX], female karyotype, positive for three copies of 1q21 including CKS1B gene. Free kappa and lambda light chain levels in urine were 39.9 (reference range 1.35–24.19) and 1.59 (0.24–6.66) with a kappa/lambda ratio of 25.09 (2.04–10.37). Free kappa and lambda light chains in serum were 12.6 (3.3–19.4) and 16.5 (5.7–26.3) with a kappa/lambda ratio of .76 (0.26–1.65). No M protein was detected in the SPEP or UPEP. The albumin level was 3.6, beta-2 microglobulin was 1.347 mg/L, and LDH was 163. The patient was diagnosed with nonsecretory multiple myeloma with extramedullary plasmacytoma (ISS stage I).

Around the time of TAH/BSO, the patient also reported progressively painful swelling on the left side of her neck accompanied with odynophagia, dysphagia, and hoarseness. CT of neck showed a left thyroid mass (7 × 5 × 7 cm) with irregular borders and a multinodular thyroid enlargement. (Figure 1(a)). Diagnostic incision biopsy demonstrated a very friable, irregular, malignant-appearing mass in the left lobe. A portion of the mass was removed and sent for analysis. Biopsy confirmed lambda-restricted plasma cell neoplasm involving the strap muscles (Figure 1(b)). The neoplastic plasma cells were positive for CD138, CD79a, CD45 (dim), MUM1, VS38C, and CD56. The patient remained clinically and biochemically euthyroid.

Whole body FDG-PET scan showed FDG uptake in a 4.4 × 4.7 cm mass with central necrosis within the left thyroid lobe (Figure 1(c)) along with mild FDG uptake within two right breast nodules. (Figure 2(a)). Breast U/S and mammography confirmed the nodules on the PET scan and showed other multiple bilateral nodules. Excision biopsy of the right breast nodule also showed lambda-restricted plasma cell neoplasm (Figure 2(b) and 2(c)) positive for CD 56, CD138, CD79a, and VS38C. The patient also started complaining of lower extremity bone pain, but skeletal survey was negative.

The patient was started on bortezomib (Velcade), cyclophosphamide, and dexamethasone (VCD). After the first cycle, lenalidomide (Revlimid) was added to the regimen (RVCD). The patient completed a total of 1 cycle of VCD and 4 cycles of RVCD. Follow-up PET-CT scan done 6 weeks after the 5th cycle showed no evidence of active lesions. The patient had a clinical complete response (CR), so she proceeded with autologous stem cell transplantation (ASCT) 8 weeks after the 5th cycle of chemotherapy with high-dose melphalan conditioning. The patient tolerated the treatment well. She will be continued indefinitely on daily lenalidomide and alternate weekly bortezomib maintenance therapy and will be followed up with PET-CT scans.

3. Discussion

This case poses multiple challenges right from its presentation to its treatment. First, profuse uterine bleeding is an extremely rare mode of initial presentation of MM [11]. Female reproductive organs, breasts, skeletal muscle, and thyroid gland, are exceedingly rare sites of EMD reported mostly in isolated case reports [11–13]. To the best of our knowledge, this is the only case report of MM with simultaneous involvement of the female reproductive system, thyroid and breasts.

Based on our current knowledge, multiple myeloma can lead to formation of soft tissue plasmacytomas most commonly from direct extension and local invasion of skeletal lesions. Rarely, MM can spread through hematogenous dissemination. Molecular mechanisms of EMD are poorly understood. However, reduced expression of cell adhesion molecules like VLA-4, CD44, P-selectin, and CD56, promotion of homing of myeloma cells by decreased expression of chemokine receptors like CCR1, CCR2, and CXCR4, and increased angiogenesis have been proposed as mechanisms [14]. In our case, the absence of bony lesions and the distance between sites of plasmacytosis points towards hematogenous spread.

Multiple studies have shown that extramedullary disease presages a poor prognosis and warrants more aggressive treatment strategies. A study of 1,003 myeloma cases by Varettoni et al. showed that EMD had an adverse prognostic impact on overall survival (hazard ratio 3.5) and progression-free survival (H.R 1.5), even more so when present at the time of diagnosis [7]. Usmani et al. also found that the 5-year overall survival in patients with extramedullary disease at diagnosis was shorter than in non-EMD patients (31% versus 59%). Presence of EMD at diagnosis was also associated with poor prognostic factors at baseline like anemia, thrombocytopenia, elevated centrosome index, and unfavorable cytogenetic abnormalities like MF molecular subtype (with translocation 14; 16 or 14; 20) and PR molecular subtype [15]. Our patient was positive for three copies of 1q21 with CKS1 gene which confers intermediate to high risk. An extra copy of 1q21 (CKS1B) is considered to be an adverse prognostic indicator. Gain/amplification of 1q21 increases the risk of MM progression, and incidence of amplification is higher in relapsed MM than in newly diagnosed patients [1, 16]. No other chromosomal abnormalities were found.

There are currently no established guidelines for the treatment of multiple myeloma with EMD. However, our current understanding is that patients with extramedullary myeloma eligible for stem cell transplantation could be treated with a triplet induction therapy followed by autologous stem cell transplantation (ASCT), triplet consolidation therapy, and maintenance with lenalidomide at least. For elderly patients not eligible for stem cell transplantation, bortezomib-melphalan-prednisone (VMP) or continuous lenalidomide-dexamethasone (Len-Dex) therapy may be done [1, 3, 16, 17]. Another treatment approach for aggressive disease with multiple plasmacytomas may be regimens like VDT-PACE (bortezomib, dexamethasone,

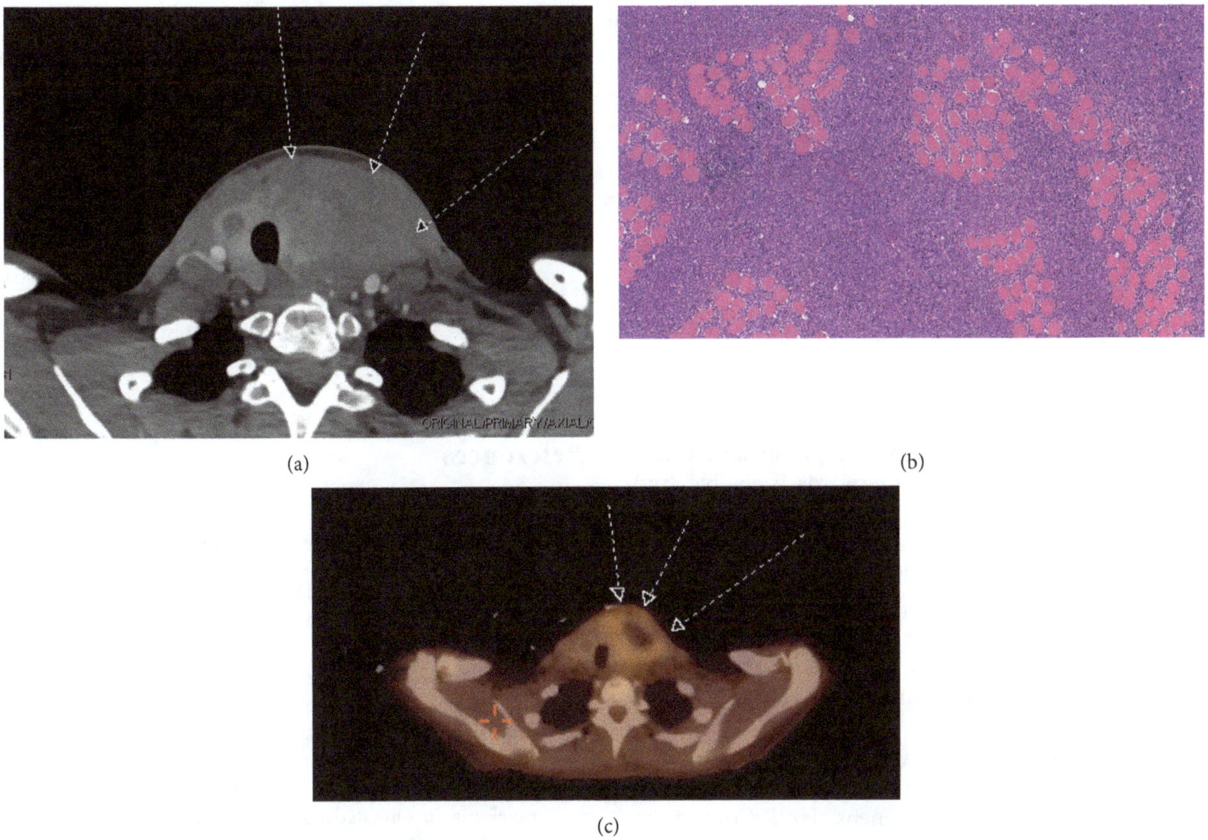

Figure 1: (a) CT scan showing thyroid gland with large left lobe mass. (b) Sheets of monoclonal plasma cells infiltrating skeletal muscle fibers, H&E. (c) PET-CT showing 4.4 × 4.7 cm mass with central necrosis within the left thyroid lobe.

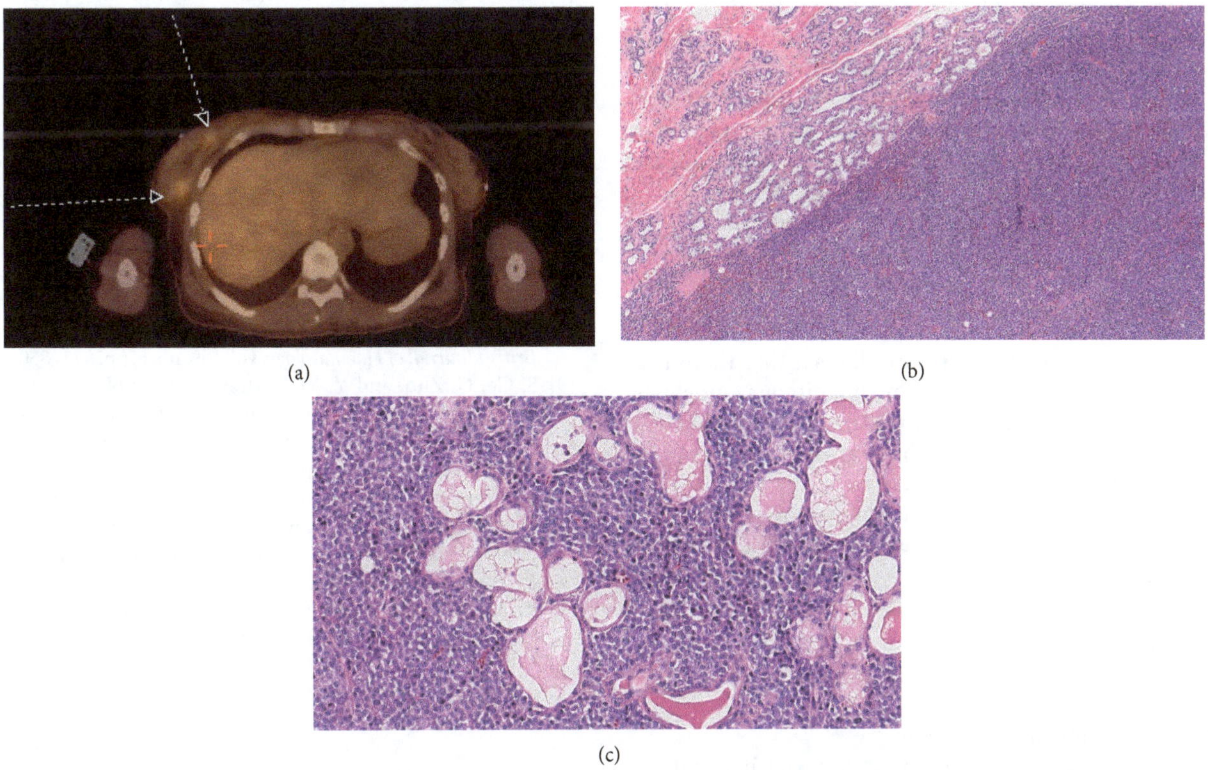

Figure 2: (a) PET-CT showing right breast nodules with FDG uptake. (b) Breast lesion consisting of monoclonal plasma cells, H&E. (c) Monoclonal plasma cells permeate the native breast lobules, H&E.

Table 1: Treatment regimens that can be used in multiple myeloma with extramedullary disease.

Stem cell transplantation eligible patients	Triplet induction therapy followed by ASCT, triplet consolidation therapy, and maintenance with lenalidomide at least
Elderly patients not eligible for stem cell transplantation	Bortezomib-melphalan-prednisone (VMP) or continuous lenalidomide-dexamethasone (Len-Dex)
Very aggressive disease especially with multiple plasmacytomas	VDT-PACE (bortezomib, dexamethasone, thalidomide, cisplatin, doxorubicin, cyclophosphamide, and etoposide) followed by ASCT if eligible and maintenance with bortezomib-based regimen
Treatment modalities under study which may be used with traditional regimens	Pomalidomide, daratumumab, elotuzumab, carfilzomib

thalidomide, cisplatin, doxorubicin, cyclophosphamide, and etoposide). ASCT may be done afterwards if eligible, and maintenance with bortezomib-based regimen will be done [1, 3, 16, 17] (see Table 1 for summary). In our case, given the aggressiveness of disease and atypical sites of involvement, a four-drug regimen (RVCD) was used, and maintenance therapy with both lenalidomide and bortezomib will be done. VDT-PACE regimen was a consideration, but our patient achieved a complete clinical response with RVCD therefore obviating its need.

As for the drugs used for treatment of MM with EMD, bortezomib has proven efficacy and may be incorporated in the multitude of treatment regimens [18]. Conversely, studies have mounted evidence against thalidomide's efficacy in treating multiple myeloma with EMD [19]. Emerging drugs include the immunomodulatory drug pomalidomide which is shown to be efficacious even against the extramedullary component [6]. Other myeloma drugs like daratumumab, elotuzumab, and carfilzomib are also being studied for their role in MM with EMD [3]. As far as the role of autologous hematopoietic stem cell transplantation (ASCT) is concerned, it provides survival advantages but is less efficacious in patients with extramedullary disease [10, 20]. In addition, with EMD, tandem ASCT does not give any survival benefit over single transplantation [21].

4. Conclusions

Our discussion should underscore the fact that there is a dearth of prospective studies and no unanimous guidelines regarding the treatment of multiple myeloma with extramedullary disease. So, there might be great subjectivity and variability based on clinician preference. With the advent of new treatment options, the need for more studies becomes even more pertinent to ensure an evidence-based approach.

Abbreviations

MM:	Multiple myeloma
EMD:	Extramedullary disease
TAH/BSO:	Total abdominal hysterectomy with bilateral salpingo-ophorectomy
ASCT:	Autologous stem cell transplantation.

References

[1] S. V. Rajkumar, "Multiple myeloma: 2018 update on diagnosis, risk-stratification, and management," *American Journal of Hematology*, vol. 93, no. 8, pp. 981–1114, 2018.

[2] S. V. Rajkumar, M. A. Dimopoulos, A. Palumbo et al., "International myeloma working group updated criteria for the diagnosis of multiple myeloma," *The Lancet Oncology*, vol. 15, no. 12, pp. e538–e548, 2014.

[3] C. Touzeau and P. Moreau, "How I treat extramedullary myeloma," *Blood*, vol. 127, no. 8, pp. 971–976, 2016.

[4] R. A. Kyle, T. M. Therneau, S. V. Rajkumar, D. R. Larson, M. F. Plevak, and L. J. Melton III, "Incidence of multiple myeloma in Olmsted county, Minnesota," *Cancer*, vol. 101, no. 11, pp. 2667–2674, 2004.

[5] R. A. Kyle, M. A. Gertz, T. E. Witzig et al., "Review of 1027 patients with newly diagnosed multiple myeloma," *Mayo Clinic Proceedings*, vol. 78, no. 1, pp. 21–33, 2003.

[6] K. D. Short, S. V. Rajkumar, D. Larson et al., "Incidence of extramedullary disease in patients with multiple myeloma in the era of novel therapy, and the activity of pomalidomide on extramedullary myeloma," *Leukemia*, vol. 25, no. 6, pp. 906–908, 2011.

[7] M. Varettoni, A. Corso, G. Pica, S. Mangiacavalli, C. Pascutto, and M. Lazzarino, "Incidence, presenting features and outcome of extramedullary disease in multiple myeloma: a longitudinal study on 1003 consecutive patients," *Annals of Oncology*, vol. 21, no. 2, pp. 325–330, 2010.

[8] C. Varga, W. Xie, J. Laubach et al., "Development of extramedullary myeloma in the era of novel agents: no evidence of increased risk with lenalidomide-bortezomib combinations," *British Journal of Haematology*, vol. 169, no. 6, pp. 843–850, 2015.

[9] S. Ge, G. Zhu, and Y. Yi, "Extramedullary plasmacytoma of the larynx: literature review and report of a case who subsequently developed acute myeloid leukemia," *Oncology Letters*, vol. 16, no. 3, pp. 2995–3004, 2018.

[10] M. Weinstock, Y. Aljawai, E. A. Morgan et al., "Incidence and clinical features of extramedullary multiple myeloma in patients who underwent stem cell transplantation," *British Journal of Haematology*, vol. 169, no. 6, pp. 851–858, 2015.

[11] A. M. Feldman, Z. Zhang, T. Buekers, and M. A. Elshaikh, "Management of gynaecologic plasmacytoma: a review

article," *Journal of Obstetrics and Gynaecology*, vol. 37, no. 1, pp. 5–10, 2017.
[12] A. Surov, H. J. Holzhausen, K. Ruschke, D. Arnold, and R. P. Spielmann, "Breast plasmacytoma," *Acta Radiologica*, vol. 51, no. 5, pp. 498–504, 2010.
[13] M. J. Hassan, S. Khans, M. Pujani, S. Jetley, P. K. Raina, and R. Ahmad, "Extramedullary plasmacytoma of the thyroid: report of a rare case," *Blood Research*, vol. 49, no. 4, pp. 280–283, 2014.
[14] J. Bladé, C. Fernández de Larrea, L. Rosiñol, M. T. Cibeira, R. Jiménez, and R. Powles, "Soft-tissue plasmacytomas in multiple myeloma: incidence, mechanisms of extramedullary spread, and treatment approach," *Journal of Clinical Oncology*, vol. 29, no. 28, pp. 3805–3812, 2011.
[15] S. Z. Usmani, C. Heuck, A. Mitchell et al., "Extramedullary disease portends poor prognosis in multiple myeloma and is over-represented in high-risk disease even in the era of novel agents," *Haematologica*, vol. 97, no. 11, pp. 1761–1767, 2012.
[16] Multiple myeloma-NCCN evidence blocks, 2018, https://www.nccn.org/professionals/physician_gls/pdf/myeloma_blocks.pdf.
[17] J. Bladé, "How I treat refractory disease and extramedullary disease," *Clinical Lymphoma Myeloma and Leukemia*, vol. 15, p. e17, 2015.
[18] P. Kapoor, V. Ramakrishnan, and S. V. Rajkumar, "Bortezomib combination therapy in multiple myeloma," *Seminars in Hematology*, vol. 49, no. 3, pp. 228–242, 2012.
[19] L. Rosiñol, M. T. Cibeira, J Bladé et al., "Extramedullary multiple myeloma escapes the effect of thalidomide," *Haematologica*, vol. 89, no. 7, pp. 832–836, 2004.
[20] L. Kumar, R. Gogi, A. K. Patel et al., "Multiple myeloma with extramedullary disease: impact of autologous stem cell transplantation on outcome," *Bone Marrow Transplantation*, vol. 52, no. 10, pp. 1473–1475, 2017.
[21] N. Gagelmann, D.-J. Eikema, S. Iacobelli et al., "Impact of extramedullary disease in patients with newly diagnosed multiple myeloma undergoing autologous stem cell transplantation: a study from the Chronic Malignancies Working Party of the EBMT," *Haematologica*, vol. 103, no. 5, pp. 890–897, 2018.

37

Myocarditis Concurrent with Sweet Syndrome: A Presentation of Acute Myeloid Leukemia

Christopher G. Burkeen, David Pottinger, Chaitanya Iragavarapu, Reshma Ramlal, and Gerhard Hildebrandt

University of Kentucky Markey Cancer Center, 800 Rose Street, Lexington, KY 40536, USA

Correspondence should be addressed to Christopher G. Burkeen; christopher.burkeen@uky.edu

Academic Editor: Sudhir Tauro

Acute myeloid leukemia (AML) is the most common acute leukemia in American adults and portends a poor prognosis if untreated. Commonly, AML presents with symptoms related to concurrent leukopenia, anemia, or thrombocytopenia; however, due to its ability to affect many organ systems in the body, AML can have a highly varied clinical presentation. One such presentation is myocarditis, which is a rarely reported manifestation of AML. Myocarditis can have a varied clinical picture and often requires exclusion of other causes of cardiac dysfunction. Sweet syndrome, also known as acute febrile neutrophilic dermatosis, is another presentation of AML; however, it is more commonly associated with AML than cardiac involvement. Sweet syndrome can occur in patients with an already established malignancy or can occur de novo in a patient with previously undiagnosed cancer and, interestingly, can also be accompanied by extracutaneous manifestations, one of which is myocarditis. Herein, we report a case of a 45-year-old male with a history of obesity and depression who presented with chest pain, a tender and diffuse rash, and pancytopenia. Heart catheterization performed at outside institution was negative for coronary artery disease. Cardiac MRI images were compatible with myocarditis. Dermal biopsy of the rash was consistent with sweet syndrome. Peripheral blood flow cytometry and bone marrow biopsy confirmed the diagnosis of AML. He was treated with an induction chemotherapy regimen of 7 days of cytarabine and 3 days of daunorubicin with resolution of his chest pain and skin lesions. The patient had persistent leukemia cells on day 14 postinduction bone marrow biopsy and was treated with high-dose cytarabine reinduction treatment. Bone marrow biopsy with count recovery after reinduction therapy revealed complete response (CR).

1. Introduction

Acute myeloid leukemia (AML) is the most common acute leukemia in American adults, accounting for 80% of all leukemia and totaling to a yearly incidence of 20,000 cases in the US [1]. AML is known to have a highly varied clinical presentation due to its ability to infiltrate and affect many organ systems in the body. One such association is a clinical entity known as sweet syndrome, which is also known as acute febrile neutrophilic dermatosis. Sweet syndrome is characterized by discrete, tender skin lesions with a heavy infiltrate of mature neutrophils and may be accompanied by extracutaneous disease. In up to 20% of cases, sweet syndrome is associated with malignancy with AML being the most frequent [2]. It can occur in patients with established diagnosis of malignancy as a paraneoplastic disorder, or it could occur prior to a formal diagnosis of malignancy. Furthermore, one potential extracutaneous manifestation of sweet syndrome is myocarditis, which is also a rare presentation of AML. Autopsies of patients who expired due to AML have shown that up to 37.1% have cardiac leukemic infiltrates [3]. However, myocarditis is a very uncommon manifestation of this, with our literature review producing only three case reports describing this association with AML. Our literature review also produced only four cases of patients with concurrent sweet syndrome and myocarditis. Here, we present a patient who presented with chest pain and increased cardiac enzymes secondary to myocarditis, a rash that was biopsy proven to be sweet syndrome, and pancytopenia secondary to new diagnosis of AML.

2. Case Presentation

A 45-year-old male with a past medical history of hypertension and depression presented to an outside hospital's emergency department with a primary complaint of chest pain of one day duration. He was in his usual state of health prior to the onset of the chest pain. This chest pain was progressively worsening, substernal, radiated to his back, and was unaffected by position. On presentation, he was found to have elevated troponins and was provided nitroglycerin, which relieved his chest pain. Initial electrocardiogram (ECG) was without any ST elevations. He was subsequently taken for left heart catheterization and found to have nonobstructive coronary artery disease. He was discharged to home on metoprolol, aspirin, statin, and a proton pump inhibitor. He was also discharged on indomethacin due to suspicion of myocarditis at that time. After discharge, however, his chest pain continued to worsen. Around that time, he also started to notice a painful dark rash on his legs.

The worsening chest pain and new onset rash prompted him to return to the ED about five days after his recent discharge, and he was subsequently transferred to our hospital's ED. On presentation, he further endorsed strong feelings of fatigue over the prior few days and was admitted to several nights of drenching sweats. He also had subjective fevers and chills. He denied any recent shortness of breath, documented fevers, changes in weight, or sensation of heart palpitations. The patient was afebrile with a heart rate of 76, blood pressure of 129/63, a respiratory rate of 18, and 99% oxygen saturation in room air. On physical exam, the patient was an obese male in no acute distress. He was observed to have a linear grouping of well-circumscribed tender papules with a deep red to purple base on his left thigh with the largest lesion being about six centimeters. He also had similar smaller lesions located on his right forearm, left upper arm, and left cheek. Cardiopulmonary exam was normal with clear lungs in all fields and no abnormal heart sounds or peripheral edema. The rest of systemic examination was normal.

Initial laboratory evaluation revealed elevated high-sensitivity troponins at 958 ng/L (<19 ng/L) and elevated NT-proBNP at 1104 pg/mL (<449 pg/mL). Repeat high-sensitivity troponin level 2 hours later was stable at 899 ng/L. His initial ECG showed no acute changes (Figure 1), and a bedside echocardiogram showed a preserved ejection fraction.

Continued workup revealed a white blood cell count of 2.20 k/μL (3.7–10.3 k/uL), an absolute neutrophil population of 0.75 k/μL, 21% peripheral blasts, hemoglobin of 8.7 g/dL (13.7–17.5 g/dL), and a platelet count of 116 k/μL (155–369 k/uL). This pancytopenia with peripheral blasts and an elevated LDH of 335 U/L (116–250 U/L) raised strong suspicion for acute leukemia. His uric acid, creatinine, and liver function tests were all within normal limits. Peripheral blood smear confirmed pancytopenia with circulating blasts. Peripheral blood flow cytometry was significant for expanded myeloid blast population with 19% of the cells. Subsequent bone marrow biopsy confirmed acute myeloid leukemia with 62% blasts by flow cytometry in a hypercellular marrow with markedly decreased background hematopoiesis. Immunophenotype showed blasts expressing CD34, CD117, partial CD13, dim CD33, HLA-DR, CD7, CD38, and moderate to dim CD45. Bone marrow aspirate smear is shown in Figure 2. Molecular testing for NPM1 and FLT3 was negative. FISH panel was positive for t(11q23) and gain of 3′KMT2A, diagnosing him with poor-risk mixed leukemia lineage- (MLL-) associated AML.

A dedicated cardiac MRI (Figure 3) demonstrated evidence of nonischaemic myocardial inflammation consistent with myocarditis. It also demonstrated multiple areas of late subepicardial gadolinium enhancement in the lateral wall and midmyocardial enhancement in the septum. Of note, the MRI showed a normal ejection fraction and no associated pericardial effusion. CMV PCR, coxsackie viral PCR, adenovirus PCR, Lyme serology, anaplasmosis serology, ehrlichiosis serology, mycoplasma PCR, influenza A and B testing, COVID-19 PCR, HIV screen, and hepatitis testing were negative. Furthermore, syphilis RPR, ANA, ANCA, and blood and urine cultures were also negative. With these negative tests, a presumptive diagnosis of AML-related myocarditis was made via exclusion. A biopsy of the patient's skin lesions was then performed, revealing for a "dense dermal infiltrate of polymorphonuclear cells in a pattern that would fit best with a neutrophilic dermatosis," qualifying a final diagnosis of sweet syndrome. The histologic image of the skin biopsy at both low and high magnification is shown in Figure 4.

The patient was started on "7 + 3" induction chemotherapy with seven days of cytarabine dosed at 100 mg/m^2 daily and three days of daunorubicin dosed at 60 mg/m^2 daily. The patient had complete resolution of his chest pain shortly thereafter and marked improvement in his skin lesions. His day 14 postinduction bone marrow biopsy showed 60% cellularity with 50% blasts consistent with prior leukemic blasts by flow cytometry. Due to persistent presence of leukemia, he was started on high-dose cytarabine (HiDAC) reinduction chemotherapy. After HIDAC, the patient had count recovery, and bone marrow biopsy at that time revealed no evidence of acute myeloid leukemia; therefore, he was determined to have complete response. He was discharged from the hospital seven weeks after his admission date. At the time of discharge, his skin lesions had healed to a significant extent.

3. Discussion

Acute myeloid leukemia has a highly variable clinical presentation with rare associations documented. AML-related myocarditis is one such poorly studied disease entity. In general, myocarditis is a disease secondary to inflammation of the cardiac muscle and has a nonspecific clinical presentation that ranges from acute chest pain to new onset heart failure to cardiogenic shock, among others. Diagnosis of clinically suspected myocarditis is based on a combination

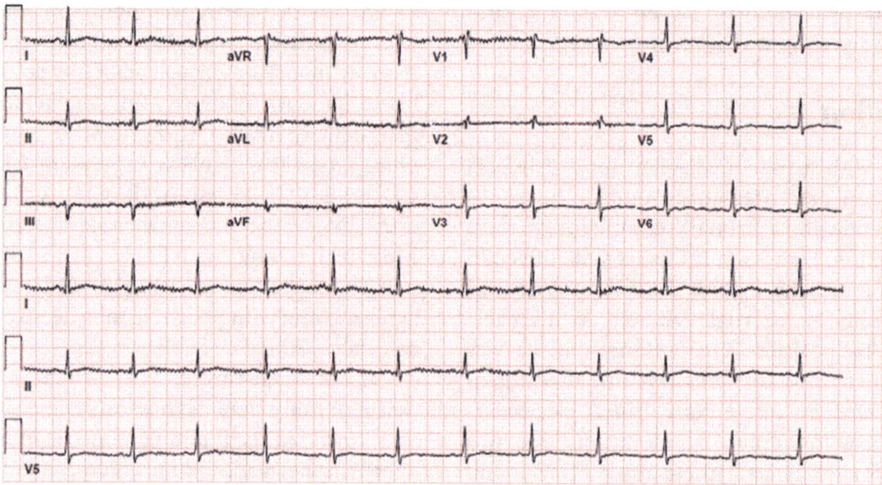

FIGURE 1: EKG performed in the ED showed a heart rate of 74 and a regular sinus rhythm, with no acute disease processes.

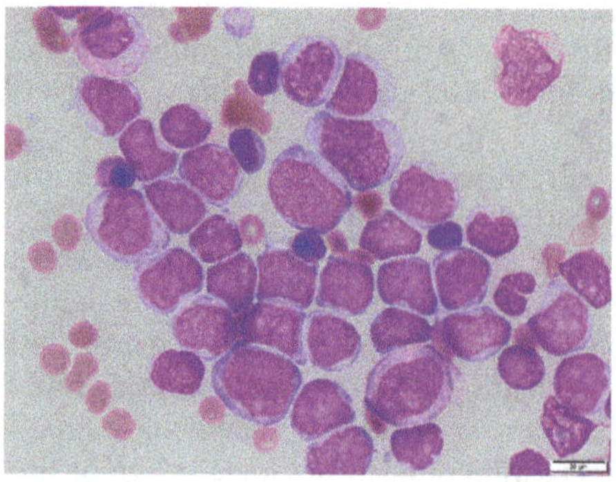

FIGURE 2: Bone marrow aspirate smears were significant for approximately 62% myeloblasts, and the background hematopoiesis was markedly decreased.

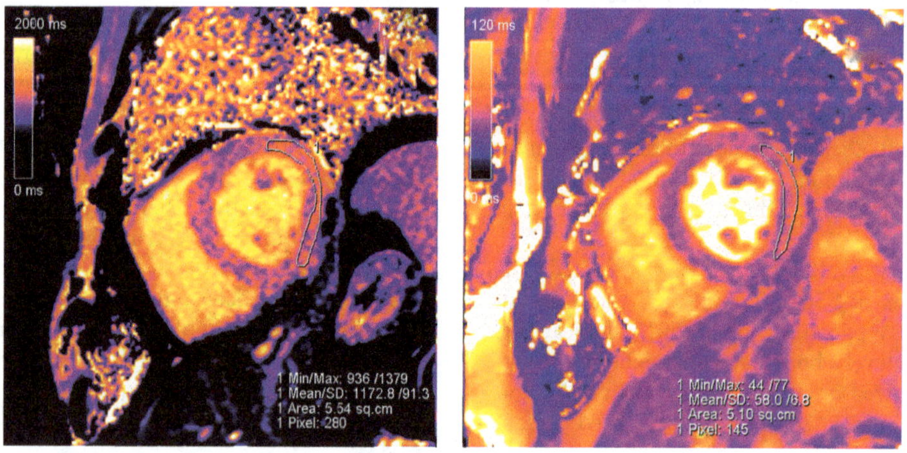

(a) (b)

FIGURE 3: Continued.

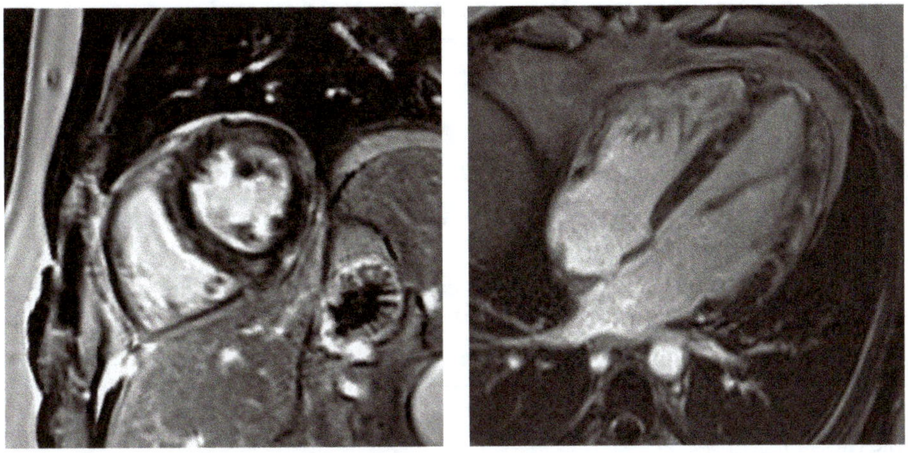

(c) (d)

Figure 3: Cardiac MRI showed features consistent with myocarditis satisfying the updated Lake Louise criteria [4], visualized in these images. (a) Mid-short-axis native T1 mapping demonstrated elevated native myocardial T1 at 1173 ms (local lab normal reference: 950–1050 ms). (b) Mid-short-axis T2 mapping demonstrated elevated myocardial T2 at 58 ms (normal reference: 40–50 ms). (c) Mid-short-axis phase-sensitive inversion recovery late gadolinium enhancement image showed multiple areas of subepicardial enhancement in the lateral wall, as well as midmyocardial enhancement in the septum. (d) Four-chamber late gadolinium enhancement image demonstrated midmyocardial enhancement in the septum and subepicardial to midmyocardial enhancement in the lateral wall.

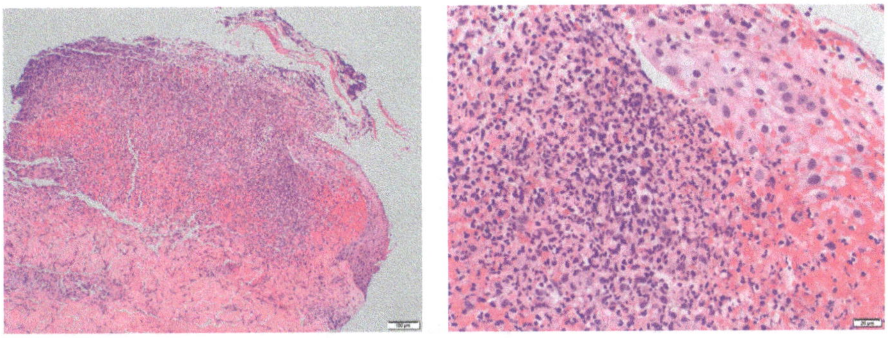

(a) (b)

Figure 4: Skin biopsy showed dense dermal infiltrate of polymorphonuclear cells at both low (a) and high (b) magnification.

of the clinical presentation and diagnostic findings, which can include characteristic tissue imaging on cardiac MRI [5]. This diagnosis via cardiac MRI is established via the updated Lake Louise criteria where both of the following criteria must be met: demonstration of edema, with regional or global myocardial signal intensity increase in T2-weighted images or with prolonged T2 relaxation times on native T2 mapping, as well as late gadolinium enhancement in a nonischaemic distribution on inversion recovery-prepared gadolinium-enhanced T1-weighted images [4]. Often, coronary arterial disease has to be ruled out via angiography. Of course, gold standard diagnosis of myocarditis is based on endomyocardial biopsy [6]. Infiltration of the heart muscle by malignant leukemia cells is a known sequela of AML, but this process is usually subclinical for unknown reasons [3]. Of 420 autopsies of myelogenous or lymphocytic leukemia patients evaluated by Roberts et al., 288 (69%) of patients had some degree of leukemic involvement of the heart. 190 of these patients had pericardial involvement, which was the most common cardiac site of involvement [3]. AML with an initial presentation of pericarditis is estimated to occur in 1-2% of cases. Myocarditis, however, is less frequently documented. In our literature review, we identified only three previous case reports documenting AML-related myocarditis, which are described in Table 1 [7–9]. Of note, pericarditis was also present in two of the three cases. Furthermore, two of the three patients had cardiac MRI with characteristic findings, and all three patients had negative coronary artery angiography.

In contrast, acute myeloid leukemia is associated with dermatologic involvement more commonly, with presence in about 10% of new cases. These skin lesions include erythematous nodules, papules, or plaques, among others [10, 11]. One of these dermatologic associations is an entity known as sweet syndrome. The classical form of sweet syndrome, also known as neutrophilic dermatosis, is a rare disorder consisting of fever, neutrophilia, and tender erythematous skin lesions characterized by mature neutrophils

Table 1: Myocarditis/myopericarditis in AML patients.

Age/sex	Presentation	Cardiac evaluation	Leukemic evaluation	Treatment	Author
37/F	Acute exertional chest pain with radiation to arms. ECG with ST elevations in leads I, aVL, V1, and V2 and PR elevation in lead AVR. Troponin elevated at 1.6 ng/mL. CBC showed WBC of 13.7 k/μL with 28% blasts, Hgb of 10.0 g/dL, and Plts 145 k/μL.	Negative coronary artery angiography. TTE: EF of 50–55% with hypokinetic right ventricle. Cardiac MRI: EF of 33% with signal changes consistent with myocarditis.	AML "confirmed on bone marrow biopsy."	Myopericarditis: colchicine and NSAIDs. AML treatment not stated.	Snavely et al. [7]
48/M	Acute substernal chest pain. Febrile (103.4°F). ECG with ST segment elevation in leads I, II, aVL, and V_5 with PR elevation and ST depression in aVR. Troponin-I was 14.8 ng/mL. CBC revealed hemoglobin of 10.8 g/dL, white cell count of 13,000/μL, 56% blasts, absolute neutrophil count of 1,430/μL, and platelet count of $83 \times 10^3/\mu$L.	Negative coronary artery angiography with an ejection fraction of 40–45%. There was mild hypokinesis in the midinferior and mid-anterolateral walls and no pericardial effusions. TTE revealed the same findings.	Bone marrow biopsy: hypercellular marrow with diffuse mononuclear infiltrates with flow cytometry consistent with AML. FISH analysis was positive for t(6; 9) (p23; q34).	Myopericarditis: colchicine 0.6 mg BID; ibuprofen 600 mg TID AML: 7 d cytarabine and 3 d idarubicin followed by salvage therapy with HIDAC and midostaurin.	Agrawal et al. [8]
62/M	Acute chest pain. ECG with ST elevation in inferior leads. Troponin of 1.5 μg/L.	TTE: normal biventricular function with inferolateral hypokinesia. Angiography: normal coronary arteries. Cardiac MRI: cardiac dysfunction with areas of myocardial edema and late enhancement.	Bone marrow biopsy: 47% blasts suggestive for AML.	Myocarditis: anti-inflammatory therapy. AML: fludarabine, steroids, and cytarabine.	De Lazzari et al. [9]

AML: acute myeloid leukemia; CBC: complete blood count; ECG: electrocardiogram; EF: ejection fraction; FISH: fluorescence in situ hybridization; Hgb: hemoglobin; HIDAC: high-dose cytarabine; Plts: platelets; TTE: transthoracic echocardiogram; WBC: white blood cells.

in the upper dermis [12]. Numerous precipitating factors have been identified, including inflammatory bowel disease, pregnancy, and administration of drugs such as G-CSF, among others. Sweet syndrome cases are very often associated with malignancy, with AML being the most common offender. Malignancy-associated sweet syndrome has been documented on numerous occasions to be the presenting symptom of previously undiagnosed neoplastic process; however, it can also occur as a paraneoplastic process in a patient with an already established diagnosis of malignancy. The exact pathogenesis of sweet syndrome is not fully understood; various proposed mechanisms have included an exaggerated hypersensitivity reaction, heritable mutations predisposing to the illness, and dysregulated cytokine (especially G-CSF) production. The lesions classically appear in multiple locations on the body, with one study suggesting that the upper and lower extremities and trunk were most commonly affected [13]. This study also found that a majority of the lesions were erythematous, with plaques being the most common morphology, but with vesicles or pustules being a known variant of the disease, appearing just under 20% of the time. The lesions were tender to palpation in 43% of cases and pruritic in 18% of cases. The gold standard for diagnosis is a biopsy showing the characteristic diffuse infiltration by mature neutrophils. First-line treatment is systemic corticosteroids, which typically cause immediate improvement in symptoms, with subsequent resolution of skin lesions [13]. Treatment of the underlying cause, if identified, is also indicated.

Our patient's presentation was consistent with malignancy-associated sweet syndrome in several ways. The papular lesions were tender, erythematous, and characteristically distributed on his lower and upper extremities. His previously undiagnosed AML is the most common malignancy associated with sweet syndrome. A skin biopsy ultimately confirmed the disease, and his rash improved with treatment of his malignancy. This patient's concurrent myocarditis diagnosis was established with cardiac MRI using the updated Lake Louise criteria [4]. His myocarditis was likely related to his diagnosis of sweet syndrome due to exclusion of other etiologies and occurring in the setting of both sweet syndrome rash and acute leukemia, two known

Table 2: Cases of sweet syndrome with concurrent myocarditis.

Age/sex	Suspected etiology	Factors supporting diagnosis of sweet syndrome	Factors supporting diagnosis of myocarditis	Therapy administered	Outcome	Author
40/F	Mesalamine (drug induced)	Edematous and erythematous plaques with some central blistering and erosions, located on the arm, neck, and palate. Biopsy: inflammatory infiltrate of the dermis, consisting of neutrophils and leukocytoclasis.	Fever, acute shortness of breath, and chest pain. Troponin T 0.12 ng/mL (elevated) and CRP 184 mg/L (elevated). ECG: diffuse ST elevations. Cardiac MRI: diffuse pericardial enhancement and edema.	Topical clobetasol cream, 6 weeks of indomethacin + colchicine, and mesalamine discontinued	Resolution of myopericarditis within 20 days; no skin lesions at 6 weeks of follow-up	Shabtaie et al. [14]
64/F	Myelodysplastic syndrome	Movable, tender, erythematous, cutaneous nodule of 1.5 cm × 1.5 cm at the inner aspect of the right lower leg. Skin biopsy demonstrated acute febrile neutrophilic dermatosis.	Clinically, the patient had symptoms consistent with myocarditis. Cardiac MRI: a small amount of pericardial effusion and slightly dilated LA. Postmortem heart biopsy: perivascular and myocardial neutrophil infiltration.	Prednisolone 30 mg/day	Death secondary to sudden cardiac arrest 3 days after presentation	Shimizu [15]
41/M	Idiopathic	Painful erythematous papules and plaques on the nape, neck, shoulders, and arms, as well as painful hyperpigmented subcutaneous nodules. Skin biopsy: subepithelial edema, dermal inflammatory infiltrate with polymorphonuclear predominance and absence of vasculitis.	EKG changes and elevated cardiac biomarkers. Cardiac MRI: patchy subepicardial enhancement and slight edema in the inferolateral wall.	Oral prednisolone 1 mg/kg/day	Complete resolution of symptoms within 4 days of presentation	Graça-Santos et al. [16]
42/M	G-CSF administration	"New skin lesions compatible with sweet syndrome reactivation." Sweet syndrome had previously been confirmed on biopsy in an episode 1 year prior.	Myocardial biopsy revealed interstitial edema and perivascular neutrophil infiltrate. Additionally, an echocardiogram with new LV systolic dysfunction and CXR with enlarged cardiac silhouette.	Hydrocortisone 1 mg/kg/day, with noninvasive ventilation and IV diuretics	Clinical parameters, invasive monitoring values, and ventricular function normalized at 48 hours	Díaz et al. [17]

CXR: chest X-ray; CRP: C-reactive protein; ECG: electrocardiogram; LA: left atrium; LV: left ventricle.

associations. The treating physicians still decided to treat with an anthracycline-based induction chemotherapy regimen despite the finding of myocarditis. This was because the patient still had preserved heart function, was hemodynamically stable, and was of young age with few comorbidities and thus would most benefit from high-intensity induction chemotherapy. Fortunately, his chest pain never recurred after treatment of his leukemia. Cases in the literature regarding the combination of sweet syndrome and myocarditis are described in Table 2 [14–17]. All four patients were treated for their sweet syndrome with some form of steroid administration. Three of the four had complete recovery from their disease; however, the fourth died due to cardiac arrest shortly after presentation. Of significance, there are no reported cases of sweet syndrome with concurrent myocarditis as symptoms of acute myeloid leukemia.

In conclusion, this patient had biopsy-proven neutrophilic dermatosis and subacute myocarditis as presenting symptoms of acute myeloid leukemia, supporting a diagnosis of sweet syndrome. Providers should be aware of this clinical syndrome, especially because it may be the first manifestation of underlying hematologic malignancy.

References

[1] I. De Kouchkovsky and M. Abdul-Hay, "Acute myeloid leukemia: a comprehensive review and 2016 update," *Blood Cancer Journal*, vol. 6, no. 7, p. e441, 2016.

[2] R. E. Isaac, D. Sinson, and S. Jones, "Sweet syndrome," *British Journal of Oral and Maxillofacial Surgery*, vol. 53, no. 9, pp. 894-895, 2015.

[3] W. C. Roberts, G. P. Bodey, and P. T. Wertlat, "The heart in acute leukemia a study of 420 autopsy cases," *The American Journal of Cardiology*, vol. 21, no. 3, pp. 388–412, 1968.

[4] M. Ferreria, "Cardiovascular magnetic resonance in non-ischemic myocardial inflammation: expert recommendations," *JACC*, vol. 72, no. 24, pp. 3158–3176, 2018.

[5] M. P. Gannon, E. Schaub, C. L. Grines, and S. G. Saba, "State of the art: evaluation and prognostication of myocarditis using cardiac MRI," *Journal of Magnetic Resonance Imaging*, vol. 49, no. 7, pp. e122–e131, 2019.

[6] A. L. P. Caforio, S. Pankuweit, E. Arbustini et al., "Current state of knowledge on aetiology, diagnosis, management, and therapy of myocarditis: a position statement of the European society of cardiology working group on myocardial and pericardial diseases," *European Heart Journal*, vol. 34, no. 33, pp. 2636–2648, 2013.

[7] C. Snavely, J. Habboushe, and C. Snavely, "A placebo-controlled trial of subcutaneous semaglutide in nonalcoholic steatohepatitis," *Journal of Emergency Medicine*, vol. 20, pp. 30343–30347, 2020.

[8] K. Agrawal, L. Miles, N. Agrawal, and A. Khan, "A typical presentation of acute myeloid leukemia," *World Journal of Oncology*, vol. 9, no. 1, pp. 29–34, 2018.

[9] M. De Lazzari, E. Hiso, M. Perazzolo Marra et al., "Myocarditis as first manifestation of acute myeloid leukemia," *European Heart Journal*, vol. 35, p. 1204, 2014.

[10] R. N. Chavan, M. A. Cappel, R. P. Ketterling et al., "Histiocytoid Sweet syndrome may indicate leukemia cutis: a novel application of fluorescence in situ hybridization," *Journal of the American Academy of Dermatology*, vol. 70, no. 6, pp. 1021–1027, 2014.

[11] S. Kaddu, P. Zenahlik, C. Beham-Schmid, H. Kerl, and L. Cerroni, "Specific cutaneous infiltrates in patients with myelogenous leukemia: a clinicopathologic study of 26 patients with assessment of diagnostic criteria," *Journal of the American Academy of Dermatology*, vol. 40, no. 1, pp. 966–978, 1999.

[12] K. V. Ratnam, C. J. L. Khor, and W. P. Daniel Su, "Leukemia cutis," *Dermatologic Clinics*, vol. 12, no. 2, pp. 419–431, 1994.

[13] P. R. Cohen, "Sweet's syndrome-a comprehensive review of an acute febrile neutrophilic dermatosis," *Orphanet Journal of Rare Diseases*, vol. 2, no. 1, p. 34, 2007.

[14] S. A. Shabtaie, N. Y. Tan, R. S. Parikh, and K. A. Papadakis, "Concurrent sweet's syndrome and myopericarditis following mesalamine therapy," *BMJ Case Reports*, vol. 85, 2018.

[15] K. Shimizu, "Neutrophilic infiltration of the myocardium in a patient with myelodysplastic syndrome," *American Journal of Hematology*, vol. 58, no. 4, pp. 337-338, 1998.

[16] L. Graça-Santos, K. Kieselova, F. Montenegro-Sá, J. Guardado, and J. Morais, "Comprometimento cardíaco na síndrome de sweet: um achado raro numa doença rara," *Arquivos Brasileiros de Cardiologia*, vol. 115, no. 1, pp. 6–9, 2020.

[17] J. M. Díaz, M. Fernández, G. Rivero, D. Hernán, C. Hernán, and C. . A. Belziti, "Sweet's syndrome with severe cardiac involvement," *Revista Argentina de Cardiología*, vol. 84, no. 3, pp. 248-249, 2016.

Keeping an Eye on Bisphosphonate Therapy in Myeloma: A Case Report of Ocular Inflammation Postzoledronic Acid Infusion

Rehman Faryal and Amjad Hayat

Haematology Department, University Hospital Galway, Galway, Ireland

Correspondence should be addressed to Rehman Faryal; rehman.faryal@hse.ie

Academic Editor: Alessandro Gozzetti

Bisphosphonates have evolved over the past decades from oral to more potent intravenous preparations. Along with significant paradigm shift in the management of myeloma over the past years, stronger nitrogen-containing bisphosphonates, due to their antiresorptive action on the bones, have found their way as a key and integral part in the management of bone disease in myeloma. Multiple randomized controlled trials have established efficacy of bisphosphonates in reducing skeletal-related events in myeloma. Some well-documented adverse events include acute-phase reactions, esophageal irritation, and osteonecrosis of the jaw. Across all clinical indications, the incidence of inflammatory eye reactions after bisphosphonate infusion ranges from 0.046% to 1%. However, data from myeloma patients are extrapolated from few reported cases in literature with varying management strategies including discontinuation, switching to different forms, and rechallenging with steroid cover. Inflammatory eye reactions can vary from self-limiting conjunctivitis and episcleritis to serious uveitis and vision-threatening orbital inflammation. We present a similar case of a patient with IgG kappa myeloma who developed flu-like symptoms followed by severe orbital inflammation within 48–72 hours after receiving zoledronic acid infusion. The patient was successfully managed with intravenous methyl prednisolone followed by oral tapering dose of steroids and discontinuation of further bisphosphonate therapy. A complete recovery was noted in a week's time.

1. Introduction

Multiple myeloma is a disorder of clonal plasma cells which are derived from postgerminal B cells. It accounts for around 1% of all cancers and 13% of hematological malignancies. Median age of diagnosis is around 70 years with 37% of myeloma patients younger than 65 years [1]. Alongside anemia, hypercalcemia, and renal impairment, lytic bone lesions are an important feature of myeloma, which can complicate the course of disease with severe pain and skeletal-related events (SREs) including pathological fractures and cord compression. Approximately 80% of multiple myeloma patients experience a pathological fracture over the course of their disease [2]. Introduction of immunomodulatory drugs, proteasome inhibitors, and monoclonal antibodies into the treatment algorithms have translated into better survival outcomes. Over the past decades, bisphosphonates have found central role in osteoporosis, malignancies, and Paget's disease, and now they are an integral part of the management of bone disease in myeloma. Bisphosphonates have evolved from oral therapies to more potent, dose-convenient, intravenous therapies. Generally, well tolerated, they are known to cause side effects ranging from mild acute-phase reactions, esophageal irritation, hypocalcemia, and atrial fibrillation to rare serious adverse events such as osteonecrosis of the jaw. Relatively rare adverse effects of bisphosphonate therapy are inflammatory eye reactions (IERs) ranging from conjunctivitis and episcleritis to vision-threatening uveitis, scleritis, and severe orbital inflammation. Due to their increasing indications, usage, and previously underreporting, more cases of ophthalmological adverse events have come to light in recent years.

2. Case Presentation

A 45-year-old man presented to the eye casualty with right-sided periorbital swelling, pain, epiphora, and chemosis three days after receiving zoledronic acid in hematology day ward. He had a history of recently diagnosis of IgG kappa myeloma, R-ISS stage I, with multiple lytic lesions on the ribs, and a bone-related plasmacytoma on the left-sided ninth rib. He was an ex-smoker with a smoking history of 15 pack years. He had no other significantly past medical history and was not on any regular medications prior to his diagnosis. He was started on bortezomib/lenalidomide/dexamethasone (VRD) therapy. At the start of the second cycle, he received zoledronic acid 4 mg intravenously. He started noticing flu-like symptoms 24 hours after infusion, along with mild joint pains and minimal right eyelid swelling. Over the next 48 hours, he reported worsening right eye swelling, pain, redness, and difficulty in opening his eye (Figure 1).

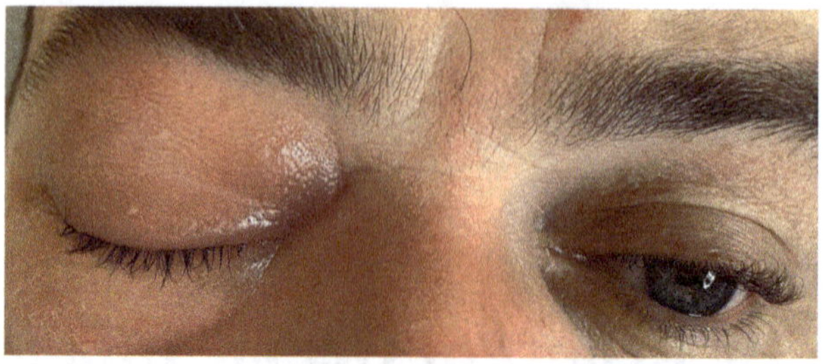

FIGURE 1: Right eyelid and periorbital swelling and redness.

On examination, his visual acuity was 6/9 bilaterally. A computed tomography (CT) scan of both orbits was requested to assess any possible retrobulbar inflammation. CT findings were suggestive of right-sided orbital cellulitis (Figure 2). On suspicion of a possible infective episode, he was empirically started on IV antibiotics. His symptoms continued to worsen over the next 12 hours, and it was decided to start on IV methyl prednisolone 500 mg once daily. By day three of IV steroids, there was a significant resolution of swelling and pain. He was discharged on oral prednisolone 60 mg which was tapered down every third day. He was followed up in day ward after a week where he reported complete recovery. Based on severity of the event and ophthalmology opinion, it was agreed to discontinue any further bisphosphonate therapy.

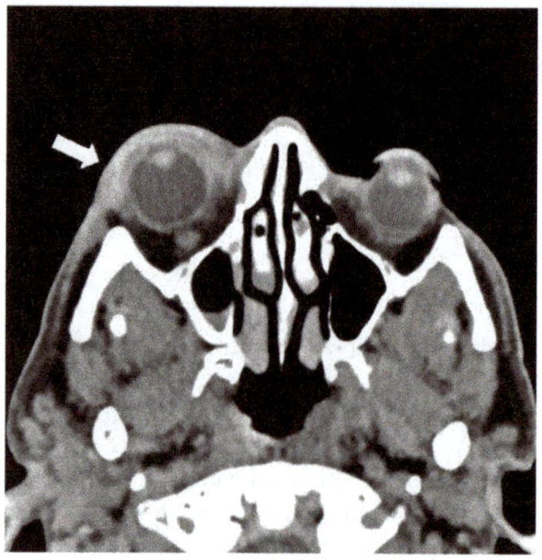

FIGURE 2: Mild right eye proptosis and soft tissue thickening overlying the right orbit (arrow). Edema of the medial and superior rectus muscles. Postseptal involvement with inflammatory fat stranding in the intraconal fat posterior to the globe.

3. Types of Bisphosphonates and Mechanism of Action

Bisphosphonates are structural analogues of naturally occurring inorganic pyrophosphates, which bind to the hydroxyapatite binding site on the exposed areas of the bone, undergoing active resorption. During the resorptive process, bisphosphonates are absorbed by the osteoclasts, eventually leading to apoptosis.

Chemically, they are classified into two categories: non-nitrogen-containing bisphosphonates that include early first-generation bisphosphonates such as clodronate and etidronate. They are structurally very similar to naturally occurring inorganic pyrophosphates. The second category consists of nitrogen-containing bisphosphonates which include second- and third-generation compounds such as alendronate, risedronate, ibandronate, pamidronate, and zoledronic acid. The addition of nitrogen/amine group to the bisphosphonate upgrades its antiresorptive potency by 10–10,000 compared to nonnitrogen-containing bisphosphonates [3, 4]. It is important to know that, along with the antiresorptive effect, pyrophosphates (including naturally occurring inorganic pyrophosphates and bisphosphonates) also inhibit calcification and mineralization of the bone. However, the potential to inhibit mineralization differs among the bisphosphonates, for example, risedronate inhibits bone resorption and mineralization at the same concentration (therapeutic index 1 : 1). In contrast, for nitrogen-containing bisphosphonates, the potential to inhibit mineralization is 1000 times less than its antiresorptive effect at the same concentration of the drug. Therefore, it renders a favorable therapeutic index to treat conditions such as myeloma-related bone disease.

Once absorbed by the osteoclasts, nonnitrogen-containing bisphosphonates are metabolized and incorporated into newly formed adenosine triphosphate (ATP) molecules. These nonhydrolysable ATPs accumulate and are unable to drive ATP-dependent cellular processes, resulting in osteoclast apoptosis. In comparison, nitrogen-containing bisphosphonates, once absorbed by the osteoclasts, inhibit the activity of farnesyl pyrophosphate synthase, a key regulatory enzyme in the mevalonic acid pathway resulting in posttranslational modifications of key proteins and eventually resulting in osteoclast apoptosis [4].

4. Pathophysiology of Ocular Inflammation

Bisphosphonate treatment has been known to trigger the release of cytokines, IL-1 and IL-6, and other acute-phase proteins. In one study, it is suggested that nitrogen-containing bisphosphonates stimulate gamma/delta T cells (γ/δ T cells) in peripheral blood. Furthermore, it is suggested that the intensity of the acute-phase reaction seemed to correlate with the magnitude of increase in γ/δ T cells [5].

The exact mechanism of underlying ocular inflammatory response largely remains unknown. One suggested mechanism is that the drug is secreted into the tears by the lacrimal gland triggering a transitory localized irritation leading to the release of cytokines and other acute-phase proteins in the eye or cause activation of gamma/delta T cells within the orbit [6–8]. Preclinical animal studies reported conjunctivitis and episcleral congestion in rabbits with very supratherapeutic doses of pamidronate (daily dose of 30 mg/kg for 6 months), and it was identified that, at these doses, pamidronate secrets tears [9, 10].

The acute cytokines or T-cell response could explain the immediate eye reactions that take place within a short window. However, it is difficult to explain very delayed reactions occurring after weeks or months. It is uncertain whether the type of bisphosphonates used or disease-related factors such as background inflammatory conditions, immune dysregulation, or progressive accumulation of bisphosphonates overtime within the eye play any possible role to illicit these delayed reactions [6].

5. Discussion

Myeloma represents a subsegment of the patients receiving bisphosphonate therapies. Over the past years, multiple randomized placebo trials have demonstrated the efficacy of clodronate, pamidronate, and zoledronic acid in reducing bone pains and skeletal-related events. One study showed zoledronic acid was found to be as effective as pamidronate in reducing pain and incidence of SREs [11]. In another study, Medical Research Council (MRC) Myeloma IX trial, it not only shows zoledronic acid to be better than clodronate in reduction of SREs but also demonstrates that addition of zoledronic acid to standard first-line myeloma treatment reduced the risk of death by 16% and prolonged median overall survival by 5.5 months compared to clodronate [12]. However, a meta-analysis from Cochrane database was not able to confirm superiority of one bisphosphonate over another, but it is important to note that zoledronic acid is the only bisphosphonate to show survival benefit in placebo-controlled trials [13, 14]. Most experts and myeloma groups recommend a 2-year duration of bisphosphonate therapy, which is extrapolated from all placebo-controlled trials, in which the maximum duration of bisphosphonate therapy was 2 years.

Overall, the incidence of IERs after bisphosphonate exposure ranges from 0.046% to 1%, with onset occurring from a few hours after exposure up to more than 3 years, with a median of 3 weeks [9]. Around 1 in 10 patients receiving bisphosphonates have flu-like symptoms such as fever, arthralgia, and myalgia following the first dose. The rate of reactions reduces to half following subsequent infusions. In one study, HORIZON trial, the rate of acute-phase reactions after the third dose was suggested to be around 2.8% [9].

Although most of the data around ocular adverse effects of bisphosphonates comes from its use in broader categories of indications such as osteoporosis, Paget's disease, and solid cancers such as breast, prostate, and lung cancers, the data of myeloma patients come from few case reports in literature with variability in the management ranging from discontinuation of bisphosphonate therapy to rechallenging with the same or different forms of bisphosphonate. Maniel et al. report a recurrence of ocular symptoms including eyelid swelling, chemosis, and diplopia on rechallenging 4 months after the first episode with the same bisphosphonate (pamidronate) [15]. Similarly, Benderson et al. reports recurrence of milder symptoms after switching from zoledronic acid to pamidronate infusion with methyl prednisolone support and continued monthly pamidronate with steroid cover thereafter with minimal symptoms [16]. Gathering data from other indications for bisphosphonate, Fraunfelder and Fraunfelder reported 17 cases of unilateral scleritis associated with intravenous pamidronate which required discontinuation of the pamidronate therapy [17].

The decisions to rechallenge should be based on the severity of the adverse event and accurate diagnosis with formal evaluation by ophthalmology. Isolated conjunctivitis or episcleritis, having good prognosis, often experiences complete resolution without specific treatment after few days. Nonspecific conjunctivitis usually decreases in intensity during subsequent exposure to a bisphosphonate [17]. In context of myeloma where benefits clearly outweigh the risks in such circumstances, retreatment with or without steroid cover is generally safe. Patients presenting with severe orbital inflammation, once septic elements are excluded, should be promptly initiated on intravenous steroids. More severe adverse events such as uveitis, scleritis, and orbital inflammation can have serious and long-lasting consequences. In case of scleritis to fully resolve, bisphosphonate must be discontinued [17]. Cases such as these should be dealt with utmost care in conjunction with ophthalmology before a decision to rechallenge is made.

6. Conclusion

Bisphosphonate therapy for myeloma patients continues to be an integral part of myeloma management. Physicians and hematologists should be aware of these uncommon adverse events, and based on the severity of the events and in collaboration with ophthalmology support, a well-informed decision should be made in best interest of the patient.

References

[1] A. Palumbo and K. Anderson, "Multiple myeloma," *New England Journal of Medicine*, vol. 364, no. 11, pp. 1046–1060, 2011.

[2] L. J. Melton, R. A. Kyle, S. J. Achenbach, A. L. Oberg, and S. V. Rajkumar, "Fracture risk with multiple myeloma: a population-based study," *Journal of Bone and Mineral Research*, vol. 20, no. 3, pp. 487–93, 2005.

[3] R. G. G. Russell, "Bisphosphonates: from bench to bedside," *Annals of the New York Academy of Sciences*, vol. 1068, no. 1, pp. 367–401, 2006.

[4] M. T. Drake, B. L. Clarke, and S. Khosla, "Bisphosphonates: mechanism of action and role in clinical practice," *Mayo Clinic Proceedings*, vol. 83, no. 9, pp. 1032–1045, 2008.

[5] V. Kunzmann, E. Bauer, and M. Wilhelm, "γ/δ T-cell stimulation by pamidronate," *New England Journal of Medicine*, vol. 340, no. 9, pp. 737-738, 1999.

[6] E. M. Clark and D. Durup, "Inflammatory eye reactions with bisphosphonates and other osteoporosis medications: what are the risks?" *Therapeutic Advances in Musculoskeletal Disease*, vol. 7, no. 1, pp. 11–16, 2015.

[7] F. W. Fraunfelder and F. T. Fraunfelder, "Adverse ocular drug reactions recently identified by the national registry of drug-induced ocular side effects," *Ophthalmology*, vol. 111, no. 7, pp. 1275–1279, 2004.

[8] J. D. Peterson and E. H. Bedrossian, "Bisphosphonate-associated orbital inflammation-a case report and review," *Orbit*, vol. 31, no. 2, pp. 119–123, 2012.

[9] M. Pazianas, E. M. Clark, P. A. Eiken, K. Brixen, and B. Abrahamsen, "Inflammatory eye reactions in patients treated with bisphosphonates and other osteoporosis medications: cohort analysis using a national prescription database," *Journal of Bone and Mineral Research*, vol. 28, no. 3, pp. 455–463, 2013.

[10] P. S. Subramanian, J. B. Kerrison, P. C. Calvert, and N. R. Miller, "Orbital inflammatory disease after pamidronate treatment for metastatic prostate cancer," *Archives of Ophthalmology*, vol. 121, no. 9, pp. 1335-1336, 2003.

[11] L. S. Rosen, D. Gordon, M. Kaminski et al., "Long-term efficacy and safety of zoledronic acid compared with pamidronate disodium in the treatment of skeletal complications in patients with advanced multiple myeloma or breast carcinoma," *Cancer*, vol. 98, no. 8, pp. 1735–1744, 2003.

[12] G. J. Morgan, F. E. Davies, W. M. Gregory et al., "First-line treatment with zoledronic acid as compared with clodronic acid in multiple myeloma (MRC Myeloma IX): a randomised controlled trial," *The Lancet*, vol. 376, no. 9757, pp. 1989–1999, 2010.

[13] R. Mhaskar, J. Redzepovic, K. Wheatley et al., "Bisphosphonates in multiple myeloma: a network meta-analysis," *Cochrane Database of Systematic Reviews*, vol. 5, Article ID 003188, 2012.

[14] E. Terpos, G. D. Roodman, and M. A. Dimopoulos, "Optimal use of bisphosphonates in patients with multiple myeloma," *Blood*, vol. 121, no. 17, pp. 3325–3328, 2013.

[15] T. P. J. Meaney, M. Musadiq, and P. G. J. Corridan, "Diplopia following intravenous administration of pamidronate," *Eye*, vol. 18, no. 1, pp. 103-104, 2004.

[16] D. Benderson, J. Karakunnel, S. Kathuria, and A. Badros, "Scleritis complicating zoledronic acid infusion," *Clinical Lymphoma and Myeloma*, vol. 7, no. 2, pp. 145–147, 2006.

[17] F. W. Fraunfelder and F. T. Fraunfelder, "Bisphosphonates and ocular inflammation," *New England Journal of Medicine*, vol. 348, no. 12, pp. 1187-1188, 2003.

Multiple Myeloma with Foamy Mott Cells

Karen Nalbandyan[1] **Daniel Benharroch**[1] **Benzion Samueli**[1]
Michael Kafka,[2] **and Anna Gourevitch**[3]

[1]*Department of Pathology, Soroka University Medical Center, Faculty of Health Sciences, Ben-Gurion University of the Negev, Beer-Sheva, Israel*
[2]*Division of Hematology, Hematology Laboratory, Soroka University Medical Center, Faculty of Health Sciences, Ben Gurion University of the Negev, Beer-Sheva, Israel*
[3]*Division of Hematology, Soroka University Medical Center, Faculty of Health Sciences, Ben-Gurion University of the Negev, Beer-Sheva, Israel*

Correspondence should be addressed to Karen Nalbandyan; nalbandyankaren@gmail.com

Academic Editor: Salah Aref

Intracytoplasmic assorted vacuoles containing immunoglobulin collections are occasionally seen in multiple myeloma. When abundant, they impart a foamy appearance to the tumor cells, which is a potential source for diagnostic pitfalls. Herein, we report the case of a patient who presented with skeletal pain and CT confirmed lytic lesions. A bone marrow biopsy revealed multiple myeloma with unusual foamy Mott cells. The patient was subsequently treated with four cycles of cyclophosphamide, bortezomib, and dexamethasone induction therapy, followed by 3 cycles of lenalidomide with dexamethasone. A biopsy performed following initial biological and immunomodulatory drugs revealed different morphological and clonal characteristics. These features were modified again, five years later, and again, after two years of close monitoring. Hematopathologists should be aware of this morphologic variant of myeloma as well as for the capacity of clonal characteristics, such as light chain monotype, to fluctuate subsequent to treatment.

1. Introduction

Multiple myeloma is a multifocal plasma cell neoplasm associated with an M-protein in the serum and/or urine [1]. Myeloma cells show a wide spectrum of morphological variation, from a near normal plasmacytic phenotype to pleomorphic multinucleated or anaplastic forms. As a rule, the tumor cells are larger than their nonneoplastic counterparts; however, normal and small cell sized variants have been described. Other variations include nuclear convolutions and Burkitt-like or blastic morphology [2]. Occasionally, intracellular immunoglobulin (Ig) accumulations are seen within variable sized vacuoles. Such inclusions are called Dutcher bodies if seemingly intranuclear and Russel bodies if intracytoplasmatic; when numerous, the cell carrying them is termed a Mott cell. Here, we report a rare case of multiple myeloma with foamy cell features. The finding may be significant as a potential source of diagnostic pitfall.

2. Case Presentation

2.1. Clinical Summary. A 65-year-old Caucasian male presented in May 2015 for evaluation of right-shoulder and upper-back pain for the preceding 6 months. Computed tomography (CT) showed a paraspinal soft tissue mass, compression of the D7 and D8 vertebrae, and lytic lesions in the right scapula and D9 vertebra. Blood tests revealed the following: hemoglobin 13.6 g/dl, creatinine 1.45 mg/dl, globulins 5.9 g/dl, with a monoclonal peak of IgG kappa of 3.9 g, free kappa light chain 165 mg/dl, and kappa/lambda ratio 22.10. Urine protein was 5.7 g/l, and Bence-Jones protein was negative. Bone marrow investigation was performed in relation with a working diagnosis of multiple myeloma.

2.2. Pathological Findings. Bone marrow biopsies obtained from the patient were fixed in 4% buffered formaldehyde (Gadot Biochemical Industries, Haifa, Israel), decalcified in 10% EDTA decalcification solution (Milestone, Italy), processed at 40°C, and embedded in paraffin blocks at 61°C in Tissue-Tek VIP6-E2 processor (Sakura), according to the standard protocol of the laboratory. Sections of 5–10 μm in thickness were stained with Mayer's hematoxylin (Pioneer/ Sigma) and eosin (Pioneer Research Chemicals, Ltd.) in Tissue-Tek Prisma E-2S automated slide stainer (Sakura). The immunostainings and chromogenic in situ hybridization (CISH) were carried out on a BenchMark XT Full System (Ventana, Tucson, AZ, USA) using antibodies to the following: CD68 clone PG-M (Dako), anti-kappa (clone L1C1) and anti-lambda (clone Lamb14), both from Cell-Marque, and anti-cytokeratin antibody clones AE1/AE3 and MNF116. Cytoplasmic kappa and lambda mRNA CISH probes were ready to use (Ventana). Histological examination was performed using an Olympus BX41 microscope (Olympus, Tokyo, Japan). Smears from bone marrow aspirates were prepared manually and stained with Wright stain by an automatic Sysmex SP50 slide stainer.

On bone marrow aspiration, cells of unequivocal plasmacytic morphology comprised 4% of all leukocytes. In addition, 20% of total leukocytes were represented by very large cells with eccentric nuclei and highly vacuolated cytoplasm. Their differential diagnosis included Mott cells and macrophages.

The bone marrow biopsy was mildly hypercellular for age (about 75%), predominantly erythroid lineage. Numerous large cells with foamy cytoplasm, resembling foamy macrophages or Gaucher cells (Figure 1(a)), were identified. The large cells stained negative for CD68 PGM1 (Figure 1(b)), periodic acid-Schiff (PAS), and both cytokeratin AE1/AE3 and MNF116. They showed strong positive cellular membrane staining for CD138 (Figure 1(c)); the staining for kappa light chain was positive, cytoplasmatic, in 60% of the marrow nucleated cells (Figure 1(d)), whereas lambda light chain was positive in isolated cells only (<1%). A FISH confirmed kappa light chain restriction, consistent with monoclonality. The patient was subsequently treated with 4 cycles of cyclophosphamide, bortezomib, and dexamethasone induction therapy, followed by 3 cycles of lenalidomide with dexamethasone (Rd), which was marked by a good partial response.

On follow-up, bone marrow biopsy was performed in December 2015 (7 months after initial presentation), the large vacuolated cells comprised only 5% of the cellular marrow (Figure 1(e)). However, the marrow showed prominent (50%) infiltration by medium sized atypical plasma cells, without vacuolization, highlighted by CD138. This population was positive for lambda light chain (Figure 1(f)). Serum immunofixation revealed a new IgG with lambda in addition to the original IgG with kappa light chains. Repeat immunofixations consistently demonstrated this biclonality. An electron microscopy study was attempted on a follow-up aspiration specimen, but it was not successful. The patient was maintained on the same treatment with a very good partial response.

In June 2016, the patient received high dose melphalan and an autologous bone marrow transplantation. The patient was treated with lenalidomide maintenance for 2 years. The patient maintained a stable partial response during that time, which lasted until January 2020. No progression was noted per serum protein electrophoresis or by repeated bone marrow examinations. In December 2020 (5 years after initial treatment), a serum protein electrophoresis and immunofixation (SPEP) disclosed an M spike which was 0.6 g/dL, IgG 1992 g/dL, kappa light chain 1825 g/dL, and free light chain ratio (FLCR) of 3.03. PET CT showed older, multiple lytic bone lesions without FDG uptake. A positive immunofixation with an elevated bone marrow monotypic kappa light chain are considered to represent progression of disease. Bone marrow biopsy taken at this time showed an interstitial infiltration comprising about 30% of the bone marrow, composed of large cells, displaying both morphology and phenotype (including kappa restriction) identical to those seen in the original biopsy (2015). In our opinion, this represented a reemergence of the initial tumor clone. At this point, continued close monitoring was applied.

In January 2021, the patient's disease was reevaluated. BMB revealed a 40% infiltration of kappa light chain monotypic plasma cells, with widespread large Mott cells. SPEP showed M spike of 0.64 g/dL, IgG 2085 g/dL, and kappa light chain 1979 g/dL with FLCR 3.97. The patient's CBC and chemistry were normal. A plan has been initiated to treat the patient with carfilzomib and daratumumab with dexamethasone.

3. Discussion

We present a case of multiple myeloma with "foamy" myeloma cells. A few conditions with similar morphology have been described in multiple myeloma. The cytoplasm of typical Mott-type plasma cells contains globules composed of retained immunoglobulins [3, 4]. However, classically the vacuoles are larger than in the present case and the residual cytoplasm is basophilic; therefore, they usually do not present a diagnostic difficulty. In contrast, large cells with a foamy cytoplasm, as in the present case, should raise suspicion of Gaucher cells. However, negative stains for CD68 PGM1 are not in favor of Gaucher cells. On the other hand, infrequently so-called Gaucher-like or pseudo-Gaucher cells have been described in multiple myeloma, corresponding to macrophages, filled with variable contents [5]. The large cells described in our case are morphologically reminiscent of these Gaucher-like cells. However, pseudo-Gaucher cells are of histiocytic lineage [6, 7], as should be confirmed by their positivity for CD68, while in our case the foamy cells were exclusively plasmacytes, confirmed by an immunophenotype which was negative for CD68 and positive for CD138 and kappa light chain. A population of large plasma cells with numerous crystalline intracytoplasmic inclusions has also been described in crystal-storing histiocytosis [8].

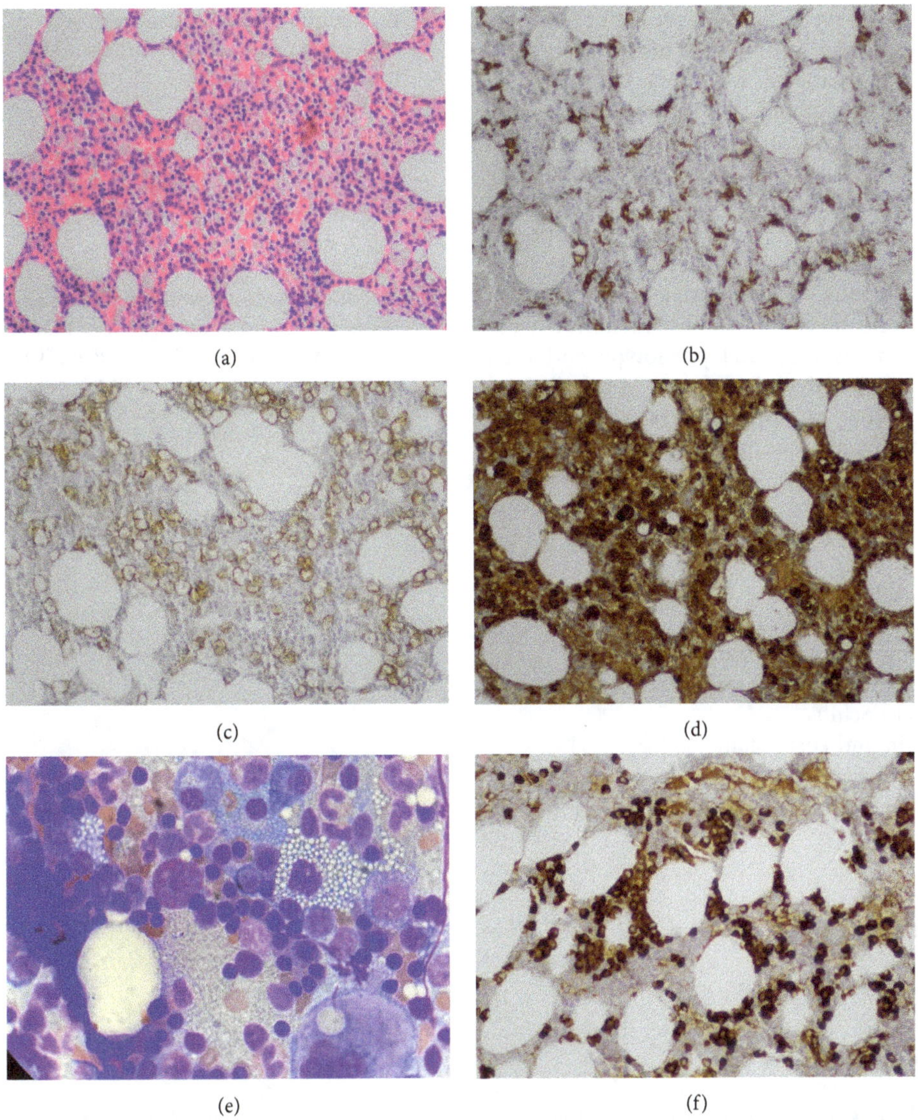

FIGURE 1: Bone marrow biopsy with foamy Mott cells on (a) H&E immunostain for (b) CD68 highlights scattered smaller cells of macrophage-monocyte lineage, but are negative in the larger foamy cells; however, they are positive for (c) CD138 and (d) kappa, confirming their plasmacytic differentiation. Note that the cytoplasmatic kappa IHC pattern matches the inclusions seen on H&E. (e) Bone marrow aspirate smear (Wright stain). (f) Posttherapy bone marrow biopsy, lambda light chain. Trephine biopsy cells original magnification 200x; aspirate smear (cell (E)) original magnification 1000x.

However, such large plasma cells are admixed with bona fide foamy histiocytes, which was not the case for our patient. In our opinion, the large cells seen in the present case were most probably a variant of Mott cells harboring numerous unusually small intracytoplasmic immunoglobulin globules. Due to this feature, the cytoplasm of Mott cells appears abundant and foamy, mimicking histiocytes seen in some storage diseases.

The findings in the follow-up biopsies seem to reflect concomitant involvement by two tumor clones of different cytological and immunohistochemical phenotypes. The initially diagnosed clone was comprised of the morphologically foamy Mott cells and was kappa light chain restricted. This clone showed partial response to treatment, at which point a second lambda light chain restricted clone emerged, which was refractory to treatment. Such an evolution probably represents an example of the so-called clonal competition with alternating dominance, previously described and discussed [9], wherein under various therapy regimens, some tumor clones are suppressed while others take proliferative advantage, becoming more dominant. This phenomenon may also explain the relapse of the kappa light chain positive, foamy Mott cell clone in 2020, confirmed and expanded in June 2021.

Multiple myelomas with predominantly mature plasma cell phenotype (so-called Marschalko subtype) show a significantly better prognosis than immature variants (e.g., plasmablastic myeloma) [5]. Nevertheless, current prognostic schemes for multiple myeloma do not include a morphological classification of the tumor [5].

In conclusion, we have described a case of multiple myeloma with the unusual morphology of the Mott cells. The unique foamy appearance was imparted by small intracytoplasmic immunoglobulin globules. These cells closely simulate foamy macrophages or Gaucher cells and may be the source of a diagnostic error. Appropriate immunohistochemistry, including CD68, CD138, kappa, and lambda, along with clinical correlation, easily resolves the diagnosis. A follow-up biopsy consequent to therapy showed a near complete response of the original tumor with emergence of a second myeloma clone with different cytological and immunohistochemical phenotype and then subsequent reemergence of the initial, foamy Mott cell clone after five years of follow-up. Such changes may represent clonal competition with alternating dominance.

Abbreviations

Ig: Immunoglobulin
EDTA: Ethylenediaminetetraacetic acid
CISH: Chromogenic in situ hybridization
CT: Computed tomography
PAS: Periodic acid-Schiff
H&E: Hematoxylin and eosin stain
IHC: Immunohistochemistry.

Consent

Consent was obtained from the patient before submission for publication.

Authors' Contributions

KN conceptualized the study, developed methodology, did investigation, provided resources, and wrote the original draft and was responsible for visualization; DB developed methodology and supervised the study; BS, MK, and DB reviewed and edited the article and were responsible for visualization; AG provided resources, developed methodology, and reviewed and edited the article.

References

[1] S. H. Swerdlow, E. Campo, N. L. Harris et al., *WHO Classification of Tumours of Haematopoietic and Lymphoid Tissues*, World Health Organization, Lyon, France, 2017.

[2] R. Gupta, N. Hussain, K. Rahman, and S. Nityanand, "Plasma cell myeloma with unusual morphology-a series of 6 cases," *European Journal of Haematology*, vol. 93, no. 2, pp. 165–170, 2014.

[3] P. Cazzini, V. E. Watson, and H. M. Brown, "The many faces of Mott cells," *Veterinary Clinical Pathology*, vol. 42, no. 2, pp. 125-126, 2013.

[4] K. A. McCormick, X. Chen, and R. B. Walter, "Mott cells," *European Journal of Haematology*, vol. 90, no. 1, p. 83, 2013.

[5] B. Ribourtout and M. Zandecki, "Plasma cell morphology in multiple myeloma and related disorders," *Morphologie*, vol. 99, no. 325, pp. 38–62, 2015.

[6] P. Shenjere, A. Roy, B. Eyden, and S. S. Banerjee, "Pseudogaucher cells in multiple myeloma," *International Journal of Surgical Pathology*, vol. 16, no. 2, pp. 176–179, 2008.

[7] V. Saroha, P. Gupta, M. Singh, and T. Singh, "Pseudogaucher cells obscuring multiple myeloma: a case report," *Cases Journal*, vol. 2, no. 1, 2009.

[8] J.-S. Lee, I. Kyongok, S. N. Park et al., "A challenging diagnosis: crystal-storing histiocytosis in plasma cell myeloma," *American Journal of Clinical Pathology*, vol. 143, no. 2, 2015.

[9] J. J. Keats, M. Chesi, J. B. Egan et al., "Clonal competition with alternating dominance in multiple myeloma," *Blood*, vol. 120, no. 5, pp. 1067–1076, 2012.

40

Hemorrhagic Cystitis Secondary to Adenovirus and BK Virus Infection in a Diffuse Large B-Cell Lymphoma Patient with Recent CAR T-Cell Therapy

Abdul Moiz Khan,[1] **Zainub Ajmal**,[1] **Fatima Tuz Zahra**,[1] **Ananthakrishnan Ramani**,[2] and **Ira Zackon**[3]

[1]*Department of Internal Medicine, Albany Medical Center, Albany, NY, USA*
[2]*Department of Infectious Diseases, Albany Medical Center, Albany, NY, USA*
[3]*New York Oncology Hematology, Albany Medical Center, Albany, NY, USA*

Correspondence should be addressed to Abdul Moiz Khan; khana13@amc.edu

Academic Editor: Chihaya Imai

Patients who undergo chimeric antigen receptor T-cell therapy (CAR T-cell therapy) are immunosuppressed due to multiple factors. While adenovirus and BK virus are well-known pathogens in the context of hematopoietic stem cell transplant, there are no detailed reports of these infections in the setting of CAR T-cell therapy. We describe a 70-year-old male who recently underwent CAR T-cell therapy for diffuse large B-cell lymphoma. He presented with intractable gross hematuria and dysuria. Workup revealed adenovirus viremia and viruria and BK virus viruria. He was treated for adenovirus hemorrhagic cystitis with intravenous cidofovir 1 mg/kg/day, every three days for three weeks, with good clinical response. We also discuss the mechanisms of immunosuppression in CAR T-cell therapy as well as the principles of treatment of adenovirus and BK virus infections in the immunosuppressed patient.

1. Introduction

Hemorrhagic cystitis (HC) is a diffuse inflammatory condition of the urinary bladder due to an infectious or noninfectious etiology resulting in bleeding from the bladder mucosa [1]. Infectious agents include bacteria, viruses (such as adenovirus and BK virus), fungi, or parasites. Noninfectious causes include medications such as cyclophosphamide, environmental toxins, and radiation [1, 2]. Prompt management of HC is vital especially in the context of immunosuppression. Chimeric antigen receptor T-cell therapy (CAR T-cell therapy) is an emerging type of immunotherapy for various hematological malignancies. Patients who undergo CAR T-cell therapy are generally immunosuppressed and prone to infections [3]. While adenovirus and BK virus are well-recognized pathogens in the context of hematopoietic stem cell transplant, only 2 cases of adenovirus viremia in CAR T-cell therapy patients have been reported by Chandorkar in a retrospective study [4]. Importantly, to the best of our literature review, there are no detailed accounts of concurrent infection with both these agents in the setting of CAR T-cell therapy.

We describe a case of HC secondary to adenovirus and BK virus in a patient with diffuse large B-cell lymphoma with recent CAR T-cell therapy. We discuss the mechanisms of immunosuppression in CAR T-cell therapy and the principles of treatment of adenovirus and BK virus infections in the immunocompromised patients.

2. Case Presentation

A 70-year-old male with diffuse large B-cell lymphoma presented with worsening dysuria, frequency, urgency, and gross hematuria along with mild suprapubic pain for 10 days. Hematuria was initially intermittent though it became persistent with infrequent passage of clots. The patient had failed an outpatient course of trimethoprim/sulfamethoxazole for a possible bacterial urinary tract infection. He denied fever, chills, flank pain, trauma, or weight loss. On our initial physical exam, he had a temperature of 37 C, blood pressure 120/55 mmHg, pulse 100 beats/min, respiratory rate 20/min, and oxygen saturation 98% on room air. He had prominent conjunctival pallor, a mildly distended abdomen with moderate tenderness in the suprapubic region. However, no flank or costovertebral angle tenderness, scrotal or penile swelling or tenderness, or cervical, axillary, or inguinal lymphadenopathy was noted.

The patient was diagnosed with diffuse large B-cell lymphoma in 2007 with multiple recurrences. Most recently, he had received lymphodepleting chemotherapy with fludarabine and cyclophosphamide followed by axicabtagene ciloleucel CAR T-cell therapy (2×10^6 cells/kg) two months before the presentation, in December 2019. He experienced grade 2 cytokine release syndrome during the treatment which warranted therapy with interleukin-6 inhibitor, tocilizumab. He had also received multiagent chemotherapeutic regimens between 2007 and 2018 for recurrences, including an autologous stem cell transplant in 2017. Additionally, he had a 60 pack-year smoking history which he quit 5 years ago. He denied any significant travel or occupational exposures.

Initial workup revealed pancytopenia with a white blood cell count of 3.2×10^3 (normal level 4–9 x 10^3 cells/μL), absolute neutrophil count 2.5×10^3 (1.5–5.2 $\times 10^3$ cells/μL), absolute lymphocyte count 0.3×10^3 (1.1–3.9 $\times 10^3$ cells/μL), hemoglobin 8.9 (13.6–16.7 g/dl), hematocrit 26.3 (40–49%), and platelet count 17×10^3 (130–350 $\times 10^3$ cells/μL). Creatinine was 1.60 (patient's baseline was 1 mg/dL) and estimated GFR 43 (normal >60 mL/min/1.73 m^2). Urinalysis showed 1+ leukocyte esterase, negative nitrite, 3+ hemoglobin, 50–100/high power field (HPF) WBCs and too numerous to count RBCs. Urine gram stain and culture had 3+ polymorphonuclear cells but no bacterial or fungal growth. Two sets of aerobic and anaerobic blood cultures were negative. On imaging, computerized tomography (CT) scan of the abdomen and pelvis showed moderate right hydroureteronephrosis with surrounding fat stranding of the kidney and ureter along its entire course. Ureteral dilation was up to 1.1 cm and bladder wall thickening with surrounding fat stranding were seen. Adenovirus and BK virus PCR were ordered.

While the results of adenovirus and BK virus PCR were awaited, supportive care was provided with intravenous fluids, phenazopyridine, and analgesics. Patient also received intravenous immunoglobulin (IVIG) for hypogammaglobulinemia. Antibiotics were held given the low likelihood of bacterial urinary tract infection. In order to rule out obstruction based on the findings of hydroureteronephrosis, rigid cystourethroscopy, bilateral retrograde pyelogram, right ureteroscopy, bladder biopsies, and fulguration were performed. Cystoscopy revealed diffuse gross cystitis with mucosal mounding. Bilateral retrograde pyelogram demonstrated poor drainage and calyceal blunting on the right-side, hence a ureteral stent was placed, whereas the left side was normal. Meanwhile, adenovirus was detected by PCR in urine as well as serum. BK virus DNA quantitation by real time PCR in urine showed 1,300,000 copies/ml (log copies 6.11), though BK viral DNA was not detected in serum. Hypogammaglobulinemia with IgG level 288.2 (667–1485 mg/dL), IgM <20 (46–216 mg/dl), and IgA 33 (63–391 mg/dL) was also seen. Bladder biopsy, urine cytology from the right kidney, and bladder washings ruled out malignancy and showed evidence of acute inflammation. Although the patient did not show any appreciable improvement in the symptoms, the renal function gradually improved to baseline.

Once the adenoviremia/viruria and BK viruria were confirmed, and the renal function improved, the patient was started on intravenous cidofovir for adenovirus HC at a dose of 1 mg/kg/day (90 mg), three times a week, for a total of three weeks. He also received probenecid and 500 ml of normal saline before and after the administration of cidofovir for renal protection. His renal function and blood counts were closely monitored and remained stable. The patient had resolution of hematuria and marked sustained improvement of lower urinary tract symptoms within 2 weeks of completion of therapy.

3. Discussion

Hemorrhagic cystitis (HC) in the setting of immunosuppression can be secondary to infectious or noninfectious causes. While adenovirus viremia and viruria and BK viruria were consistent with viral HC in our case, cyclophosphamide induced HC was also considered. Early-onset HC within the first few days of cyclophosphamide administration is linked to acrolein, a urotoxic metabolite of cyclophosphamide. However, HC can develop weeks to months after treatment in patients who receive high dose of cyclophosphamide [5, 6]. Late HC is most often secondary to adenovirus and BK virus infections in the setting of immunosuppression from the cyclophosphamide rather than a direct toxic effect [6–8]. In our patient, onset of symptoms almost 2 months after cyclophosphamide administration and persistent lymphodepletion supports an indirect role of cyclophosphamide.

Patients receiving CD 19 CAR T-cell therapy are immunosuppressed for multiple reasons. Effects of malignancy itself, prior cytotoxic treatments, and lymphodepleting chemotherapy, given immediately before CAR T-cell therapy, lead to cytopenias and may disrupt mucosal barriers. CAR T-cell therapy can be complicated by cytokine release syndrome (CRS) or neurotoxicity which may necessitate the use of immunosuppressive agents such as corticosteroids and tocilizumab. In addition, CD19 CAR T-cells cause depletion of normal CD19+ B-cells which may lead to hypogammaglobulinemia [3, 9]. Our patient had all these risk factors that may have compounded the risk of adenovirus and BK virus infection. However, the persistent lymphodepletion and suppressed cellular immunity from the chemotherapy given prior to the CAR T-cell therapy likely had the highest role in development of the infections.

Human adenovirus (AdV) is a nonenveloped, double-stranded, linear DNA virus that causes a wide array of diseases in both immunocompetent and immunocompromised patients, although fulminant manifestations such as HC are more common in immunocompromised population [10]. Disseminated disease carries a high mortality rate [11]. BK virus belongs to the *Polyomaviridae* family of non-enveloped, double-stranded DNA viruses. Unlike adenovirus, BK virus infections manifest through reactivation of latent virus in the setting of immunosuppression, and clinically significant infections are less frequent in immunocompetent hosts [12, 13]. In addition to the potential of causing HC by itself, BK virus may have an augmenting role since studies have shown that BK virus increases the risk of adenovirus co-infection and contributes to enhanced Adenovirus replication [14, 15].

Treatment options for treating adenovirus HC are limited. Intravenous (IV) cidofovir appears to be the most promising drug for adenovirus infection. Close monitoring and preventive strategies are required for cidofovir-associated nephrotoxicity [11, 16]. European Conference on Infections in Leukemia (ECIL) guidelines (2011) support the treatment of human adenovirus disease with IV cidofovir along with renal protective measures such as hyperhydration and oral probenecid. The recommended dosage is 5 mg/kg/week for 2 weeks and 5 mg/kg every 2 weeks thereafter, given the lack of data on other dosage schedules [17]. However, Nagafuji described treating 16 patients with adenovirus HC following hematopoietic stem cell transplant (HSCT) with IV cidofovir (CDV) at 1 mg/kg/day, three times weekly for 3 weeks. CDV therapy cleared adenovirus from urine in 86% and led to clinical improvement in HC in 71% of the evaluated patients [18]. Yoshimura and Bordigoni have also reported encouraging results with IV cidofovir for treatment of adenovirus infections in patients with allogeneic HSCT [19, 20]. Given the acute kidney injury in our patient, a dose of 1 mg/kg/day, three times weekly for 3 weeks, was used with hyperhydration and probenecid. In addition, there are some reports of intravesical cidofovir, brincidofovir, ribavirin, and vidarabine used successfully for adenovirus infections, though further investigations are needed to establish their role [11, 21–24].

ECIL guidelines (2017) also provide a framework for the treatment of BK virus HC, which mostly relies on supportive measures such as hyperhydration, bladder irrigation, platelet transfusions as needed, and pain management. Some studies have reviewed intravenous cidofovir as an effective therapy, although there is no consensus on best dose schedule, and adverse effects mainly nephrotoxicity should be considered on a case-by-case basis [25, 26]. Overall, antiviral treatment with cidofovir remains controversial and of uncertain efficacy due to a lack of randomized controlled trials [26].

4. Conclusions

Patients undergoing CAR T-cell therapy are immunosuppressed and prone to pathogens including adenovirus and BK virus. Intravenous cidofovir has proven to be an effective treatment for adenovirus infections in the setting of immunosuppression. Renal function should be closely monitored and measures such as hyperhydration and probenecid should be employed to reduce the risk of cidofovir nephrotoxicity.

Disclosure

The authors declare that this research did not receive any grant from funding agencies in the public, commercial, or not-for-profit sectors.

References

[1] R. Manikandan, S. Kumar, and L. N. Dorairajan, "Hemorrhagic cystitis: a challenge to the urologist," *Journal of the Urological Society of India*, vol. 26, no. 2, pp. 159–166, 2010.

[2] S. Haldar, C. Dru, and N. A. Bhowmick, "Mechanisms of hemorrhagic cystitis," *American Journal of Clinical and Experimental Urology*, vol. 2, no. 3, pp. 199–208, 2014.

[3] J. A. Hill, D. Li, K. A. Hay et al., "Infectious complications of CD19-targeted chimeric antigen receptor-modified T-cell immunotherapy," *Blood*, vol. 131, no. 1, pp. 121–130, 2018.

[4] A. A. Riddell, A. D. Anderson, M. I. Morris, Y. Natori, K. V. Komanduri, and J. F. Camargo, "Viral kinetics and outcomes of adenovirus reactivation following allogeneic hematopoietic cell transplant or CAR-T cell therapy," *Biology of Blood and Marrow Transplantation*, vol. 26, no. 3, p. S331, 2020.

[5] A. Thompson, A. Adamson, A. Bahl et al., "Guidelines for the diagnosis, prevention and management of chemical- and radiation-induced cystitis," *Journal of Clinical Urology*, vol. 7, no. 1, pp. 25–35, 2014.

[6] A. Huddart, R. J. Jones, and R. A. Brodsky, "Cyclophosphamide and cancer: golden anniversary," *Nature Reviews Clinical Oncology*, vol. 6, no. 11, pp. 638–647, 2009.

[7] J. F. Apperley, S. J. Rice, J. A. Bishop et al., "Late-onset hemorrhagic cystitis associated with urinary excretion of polyoma viruses after bone marrow transplantation," *Transplantation*, vol. 43, no. 1, pp. 108–112, 1987.

[8] R. R. Goldman, K. V. Shah, S. J. Baust, G. W. Santos, and R. Saral, "Association of BK viruria with hemorrhagic cystitis in recipients of bone marrow transplants," *New England Journal of Medicine*, vol. 315, no. 4, pp. 230–234, 1986.

[9] J. N. Brudno and J. N. Kochenderfer, "Toxicities of chimeric antigen receptor T cells: recognition and management," *Blood*, vol. 127, no. 26, pp. 3321–3330, 2016.

[10] T. Lion, "Adenovirus infections in immunocompetent and immunocompromised patients," *Clinical Microbiology Reviews*, vol. 27, no. 3, pp. 441–462, 2014.

[11] S. Cesaro, M. Berger, M. Berger et al., "A survey on incidence and management of adenovirus infection after allogeneic HSCT," *Bone Marrow Transplantation*, vol. 54, no. 8, pp. 1275–1280, 2019.

[12] G. R. Ljungman, R. S. Francis, M. J. Smyth, C. Smith, and R. Khanna, "BK polyomavirus: clinical aspects, immune regulation, and emerging therapies," *Clinical Microbiology Reviews*, vol. 30, no. 2, pp. 503–528, 2017.

[13] M. D. Reploeg, G. A. Storch, and D. B. Clifford, "BK virus: a clinical review," *Clinical Infectious Diseases*, vol. 33, no. 2, pp. 191–202, 2001.

[14] I. Bil-Lula and M. Woźniak, "Co-infection with human polyomavirus BK enhances gene expression and replication of human adenovirus," *Archives of Virology*, vol. 163, no. 7, pp. 1841–1849, 2018.
[15] I. Bil-Lula, M. Ussowicz, B. Rybka et al., "PCR diagnostics and monitoring of adenoviral infections in hematopoietic stem cell transplantation recipients," *Archives of Virology*, vol. 155, no. 12, pp. 2007–2015, 2010.
[16] C. A. Kałwak, A. M. Leen, and J. J. Boelens, "How I treat adenovirus in hematopoietic stem cell transplant recipients," *Blood*, vol. 116, no. 25, pp. 5476–5485, 2010.
[17] S. Matthes-Martin, T. Feuchtinger, P. J. Shaw et al., "European guidelines for diagnosis and treatment of adenovirus infection in leukemia and stem cell transplantation: summary of ECIL-4 (2011)," *Transplant Infectious Disease*, vol. 14, no. 6, pp. 555–563, 2012.
[18] K. Ljungman, K. Aoki, H. Henzan et al., "Cidofovir for treating adenoviral hemorrhagic cystitis in hematopoietic stem cell transplant recipients," *Bone Marrow Transplantation*, vol. 34, no. 10, pp. 909–914, 2004.
[19] T. Nagatoshi, M. Nishimoto, T. Nakane et al., "Cidofovir treatment for adenovirus-associated hemorrhagic cystitis in adult recipients of allogeneic hematopoietic stem cell transplantation: a retrospective comparative study," *Biology of Blood and Marrow Transplantation*, vol. 23, no. 3, p. S202, 2017.
[20] P. Nakamae, A.-S. Carret, V. Venard, F. Witz, and A. Le Faou, "Treatment of adenovirus infections in patients undergoing allogeneic hematopoietic stem cell transplantation," *Clinical Infectious Diseases*, vol. 32, no. 9, pp. 1290–1297, 2001.
[21] K. Miyamura, M. Hamaguchi, H. Taji et al., "Successful ribavirin therapy for severe adenovirus hemorrhagic cystitis after allogeneic marrow transplant from close HLA donors rather than distant donors," *Bone Marrow Transplantation*, vol. 25, no. 5, pp. 545–548, 2000.
[22] M. Saito, S. Ueda, T. Maeda et al., "Vidarabine therapy for virus-associated cystitis after allogeneic bone marrow transplantation," *Bone Marrow Transplantation*, vol. 20, no. 6, pp. 485–490, 1997.
[23] M. Nakamura, T. Kondo, M. Umeda, H. Kawabata, K. Yamashita, and A. Takaori-Kondo, "Successful treatment with intravesical cidofovir for virus-associated hemorrhagic cystitis after allogeneic hematopoietic stem cell transplantation: a case report and a review of the literature," *Journal of Infection and Chemotherapy*, vol. 22, no. 7, pp. 495–500, 2016.
[24] I. D. Ramsay, C. Attwood, D. Irish, P. D. Griffiths, C. Kyriakou, and D. M. Lowe, "Disseminated adenovirus infection after allogeneic stem cell transplant and the potential role of brincidofovir-case series and 10 year experience of management in an adult transplant cohort," *Journal of Clinical Virology*, vol. 96, pp. 73–79, 2017.
[25] M. Philippe, F. Ranchon, L. Gilis et al., "Cidofovir in the treatment of BK virus-associated hemorrhagic cystitis after allogeneic hematopoietic stem cell transplantation," *Biology of Blood and Marrow Transplantation*, vol. 22, no. 4, pp. 723–730, 2016.
[26] S. Labussiere-Wallet, T. Dalianis, C. Hanssen Rinaldo et al., "ECIL guidelines for the prevention, diagnosis and treatment of BK polyomavirus-associated haemorrhagic cystitis in haematopoietic stem cell transplant recipients," *Journal of Antimicrobial Chemotherapy*, vol. 73, no. 1, pp. 12–21, 2018.

41

Postsurgical Diagnosis of an Unusual Case of Primary Hepatic Lymphoma Presenting as Liver Abscess with an Uncommon Complication: A Hepatogastric Fistula

Mbarek Yaka,[1] Farid Chehab,[2] Mohmed Allaoui,[3] Abdelmonaim Ait Ali,[4] and Aziz Zentar[4]

[1]*Department of Surgery, Military University Hospital Med V, University Hassan II of Casablanca, Casablanca, Morocco*
[2]*Department of Surgery, Ibn Rochd University Hospital, University Hassan II of Casablanca, Casablanca, Morocco*
[3]*Department of Pathology, Military University Hospital Med V, Rabat, Morocco*
[4]*Department of Surgery, Military University Hospital Med V, Rabat, Morocco*

Correspondence should be addressed to Mbarek Yaka; mbarekyaka@yahoo.fr

Academic Editor: Kostas Konstantopoulos

Primary hepatic lymphoma (PHL) is a very rare malignancy and constitutes 0.016% of all cases of non-Hodgkin's lymphoma and 0.4% of extranodal non-Hodgkin's lymphoma. We describe a rare case of primary hepatic lymphoma presenting as liver abscess which was complicated with the development of a hepatogastric fistula. A 58-year-old man presented with clinical signs of sepsis, high-grade fever, right upper abdominal pain, and weight loss which had progressed in the past 8 months. Noncontrast abdominal computed tomography (CT) revealed a heterogeneously hypodense lesion in the left lobe of the liver with multiple air foci within, which are seen to extend into the body of the stomach. The patient was initially misdiagnosed as a case of rupture of liver abscess into the stomach. Postoperative liver biopsy examination confirmed a diagnosis of diffuse large B-cell lymphoma. Systemic staging revealed no evidence of nodal or bone marrow involvement, so PHL was diagnosed. Chemotherapy was initiated, but discontinued due to the patient's general condition. Finally, the patient succumbed to neutropenic fever following chemotherapy. Here, we present the exceptional case of a primary hepatic lymphoma with an unusual complication, a hepatogastric fistula, and try through the existing literature to show the difficulties involved in diagnosis and treatment.

1. Introduction

PHL is a rare form of non-Hodgkin lymphoma (NHL), and it is a tumor confined to the liver without evidence of lymphomatous involvement of the lymph nodes, spleen, bone marrow, or other lymphoid structures. The vast majority of PHL is NHL, most often a diffuse large B-cell lymphoma type. PHL was often misdiagnosed as some other tumor and frequently diagnosed intra- or postoperatively. We report an interesting case of PHL that was difficult to discriminate from a liver abscess, with an unusual complication, hepatogastric fistula, diagnosed after postoperative biopsy report, and try through the existing literature to show the difficulties involved in diagnosis and treatment.

2. Case Report

A 58-year-old male with no significant past medical history presented to our emergency department with fever, right upper abdominal pain, vomiting, hematemesis, anorexia, night sweats, and unexplained weight loss. Physical examination revealed an asthenic patient with mild mucocutaneous pallor, a temperature of 38°C, pulse rate of 110/min, blood pressure of 90/60 mmHg, and respiratory rate of 17/min. There was no clinical jaundice. Per abdominal examination revealed mild tenderness in the epigastric and right hypochondriac regions, with palpable liver extending one cm below the right subcostal margin, rounded margin. The spleen and superficial lymph nodes were not palpable. Initial investigations showed hemoglobin of 7.3 g/dl, total leukocyte count of 22,000 cells/mm^3 (neutrophils 82%), and platelet counts (139,000 cells/mm^3). Serum lactate dehydrogenase (LDH), C-reactive protein (CRP), and procalcitonin levels were elevated, but the levels of other tumor markers, such as alpha-fetoprotein (AFP) and carcinoembryonic antigen (CEA), were normal. Serology was negative for hepatitis B virus (HBV) surface antigen, HCV, and human immunodeficiency virus. An urgent noncontrast computed tomography (CT) examination of the abdomen and pelvis was performed which showed a heterogeneously hypodense lesion in the left lobe of the liver with multiple air foci within. The liver lesion was extending directly into the body of the stomach (Figure 1). The walls of the fundus and lesser curvature of the stomach could not be defined. These features were suggestive of rupture of left lobe liver abscess into the stomach. The spleen was remarkably normal, and the mesenteric, para-aortic, and retroperitoneal lymph nodes were not enlarged. Based on a presumptive diagnosis of liver abscess, the patient was initially treated with broad-spectrum antibiotics. The patient's clinical condition deteriorated, and a decision of surgical exploration was made. Intraoperative findings revealed dense adhesions of the left lobe of the liver with the anterior wall of the stomach and diaphragmatic surface. There was a 2 cm × 1 cm defect on the anterior wall of the stomach, and it was communicating with the abscess cavity in the left lobe of the liver. There was no peritoneal soiling. Necrosis tissues were removed from the liver, we drained the abscess cavity, and subhepatic drain was placed. The margins of the gastric perforation were freshened and primarily repaired (Figure 2). The patient was kept on nasojejunal tube for one week with broad-spectrum antibiotics and total parenteral nutrition. Histopathology of the surgical liver biopsy revealed a hepatic diffuse infiltration of large typical lymphoid B-cells, with necrosis. Immunohistochemistry was positive for CD20 and Ki-67 (80%) (Figure 3).

Postoperative investigations for disseminated non-Hodgkin lymphoma (NHL) by CT scan of the thorax did not reveal any lymphadenopathy or mass lesion. FDG-PET scan and bone marrow biopsy were negative. Thus, a diagnosis of primary non-Hodgkin lymphoma of the liver, large cell type, was confirmed. The patient condition did not allow additional complementary surgery, and he was managed with six cycles of R-CHOP regimen, rituximab, cyclophosphamide, doxorubicin, vincristine, and prednisone. However, a persistent fever occurred 1 month after three cycles of chemotherapy. The patient succumbed to neutropenic fever following chemotherapy.

3. Discussion

PHL and hepatogastric fistula are extremely rare. To our knowledge, this is the first report on a primary hepatic lymphoma invading the adjacent stomach, which was complicated with the development of a hepatogastric fistula. PHL was first described in 1965 by Ata and Kamel [1]. Some authors defined primary hepatic lymphoma as a very rare malignant tumor with the features of liver involvement and without involvement of other organs and tissues including the bone marrow, lymph nodes, spleen, and peripheral blood until at least 6 months after diagnosis [2, 3].

Primary hepatic lymphoma is very rare and constitutes about 0.0016% of all cases of non-Hodgkin's lymphoma (NHL) [4]. Extranodal lymphomas account for 10%–25% of non-Hodgkin's lymphomas, in which PHL is responsible for less than 1% [5].

PHL can occur at any age, and the average age of the reported patients is the fifth or sixth decade of life. It affects preferentially men with a male/female ratio of 2–3/1 [6]. PHL may be Hodgkin's or non-Hodgkin's; however, the latter is more common. Immunophenotypically, the B-cell is commoner than T-cell type [5]. The etiology of PHL is uncertain, and it may be associated with HIV, AIDS, hepatitis B and C, Epstein–Barr virus, liver cirrhosis, primary biliary cirrhosis, immunosuppressive therapy, and autoimmune diseases [7]. However, our case did not have any of the above conditions.

Symptoms are usually nonspecific and include hepatomegaly, gastrointestinal symptoms (abdominal pain, vomiting, and loss of appetite), right upper quadrant, and epigastric pain. Many cases are diffuse large B-cell lymphoma, and the patients show B-symptomatology of weight loss, fever, and night sweats, as well as fatigue and lethargy. Other rare clinical manifestations include pleural effusion, jaundice, thrombocytopenia, metabolic acidosis, and hypercalcemia [8]. Laboratory abnormalities associated with PHL include anaemia, neutropenia, hypercalcemia, and variably raised LDH, one serum alkaline phosphatase, b-microglobulin, and aminotransferase activities. The tumor markers AFP and CEA are found within normal range, in almost all cases of PHL [2].

On ultrasound imaging, majority are hypoechoic as compared to surrounding normal liver parenchyma. Radiological features of PHL are usually nonspecific, and the most common presentation on the computed tomography (CT) scan is a solitary hypoattenuating lesion, which may have a central area of low intensity indicating necrosis. Other less common radiological findings are multiple lesions and diffuse infiltration patterns [9]. On MRI, the lesion appears hypointense on T1-weighted and mildly hyperintense on T2-weighted images. However, it is often difficult to distinguish hepatic lymphoma from hepatocarcinoma or gastrointestinal tract metastasis because of the rarity of this disease and the nonspecific clinical presentation, laboratory, and radiologic features [10].

Diagnosis is often made upon histopathological and immunohistochemical investigation of the liver biopsy by using percutaneous needle aspiration, laparoscopy, or laparotomy [11]. In our case, liver biopsy was performed preoperatively because the lesion was profoundly symptomatic, and due to the rarity of the disease, we considered liver abscess with hepatogastric fistula in our first diagnosis.

Treatment modalities include surgical resection, chemotherapy, and radiotherapy alone or in combination. Most of the reported cases are diffuse large B-cell lymphomas, but this type is usually aggressive with a relatively poor prognosis [5]. Current literature favors combination

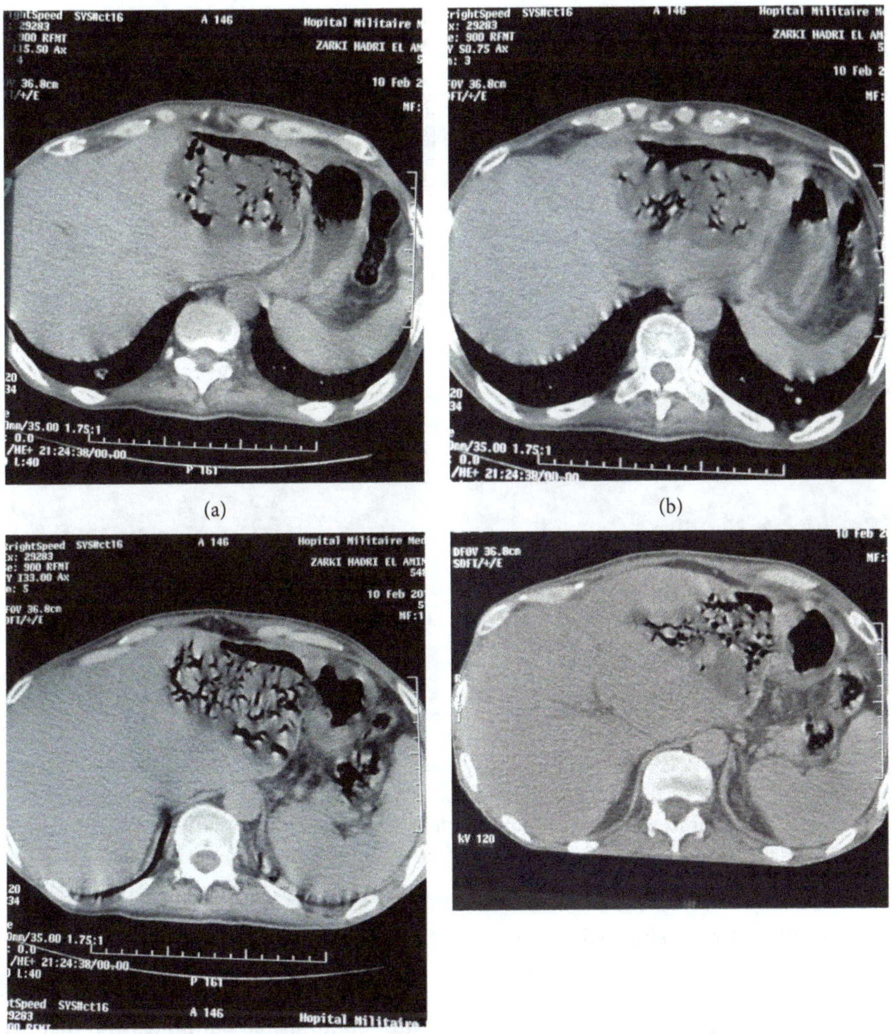

(a) (b) (c) (d)

FIGURE 1: Preoperative CT scan showing (a, b) liver cystic mass containing multiple air foci; (c, d) hepatogastric fistula.

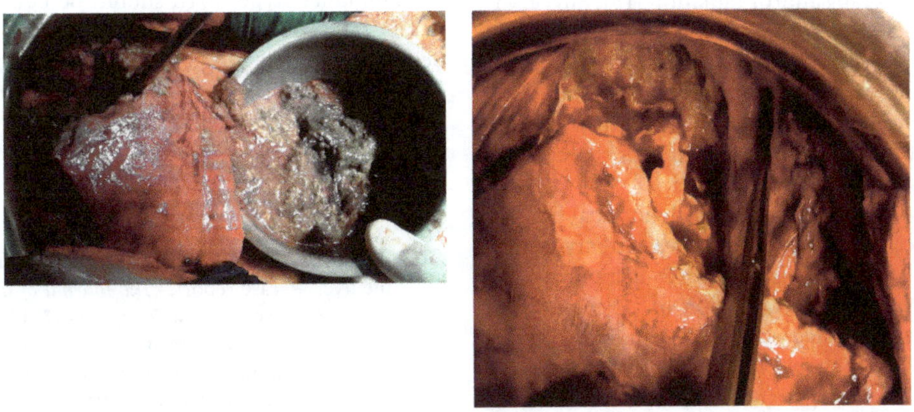

(a) (b)

FIGURE 2: Operative view of the anterior surface of the left lobe of the liver showing (a) necrotic area of liver lymphoma and (b) hepatogastric fistula.

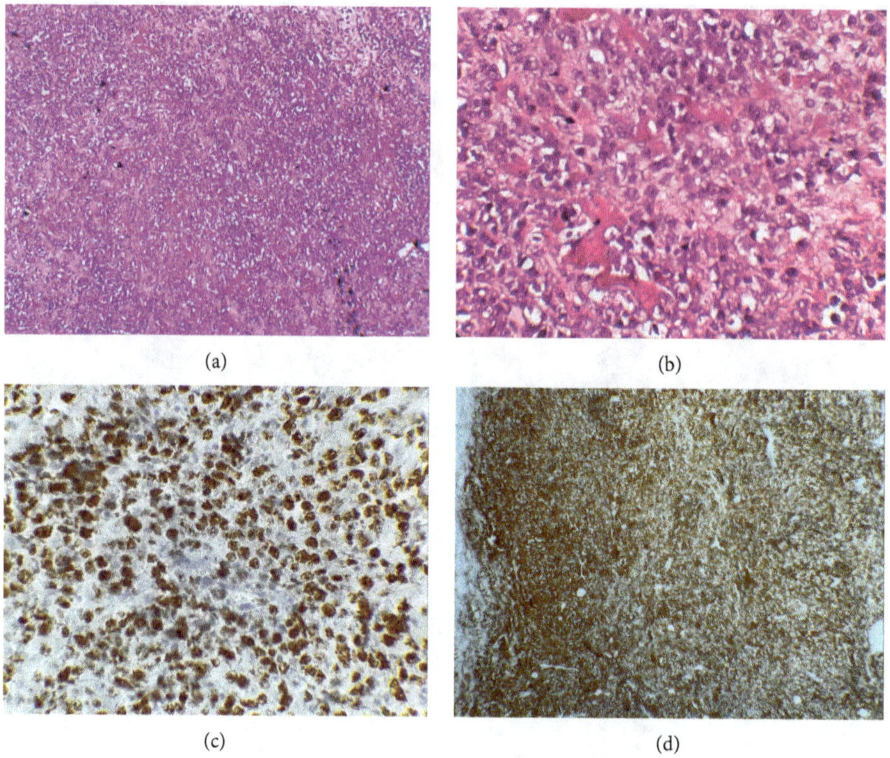

Figure 3: Histopathological examination. (a) Diffuse proliferation of atypical lymphoid cells (HE, GX 40). (b) Large numbers of lymphocytes ranging in size from medium to large, with oval or round nuclei containing fine chromatin and scanty cytoplasm (HE, GX 200). (c) Immunohistochemical staining was positive for CD20 (a B-cell marker). (d) The Ki-67 index was positive in 80%.

chemotherapy as the frontline treatment owing to its noninvasive nature and improved survival outcomes. The standard treatment for patients with diffuse large B-cell lymphoma is CHOP. The addition of rituximab, a monoclonal antibody targeting the pan-B-cell antigenic marker CD20, to the CHOP regimen augments the complete response rate and prolongs overall survival [11, 12]. Optimal treatment is not yet defined. However, recent series reported favorable short and midterm outcomes and longer survival rates with the use of liver resection followed by adjuvant chemotherapy and/or radiation [13]. Surgery is a better option for localized disease with adequate normal liver volume, and preoperative chemotherapy can be tried with an attempt to reduce the tumor volume [5, 14]. However, because our patient's general condition did not permit, we did not proceed with a formal liver resection as indicated in this setting.

The clinical case we present is extremely unusual because there is a coincidence of two very rare features, primary hepatic lymphoma and hepatogastric fistula. Direct invasion to the gastric wall is the basis of the formation of a hepatogastric fistula. Nevertheless, a hepatogastric fistula is a rare complication, even more so for primary liver lymphoma. Such a fistula has been described following transarterial embolization, radiotherapy for hepatocellular carcinoma, percutaneous radiofrequency of hepatocellular carcinoma, pyogenic liver abscess, iatrogenic injury of the stomach, percutaneous catheter drainage of the liver abscess, or by direct infiltration of the stomach by hepatocellular carcinoma [15].

4. Conclusion

In conclusion, we have reported an exceptional case of PHL with an unusual complication that was difficult to discriminate from a liver abscess with a hepatogastric fistula. The preoperative diagnosis was difficult due to the rarity of the disease, the clinical and imaging manifestations of PHL were nonspecific, and levels of alpha-fetoprotein and carcinoembryonic antigen (CEA) were normal. The diagnosis of PHL should be strictly based on histopathology and immunophenotype. PHL should be considered in the differential diagnosis in a patient with space-occupying liver lesions. Favorable prognosis of PHL can be obtained by early surgery combined with chemotherapy in strictly selected patients.

References

[1] A. A. Ata and I. A. Kamel, "Primary reticulum cell sarcoma of the liver. A case report," *The Journal of the Egyptian Medical Association*, vol. 48, no. 7, pp. 514–521, 1965.

[2] A. Mastoraki, M. I. Stefanou, E. Chatzoglou et al., "Primary hepatic lymphoma: dilemmas in diagnostic approach and therapeutic management," *Indian Journal of Hematology and Blood Transfusion*, vol. 30, no. 3, pp. 150–154, 2014.

[3] D. Caccamo, N. K. Pervez, and A. Marchevsky, "Primary lymphoma of the liver in the acquired immunode ciency syndrome," *Archives of Pathology and Laboratory Medicine*, vol. 110, pp. 553–555, 1986.

[4] X. W. Yang, W. F. Tan, W. L. Yu et al., "Diagnosis and surgical treatment of primary hepatic lymphoma," *World Journal of Gastroenterology*, vol. 16, no. 47, pp. 6016–6019, 2010.
[5] K. Lei, "Primary non-hodgkin's lymphoma of the liver," *Leukemia & Lymphoma*, vol. 29, no. 3-4, pp. 293–299, 1998.
[6] V. S. Avlonitis and D. Linos, "Primary hepatic lymphoma: a review," *The European Journal of Surgery=Acta Chirurgica*, vol. 165, no. 8, pp. 725–729, 1999.
[7] N. Takeuchi and K. Naba, "Primary hepatic lymphoma is difficult to discriminate from a liver abscess," *Case reports in Gastrointestinal Medicine*, vol. 2014, Article ID 925307, 6 pages, 2014.
[8] F. Xiong and Y.-S. Guan, "Primary hepatic lymphoma: is it a disease entity?" *Hepatoma Research*, vol. 3, no. 5, pp. 73–78, 2017.
[9] N. Mehta, L. Jayapal, M. Goneppanavar, and V. P. Nelamangala Ramakrishnaiah, "Primary hepatic lymphoma: a rare case report," *JGH Open*, vol. 3, no. 3, pp. 261–263, 2019.
[10] M. M. Maher, S. R. McDermott, H. M. Fenlon et al., "Imaging of primary non-hodgkin's lymphoma of the liver," *Clinical Radiology*, vol. 56, no. 4, pp. 295–301, 2001.
[11] G. Tatsumi, N. Ukyo, H. Hirata, and M. Tsudo, "Primary hepatic lymphoma in a patient with rheumatoid arthritis treated with methotrexate," *Case Reports in Hematology*, vol. 2014, Article ID 460574, 2014.
[12] A. Masood, S. Kairouz, K. H. Hudhud et al., "Primary non-Hodg-kin lymphoma of liver," *Current Oncology*, vol. 16, pp. 74–77, 2009.
[13] Y.-D. Yu, D.-S. Kim, G.-Y. Byun et al., "Primary hepatic marginal zone B cell lymphoma: a case report and review of the literature," *Indian Journal of Surgery*, vol. 75, no. S1, pp. 331–336, 2013.
[14] A. Zentar, M. Tarchouli, H. Elkaoui et al., "Primary hepatic lymphoma," *Journal of Gastrointestinal Cancer*, vol. 45, no. 3, pp. 380–382, 2014.
[15] V. S. Gandham, B. Pottakkat, L. C. Panicker, and R. V. Hari, "Hepatogastric fistula: a rare complication of pyogenic liver abscess," *BMJ Case Reports*, vol. 2014, 2014.

42

A Case Report with Severe Thrombocytopenia Induced by Axitinib

Ulkuhan I. Koksal, Janeiro Valle Goffin, Brian Lewis, Oliver A. Sartor, Elizaveta Belyaeva, Francisco Socola, and Pedro C. Barata

Tulane Cancer Center, School of Medicine, Tulane University, New Orleans, LA, USA

Correspondence should be addressed to Pedro C. Barata; pedrobaratamd@gmail.com

Academic Editor: Håkon Reikvam

Axitinib is an oral, second-generation tyrosine kinase inhibitor that is selective for vascular endothelial growth factor receptors (VEGFR). This agent is approved as monotherapy or in combination with immune checkpoint inhibitors for the treatment of metastatic renal cell carcinoma. Axitinib is associated with a safety profile very similar to other anti-VEGFR inhibitors but usually with fewer hematologic adverse events, due to the selectivity for VEGF. In this report, we presented a rare case of grade 4 axitinib-induced thrombocytopenia, not observed with other antiangiogenic therapies. We discuss the differential diagnostic work-up, the necessary multidisciplinary approach, and the successful management of the case.

1. Introduction

Renal cell carcinoma (RCC) is the sixth most common cancer for men and eighth most common cancer for women in the USA [1]. Immunotherapies and antiangiogenic drugs are the main treatment options for patients who present with advanced and/or unresectable disease [2]. In most cases, metastatic RCC progresses despite first-line treatment, and usually a sequence of different anti-vascular endothelial growth factor (VEGF) targeted therapies control the disease for a few years [3].

Axitinib is an oral and selective second-generation inhibitor of vascular endothelial growth factor receptor (VEGFR) 1, 2, and 3 [4]. It was approved in January 2012 for the treatment of metastatic RCC after failure of one systemic therapy and more recently in combination with pembrolizumab and avelumab for front-line treatment of metastatic RCC by the Food and Drug Administration [5–7].

Axitinib is in general well tolerated with approximately 30% of any adverse events of any grade, but with low frequency of significant myelosuppression including anemia (<1%), neutropenia (1%), thrombocytopenia (<1%), and lymphopenia (3%), when compared with other anti-VEGFR inhibitors (Tables 1 and 2) [5–14]. However, when they occur, they pose a significant challenge to treating physicians.

Herein, we present a patient with significant axitinib-induced thrombocytopenia; we discuss the differential diagnostic work-up and multidisciplinary management.

2. Case Presentation

In July 2008, a 70-year-old Caucasian man, who had Karnofsky performance score of 70%, with a significant medical history of grade 2 diastolic dysfunction, hyperlipidemia, hypertension, abdominal aortic aneurysm, coronary artery disease, esophagus stenosis, and hiatal hernia, all controlled with medication, presented with a 5 cm left renal mass of approximately invading the renal capsule, compatible with left RCC. The patient had no family history of cancer. The other drugs used by the patient were tadalafil, levothyroxine sodium, losartan potassium, amlodipine besylate, metoprolol, febuxostat, atorvastatin calcium, oxycodone HCl as needed, and acetylsalicylic acid. His social habits included sporadic alcohol consumption.

The patient underwent a left radical nephrectomy (08/2008); pathology revealed a pT1b clear cell renal cell carcinoma, nuclear grade II, without perirenal fat extension,

Table 1: Hematologic adverse effects in major trials of Axitinib.

	Axi vs Placebo (Atlas) [8]	Axi vs. sorafenib (Front-line) [9]	Axi + pembrolizumab (KEYNOTE 426) [7]	Axi + avelumab (JAVELIN 101) [5]		Axi vs. sorafenib (AXIS) [6]	
	Any grade	Any grade	Any grade	Grade ≥3	All grades	Grade ≥3	Grade ≥3
Anemia	NR*	NR	7.9	0.7	6	1.6	<1
Neutropenia	2	NR	1.9	0.2	1.4	0.2	1
Lymphopenia	NR*	NR	NR	NR	NR	NR	3
Thrombocytopenia	2	NR	2.6	0	3.5	0.2	<1

NR: not reported; *<2%.

Table 2: Thrombocytopenia induced by VEGFR TKIs in RCC.

	Thrombocytopenia	
	All grades (%)	Grade III or IV (%)
Axitinib [6]	15	<1
Pazopanib [10]	41	3–1
Sunitinib [11]	65	8
Cabozantinib [12]	39.7	1.3
Sorafenib [6]	14	0
Tivozanib [13]	18	<1
Lenvatinib* [14]	NR	5

NR: not reported. *lenvatinib plus everolimus.

and no adrenal gland involvement and negative margins (pT1b Nx Mx).

Approximately 6 years after his renal surgery (07/2014), the patient developed bilateral lower extremity weakness and walking difficulty, and diagnostic imaging revealed recurrent disease with thoracic spinal metastases (T6 and T7), causing cord compression at this level. He subsequently underwent corpectomy (T2–T9) and decompressive laminectomy (T6, T7, with a partial T5), and radiation therapy (XRT) was completed by August 2014. Pathology confirmed metastatic clear cell renal cell carcinoma. After radiation therapy, systemic treatment with pazopanib was initiated (09/2014).

The patient was on pazopanib 800 mg/day for two years with overall good tolerance including mild anemia and thrombocytopenia (grade I-II), but pazopanib dose was eventually decreased due to significant fatigue, diarrhea, and abdominal pain. Until June 2016, the patient was on pazopanib intermittently with GI toxicities and fatigue and eventually discontinued (06/2016) due to persistent toxicity.

He then received second-line nivolumab for a total of sixteen months but developed spinal progression at T5–T7 requiring decompressing surgery (04/2017) followed by XRT.

The patient was then successfully rechallenged with pazopanib from 06/2017 to 01/2019, with good tolerance on a lower dose of 600 mg/day and overall stable disease.

In January 2019, he again developed the progressive spinal disease at T5–T7 and underwent repeated surgical decompression. The patient was successfully treated with corticosteroids and was started on axitinib 5 mg BID.

After 10 days of starting axitinib, the patient developed severe fatigue (grade 4). He was observed in the outpatient clinic, and his complete blood count (CBC) revealed a platelet (Plt) count of 4×10^9/liter. The baseline platelet count before treatment with axitinib was 245×10^9/liter. Axitinib treatment was stopped, and the patient was admitted to the hospital for supportive therapy and work-up studies.

At this time, viral serology (hepatitis, CMV, and HIV) tests were tested negative. The patient's renal and hepatic function tests were in normal limits. Prothrombin time, INR and activated partial thromboplastin time, fibrinogen, and D-dimer levels were normal, and direct and indirect Coombs tests were negative. ADAMTS13 (a disintegrin and metalloprotease domain, with thrombospondin type 1 motif 13) activity test resulted 42.5% (normal greater than 10%), and the serotonin release assay was normal (<1). Disseminated intravascular coagulation (DIC), thrombotic thrombocytopenic purpura (TTP), and heparin-induced thrombocytopenia were excluded diagnoses.

Abdominal ultrasound showed normal spleen dimensions. Bone marrow biopsy was performed which was normocellular, without metastatic disease, no increase blast (<1%), and no significant dysplasia. Megakaryocytes were in normal proportion (Figure 1).

The patient received supportive treatment with platelet transfusion (six units in total) with a good platelet transfusion response. Despite axitinib discontinuation, his platelet counts did not recover ($12–15 \times 10^9$/liter), and approximately one week later, he was started on a 4-day pulse of dexamethasone for possible immune thrombocytopenia, with an improvement of his platelet count to above 30×10^9/liter after two days. His platelet counts continued to recover but stabilized at 88×10^9/liter after 2 weeks of treatment. The second course of high-dose steroids was repeated to allow starting a new TKI for RCC.

The patient was eventually started on cabozantinib 40 mg with good tolerance and no worsening of thrombocytopenia. Interestingly, after two months of holding axitinib and while on cabozantinib, the platelet count increased to 136×10^9/Liter. At the last visit, the patient was still on cabozantinib with clinical response and no other hematological events were observed.

3. Discussion

Herein, we describe a rare event of grade IV axitinib-induced thrombocytopenia, which was partially resolved with therapy discontinuation and high-dose steroids and not associated with exposure to other anti-VEGF inhibitors.

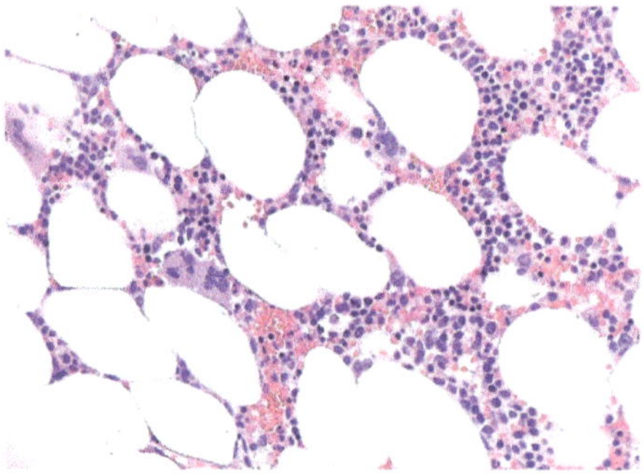

Figure 1: Biopsy shows normocellular bone marrow for age ~30–40% with trilineage hematopoiesis without evidence of involvement by metastatic carcinoma or hematopoietic neoplasm. Megakaryocytes are normal in numbers and do not show significant atypia.

Thrombocytopenia in solid tumors can occur from bone marrow involvement with cancer, toxicity of anticancer treatments, or platelet consumption by DIC or TTP. Immune-related thrombocytopenia is rare in solid tumors [15]. Tumor cells can produce substances that induce platelet aggregation, and this aggregation causes immune-mediated destruction of platelets. Of note, there are few cases with RCC related ITP in literature. Furthermore, paraneoplastic syndrome can cause ITP in RCC patients regardless of stage [15]. The diagnosis of paraneoplastic ITP is one of the exclusion criteria supported by a normocellular bone marrow biopsy and platelet response after definitive treatment of the underlying RCC. In our case, thrombocytopenia occurred after starting a new drug and recovered after discontinuing the therapy and high-dose steroids, favoring the diagnosis of a drug-induced thrombocytopenia over a paraneoplastic syndrome.

In metastatic RCC, antiangiogenic TKIs are standard-of-care. VEGF-induced thrombocytopenia is rare reported in less than 10% with sunitinib and even less with newer generation TKIs [16]. There are several possible etiologies for TKI-induced thrombocytopenia, including the inhibition of KIT signaling, which is important for erythropoiesis, lymphopoiesis, and megakaryopoiesis; inhibition of VEGF, FLT-3, and PDGFR; and microangiopathy due to hypertension [16,17].

In a phase II trial in cytokine refractory RCC patients, there was no hematologic toxicity related with axitinib [18]. In another phase II trial, sorafenib refractory patients were also treated with axitinib. Grade I-II thrombocytopenia was reported in 19.6% of patients, and no grade ≥3 thrombocytopenia was reported in this study either [19]. Finally, in the AXIS trial, hematologic side effects were less frequent in axitinib arm when compared with sorafenib. Grade I-II thrombocytopenia occurred in 15% of patients, and only one patient had grade ≥3 thrombocytopenia [6]. Altogether in RCC studies with axitinib ($N = 672$), all grade thrombocytopenia occurred in about 1.6% of cases, grade 3 in 0.1%, and grade 4 in 0% [20].

Data reported in clinical trials are often not representative of the safety profile observed in real-world data. The exclusion criteria used in clinical studies of axitinib included ECOG ≤2 or Karnofsky performance score >70, grade III or IV heart failure, uncontrolled hypertension, active central nervous system metastasis, autoimmune disease, inadequate renal, hepatic, or hematologic organ function. Of note, our patient had none of these conditions. In addition, axitinib was not the first- or second-line treatment for this patient after prior-TKI. It is possible that prior angiogenic therapies may have caused thrombocytopenia, yet it did not occur with subsequent treatment with cabozantinib.

Drug-induced thrombocytopenia can be clinically significant, and significant thrombocytopenia has been previously reported with sunitinib in combination with trastuzumab in a patient with metastatic breast cancer after three weeks on treatment with both agents [17].

Other causes of thrombocytopenia have to be excluded for the final diagnosis of drug-induced thrombocytopenia. There is no test to confirm or rule out that the patient had ITP versus drug-induced thrombocytopenia. The treatment for drug-induced thrombocytopenia is to stop the culprit drug; however, steroids may be given to improve the total platelet count.

In this particular case, drug-induced thrombocytopenia is the most likely diagnosis because (1) there was a platelet count decrease (from normal to 4×10^9/Liter) after 10 days of starting axitinib; (2) there was no interaction between axitinib and other drugs that are used by the patient [21] and (3) other causes such as infections, DIC, TTP, and bone marrow involvement were ruled out. In addition, after 2 months of discontinuation of axitinib and after a pulse of steroids, platelets increased to 136×10^9/liter.

In conclusion, severe thrombocytopenia induced by axitinib is a rare but potentially life-threatening event and may be drug-specific rather than class-specific effect. A short-term pulse of corticosteroids and therapy discontinuation was associated with a clinical improvement and allowed further treatment with a different anti-VEGF therapy.

References

[1] R. L. Siegel, K. D. Miller, and A. Jemal, "Cancer statistics, 2019," *CA: A Cancer Journal for Clinicians*, vol. 69, no. 1, pp. 7–34, 2019.

[2] T. K. Choueiri and R. J. Motzer, "Systemic therapy for metastatic renal-cell carcinoma," *New England Journal of Medicine*, vol. 376, no. 4, pp. 354–366, 2017.

[3] K. Zarrabi, C. Fang, and S. Wu, "New treatment options for metastatic renal cell carcinoma with prior anti-angiogenesis therapy," *Journal of Hematology & Oncology*, vol. 10, no. 1, 2017.

[4] D. D. Hu-Lowe, H. Y. Zou, M. L. Grazzini et al., "Nonclinical antiangiogenesis and antitumor activities of axitinib (AG-013736), an oral, potent, and selective inhibitor of vascular endothelial growth factor receptor tyrosine kinases 1, 2, 3," *Clinical Cancer Research*, vol. 14, no. 22, pp. 7272–7283, 2008.

[5] R. J. Motzer, K. Penkov, J. Haanen et al., "Avelumab plus axitinib versus sunitinib for advanced renal-cell carcinoma,"

New England Journal of Medicine, vol. 380, no. 12, pp. 1103–1115, 2019.

[6] B. I. Rini, B. Escudier, P. Tomczak et al., "Comparative effectiveness of axitinib versus sorafenib in advanced renal cell carcinoma (AXIS): a randomised phase 3 trial," *The Lancet*, vol. 378, no. 9807, pp. 1931–1939, 2011.

[7] B. I. Rini, E. R. Plimack, V. Stus et al., "Pembrolizumab plus axitinib versus sunitinib for advanced renal-cell carcinoma," *New England Journal of Medicine*, vol. 380, no. 12, pp. 1116–1127, 2019.

[8] M. Gross-Goupil, T. G. Kwon, M. Eto et al., "Axitinib versus placebo as an adjuvant treatment of renal cell carcinoma: results from the phase III, randomized ATLAS trial," *Annals of Oncology*, vol. 29, no. 12, pp. 2371–2378, 2018.

[9] T. E. Hutson, V. Lesovoy, S. Al-Shukri et al., "Axitinib versus sorafenib as first-line therapy in patients with metastatic renal-cell carcinoma: a randomised open-label phase 3 trial," *The Lancet Oncology*, vol. 14, no. 13, pp. 1287–1294, 2013.

[10] R. J. Motzer, T. E. Hutson, D. Cella et al., "Pazopanib versus sunitinib in metastatic renal-cell carcinoma," *New England Journal of Medicine*, vol. 369, no. 8, pp. 722–731, 2013.

[11] R. J. Motzer, T. E. Hutson, P. Tomczak et al., "Sunitinib versus interferon alfa in metastatic renal-cell carcinoma," *New England Journal of Medicine*, vol. 356, no. 2, pp. 115–124, 2007.

[12] T. K. Choueiri, B. Escudier, T. Powles et al., "Cabozantinib versus everolimus in advanced renal-cell carcinoma," *New England Journal of Medicine*, vol. 373, no. 19, pp. 1814–1823, 2015.

[13] R. J. Motzer, D. Nosov, T. Eisen et al., "Tivozanib versus sorafenib as initial targeted therapy for patients with metastatic renal cell carcinoma: results from a phase III trial," *Journal of Clinical Oncology*, vol. 31, no. 30, pp. 3791–3799, 2013.

[14] R. J. Motzer, T. E. Hutson, H. Glen et al., "Lenvatinib, everolimus, and the combination in patients with metastatic renal cell carcinoma: a randomised, phase 2, open-label, multicentre trial," *The Lancet Oncology*, vol. 16, no. 15, pp. 1473–1482, 2015.

[15] E. J. Cho, H. J. Lee, K. U. Park, U.-Y. Kim, H. J. Lee, and S. M. Bang, "Immune thrombocytopenic purpura in a patient with renal cell carcinoma," *The Korean Journal of Internal Medicine*, vol. 29, no. 5, pp. 671–674, 2014.

[16] M. Schmidinger, "Understanding and managing toxicities of vascular endothelial growth factor (VEGF) inhibitors," *European Journal of Cancer Supplements*, vol. 11, no. 2, pp. 172–191, 2013.

[17] M. Trinkaus, M. Trudeau, and J. Callum, "Drug-induced immune thrombocytopenic purpura secondary to sunitinib," *Current Oncology*, vol. 15, no. 3, pp. 152–154, 2008.

[18] O. Rixe, R. M. Bukowski, M. D. Michaelson et al., "Axitinib treatment in patients with cytokine-refractory metastatic renal-cell cancer: a phase II study," *The Lancet Oncology*, vol. 8, no. 11, pp. 975–984, 2007.

[19] B. I. Rini, G. Wilding, G. Hudes et al., "Phase II study of axitinib in sorafenib-refractory metastatic renal cell carcinoma," *Journal of Clinical Oncology*, vol. 27, no. 27, pp. 4462–4468, 2009.

[20] https://www.medicines.org.uk/emc/product/4325/smpc.

[21] https://www.drugs.com/drug-interactions/axitinib.html.

43

Myeloid Disease with the CSF3R T618I Mutation after CLL

Maria Eduarda Couto,[1] **Susana Bizarro**,[2] **Domingos Sousa**,[3] **Nelson Domingues**,[1] **Isabel Oliveira**,[1] **Gabriela Martins**,[4] **Manuel R. Teixeira**,[2,5] **and Mário Mariz**[1]

[1]*Onco-hematology Department, Instituto Português de Oncologia Do Porto F.G. E.P.E., Porto, Portugal*
[2]*Genetics Department, Instituto Português de Oncologia Do Porto F.G. E.P.E., Porto, Portugal*
[3]*Internal Medicine Department, Centro Hospitalar e Universitário Do Algarve E.P.E., Porto, Portugal*
[4]*Immunology Department, Instituto Português de Oncologia Do Porto F.G. E.P.E., Porto, Portugal*
[5]*Biomedical Sciences Institute, University of Porto, Porto, Portugal*

Correspondence should be addressed to Maria Eduarda Couto; eduarda.scouto@gmail.com

Academic Editor: Stephen E. Langabeer

Chronic lymphocytic leukemia (CLL) is frequently an indolent diagnosis, with most of the patients being under surveillance for long time. There is an increased risk of a second neoplasia in CLL, rarely hematological (in the myeloid lineage is even rarer). A 58-year-old male was diagnosed with CLL in 2012, remaining in regular surveillance until 2014. Then, the CLL progressed, and 6 cycles of rituximab, fludarabine, and cyclophosphamide were prescribed with partial response. He remained in surveillance and suffered 2 episodes of autoimmune hemolytic anemia until 2019. Then, the hemolytic anemia relapsed and a neutrophilia became evident (progressing slowly), as well as a thrombocytopenia and splenomegaly without adenopathy were found. The bone marrow aspirate showed a chronic myeloproliferative disease without dysplasia. A peripheral blood search for the *CSF3R* mutation (T618I) was positive, also suggesting Chronic Neutrophilic Leukemia (CNL). For a discrete monocytosis, a chronic myelomonocytic leukemia (CMML) was also considered. Hydroxyurea was then prescribed. The T618I CSF3R mutation is highly suggestive of CNL (being diagnostic criteria for CNL); however, this case may also suggest CMML as a possible diagnosis (there are other mutations in the CSF3R gene described for CMML, but not the T618I, which is highly exclusive of CNL according to the literature). To our knowledge, this is the first report of a possible CNL in a CLL patient (the opposite was already described in 1998).

1. Introduction

Chronic lymphocytic leukemia (CLL) is a very common and usually indolent lymphoid malignancy. Most patients remain in surveillance for a long time. CLL increases the risk of secondary malignancies, mainly in the skin and digestive tract, by diminishing the humoral and cellular responses of the immune system.

A Chronic Neutrophilic Leukemia (CNL) is defined by persistent neutrophilic proliferation (mainly mature forms), hyperplasia of the bone marrow granulocyte lineage, and usually splenomegaly. [1] It is a BCR-ABL negative myeloproliferative neoplasm, named in 1964 for the first time. It is a rare event typically found in elderly people, more frequently males [1]. Patients are usually asymptomatic, but there is a hemorrhagic tendency probably caused by the neutrophilia and vascular infiltration by the disease [1]. The recent finding of the activating mutations of the gene *CSF3R*, the T618I (found in 80% of the cases), revolutionized the understanding of the pathogenesis of this disease, nowadays being an important diagnosis criterion [1–6]. However, CNL still is an exclusion diagnosis.

The diagnosis of a chronic myeloid neoplasia as CNL in a patient with a chronic lymphoid neoplasia is a rare phenomenon, mainly when the first diagnosis is CLL [7–8]. As far as we know, there is only one case report describing a CLL after a CNL, published in 1998 [7].

2. Case Report

A 58-year-old male was diagnosed with CLL Rai 1 in 2012, remaining in regular surveillance. He had a past medical history of hyperuricemia, hypertension, hypothyroidism, prostate benign hyperplasia, biliary calculus, and clear cells carcinoma of the right kidney (submitted to partial nephrectomy).

In 2014, the CLL progressed with anemia, growing adenopathy, and fast doubling of the leucocyte count. Rituximab, fludarabine, and cyclophosphamide were prescribed for 6 cycles, and the patient achieved a partial response, remaining in surveillance afterwards.

One year later, he was hospitalized for febrile neutropenia caused by right base pneumonia, in septic shock and multiorganic failure (being admitted in the ICU). This episode was followed by another admittance for febrile neutropenia with respiratory symptoms in 6 months.

In 2016, the patient developed autoimmune hemolytic anemia. Prednisolone 1 mg/kg and folic acid were prescribed, being stopped in 3 months with a fast relapse of the hemolysis. A second treatment course was performed for 7 months, with stabilization of the hemoglobin levels around 11-12 g/dL.

Suddenly in the end of 2018, there was a significant increase in the leucocyte count, mainly caused by a neutrophilia (Table 1). The previous kidney cancer had no signs of relapse, and there was no infectious process in the course. There was a soft decrease in the hemoglobin level, but the increase in the leucocyte and neutrophil counts persisted, with the identification of immature myeloid forms in the peripheral blood smear and 0.31×10^9/L of blast cells. A leukemic reaction was suspected. In three months, the hemolytic anemia relapsed, preceded by a dental abscess. The patient complained about asthenia, loss of weight (5 kg in 5 months), bone pain, and nausea. He denied other symptoms. The leukocytosis and neutrophilia became even more evident, as well as the thrombocytopenia. The direct coombs test was positive for complement and IgG (1 : 30). An abdominal echography showed homogeneous splenomegaly (15.8 cm). The flow cytometer of the peripheral blood showed polyclonal B lymphocytes circulating. The bone marrow aspirate was morphologically suggestive of a chronic myeloproliferative disease without dysplasia. The del17p was found by FISH (fluorescence in situ hybridization) in the bone marrow aspirate. The flow cytometer of the bone marrow aspirate identified a major population of the neutrophilic lineage in different stages of maturation, without blasts; no signs of the CLL were found at this point. One month later, a second bone marrow aspirate showed the same morphological results; the karyotype analysis of the bone marrow aspirate identified an isochromosome 17q. Prednisolone was restarted 1 mg/kg with improvement of the anemia but worsening of the thrombocytopenia (to values inferior to 100×10^9/L). The search for the *CSF3R* gene mutations in the peripheral blood was positive for the most common mutation (T618I), which is a defining criterion for CNL. After 3 months, the patient became clinically asymptomatic with reduction of the leucocyte count and splenomegaly with hydroxyurea 5 gr/week, also under prednisolone 20 mg daily for the hemolytic anemia. After 12 months, the leukocytosis with neutrophilia increased, blasts were identified in the peripheral blood, and a splenomegaly became evident. The patient was not eligible for bone marrow transplant, becoming a palliative case. Multiple nodules were found in a cerebral CT scan (requested for neurologic complains), possibly due to kidney cancer relapse, which were never biopsied for the severe thrombocytopenia.

3. Discussion

It is well known that CLL is a disease that remains in constant clonal evolution [9]. The CLL is commonly associated with an increased risk of a second neoplasia, but rarely hematologic (and even rarer a myeloid event) as we report here. As far as we know, there is only one similar case, in which the CNL preceded the CLL diagnosis, in an era when genomics were not part of the diagnosis criteria for CNL [7]. Besides being rare, CNL must be considered in this clinical case, as well as a CMML.

The clinic signs, blood counts, bone marrow results, and molecular biology studies were highly suggestive of a myeloproliferative malignancy. The thrombocytopenia could be explained by the increasing spleen, often heralding a blast crisis. LDH and B12 vitamin levels are typically high in a leukemoid reaction, with low levels of G-CSF [1].

There are many findings suggestive of CNL in this clinical case: a high and persistent neutrophilia without any other explanation for happening; a nearly normal monocyte count (an increase in leucocytes could have caused an increase in the absolute value of monocytes); the bone marrow studies (conducted in two different occasions) evidencing a myeloproliferative process; and the flow cytometry identifying a major population of the neutrophilic lineage in different stages of maturation, without blasts. The search for the activating mutation T618I of the CSF3R gene is essential for the final diagnosis of CNL. This gene is related to other disorders apart from CNL, such as CMML, severe congenital neutropenia, hereditary chronic neutrophilia, and rarely myeloid leukemia, and recently, it was described in the literature also in atypical CML [10]. However, the specific T168I mutation was never described in CMML [11]. CNL is not associated with lymphoproliferative neoplasms other than CLL (there is only one case report of a CLL after a CNL, but not the opposite) [7].

CMML should be considered too. Apart from the neutrophilia, this patient also had a monocyte count in the upper limit of normal values (absolute counts regularly between 0.94 and $1{,}94 \times 10^9$/L, having one episode with 0.39×10^9/L), a persistent monocytosis. CMML is a more common diagnosis compared with CNL.

The loss of the short arm of chromosome 17 (where the TP53 gene is located) identified in the bone marrow aspirate is a genetic abnormality typically found in CLL (as well as the hemolytic events) but not in myeloproliferative diseases. However, there were no signs of CLL in the flow cytometry at the myeloid diagnosis time. The archival cytogenetic sample did not have sufficient quality to allow the study for the CSF3R mutation or p53 mutation.

In what refers to the therapeutic approach, a cytoreduction with hydroxyurea is usually successful in the leukocytosis control and splenomegaly (25% of the patients are refractory) for both CNL and CMML [3, 11].

Table 1: Blood counts obtained in a temporal line (from the left to the right; time 0 is the moment of the myeloid diagnosis and the beginning of hydroxyurea).

	17 months before	16 months before	12 months before	7 months before	5 months before	3 months before	2 months before	1 month before	Time 0 (HU started)	1 month later	2 months later	3 months later	4 months later	6 months later	12 months later
Hemoglobin g/dl	10.7	11.6	12.1	11.4	11.4	9.4	8.9	11.3	11.5	9,5	12,4	11,1	11,4	9,4	8,2
Leucocytes × 10^9/L	9.96	8.33	11.59	13.81	24.82	62.71	77.8	81.7	84.01	21,15	38,61	14,91	61,48	71,77	117,01
Neutrophils × 10^9/L	5.94	5.03	7.74	10.21	19.94	51.23	63.8	69.48	72.67	15,69	34,77	13,08	53,96	63,02	94,78
Eosinophils × 10^9/L	0.34	0.18	0.20.18	0.14	0.22	0.63	0.78	0.03	0	0,03	0.02	0	0,03	0	0
Basophils × 10^9/L	0.05	0.05	0.1	0.07	0.18	0.63	0	0.05	0.34	0,08	0,12	0,04	0,03	0	0,59
Lymphocytes × 10^9/L	2.3	2	2.24	2.09	1.96	2.76	3.11	2.01	1.01	1,11	1,96	1,11	1,98	6,48	2,34
Monocytes × 10^9/L	1.23	1.02	1.07	1.12	1.23	0.94	0.39	1.94	1.09	2,65	0,53	0,45	1,03	1,09	9,95
Immature granulocytes × 10^9/L	0.1	0.05	0.16	0.18	1.29	Metamielocytes 2,76 × 10^9/L, mielocytes 2,20 × 10^9/L, promielocytes 1,25 × 10^9/L	Metamielocytes 5,45 × 10^9/L, mielocytes 4,28 × 10^9/L	8.19	Metamielocytes 2,86 × 10^9/L, mielocytes 4,62 × 10^9/L, promielocytes 1,43 × 10^9/L	1,59	1,21	0,23	4,45	Metamielocytes 1,82 × 10^9/L, mielocytes 0,36 × 10^9/L	Metamielocytes 4,1 × 10^9/L, mielocytes 1,76 × 10^9/L, promielocytes 1,76 × 10^9/L, blasts 1,76 × 10^9/L
Platelets × 10^9/L	263	189	228	211	193	204	147	117	96	77	50	66	67	86	14
Blasts × 10^9/L						0.31									
Sedimentation velocity							20/45								

The main therapeutic options for CNL are interferon, hypometlylating agents, ruxolitinib, thalidomide, and cladribine [3]. TKI therapy was experimented successfully in a CNL patient for the first time in 2004, for the CSF3R mutation [12]. Treatment with the SRC kinase inhibitor dasatinib and the JAK1/2 kinase inhibitor ruxolitinib also have shown efficacy for CNL with membrane proximal mutations and truncation mutations, respectively [3, 12, 13]. Most of the agents proposed for CNL treatment are palliative, not achieving remission of the disease. There is little role for bone marrow transplantation (the only curative option) or induction regimens, given the bad results obtained [1]. The prognosis of CNL is not favorable nowadays: between 20–30 months of median survival and a transformation rate to AML between 10 and 21. 2% in a median time of 21 months. Due to the rarity of the disease, there is no prognostic scoring system approved to guide treatment options and follow-up [1, 3, 8].

The main treatment options for CMML are hypomethylating agents (such as 5-azacitidine or decitabine), with an overall response rate of ~30–40% and complete remission rate of ~7–17%, with no impact on mutational allele burdens. Allogeneic stem cell transplant is the only potentially curative option, but it is associated with significant morbidity and mortality [11].

The authors emphasize the importance of the T618I mutation in the CNL diagnosis, and they wonder whether it is enough to exclude the CMML diagnosis. A wider targeted genotyping could be appropriate to better clarify the etiology of this disease. Future investigations should address the T618I mutation presence in a broad group of CMML patients, in order to strengthen its specificity. Furthermore, the impact of this mutation in selecting treatment options for CNL should also be better understood.

References

[1] N. Szuber and A. Tefferi, "Chronic neutrophilic leukemia: new science and new diagnostic criteria," *Blood Cancer Journal*, vol. 8, p. 19, 2018.

[2] J. E. Maxson and J. W. Tyner, "Genomics of chronic neutrophilic leukemi," *Blood*, vol. 129, no. 6, pp. 715–722, 2017.

[3] M. A. Elliott and A. Tefferi, "Chronic neutrophilic leukemia: 2018 update on diagnosis, molecular genetics and management," *American Journal of Hematology*, vol. 93, no. 4, pp. 578–587, 2018.

[4] Y. Ouyang, C. Qiao, Y. Chen, and S.-J. Zhang, "Clinical significance of CSF3R, SRSF2 and SETBP1 mutations in chronic neutrophilic leukemia and chronic myelomonocytic leukemia," *Oncotarget*, vol. 8, no. 13, pp. 20834–20841, 2017.

[5] A. Pardanani, T. L. Lasho, R. R. Laborde et al., "CSF3R T618I is a highly prevalent and specific mutation in chronic neutrophilic leukemia," *Leukemia*, vol. 27, no. 9, pp. 1870–1873, 2013.

[6] J. E. Maxson, J. Gotlib, D. A. Pollyea et al., "Oncogenic CSF3R mutations in chronic neutrophilic leukemia and atypical CML," *New England Journal of Medicine*, vol. 368, no. 19, pp. 1781–1790, 2013.

[7] K. Ito, K. Usuki, S. Iki, and A. Urabe, "Chronic neutrophilic leukemia associated with chronic lymphocytic leukemia," *International Journal of Hematology*, vol. 68, no. 1, pp. 87–94, 1998.

[8] N. Szuber, "CSF3R-muated chronic neutrophilic leukemia: long-term outcome in 19 consecutive patients and risk model for survival," *Blood Cancer Journal*, vol. 8, p. 21, 2018.

[9] Q.-G. Zhang, J. Wang, W.-Y. Gong, and Q.-C. Jin, "Clonal evolution in a chronic neutrophilic leukemia patient," *Hematology*, vol. 24, no. 1, pp. 455–458, 2019.

[10] S. Kim, "PB2077. The CSF3R T618I mutation is highly prevalent among atypical chronic myeloid leukemia patients from South Korea: a single center experience," in *Proceedings of the European Hematology Associatio 24th Congress*, Amsterdam, The Netherlands, July 2019.

[11] M. M. Patnaik and A. Tefferi, "Chronic myelomonocytic leukemia: 2018 update on diagnosis, risk stratification and management," *American Journal of Hematology*, vol. 93, no. 6, pp. 824–840, 2018.

[12] I. K. Choi, B.-S. Kim, K.-A. Lee et al., "Efficacy of imatinib mesylate (STI571) in chronic neutrophilic leukemia with t (15; 19): case report," *American Journal of Hematology*, vol. 77, no. 4, pp. 366–369, 2004.

[13] K.-H. T. T. Dao, J. Gotlib, M. M. N. Deininger et al., "Efficacy of ruxolitinib in patients with chronic neutrophilic leukemia and atypical chronic myeloid leukemia," *Journal of Clinical Oncology*, vol. 38, no. 10, pp. 1006–1018, 2020.

44

Methotrexate-Associated Lymphoproliferative Disorder in a Patient with Psoriasis: A Case Report and Review of the Literature

Carolina Afonso ,[1] Adriana Roque ,[1] Cátia Almeida ,[1] Maria Beatriz Pimentão,[2] Maria José Julião ,[2] Rodolfo Silva ,[3] Catarina Geraldes ,[1] and Marília Gomes [1]

[1]*Hematology Unit, Hospitais da Universidade de Coimbra, Centro Hospitalar e Universitário de Coimbra, Coimbra, Portugal*
[2]*Pathology Unit, Hospitais da Universidade de Coimbra, Centro Hospitalar e Universitário de Coimbra, Coimbra, Portugal*
[3]*Nuclear Medicine Unit, Hospitais da Universidade de Coimbra, Centro Hospitalar e Universitário de Coimbra, Coimbra, Portugal*

Correspondence should be addressed to Carolina Afonso; 11138@chuc.min-saude.pt

Academic Editor: Pier Paolo Piccaluga

Iatrogenic immunodeficiency-associated lymphoproliferative disorders (LPDs) are heterogeneous clinicopathological entities developing in patients receiving immunosuppression. Outside the posttransplant setting, methotrexate (MTX), a drug commonly used for the treatment of autoimmune diseases, is an immunosuppressive agent frequently reported to be associated with LPD. MTX-associated LPD (MTX-LPD) includes a spectrum of lymphocytic proliferations, ranging from polyclonal hyperplasia to malignant lymphoma. MTX-LPD diagnosis can be challenging, as signs and symptoms are often nonspecific and may overlap with those of several other conditions, including exacerbation of the underlying autoimmune disease. Spontaneous regression of LPD after MTX discontinuation is characteristic of MTX-LPD, therefore avoiding chemotherapeutic intervention in a significant proportion of patients. Other cases, however, should receive chemotherapy.

1. Introduction

Autoimmune and inflammatory rheumatic diseases have been associated with an increased risk of LPD, related to the chronic antigenic stimulation and immune dysregulation underlying those diseases [1]. Additionally, immunosuppressive agents frequently used to treat these diseases, such as MTX, have also been suggested to play a role in lymphomagenesis [2–4]. As a result, the World Health Organization (WHO) recognizes lymphoproliferative disorders arising in patients treated with immunosuppressive drugs for autoimmune disease as a separate nosological entity classified as "other iatrogenic immunodeficiency-associated LPDs" (OIIA-LPD) in the revised 4th edition of the WHO Classification of Tumors of Hematopoietic and Lymphoid Tissues [4].

Most OIIA-LPD develop in patients treated with MTX for autoimmune diseases [5]. Therefore, MTX may further increase the risk of LPD in this population. Regarding rheumatoid arthritis (RA), for example, it is estimated that patients undergoing treatment with MTX are 1.7 times more likely to develop LPD than those not treated with this drug [6, 7].

Most MTX-LPD cases are diffuse large B cell lymphoma (DLBCL; 35–60%), followed by classical Hodgkin lymphoma (CHL; 12–25%), while other lymphoma subtypes are rare [4, 8]. Their histopathological features are similar to those found in immunocompetent patients with equivalent lymphoma subtypes [8]. Polymorphic or lymphoplasmacytic infiltrates have been described in as many as 20% of cases of MTX-LPD [4].

The pathogenesis of these entities is not entirely understood; studies suggest that the suppression of immune surveillance by MTX, due to excessive inhibition of T helper 1 CD4+ T cells and effector memory CD8+ T cells, plays an important role [3]. In addition, by inhibiting CD8+ Epstein-

Barr virus (EBV)-specific T cells, MTX indirectly promotes proliferation of latent EBV-infected B cells, which are normally suppressed [3, 9, 10]. Indeed, these MTX-LPD are often EBV related: EBV is almost always found in polymorphic infiltrates, in approximately 80% of MTX-CHL and in 25–60% of MTX-DLBCL. [4].

Spontaneous regression of LPD after MTX discontinuation is characteristic of MTX-LPD, occurring in approximately 50% of cases [3, 11]. Patients with nonregressive lymphomas and those with relapse/regrowth (R/R) events require histology-adjusted chemotherapy [5].

2. Case Report

A 56-year-old male patient diagnosed with moderate-to-severe plaque psoriasis at the age of 14 had been receiving treatment with low-dose MTX (15 mg per week) for more than one decade when he developed constitutional symptoms of fatigue and unintentional weight loss (approximately 20% of his normal bodyweight). Physical examination revealed multiple palpable bilateral supraclavicular and cervical lymph nodes, as well as a palpable spleen 3 cm below the costal margin. Laboratory investigation revealed white blood cell and platelet count, mild anemia (hemoglobin 11.1 g/dL), elevated lactate dehydrogenase (314 U/L, normal range (NR) < 250), and increased cholestatic enzymes (γ-glutamyltransferase 192 U/L, NR < 55 U/L; alkaline phosphatase 237 U/L, NR 30–120 U/L). Microbiological and serological tests did not reveal active infection.

Computed tomography (CT) scan of the chest, abdomen, and pelvis showed mediastinal and paraaortic lymphadenopathy (the short-axis of the largest lymph node was 29 mm) and splenomegaly (with a 210 mm longitudinal axis). Additionally, the patient performed a ^{18}F fluorodeoxyglucose positron emission tomography/CT (^{18}F-FDG PET/CT) which revealed extensive hypermetabolic involvement of the spleen (with a maximum standardized uptake value, SUV max, of 16.7) and lymph nodes above (cervical, supraclavicular and mediastinal lymphadenopathy) and below the diaphragm (paraaortic, celiac, hepatic hilar, and peripancreatic); additionally, there was evidence of small, ^{18}F-FDG-avid pulmonary nodules and focal skeleton/bone marrow hypermetabolic involvement (Figure 1).

As most lymph nodes were either small or not easily accessible for biopsy, a CT-guided percutaneous core biopsy of focal splenic lesion was performed; however, histologic examination found normal splenic tissue. Bone marrow biopsy aspiration and trephine biopsy also did not detect clonal lymphoid infiltration. Given the high clinical suspicion of MTX-LPD (and despite the absence of histological confirmation), MTX was discontinued, and a watch-and-wait strategy was adopted. Constitutional symptoms progressively improved, reinforcing the diagnostic hypothesis. Since then, psoriasis was managed with combinations of topical agents and psoralen plus ultraviolet A (PUVA) therapy.

Four months after MTX discontinuation, a new PET/CT scan was performed, showing a decrease in size and

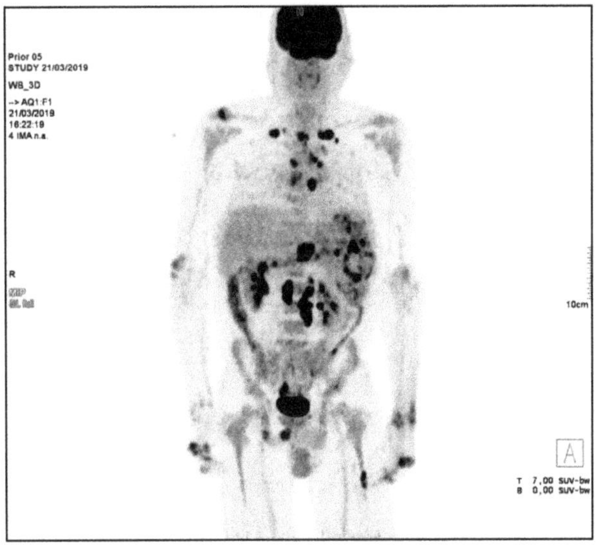

FIGURE 1: 18F-FDG PET/CT performed at initial presentation showing hypermetabolic involvement of the spleen and lymph nodes above and below the diaphragm, as well as small, 18F-FDG-avid pulmonary nodules and focal skeleton/bone marrow hypermetabolic involvement.

metabolic activity of supra and infradiaphragmatic lymphadenopathy, a reduction of the hypermetabolic activity in the spleen (SUX max of 9.5), and a spontaneous resolution of the hypermetabolic involvement of the lungs and bone marrow (Figure 2). Given the partial regression of the disease and the absence of constitutional symptoms since MTX was withdrawn, close surveillance was maintained.

A PET/CT scan performed five months later (nine months after MTX cessation) revealed an increase of the hypermetabolic activity in several supra and infradiaphragmatic lymphadenopathies accompanied by a paradoxical reduction in the size of the lymph nodes; there was also evidence of multiple splenic lesions with an increased hypermetabolic activity (SUV max of 13.2). Given the imagiologic evidence of progressive disease, a CT-guided percutaneous core biopsy of the spleen was repeated, but a definite diagnosis could not be established due to unrepresentative tissue sampling. Since the patient was asymptomatic at the time, a watchful waiting approach was maintained.

Six months later (15 months after MTX cessation), another PET/CT scan was consistent with progressive disease, with development of a new hypermetabolic lesion involving the L4 vertebral body, as well as an increased hypermetabolic activity in the spleen (SUV max of 15.9) (Figure 3).

The patient was then proposed for diagnostic splenectomy. At macroscopic examination, the splenic parenchyma showed multiple nodules, the largest one with approximately 4 cm diameter, located near the splenic hilum. Histopathological analysis revealed multiple parenchymatous nodules composed by numerous Hodgkin and Reed-Sternberg (HRS) cells positive for CD30 and CD15, with dim

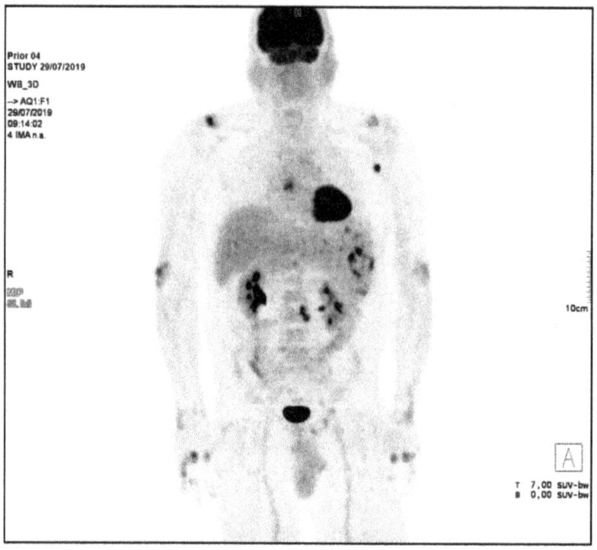

Figure 2: 18F-FDG PET/CT performed four months after MTX discontinuation, showing a reduction of the hypermetabolic activity of spleen and lymph nodes, and a spontaneous resolution of the hypermetabolic involvement of lungs and bone marrow.

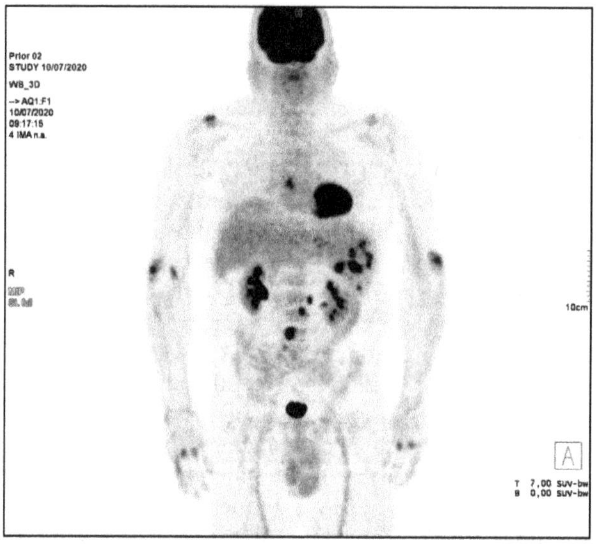

Figure 3: 18F-FDG PET/CT performed 15 months after MTX withdrawal with an increased hypermetabolic activity in the spleen and a new hypermetabolic lesion involving the L4 vertebral body, consistent with progressive disease.

expression of PAX5, and negative for CD45, CD20, CD10, and ALK; these cells were also positive for EBV-encoded RNA (EBER) (Figure 4). Immunoglobulin heavy chain (IGH) clonality testing was not performed.

A diagnosis of MTX-associated CHL (MTX-CHL), Ann Arbor stage IV-BS, advanced stage by the German Hodgkin Study Group (GHSG), International Prognostic Score (IPS) 3, was established. The patient started treatment according ABVD protocol (adriamycin, bleomycin, vinblastine, and dacarbazine). An interim PET/CT scan (after two cycles) showed a complete metabolic response (Deauville score 3), and the patient proceeded to four additional cycles of chemotherapy with omission of bleomycin (AVD), as per protocol. End-of-treatment PET/CT was consistent with a complete metabolic response (Deauville score 1). At the time of writing (eight months after completing the treatment), the patient does not show evidence of relapse and/or late treatment-related toxicity.

3. Discussion

Patients with autoimmune diseases, such as rheumatoid arthritis and psoriasis, are at increased risk of developing LPD [12]. For RA, for example, the risk of lymphoma is 2–4 times higher than that observed in the general population,

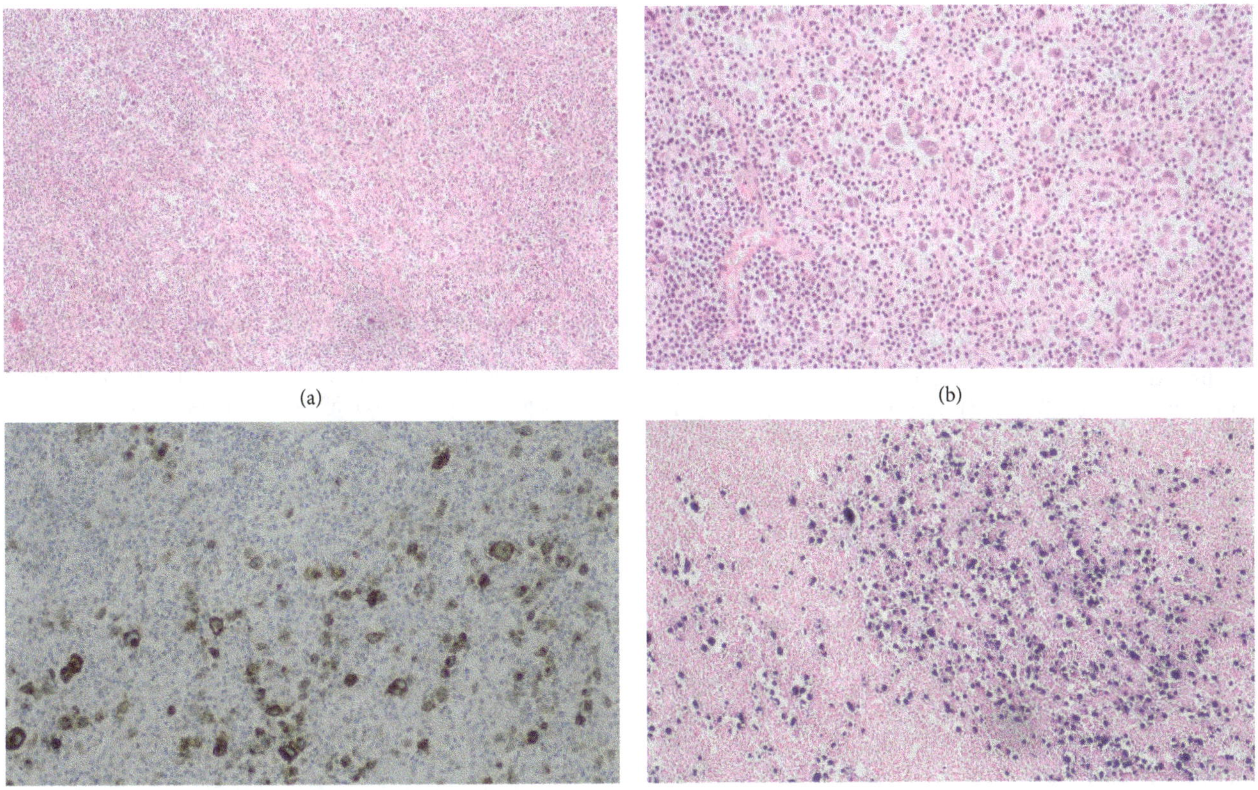

(a) (b) (c) (d)

FIGURE 4: Histopathological examination of splenectomy specimen. Infiltration of the splenic tissue by large pleomorphic neoplastic cells resembling HRS cells: (a) H&E stain, 100x magnification; b) H&E stain, 200x magnification]. These cells were positive for CD30 (c) and EBER (d).

and this risk that may be slightly increased by treatment with MTX [6, 7].

Diagnosis of MTX-LPD can be challenging, given that patients may present with nonspecific constitutional symptoms, which can arise from a variety of conditions, including exacerbation of the underlying autoimmune disease, infections, and malignancies. Additionally, given the heterogeneous pathology of MTX-LPD, multiple or repeated biopsy may be needed to establish a diagnosis [13]. Importantly, no association has been found between the duration and/or dose of MTX and MTX-LPD development [14].

In the case described above, although there was already a high index of suspicion of MTX-LPD (given the improvement of clinical symptoms and regression of disease after MTX withdrawal), histological confirmation took 21 months, mainly due to repeated nondiagnostic biopsies.

In our case, EBV was detected by in situ hybridization, in accordance with previous studies which report a high incidence (approximately 80%) of EBV positivity in CHL-LPD [4, 15].

Approximately 40–50% of MTX-LPD cases occur at extranodal sites such as the skin, digestive tract, liver, spleen, lung, bone marrow (BM), and central nervous system (CNS) [4, 11]. Regarding MTX-CHL, several studies reported higher rates of advanced-stage disease and extranodal disease when compared to sporadic CHL [8, 16–18]. Indeed, our patient presented advanced-stage disease with extranodal involvement, including the spleen, lungs, and BM.

In patients with sustained regression of MTX-LPD after immunosuppression withdrawal, chemotherapy may be avoided [11, 19]. Therefore, the first step if MTX-LPD is suspected is MTX discontinuation [18]. For most patients achieving complete remission (CR), this is expected to occur within a time interval of 4 weeks after discontinuation of immunosuppressant; conversely, for patients experiencing a partial remission (PR), the time interval between discontinuation of immunosuppressive treatment and clinical response is usually longer, often occurring about 2-3 months later [20]. In a retrospective study, the EBV-positive rate in MTX-LPD patients exhibiting spontaneous regression of LPD was higher than that observed in MTX-LPD patients without tumor regression (54.5% vs. 21.1%, respectively), suggesting that EBV may be involved not only in the development of MTX-LPD but also in its regression after MTX withdrawal [21]. Histology may also influence regression rates after MTX cessation, which are reported to be lower in MTX-CHL than in MTX-DLBCL [8, 10, 22].

Even in cases of spontaneous remission, careful observation is important, as R/R of MTX-LPD has been reported in 18–45% of patients, with a reported median duration until R/R of 10.6 months (0.7–35.6) [11, 18]. In the case described above, a partial remission of LPD was observed 4 months after MTX withdrawal, but regrowth was documented after an additional 12 months off treatment.

In cases with nonregressive LPD after MTX withdrawal and in those with R/R events, chemotherapy is the treatment of choice [5]. Regarding MTX-CHL, although there is no established standard chemotherapy regimen, most reported cases were treated with ABVD, which is considered the standard treatment for sporadic CHL [13, 23]. MTX-CHL seems to have identical response rates to chemotherapy, progression-free survival (PFS), or overall survival (OS) to sporadic CHL [16].

In recent years, an increasing number of case reports regarding the use of brentuximab vedotin (BV) in combination with AVD (BV+AVD) in front-line treatment of MTX-CHL has been published, with favorable responses and an acceptable toxicity profile [22, 23]. Although it is unknown whether MTX-CHL patients are particularly susceptible to bleomycin-induced lung toxicity, this bleomycin-free regimen represents an alternative for these patients who may have underlying pulmonary complications related to their autoimmune disease [22, 23]. Although immune checkpoint inhibitors may also be suitable for patients with MTX-CHL, their safety in patients with preexisting autoimmune disease remains controversial, particularly due to the risk autoimmune disease flare [24].

4. Conclusion

We herein report a rare case of LPD in a patient with a past long-term oral MTX administration, who successfully attained complete remission following treatment with ABVD/AVD. The case illustrates the difficulty in establishing a diagnosis of MTX-LPD. When suspected, MTX should be discontinued, as this may lead to an improvement of clinical symptoms and a spontaneous regression of disease. The case also highlights the importance of careful observation, even in cases of spontaneous remission after MTX cessation, due to possible occurrence of R/R events, which require chemotherapeutic intervention.

Consent

The patient provided the consent for the publication of the case.

Authors' Contributions

All authors have made a significant scientific contribution to the research and read and approved the article.

Acknowledgments

The authors would like to thank the patient for giving consent for the publication of the case.

References

[1] S. Yadlapati, S. Yadlapati, and P. Efthimiou, "Autoimmune/Inflammatory arthritis associated lymphomas: who is at risk?" *BioMed Research International*, vol. 2016, Article ID 8631061, 11 pages, 2016.

[2] W. M. Claudino, B. Gibson, W. Tse, M. Krem, and J. Grewal, "Methotrexate-associated primary cutaneous CD30-positive cutaneous T-cell lymphoproliferative disorder: a case illustration and a brief review," *American journal of blood research*, vol. 6, no. 1, pp. 1–5, 2016.

[3] S. Saito and T. Takeuchi, "Immune response in LPD during methotrexate administration (MTX-LPD) in rheumatoid arthritis patients," *Journal of Clinical and Experimental Hematopathology*, vol. 59, no. 4, pp. 145–155, 2019.

[4] P. Gaulard, S. H. Swerdlow, and N. L. Harris, "Other iatrogenic immunodeficiency-associated lymphoproliferative disorders," in *WHO Classification of Tumors of Haematopoietic and Lymphoid Tissues. Revised*, S. H. Swerdlow, E. Campo, and N. L. Harris, Eds., pp. 462–464, IARC publications, Lyon, France, 4th edition, 2017.

[5] M. Tokuhira, J.-i. Tamaru, and M. Kizaki, "Clinical management for other iatrogenic immunodeficiency-associated lymphoproliferative disorders," *Journal of Clinical and Experimental Hematopathology*, vol. 59, no. 2, pp. 72–92, 2019.

[6] S. Shiraiwa, Y. Y. Kikuti, J. Carreras et al., "Clinicopathological evaluation of methotrexate-associated lymphoproliferative disorders with special focus on Epstein-Barr virus-positive mucocutaneous lesions," *Journal of Clinical and Experimental Hematopathology*, vol. 60, no. 4, pp. 159–168, 2020.

[7] F. Wolfe and K. Michaud, "Lymphoma in rheumatoid arthritis: the effect of methotrexate and anti-tumor necrosis factor therapy in 18,572 patients," *Arthritis & Rheumatism*, vol. 50, no. 6, pp. 1740–1751, 2004.

[8] Y. Gion, N. Iwaki, K. Takata et al., "Clinicopathological analysis of methotrexate-associated lymphoproliferative disorders: comparison of diffuse large B-cell lymphoma and classical Hodgkin lymphoma types," *Cancer Science*, vol. 108, no. 6, pp. 1271–1280, 2017.

[9] K. Obata, T. Okui, S. Ono et al., "Comparative study on epstein-barr virus-positive mucocutaneous ulcer and methotrexate-associated lymphoproliferative disorders developed in the oral mucosa: a case series of 10 patients and literature review," *Diagnostics*, vol. 11, no. 8, p. 1375, 2021.

[10] A. Satou and S. Nakamura, "EBV-positive B-cell lymphomas and lymphoproliferative disorders: review from the perspective of immune escape and immunodeficiency," *Cancer Medicine*, vol. 10, no. 19, pp. 6777–6785, 2021.

[11] H. Toyonaga, M. Fukushima, N. Shimeno, and T. Inokuma, "Methotrexate-associated lymphoproliferative disorder in the stomach and duodenum: a case report," *BMC Gastroenterology*, vol. 19, no. 1, p. 62, 2019.

[12] S.-C. Hsiao, R. Ichinohasama, S.-H. Lin et al., "EBV-associated diffuse large B-cell lymphoma in a psoriatic treated with methotrexate," *Pathology, Research & Practice*, vol. 205, no. 1, pp. 43–49, 2009.

[13] K. Moriya, Y. Y. Kikuti, J. Carreras, Y. Kondo, S. Shiraiwa, and N. Nakamura, "Methotrexate-associated lymphoproliferative disorder demonstrating composite lymphoma of EBV-negative diffuse large B-cell lymphoma and EBV-positive mucocutaneous ulcer," *Journal of Clinical and Experimental Hematopathology*, vol. 60, no. 1, pp. 11–16, 2020.

[14] M. Tsuruoka, J. Inoue, E. Kakazu et al., "Methotrexate-associated lymphoproliferative disorder in the liver resembling

hepatocellular carcinoma treated with transarterial chemoembolization," *Internal Medicine*, vol. 59, no. 18, pp. 2255–2260, 2020.

[15] K. Fujimoto, K. C. Hatanaka, Y. Hatanaka et al., "Association of Epstein-Barr virus with regression after withdrawal of immunosuppressive drugs and subsequent progression of iatrogenic immunodeficiency-associated lymphoproliferative disorders in patients with autoimmune diseases," *Hematological Oncology*, vol. 38, no. 5, pp. 799–807, 2020.

[16] K. Yoshifuji, Y. Umezawa, A. Ichikawa, K. Watanabe, O. Miura, and M. Yamamoto, "Methotrexate-associated classical Hodgkin lymphoma shows distinct clinicopathological features but comparable clinical outcomes with sporadic cases," *In Vivo*, vol. 33, no. 5, pp. 1599–1604, 2019.

[17] E. Y. Loo, L. J. Medeiros, T. N. Aladily et al., "Classical Hodgkin lymphoma arising in the setting of iatrogenic immunodeficiency," *The American Journal of Surgical Pathology*, vol. 37, no. 8, pp. 1290–1297, 2013.

[18] M. Tokuhira, S. Saito, A. Okuyama et al., "Clinicopathologic investigation of methotrexate-induced lymphoproliferative disorders, with a focus on regression," *Leukemia & Lymphoma*, vol. 59, no. 5, pp. 1143–1152, 2018.

[19] S. Takanashi, Y. Aisa, C. Ito et al., "Clinical characteristics of methotrexate-associated lymphoproliferative disorders: relationship between absolute lymphocyte count recovery and spontaneous regression," *Rheumatology International*, vol. 37, no. 10, pp. 1629–1633, 2017.

[20] R. Rizzi, P. Curci, M. Delia et al., "Spontaneous remission of "methotrexate-associated lymphoproliferative disorders" after discontinuation of immunosuppressive treatment for autoimmune disease. Review of the literature," *Medical Oncology*, vol. 26, no. 1, pp. 1–9, 2009.

[21] Y. Hoshida, J. X. Xu, S. Fujita et al., "Lymphoproliferative disorders in rheumatoid arthritis: clinicopathological analysis of 76 cases in relation to methotrexate medication," *Journal of Rheumatology*, vol. 34, no. 2, pp. 322–331, 2007.

[22] S. Ichikawa, N. Fukuhara, K. Saito et al., "Successful treatment of methotrexate-associated classical Hodgkin lymphoma with brentuximab vedotin-combined chemotherapy: a case series," *International Journal of Hematology*, vol. 111, no. 5, pp. 667–672, 2020.

[23] Y. Sekiguchi, H. Iizuka, H. Takizawa et al., "Methotrexate-associated Hodgkin lymphoma in a patient with rheumatoid arthritis successfully treated with brentuximab vedotin in combination with doxorubicin, vinblastine, and dacarbazine (BV+AVD)," *Internal Medicine*, vol. 59, no. 17, pp. 2165–2171, 2020.

[24] K. Tanaka, M. Kuboki, S. Koi, and S. Toyota, "Nivolumab for methotrexate-associated classic Hodgkin's lymphoma in a rheumatoid arthritis patient," *Internal Medicine*, vol. 59, no. 6, pp. 829–833, 2020.

Diagnostic Challenges of Anaplastic Large Cell Lymphoma in a Resource-Limited Setting: A Case Report and Literature Review

Oluomachi Charity Nnachi,[1] **Innocent Paul Ezenwenyi**,[1] **Augustine Ejike Okoye**,[1] **Chinedu Obasi Akpa**,[1] **Chukwuma Joseph Uzoigwe**,[2] **and Gabriel Chima Ugwu**[1]

[1]*Department of Haematology, Alex Ekwueme Federal University Teaching Hospital, Abakaliki, Ebonyi, Nigeria*
[2]*Department of Histopathology, Alex Ekwueme Federal University Teaching Hospital, Abakaliki, Ebonyi, Nigeria*

Correspondence should be addressed to Oluomachi Charity Nnachi; obotican@gmail.com

Academic Editor: Pier Paolo Piccaluga

Anaplastic large cell lymphoma (ALCL) is a rare variety of non-Hodgkin's lymphoma with diverse morphologic variants. Due to the similarity of the different variants with other lymphoma entities, misdiagnosis may be inevitable when immunohistochemical and cytogenetic techniques are not available and histology alone is employed. We report a case of a 43-year-old woman with a seven-month history of neck swelling which was complicated by ulceration of the mass and pathological fracture of the right clavicle after two months delay in arriving at a correct diagnosis. Several attempts to arrive at definitive diagnosis using histology alone gave divergent reports which all misdiagnosed the case until it was sent to a facility outside the country. Our report highlights the limitations and challenges of histology in making a definitive diagnosis of ALCL and the overt importance of immunohistochemical and cytogenetic techniques which are largely unavailable in resource-constrained environment typical of tertiary centers in Nigeria and most sub-Saharan Africa countries.

1. Introduction

Anaplastic large cell lymphoma (ALCL) is a unique variety of non-Hodgkin's lymphoma. They are defined as a CD30-positive neoplasm of T-cell or null cell lineage and present clinically in two forms as a primary cutaneous or systemic disease with involvement of the skin, lungs, liver, soft tissues, and rarely bone [1]. ALCL has a broad morphologic spectrum with five or more variants of the disease [2, 3]. Diagnosis of ALCL is often a dilemma, and misdiagnosis may be inevitable when histology with haematoxylin and eosin alone is employed [4]. The incorporation of immunohistology has made diagnosis straightforward, but unfortunately, such techniques are still largely unavailable in our environment. We present a case highlighting the challenges encountered in the diagnosis of ALCL using histology alone.

2. Case Report

A 42-year-old female Nigerian civil servant presented to the adult haematology unit of Alex Ekwueme Federal University Teaching Hospital, a tertiary health facility in Ebonyi State, South-East Nigeria, in January 2019 with a seven-month history of painless right-sided neck swelling (Figure 1), fever, general body weakness, drenching night sweats, and weight loss. According to medical history, she had sought care at the internal medicine unit of our facility where she received prescription of several antibiotics, antiviral, and antituberculosis medication following a biopsy of the mass and histology report of reactive lymphadenopathy. After completing her medications, the neck swelling regressed partially. Four months later, she returned to her physician with complaints of weakness, resurgence, and rapid progression of the neck mass. On further interrogation, she was noted to be anaemic, hence necessitating referral to the haematology clinic. On presentation at our clinic, clinical examination revealed a neck mass measuring 8×6 cm (Figure 1) at the right supraclavicular region. The patient reported no pain related to the mass. There was generalized lymphadenopathy involving cervical, supraclavicular, and axillary lymph nodes (largest measuring 5×3 cm). Two months after presentation at the haematology clinic, the right supraclavicular mass

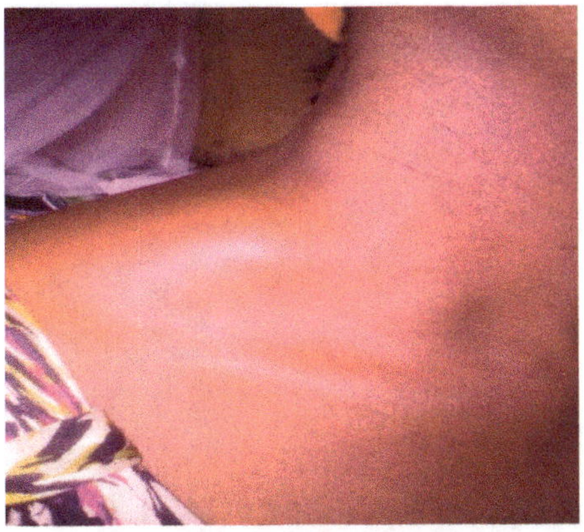

Figure 1: Photograph of neck mass at the first presentation.

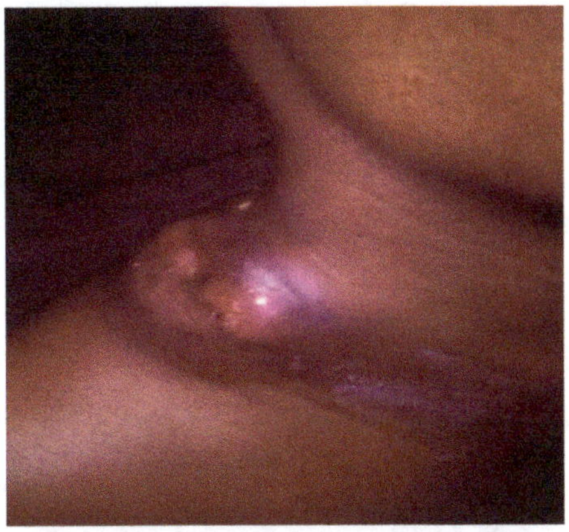

Figure 2: Ulceration of neck mass.

ulcerated with exudation of straw-colored fluid and development of a pathological fracture of the right clavicle (Figures 2–4).

Laboratory tests revealed a complete blood count with haemoglobin of 5 g/dl, with normal white blood cell and platelet parameters. ESR was 95 mm/1st hour. Peripheral blood film showed few small- and medium-sized matured lymphocytes with nuclei cleave. HIV, hepatitis B surface antigen, and hepatitis C tests were negative. An acid-fast bacilli test for the fluid from the ulcerated mass and Mantoux test were negative, while chest X-ray showed no abnormality. Renal and liver function tests had normal values. Neck ultrasound scan revealed cervical, supra-, and infraclavicular lymph node enlargements. Abdominal ultrasound showed hepatomegaly (17.2 cm), intra-, and retroperitoneal lymph node enlargement (largest measuring 4.2 cm by 1.1 cm).

The previous biopsy block of the neck mass was retrieved, and a repeat biopsy was also done and both were sent for another histology opinion. This second request made a diagnosis of small lymphocytic lymphoma (SLL) with microscopy showing sections of diffused sheets of matured lymphocytes growing in solid sheets and effacing the lymph node architecture without necrosis. Immunohistochemistry could not be done because it was not available.

The diagnosis of SLL was refuted by the managing haematologists. They argued that the patient's clinical course, especially the clavicle fracture, was uncommon in SLL. Due to this dilemma, a third histology opinion was requested from another referral pathology facility. This report noted the presence of numerous mononuclear and classic variants of Reed–Sternberg with prominent inflammatory cell components particularly eosinophils and neutrophils. Hence, a diagnosis of Hodgkin's lymphoma, mixed cellularity variant, was made (Figure 5).

Occasioned by divergent histology diagnoses from three different referral facilities, unavailability of immunohistochemical techniques, and rapid deterioration of patient's clinical condition, the specimen had to be shipped to another facility outside the country for repeat histology and immunohistochemistry. After a period of four weeks, the report of the fourth histology request was received. The

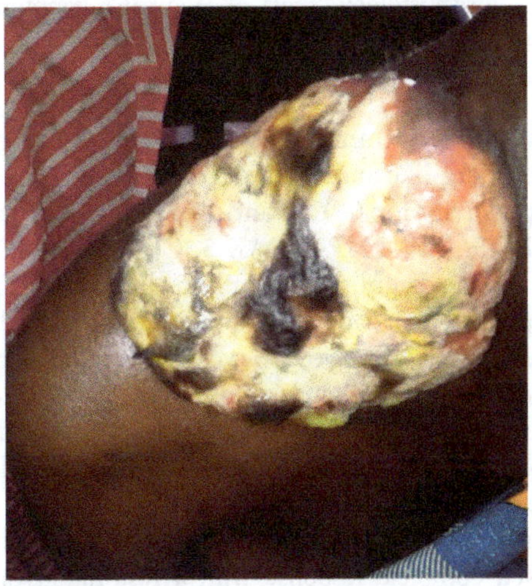

Figure 3: Extensive ulceration of neck mass while a diagnosis is awaited.

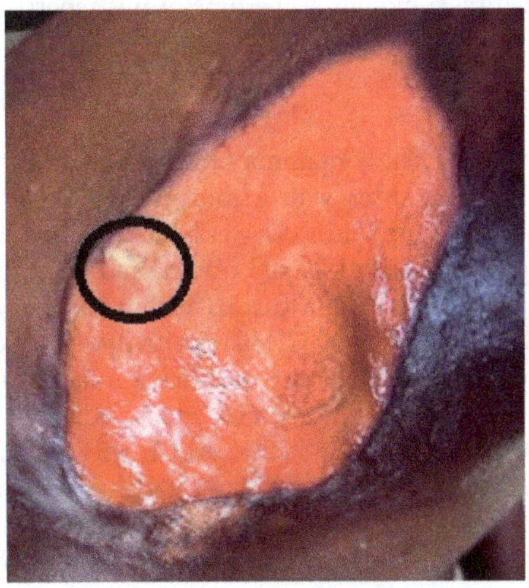

Figure 4: Protrusion of clavicular fracture end from the ulcer surface.

microscopic findings revealed significant plasmacytic infiltrate with some of the cells having a resemblance to Reed–Sternberg cells and many others that have nuclei with

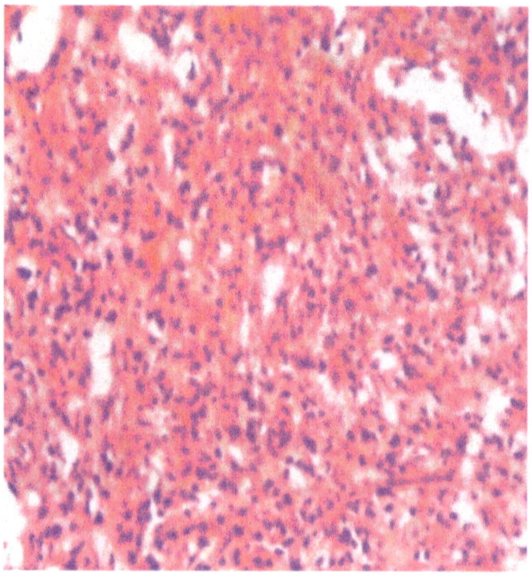

Figure 5: Third histology report of Hodgkin's lymphoma (haematoxylin and eosin stain).

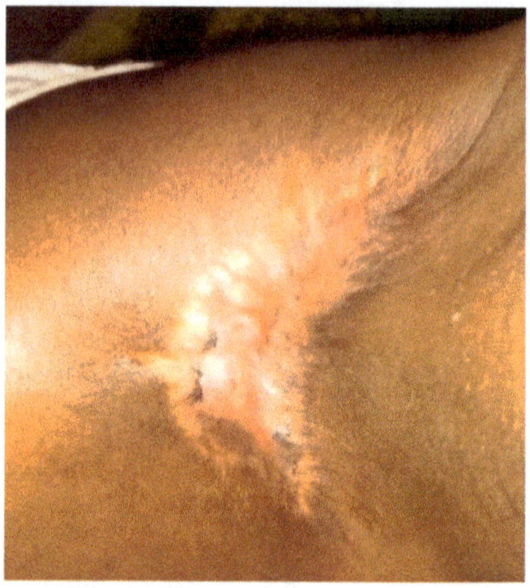

Figure 6: Postchemotherapy and radiotherapy aspect showing total regression of neck mass, fracture, and wound healing.

embryonic shape. Immunohistochemical staining of the Reed–Sternberg-like and cells with embryonic shaped nuclei showed positivity for CD 30 and ALK but are negative for EMA, CD 45, EBV-LMP 1, PAX 5, CD15, and CD 3. This report led to the diagnosis of anaplastic large cell lymphoma.

The patient was counseled and prescription ordered for chemotherapy. She received 9 cycles of cyclophosphamide, doxorubicin, vincristine, and prednisolone, wound dressing, physiotherapy, and involved-field radiotherapy. Blood parameters were monitored throughout the treatment period. During chemotherapy and radiotherapy, tumour regression was observed and total ulcer healing achieved after the ninth course. She showed complete response with a restoration of normal haemoglobin, ESR values ranging between 3 and 8 mm/1st hour, clavicle fracture and wound healing (Figure 6). Right upper limb movement has also been restored, and the patient is currently in remission (twelve months at the time of this report).

3. Discussion

Anaplastic large cell lymphoma (ALCL) is a malignancy of mature T lymphocytes with a morphologic expression of large atypical lymphoid cells with abundant cytoplasm, pleomorphic horseshoe-shaped nuclei, and prominent nucleoli [5]. This lymphoma carries malignant clones characterized by membrane CD30 positivity as a constant immunophenotypic signature and has a duality of clinical manifestation, namely, primary cutaneous ALCL with a sole skin manifestation and systemic ALCL with a multiorgan manifestation involving soft tissues and lungs, while bone involvement is rare [6]. The presence or absence of anaplastic lymphoma kinase (ALK) expression further classifies the ALCL into ALK-positive or ALK-negative which has prognostic significance. ALK-positive and ALK-negative lymphoma are morphologically similar but distinguishable on immunostaining. ALK-positive cases have translocation involving the ALK gene and expression of ALK protein. Cutaneous ALCL is mostly T-cell-derived but differs from systemic ALCL because it is always ALK-negative [7, 8].

Systemic ALK-positive ALCL is a disease with complex morphological heterogeneity that stems from its eclectic tumour cell cytology. The histologic variants include the common, lymphohistiocytic, small cell, Hodgkin-like, and composite patterns [7, 8].

Typically, ALCL evolves histologically in a manner that brings about incomplete effacement of the lymph node architecture with a proclivity of the tumour cells to make incursions into the lymph node sinuses mimicking a metastatic pattern. In the background, there is a potpourri of inflammatory cells comprising plasma cells, histiocytes, and eosinophils in the company of the malignant clones. Sometimes, the inflammatory cells are preponderant and may obscure the tumour cell population making diagnosis even more cumbersome.

The common type consists of sheets of large pleomorphic tumour cells with horseshoe-shaped or kidney-shaped nuclei, while the small cell type is characterized by small- and medium-sized pleomorphic tumour cells. The lymphohistiocytic variant consists of both small and large tumour cells forming rosettes around blood vessels in a background replete with reactive histiocytes. This background creates a diagnostic hurdle with a tendency for misdiagnosis of this subtype as atypical inflammatory lesion or haemophagocytic syndrome. The Hodgkin-like ALCL is morphologically characterized by the presence of Reed–Sternberg-like cells and shows lymph node capsular thickening and nodular fibrosis.

These morphological features that typify the different forms of ALCL were highlighted in one report or the other of the histological diagnoses made in the index case by the anatomical pathologists. Despite that, the precise disease entity was not identified due to the limitations posed by the use of haematoxylin and eosin as the sole diagnostic technique.

The clinical course of disease in the index case was not in tandem with the various histological diagnoses made, and this was further complicated by the bone involvement which is uncommon in non-Hodgkin's lymphoma. The danger of the employment of morphology alone in diagnosis lies in its inability to highlight the nuances inherent in the various lymphoma types with morphologic similarity, and further techniques are requisite for diagnostic precision.

Immunohistochemistry is invaluable in the differential diagnosis of lymphoma entities with cytomorphologic similarity to ALCL [9, 10].

Currently, diagnosis, classification, and proper treatment of lymphoma deeply depend on the detection of cellular markers and the use of genetic analysis of tissue samples to support histologic and clinical findings. These diagnostic modalities include immunohistochemistry (IHC) and/or flow cytometry, cytogenetic, and molecular analyses [8]. These techniques have become the crux of diagnostic management of lymphoma in recent times.

ALCL, though mostly T-cell-derived, displays T, B, and null immunophenotypes. Immunohistochemical staining for the following markers: ALK, CD30, CD5, CD3, CD7, CD2, CD4, CD15, CD20, EMA, and cytotoxic markers (TIA1, granzyme B, PAX5, PGMI, EBV, and perforin) is vital in the differential diagnosis of ALCL.

Consistent immunophenotypic features of most cases of ALCL include positivity to CD30, ALK, granzyme B, TIA-1, and perforin and negativity to CD20, EMA (positive in diffuse large B-cell lymphoma), CDI5 (positive in Hodgkin's lymphoma), and CD3 (positive in peripheral T-cell lymphoma).

Cytogenetic and molecular analyses in ALCL detect molecular defects which may be translocations, gene rearrangements, or recurrent genetic abnormalities. ALK protein is a normal protein coded for by the ALK gene located in chromosome 2. However, with a chromosomal translocation between chromosome 2 and chromosome 5 (t (2 : 5) (p23 : q35)), the ALK gene is brought in proximity with the nucleophosmin (NPM) gene. The NPM-ALK fusion gene formed confers constitutive activity on the tyrosine kinase receptor.

TP63 rearrangement along with the coexpression of CRBB4 and COL29AL is another molecular abnormality that is noted in ALCL. Experimental data suggest that targeted drug therapy against the coexpressed factors inhibits tumour growth and slows disease progression.

Moreover, recurrent chromosomal aneuploidies with additional 17q, 5q, 6p, 8q, 12q, Iq or loss of 4q, 1 Iq, or 13q and defects of the JAK-STAT pathway have also been implicated in the pathogenesis of ALCL.

This case report exposes the inadequacy of H&E alone in the diagnosis of lymphoma cases, but unfortunately, it is the readily available technique in our environment. More advanced techniques such as IHC, fluorescence in-situ hybridization (FISH), and reverse transcriptase-polymerase chain reaction (RT-PCR) are not common in many tertiary or referral health institutions in Nigeria and sub-Saharan Africa at large [11, 12]. This has brought about a humongous limitation to accurate diagnosis and classification of diseases and has made treatment prone to error.

The 2011 report of the International Network for Cancer Treatment and Research on the evaluation of infrastructure for lymphoma corroborated the fact that IHC, cytogenetics, and FISH techniques are unavailable in most parts of Nigeria and other sub-Saharan African countries [13].

Incidence of non-Hodgkin's lymphoma in sub-Saharan Africa is reported to be as low as 30,000 and as high as 278,000 cases each year [14, 15]. The growing burden of lymphoma fostered by population growth and human immunodeficiency virus infection is projected to be detrimental on the continent with grossly limited current diagnostic services. The burden of lymphoma may be detrimental on the continent with grossly limited current diagnostic services. In order to circumvent the diagnostic challenges posed by infrastructural inadequacy, most sub-Saharan African nations resort to sending tissue samples abroad for holistic analysis and accurate diagnosis. This approach is marred by extra cost, tissue loss in transit, increased turn-around time, delay in treatment, disease progression, loss of learning opportunity, and diminished academic interaction.

4. Conclusion

The diagnostic quagmire posed by the broad morphologic spectrum of ALCL is magnified in the setting of inadequate diagnostic techniques as found in our setting and also in most tertiary treatment centers in sub-Saharan African countries. Efforts should be geared towards the provision of these techniques, manpower training, and collaboration to strengthen our treatment centers to be better equipped to diagnose, classify, and institute appropriate timely treatment for lymphoma.

Consent

The written informed consent about the use of case details and images was obtained from the patient before the submission of this manuscript for publication.

References

[1] H. Stein, H. D. Foss, H. Durkopp et al., "CD30 (+) anaplastic large cell lymphoma: a review of its histopathologic, genetic and clinical features," *Blood*, vol. 96, pp. 3681–3695, 2000.

[2] A. Rapkiewicz, H. Wen, F. Sen, and K. Das, "Cytomorphologic examination of anaplastic Large cell lymphoma by fine-needle aspiration cytology," *Cancer*, vol. 111, no. 6, pp. 499–507, 2007.

[3] P. Das, V. K. Iyer, S. R. Mathur, and R. Ray, "Anaplastic large cell lymphoma: a critical evaluation of cytomorphological features in seven cases," *Cytopathology: Official Journal of the British Society for Clinical Cytology*, vol. 21, no. 4, pp. 251–258, 2010.

[4] D. Das, "Anaplastic large cell lymphoma: the evolution continues," *Journal of Cytology*, vol. 28, no. 4, pp. 233-234, 2011.

[5] G. Hapgood and K. J. Savage, "The biology and management of systemic anaplastic Large cell lymphoma," *Blood*, vol. 126, no. 1, pp. 17–25, 2015.

[6] Y. Yuang, X. Qibing, L. Yi, C. Yuehong, and Y. Geng, "ALK-positive anaplastic large cell lymphoma with multiple bone involvements:a case report and review of literature," *International Journal of Clinical and Experimental Medicine*, vol. 11, no. 3, pp. 2745–2751, 2018.
[7] S. Kuruba and B. D. Nah, "Anaplastic large cell lymphoma. A cytological masquerade," *The Internet Journal of Pathology*, vol. 11, no. 1, 2009.
[8] B. Falini, "Anaplastic large cell lymphoma: pathological, molecular and clinical features," *British Journal of Haematology*, vol. 114, no. 4, pp. 741–760, 2001.
[9] N. Bennani-Baiti, S. Ansell, and A. L. Feldman, "Adult systemic anaplastic large cell lymphoma: recommendations for diagnosis and management," *Expert Review of Hematology*, vol. 9, no. 2, pp. 137–150, 2015.
[10] R. A. Higgins, J. E. Blankenship, and M. C. Kinney, "The application of immunohistochemistry in the diagnosis of non-hodgkin and hodgkin lymphoma," *Archives of Pathology & Laboratory Medicine*, vol. 132, no. 3, pp. 441–461, 2008.
[11] A. O. Oluwasola, J. Olaniyi, J. A. Otegbayo et al., "A fifteen year review of lymphomas in a Nigerian healthcare centre," *Journal of Health, Population and Nutrition*, vol. 29, no. 4, pp. 310–316, 2011.
[12] O. Akinde, C. Anunobi, O. Osunkalu, A. Phillips, and O. Afolayan, "The challenges of lymphoma diagnosis in a tertiary hospital in Lagos, Nigeria," *Journal of Clinical Sciences*, vol. 13, no. 2, pp. 58–71, 2016.
[13] K. N. Naresh, M. Raphael, L. Ayers et al., "Lymphomas in sub-Saharan Africa-what can we learn and how can we help in improving diagnosis, managing patients and fostering translational research?" *British Journal of Haematology*, vol. 154, no. 6, pp. 696–703, 2011.
[14] F. Giu Lia De, E. A. Rogena, K. Naresh, M. Rapheal, I. Magrath, and L. Lorenzo, "Managing lymphomas in African settings: improving diagnostic accuracy and carryout research projects," *Cancer Control*, vol. 2103, pp. 75–82, 2011.
[15] P. kleihues and B. W. Stewart, *World Cancer Report*, International Agency for Research on Cancer IARC Press, Lyon, France, 2003.

46

A Rare Case of Hemophagocytic Lymphohistiocytosis in an Adult with Diffuse Large B-Cell Lymphoma

Chimezie Mbachi,[1] **Rita Igwilo**,[2] **Estefania Flores**,[1] **Ezekiel Chukwujindu**,[2] **and Benjamin Mba**[1]

[1]*Internal Medicine, John H. Stroger Jr. Hospital of Cook County, Chicago, IL 60612, USA*
[2]*Internal Medicine, University of Nigeria Teaching Hospital, Ituku-Ozalla, Enugu, Nigeria*

Correspondence should be addressed to Chimezie Mbachi; chimeziembachi@gmail.com

Academic Editor: Takashi Sonoki

A 71-year-old Indian female presented with a 3-month history of weight loss and fatigue. Further review confirmed a histological diagnosis of diffuse large B-cell lymphoma. Although bone marrow analysis did not reveal hemophagocytosis, she had some clinical and laboratory pointers to hemophagocytic lymphohistiocytosis (HLH). Her clinical state deteriorated rapidly with development of acute respiratory distress syndrome, diffuse alveolar hemorrhage, and subsequently death.

1. Background

This is a rare case of hemophagocytic lymphohistiocytosis in an elderly woman with diffuse large B-cell lymphoma. This case, culminating in the patient's demise, highlights the nonspecific, varied presentation and rapidly progressive nature of untreated HLH.

2. Case Presentation

The patient was a 71-year-old woman, originally from India, who came to the United States two weeks prior to presentation to our facility's outpatient clinic with a 3-month history of weight loss, dyspepsia, and fatigue. Initial workup showed a hemoglobin level (Hb) of 9.3 g/dl (12.9–16.8 g/dl) and atrophic gastritis on esophagogastroduodenoscopy (EGD). Hemoglobin estimation done at a follow-up visit with her primary care physician 2 weeks later was found to be 5 g/dl, and hospital admission for further evaluation and treatment was recommended. She was admitted the next day through the Emergency Department of a facility closer to her home of residence where she was found to have normal vital signs; a computed tomography (CT) scan of her abdomen and pelvis showed multiple abdominal and retroperitoneal lymph nodes but none greater than 1 cm, and it also revealed multiple hypodensities in the spleen and hepatomegaly. Hemoglobin and platelet levels had a nadir of 4.6 g/dl and 1000 cells/Ul (161,000–369,000 cells/Ul), respectively, requiring several packed red cells and platelet transfusions. Other significant investigation findings were new alanine aminotransferase (ALT) and aspartate aminotransferase (AST) elevations from 31 U/l to 144 U/l (5–35 IU/l) and 52 U/l to 106 U/l (0–40 IU/l), respectively, lactate dehydrogenase (LDH) of 472 U/l (85–210 U/l), ferritin of 2,604 ng/ml (11–206 ng/dl), haptoglobin of 22 mg/dl (43–215 mg/dl), and triglycerides of 489 mg/dl (30–150 mg/dl). Hepatitis B, C, and human immunodeficiency virus (HIV) antibodies were negative. Also, anti-nuclear antibody (ANA) and Coombs' test were negative. The bilirubin level was within the reference range. Similarly, serum electrophoresis was normal. Bone marrow biopsy done at this hospital before transfer to our facility showed B cells with no evidence of monoclonality, T cells with a normal CD4 : CD8 ratio, and no diagnostic aberrant antigenic expression; blasts were not increased.

The patient was subsequently transferred to our hospital ten days after the first admission for further management. Vital signs on admission were Bp 138/73, PR 78, RR 20, and

T 98.2°F. Examination revealed multiple nontender cervical lymphadenopathy. Investigations showed Hb 5 gm/dl, white blood cell (WBC) 4,200 cells/Ul, ferritin 2331 ng/ml, platelets 19,000 cells/Ul, and triglycerides 489 mg/dl. Given the high suspicion of a lymphoproliferative disorder, pathology slides (from same bone marrow biopsy done in the previous facility) were sent to a tertiary hospital for further analysis).

3. Outcome and Follow-Up

Hospital course was eventful as the patient became febrile on day 2 of admission, T-max 103°F. On day 3, she was started on dexamethasone due to the high suspicion of HLH at this time. On day 4 of admission, pathology results from the tertiary hospital showed CD 20+ diffuse large B-cell lymphoma. On day 6 of admission, she became progressively dyspnoeic with respiratory rate (RR) 40 cycles/min and SaO_2 78% on room air with increasing oxygen requirement, requiring transfer to the MICU where she was subsequently intubated with large amounts of blood exuding from the endotracheal tube after intubation. Patient's clinical status continued to deteriorate, and after careful considerations and discussions with her family, her code status was changed to "do not resuscitate" (DNR). She was subsequently extubated after which she expired on day 7 of admission.

4. Discussion

Hemophagocytic lymphohistiocytosis (HLH) is a life-threatening syndrome of multiorgan clinical and laboratory abnormalities due to abnormal immune activation [1]. The primary form, more common in children, is caused by mutations that affect lymphocyte cytotoxicity and the regulation of the immune system. The secondary form, also called acquired HLH, most frequently occurs in adults [2]. Triggers of the acquired form include infections (especially Epstein–Barr virus infection), immune deficiency states, lymphomas, and other malignancies [1]. Sometimes, specific genetic mutations may be found in patients with HLH. The underlying feature is immune dysregulation which results in impaired function of cytotoxic T lymphocytes (CTL) and natural killer (NK) cells, leading to an excess of activated macrophages and, consequently, a cytokine storm. Cytokines that have been implicated include interferon gamma (IFN-gamma), tumor necrosis factor alpha (TNF-alpha), and interleukins (IL) such as IL-2, IL-6, IL-10, IL-12, and IL-16 [3–5]. These lead to destruction of both diseased and normal host cells and tissues.

The clinical features of HLH are quite diverse, but it generally presents as a febrile illness associated with multiple organ involvement. HLH can be diagnosed if 5 out of these 8 diagnostic criteria are met: fever (temperature ≥38.5°C), splenomegaly, low or absent NK activity, peripheral cytopenia (at least two of the following: Hb <9 g/dl, platelet count <100,000/Ul, and absolute neutrophil count <1000/Ul), hypertriglyceridemia (fasting triglycerides >265 mg/dl) or hypofibrinogenemia (<150 mg/dl), hyperferritinemia (>500 ng/ml), sIL2R ≥2,400 U/ml, and hemophagocytosis in the spleen, liver, bone marrow, or lymph. In adults, it is not always required that these criteria be met before initiation of treatment due to the high mortality of HLH [1]. Hemophagocytosis is neither pathognomonic of nor required for the diagnosis of HLH. This feature was absent in the bone marrow biopsy result of our patient. Following serial bone marrow evaluations, however, hemophagocytosis may eventually be seen. Other sites such as the spleen, liver, and lymph nodes should also be assessed for hemophagocytosis [1]. Prior to being transferred to our facility, our patient had 4 out of 8 criteria (bicytopenia, hyperferritinemia, hypertriglyceridemia, and hepatomegaly). On the 2nd day of admission in our facility, she developed the 5th (fever) diagnostic criteria and was started on dexamethasone, but soon after, she developed fatal acute respiratory distress syndrome with diffuse alveolar hemorrhage. HLH can affect any organ including the lungs, liver, kidneys, and brain. In our patient, lung parenchymal injury resulted in diffuse alveolar hemorrhage which manifested as acute respiratory distress syndrome, hemoptysis, and diffuse patchy opacities on lung imaging. Similarly, she had liver involvement with hepatomegaly and deranged liver enzymes.

The H-score is an attempt to improve diagnosis of HLH. Points are given for immunosuppression; fever; organomegaly; levels of triglycerides, ferritin, alanine aminotransferase, and fibrinogen; degree of cytopenia; and presence of hemophagocytosis on the bone marrow aspirate. An H-score ≥250 confers a 99 percent probability of HLH, whereas a score of ≤90 confers a <1 percent probability of HLH [6]. Our patient's H-Score was 221, with a 96.5% probability of HLH. Also, in adult patients with a high clinical suspicion for HLH, sIL2R levels ≥2400 U/ml have been found to have an 83% sensitivity and a 100% specificity for HLH diagnosis [7], and an elevated sIL2R/ferritin ratio is also highly predictive of lymphoma-associated HLH. Although these markers are invaluable in HLH diagnosis, they are not, per se, diagnostic confirmation for HLH and must be interpreted in the right clinical context.

This case highlights the need for a high index of suspicion for HLH. Prompt treatment is critical, but the greatest barrier to a successful outcome is a delay in diagnosis due to the rarity of this syndrome, variable clinical presentation, and lack of specificity of the clinical and laboratory findings. Aggressive courses of immunosuppressants and anti-inflammatory agents (such as glucocorticoids) are used to quell the widespread inflammation. In retrospect, the index patient may have benefited from HLH-specific therapy early on in her presentation, given the suspicion of a lymphoproliferative disorder—despite initial negative biopsy results—and evidence of organ failure. In addition, employment of the sIl2R/ferritin ratio may have aided more prompt diagnosis as it has been shown to be elevated in lymphoma-associated cases of HLH. Antimicrobials are also given for the opportunistic infections that are common in these patients. Patients with lymphoma-associated HLH, as in this case, benefit the most from etoposide-containing regimens and steroids [8–10]. Etoposide selectively depletes activated T cells [11]. On November 20, 2018, the FDA approved the anti-IFN-gamma monoclonal antibody, emapalumab (proprietary name Gamifant), for salvage treatment of primary HLH in pediatric and adult HLH patients [12]. Further guidance on HLH diagnosis and treatment in adults can be seen in the recent Histiocyte Society guideline for HLH in adults [2].

Prognosis of HLH varies. Survival is dependent upon prompt recognition and treatment. Bone marrow transplant can be curative.

Additional Points

(i) The mortality rate of HLH without treatment is high, and HLH patients with associated malignancy suffer worse prognosis. (ii) High index of suspicion, early diagnosis, and early commencement of treatment are key to survival. (iii) Therapy is both supportive and definitive, targeted at the specific organ(s) involved and the underlying condition (for example, specific treatment for malignancy). (iv) Targeted HLH therapy with emapalumab has been approved for salvage treatment of primary HLH in both adult and pediatric patients. (v) HLH therapy, including stem cell transplant, has revolutionalized treatment and can result in long-term survival and cure.

Disclosure

All authors had access to the case and a role in writing the case report.

References

[1] K. L. McClain, "Clinical features and diagnosis of hemophagocytic lymphohistiocytosis," 2018, https://www.uptodate.com/contents/clinical-features-and-diagnosis-of-hemophagocytic-lymphohistiocytosis.

[2] P. La Rosée, A. Horne, M. Hines et al., "Recommendations for the management of hemophagocytic lymphohistiocytosis in adults," *Blood*, vol. 133, no. 23, pp. 2465–2477, 2019.

[3] M. Arico, C. Danesino, D. Pende, and L. Moretta, "Pathogenesis of haemophagocytic lymphohistiocytosis," *British Journal of Haematology*, vol. 114, no. 4, pp. 761–769, 2001.

[4] D. M. Komp, J. McNamara, and P. Buckley, "Elevated soluble interleukin-2 receptor in childhood hemophagocytic histiocytic syndromes," *Blood*, vol. 73, no. 8, pp. 2128–2132, 1989.

[5] Y. Tang, X. Xu, H. Song et al., "Early diagnostic and prognostic significance of a specific Th1/Th2 cytokine pattern in children with haemophagocytic syndrome," *British Journal of Haematology*, vol. 143, no. 1, pp. 84–91, 2008.

[6] L. Fardet, L. Galicier, O. Lambotte et al., "Development and validation of the HScore, a score for the diagnosis of reactive hemophagocytic syndrome," *Arthritis & Rheumatology*, vol. 66, no. 9, pp. 2613–2620, 2014.

[7] A. Hayden, M. Lin, S. Park et al., "Soluble interleukin-2 receptor is a sensitive diagnostic test in adult HLH," *Blood Advances*, vol. 1, no. 26, pp. 2529–2534, 2017.

[8] H. Trottestam, A. Horne, M. Arico et al., "Chemoimmunotherapy for hemophagocytic lymphohistiocytosis: long-term results of the HLH-94 treatment protocol," *Blood*, vol. 118, no. 17, pp. 4577–4584, 2011.

[9] S. Imashuku, K. Kuriyama, R. Sakai et al., "Treatment of Epstein-Barr virus-associated hemophagocytic lymphohistiocytosis (EBV-HLH) in young adults: a report from the HLH study center," *Medical and Pediatric Oncology*, vol. 41, no. 2, pp. 103–109, 2003.

[10] J.-I. Henter, A. Samuelsson-Horne, M. Aricò et al., "Treatment of hemophagocytic lymphohistiocytosis with HLH-94 immunochemotherapy and bone marrow transplantation," *Blood*, vol. 100, no. 7, pp. 2367–2373, 2002.

[11] A. M. Schram and N. Berliner, "How i treat hemophagocytic lymphohistiocytosis in the adult patient," *Blood*, vol. 125, no. 19, pp. 2908–2914, 2015.

[12] FDA, US Food and Drug Administration.

47

Hemophagocytic Lymphohistiocytosis in an AIDS Patient with Kaposi Sarcoma: A Treatment Dilemma

Oluwadunni E. Emiloju,[1] **Sorab Gupta**,[2] **Vivian Arguello-Guerra**,[3] **and Claudia Dourado**[2]

[1]*Department of Medicine, Einstein Medical Center, Philadelphia, PA 19141, USA*
[2]*Department of Hematology and Medical Oncology, Einstein Medical Center, Philadelphia, PA 19141, USA*
[3]*Department of Pathology and Laboratory Medicine, Einstein Medical Center, Philadelphia, PA 19141, USA*

Correspondence should be addressed to Oluwadunni E. Emiloju; emilojuo@einstein.edu

Academic Editor: Tatsuharu Ohno

Hemophagocytic lymphohistiocytosis (HLH) is a result of an abnormal activation of immune cells (T lymphocytes, natural killer cells, and macrophages) resulting in cytokine overproduction and immune destruction of cells, eventually resulting in multiorgan failure. Genetic causes are responsible for primary hemophagocytosis, but malignancies, infections, and autoimmunity underlie most of the secondary cases. We present an unusual case of a patient with AIDS and disseminated Kaposi sarcoma who was commenced on highly active antiretroviral therapy (HAART) but developed HLH secondary to immune reconstitution inflammatory syndrome (IRIS). We report this case to highlight the difficulty in managing this patient given the complex interplay of immunosuppression due to AIDS, immune reconstitution following initiation of HAART, and immune overdrive manifesting as HLH.

1. Introduction

Hemophagocytic lymphohistiocytosis (HLH) is a result of an abnormal activation of immune cells (T lymphocytes, natural killer cells, and macrophages) resulting in cytokine overproduction and immune destruction of cells, eventually resulting in multiorgan failure. Primary HLH is due to genetic defects and usually presents in childhood and very rarely in adults. However, secondary HLH can be triggered by a number of conditions including infections (viral, bacterial, fungal, and parasitic infections), malignancies (particularly lymphomas), immunodeficiencies, and autoimmune conditions.

Kaposi sarcoma is an AIDS-defining illness, and the cornerstone of AIDS-related Kaposi sarcoma treatment is highly active antiretroviral therapy (HAART).

We present a case of a patient with disseminated Kaposi sarcoma who was commenced on HAART but developed fatal hemophagocytosis secondary to immune reconstitution inflammatory syndrome (IRIS). We report this case to highlight the difficulty in managing this patient given the complex interplay of immunosuppression due to AIDS, immune reconstitution following initiation of HAART, and immune overdrive manifesting as HLH.

2. Case Description

A 59-year-old female with a past medical history of hypothyroidism presented with a rash involving her scalp, neck, torso, and vagina. She denied taking any new medication and had been on levothyroxine replacement for about 12 years: she had no known allergies. There was no significant family history; she was an ex-cigarette smoker with a 20-pack-year smoking history. Physical examination was significant for diffuse purplish plaques over the torso. Human immunodeficiency virus (HIV) viral load was 196,000 copies/ml with CD4 count 76/μL. Biopsy of the rash revealed Kaposi sarcoma, and she was commenced on HAART (emtricitabine, tenofovir alafenamide, and dolutegravir), trimethoprim-sulfamethoxazole, and fluconazole prophylaxis for opportunistic infections.

She re-presented two weeks later with fever. Physical examination revealed a maximum temperature of 38.8°C and tachycardia (pulse rate 108/min), and previously noted cutaneous Kaposi lesions were still present. She was worked up with appropriate cultures and serological testing, but no opportunistic infection was found. Further workup of her Kaposi sarcoma including upper gastrointestinal endoscopy and CT scan of her thorax, abdomen, and pelvis revealed no visceral involvement, but splenomegaly was present (Figure 1). Her fever resolved without antibiotics, but fatigue persisted, and this was attributed to HIV-associated cytopenias (platelet count 86,000/μL and hemoglobin 6.6 g/dl) for which she received red cell transfusion with improvement in her hemoglobin level (hemoglobin 9.0 g/dl after receiving 2 units of red blood cells). Her HAART regimen remained uninterrupted, and she was discharged. Follow-up labs 1 week after discharge showed worsening cytopenia (platelet count 50,000/μL and hemoglobin 8.4 g/dl), and she was referred to the Hematology office for evaluation.

She again presented 1 month from AIDS diagnosis with severe fatigue and diarrhea to another hospital. She was found to be hypotensive (systolic blood pressure 80 mmHg), necessitating intravenous fluids and a brief course of vasopressors before she was transferred to our institution. Initial labs showed pancytopenia (platelet count 6,000/μL, hemoglobin 4.3 g/dl, and leucocytes 1,900/μL). Her HIV viral load had improved from 196,000 copies/ml to 670 copies/ml, CMV antibody and parvovirus IgM were negative, and no bacterial or fungal infections were detected on cultures. She was supported with transfusions of red blood cells and platelets, but her response to transfusion was suboptimal, necessitating multiple transfusions. She also received intravenous immunoglobulin (1 g/kg), but her cytopenias persisted. She continued to receive intravenous immune globulin (IVIG) and high-dose steroids, but her pancytopenia worsened necessitating a bone marrow biopsy. Her bone marrow aspirate showed hemophagocytosis (Figure 2). Further testing revealed splenomegaly on CT scan of her abdomen, ferritin of 2,568 ng/mL, triglycerides of 151 mg/dL, and fibrinogen of 279 mg/dL. Consideration was given to discontinuing her HAART because she was undergoing immune reconstitution leading to hemophagocytosis, but the need for treating her widespread Kaposi prevailed and HAART was continued. Cytopenia progressively worsened, and she developed liver, kidney, bone marrow, respiratory, and heart failure which led to her death.

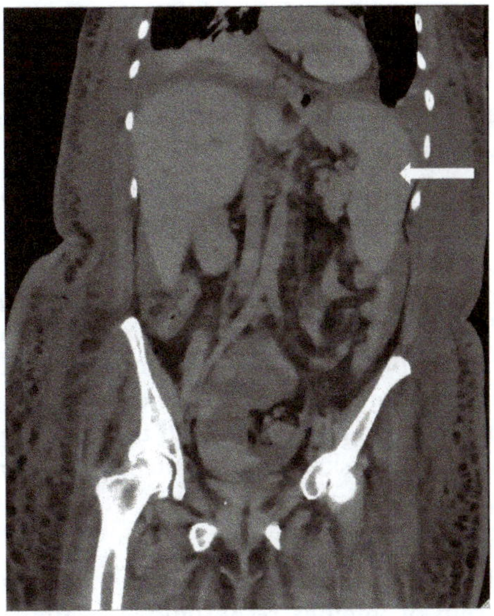

FIGURE 1: CT scan of the abdomen and pelvis. Abdominal CT scan showing splenomegaly. The spleen was enlarged and was 14 cm in length (white arrow pointing to the enlarged spleen).

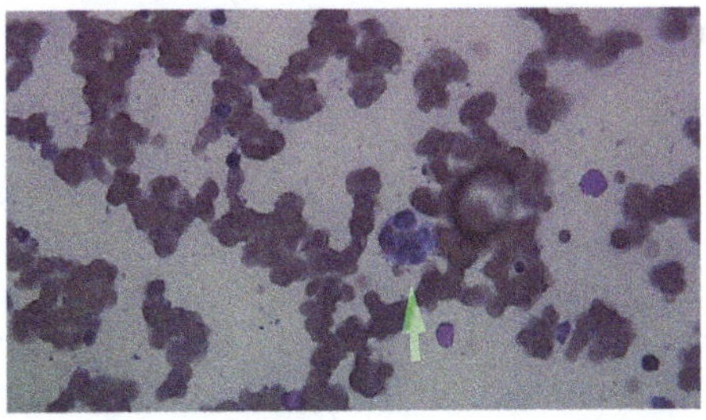

FIGURE 2: Bone marrow aspirate smear. The Wright Giemsa stain of the patient's bone marrow aspirate with an arrow highlighting a macrophage phagocytizing red blood cells, lymphocytes, and neutrophils (arrow pointing to the macrophage).

3. Discussion

Hemophagocytic lymphohistiocytosis (HLH) is a fulminant disorder resulting in unbridled activation of immune cells, resulting in death if untreated [1]. Primary HLH is due to genetic defects and usually presents in childhood and very rarely in adults. However, secondary HLH can be triggered by a number of conditions including infections (viral, bacterial, fungal, and parasitic infections), malignancies (particularly lymphomas), immunodeficiencies, and autoimmune conditions [2]. Of the recognized secondary causes of HLH, viral infections such as EBV, herpesviruses, including human herpesvirus 8 (HHV8), HIV, influenza, parvovirus, and hepatitis viruses are recognized causes [3]. A retrospective study of hemophagocytic syndrome in patients living with HIV revealed that the commonly found triggers in HIV-associated HLH were mycobacterium, CMV, cryptococcus infections, and malignancy [4].

Although she had a high HIV viremia and HHV8 (Kaposi-associated herpesvirus) infection at diagnosis, hemophagocytosis was not manifest until 6 weeks after HAART was initiated: the temporal association between HAART and hemophagocytosis makes immune reconstitution inflammatory syndrome (IRIS) the most probable trigger of her hemophagocytosis.

IRIS is the restoration of the immune response to pathogen-specific antigens, resulting in unmasking of previously subclinical opportunistic infections and nonpathogen-specific response manifesting as autoimmune conditions such as Graves' disease [5]. It is not uncommon for IRIS to develop after initiation of HAART, but its exact incidence is not known [6]. In a retrospective study, 25% of HIV patients manifested opportunistic infections after commencement of HAART [7].

Patients with IRIS manifest clinical worsening despite improvement in their immune function as evidenced by improving HIV viremia and/or CD4 count. Our patient responded to HAART as evidenced by a reduction in her viremia from 196,000 RNA/mL to 670 RNA/mL, signifying a recovery of her immune system. In our patient, she already had clinically apparent extensive cutaneous Kaposi sarcoma before the initiation of HAART, and there was no clinical worsening of her skin lesions after the commencing HAART. Her clinical deterioration was secondary to hemophagocytosis.

In the medical literature, HLH is not described as part of the spectrum of immune reconstitution in the setting of HIV/AIDS. There have however been a few case reports suggesting that hemophagocytosis secondary to IRIS can occur. Two cases of hemophagocytosis secondary to IRIS in AIDS patients with lymphoma as well as an additional 2 cases of IRIS-associated hemophagocytosis in the absence of lymphoma have been reported [8–11].

Treatment modalities in HLH include immunosuppressants such as high-dose steroids, intravenous immunoglobulin, chemotherapeutic agents such as etoposide, and allogeneic hemopoietic stem cell transplant [1]. There are no established guidelines for the treatment of IRIS-associated HLH, but previous case reports have employed continued HAART, steroids, and intravenous immunoglobulin (IVIG) [8–11]. In a retrospective review of HIV-associated hemophagocytosis, patients were also continued on HAART [12].

Given the heterogeneity of the clinical manifestations of IRIS, treatment strategies also vary and are usually aimed at the underlying infection or autoimmune condition. If patients have multiple risk factors for the development of IRIS following initiation of HAART, clinicians sometimes commence treatment for the underlying opportunistic infection first with a lag period before initiating HAART [6]. In most cases of IRIS, HAART is continued while disease-specific treatment along with anti-inflammatory therapy (nonsteroidal anti-inflammatory drugs and steroids) is used [13, 14]. In severe, life-threatening IRIS, however, some clinicians are of the opinion that there may be a need for temporary discontinuation of HAART [6]. In a patient like ours, with coexisting IRIS and HLH, there may be a role for temporary discontinuation of HAART until the HLH resolves. The other important question to answer would be to determine if there is a role for the initiation of etoposide in the setting of IRIS-associated hemophagocytosis. There are however no studies that have addressed these specific questions.

In a consensus guideline issued by members of the adult HLH working group of the Histiocyte Society, etoposide is recommended for treating adult HLH, but the duration and intensity of treatment should be tailored to the severity of HLH on a case-by-case basis. In refractory HLH, combination chemotherapy and allogenic stem cell transplantation is recommended [15].

Furthermore, due to the rarity of IRIS-associated HLH, affected patients may not be diagnosed early enough. With the benefit of hindsight, our patient had bicytopenia, fever, and splenomegaly at her prior presentation, and an earlier bone marrow biopsy might have been warranted. Although there are certain criteria that must be met to diagnose HLH, patients may not develop all these features at once, and this may lead to a delay in diagnosis and treatment. One of such criteria is elevated soluble interleukin-2 receptor (sIL-2r), also referred to as soluble CD 25 (sCD 25). Although sIL-2r of at least 2400 U/mL has a high sensitivity for HLH, it was only 63% specific in the adult cohort studied by Hayden et al. [16]. Values above 10,000 U/mL had 93% specificity for ruling in HLH [16].

The commonly used criteria were developed by the HLH-2004 study group who only studied the pediatric population [17]. Other scoring systems have also been developed. A more applicable scoring system for the diagnosis of secondary HLH in adults is the HScore, given that it was developed by studying a cohort of adult patients. HScore is calculated by adding scores for several criteria including underlying immunosuppression, fever, hepatosplenomegaly, cytopenias, hyperferritinemia, hypertriglyceridemia, hypofibrinogenemia, aspartate aminotransferase level, and hemophagocytosis on bone marrow aspirate [18]. The best cutoff HScore was 169 which had 93% sensitivity and 86% specificity for diagnosing HLH in 90% of the patients in the cohort [18]. Our patient had an HScore of 241 which corresponds to 99% probability of having HLH [18]. In a retrospective study of hemophagocytic syndrome in patients living with HIV, bone marrow aspirate had 93% specificity for diagnosis, while ferritin levels greater than 5000 ng/mL correlated with increased likelihood of death [4].

There remains the need to conduct a prospective study to evaluate the efficacy of the various treatment modalities for HLH in adults.

4. Conclusion

Clinicians need to maintain a high index of suspicion for HLH in the appropriate clinical setting. This is because an early diagnosis will aid the prompt initiation of treatment, and this can improve patient outcomes. Regarding our patient presented here, the most challenging aspect of her care was how to manage her as there are currently no treatment guidelines for IRIS-associated HLH in the setting of AIDS.

Future efforts need to be directed primarily towards conducting prospective studies to evaluate the efficacy of the various treatment modalities for HLH in adults. The specific subset of adults with IRIS, AIDS, and HLH can then be studied secondarily. We believe that by reporting this case, clinicians will be more aware of the possibility of HLH developing after initiating HAART in AIDS patients.

Acknowledgments

The authors acknowledge the contribution of Dr Jody Borgman (HIV medicine specialist, Einstein Medical Center) and Dr Manju Balasubramanian (Chief of the Department of Pathology and Laboratory Medicine, Einstein Medical Center) in the care of the patient.

References

[1] H. Al-Samkari and N. Berliner, "Hemophagocytic lymphohistiocytosis," *Annual Review of Pathology: Mechanisms of Disease*, vol. 13, no. 1, pp. 27–49, 2018.

[2] A. Hayden, S. Park, D. Giustini, A. Y. Y. Lee, and L. Y. C. Chen, "Hemophagocytic syndromes (HPSs) including hemophagocytic lymphohistiocytosis (HLH) in adults: a systematic scoping review," *Blood Reviews*, vol. 30, no. 6, pp. 411–420, 2016.

[3] N. G. Rouphael, N. J. Talati, C. Vaughan, K. Cunningham, R. Moreira, and C. Gould, "Infections associated with haemophagocytic syndrome," *The Lancet Infectious Diseases*, vol. 7, no. 12, pp. 814–822, 2007.

[4] J. P. Telles, M. de Andrade Perez, R. Marcusso, K. Correa, R. F. A. Teixeira, and W. M. Tobias, "Hemophagocytic syndrome in patients living with HIV: a retrospective study," *Annals of Hematology*, vol. 98, no. 1, pp. 67–72, 2019.

[5] M. A. French, "HIV/AIDS: immune reconstitution inflammatory syndrome: a reappraisal," *Clinical Infectious Diseases*, vol. 48, no. 1, pp. 101–107, 2009.

[6] D. M. Murdoch, W. D. F. Venter, A. Van Rie, and C. Feldman, "Immune reconstitution inflammatory syndrome (IRIS): review of common infectious manifestations and treatment options," *AIDS Research and Therapy*, vol. 4, no. 1, p. 9, 2007.

[7] M. A. French, N. Lenzo, M. John et al., "Immune restoration disease after the treatment of immunodeficient HIV-infected patients with highly active antiretroviral therapy," *HIV Medicine*, vol. 1, no. 2, pp. 107–115, 2000.

[8] M. Kanıtez, M. Kapmaz, N. Alpay, F. Selcukbiricik, A. Çağatay, and R. Diz-Küçükkaya, "Hemophagocytic syndrome associated with immune reconstitution inflammatory syndrome in a patient with AIDS related Burkitt's leukemia/lymphoma," *Case Reports in Medicine*, vol. 2014, Article ID 308081, 3 pages, 2014.

[9] S. M. Safdar, J. U. Rehman, E. M. Samman, and N. M. Bahabri, "Fatal hemophagocytic syndrome as a manifestation of immune reconstitution syndrome in a patient with acquired immunodeficiency syndrome," *Saudi Medical Journal*, vol. 34, no. 8, pp. 861–864, 2013.

[10] M.-P. Zorzou, M. Chini, A. Lioni et al., "Successful treatment of immune reconstitution inflammatory syndrome-related hemophagocytic syndrome in an HIV patient with primary effusion lymphoma," *Hematology Reports*, vol. 8, no. 4, p. 6581, 2016.

[11] M. Cuttelod, A. Pascual, A. S. Baur Chaubert et al., "Hemophagocytic syndrome after highly active antiretroviral therapy initiation: a life-threatening event related to immune restoration inflammatory syndrome?," *AIDS*, vol. 22, no. 4, pp. 549–551, 2008.

[12] L. Fardet, O. Lambotte, J.-L. Meynard et al., "Reactive haemophagocytic syndrome in 58 HIV-1-infected patients: clinical features, underlying diseases and prognosis," *AIDS*, vol. 24, no. 9, pp. 1299–1306, 2010.

[13] G. Meintjes and L. Lynen, "Prevention and treatment of the immune reconstitution inflammatory syndrome," *Current Opinion in HIV and AIDS*, vol. 3, no. 4, pp. 468–476, 2008.

[14] Y. C. Manabe, J. D. Campbell, E. Sydnor, and R. D. Moore, "Immune reconstitution inflammatory syndrome: risk factors and treatment implications," *JAIDS Journal of Acquired Immune Deficiency Syndromes*, vol. 46, no. 4, pp. 456–462, 2007.

[15] P. La Rosée, A. Horne, M. Hines et al., "Recommendations for the management of hemophagocytic lymphohistiocytosis in adults," *Blood*, vol. 133, no. 23, pp. 2465–2477, 2019.

[16] A. Hayden, M. Lin, S. Park et al., "Soluble interleukin-2 receptor is a sensitive diagnostic test in adult HLH," *Blood Advances*, vol. 1, no. 26, pp. 2529–2534, 2017.

[17] J.-I. Henter, A. Horne, M. Aricó et al., "HLH-2004: diagnostic and therapeutic guidelines for hemophagocytic lymphohistiocytosis," *Pediatric Blood & Cancer*, vol. 48, no. 2, pp. 124–131, 2007.

[18] L. Fardet, L. Galicier, O. Lambotte et al., "Development and validation of the HScore, a score for the diagnosis of reactive hemophagocytic syndrome," *Arthritis & Rheumatology*, vol. 66, no. 9, pp. 2613–2620, 2014.

48

An Unusual Case of Multiple Myeloma with Light-Chain Cast Nephropathy Secondary to a Very Large Plasmacytoma without Bone Marrow Involvement

Justin Komisarof,[1] **Jodi Lipof**,[2] **Joseph DiTursi**,[1] **Amit Chowdhry**,[3] **Hae Yoon Grace Choung**,[4] **W. Richard Burack**,[4] **Louis Constine**,[3] **and Frank Passero**[2]

[1]*Department of Medicine, University of Rochester Medical Center, 601 Elmwood Avenue, Rochester, NY 14642, USA*
[2]*Department of Hematology and Oncology, Wilmot Cancer Institute, 601 Elmwood Avenue, Rochester, NY 14642, USA*
[3]*Department of Radiation Oncology, Wilmot Cancer Institute, 601 Elmwood Avenue, Rochester, NY 14642, USA*
[4]*Department of Pathology and Laboratory Medicine, University of Rochester Medical Center, 601 Elmwood Avenue, Rochester, NY 14642, USA*

Correspondence should be addressed to Justin Komisarof; justin_komisarof@urmc.rochester.edu

Academic Editor: Pier Paolo Piccaluga

Here, we report a case of a patient who presented to Strong Memorial Hospital with new-onset renal failure and anemia and was found to have multiple myeloma with lambda light-chain cast nephropathy secondary to a very large (14 cm × 14 cm × 12 cm) plasmacytoma without bone marrow involvement. This case is notable as solitary plasmacytomas are almost never seen with concomitant myeloma-defining CRAB criteria or significantly elevated serum free light-chain ratios. Although solitary plasmacytomas are typically definitively treated with radiation, this case highlights that systemic treatment may be helpful in certain clinical scenarios.

1. Introduction

Multiple myeloma is a plasma cell dyscrasia characterized by clonal plasma cells >10% on bone marrow biopsy or the presence of a plasmacytoma in the setting of clinical features known as "CRAB criteria," which include hypercalcemia, renal insufficiency, anemia, or the presence of lytic bone lesions [1]. In the absence of CRAB criteria, a diagnosis of multiple myeloma can also be made by biomarker criteria including a free light chain ratio greater than 100, bone marrow plasma cell clonality greater than 60%, or multiple focal lesions on magnetic resonance imaging (MRI) [1]. Plasmacytomas are usually found within osseous structures but have been described in a wide range of extramedullary locations, including the liver, upper respiratory tract, gastrointestinal tract, soft tissues, and kidneys, among others [2–8]. A single plasmacytoma with minimal (<10%) or absent clonal marrow plasma cell involvement is a separate disease entity from multiple myeloma classified as a solitary plasmacytoma [9]. Solitary plasmacytomas are often treated with definitive radiation, although patients have a significant risk of progression to multiple myeloma at about 30% within 10 years of diagnosis [10–12]. The risk of progression is greater in patients with solitary plasmacytoma of bone than in patients with extramedullary plasmacytoma. Occasionally, solitary plasmacytomas may produce detectable and quantifiable monoclonal paraprotein that can be found on serum protein electrophoresis (SPEP), on serum immunofixation (IFE), or by an excess of kappa or lambda serum free light chains (sFLCs), resulting in an abnormal kappa-to-lambda ratio [13]. However, solitary plasmacytomas with low levels or undetectable disease in the bone marrow are very rarely reported with concomitant myeloma-defining CRAB criteria or a significantly elevated sFLC ratio. Here, we report a case of a patient who presented to Strong Memorial Hospital with new-onset renal failure and anemia and was found to have multiple myeloma with light-chain cast nephropathy secondary to a very large plasmacytoma without any other signs of end-organ damage or bone marrow plasma cell involvement.

2. Case Report

A 57-year-old male with a past medical history significant for papillary thyroid cancer treated definitively with thyroidectomy presented to his primary care physician with progressive fatigue, headache, and abdominal cramping. He reported dramatically decreased urine output starting two days prior to presentation, despite aggressive hydration. Initial workup revealed a markedly elevated creatinine level at 4.68 mg/dL. The patient had no prior history of kidney disease. His last known creatinine level, obtained 8 months prior, was 1.04 mg/dL. Initial laboratory studies also revealed new mild anemia with a hemoglobin level of 11.1 g/dL. He was sent to the emergency department for further evaluation. Additional lab studies on presentation revealed worsening renal function with a creatinine level of 7.72 mg/dL and hyponatremia with sodium of 127 mmol/L and normal serum osmolality of 285 mOsm. The 24-hour urine protein level was 750 mg. Renal ultrasound showed no evidence of hydronephrosis and normal-sized kidneys (11.4 cm for the R kidney and 12.3 cm for the L kidney). A chest X-ray was obtained due to decreased right-sided breath sounds on exam, which showed a large right hemithorax opacification. Follow-up CT chest revealed a $14.0 \times 14.0 \times 12.0$ cm mass in the lower lobe of the right lung (Figure 1) as well as an adjacent 1.1 cm lytic lesion in the proximal right 11th rib. The patient denied any pulmonary symptoms.

The patient's kidney function continued to worsen, and despite receiving fluids, he remained oliguric, requiring initiation of emergent hemodialysis. He underwent a kidney biopsy that revealed light-chain cast nephropathy, lambda type, with diffuse acute tubular injury (Figure 2). This finding raised suspicion for multiple myeloma. An M spike was detected on SPEP with a quantifiable paraprotein level of 0.4 g/dL, and lambda light-chain monoclonal protein was detected on serum immunofixation. The serum lambda free light-chain (FLC) level was 776 mg/dL, with an involved (lambda)-to-uninvolved (kappa) sFLC ratio of 160.3. A skeletal survey showed no additional sites of osteolytic lesions. Bone marrow biopsy revealed a slight increase in plasma cells (5%) but did not show any evidence of clonality by flow cytometry or fluorescence in situ hybridization (FISH) (Figure 3). The patient was urgently started on cyclophosphamide (300 mg/m^2 orally on days 1, 8, and 15), bortezomib (1.3 mg/m^2 subcutaneously on days 1, 4, 8, and 11), and dexamethasone (40 mg orally on days 1, 4, 8, and 11) (CyBorD) chemotherapy as well as plasmapheresis. Biopsy of the lung mass was performed, and the pathology was consistent with plasmacytoma, with lambda-restricted clonal plasma cells (Figure 4). As there were no clonal plasma cells on the bone marrow sample to perform CD138-directed FISH, the sample from the lung plasmacytoma was sent for myeloma FISH analysis, and this revealed a plasma cell clone with 13q deletion and monosomy 14. The patient initially responded well to chemotherapy and four sessions of plasmapheresis, with a reduction in lambda FLC level to 87 mg/dl. He was discharged from the hospital to continue treatment as an outpatient.

In the outpatient setting, the patient achieved at least a very good partial response (VGPR) with continued chemotherapy. The patient's kidney function continued to improve, and he was able to discontinue dialysis within one month of initiation, although his kidney function did not recover to his previous baseline. Positron emission tomography/computed tomography (PET/CT) scan performed after one cycle of chemotherapy did not show any evidence of osseous disease or additional plasmacytomas. A repeat chest CT after 4 cycles of treatment demonstrated an interval decrease in the size of the plasmacytoma to $13.0 \times 11.0 \times 10.0$ cm. Due to the development of mild neuropathy and a relative plateau in levels of FLC, his chemotherapy was switched to lenalidomide 10 mg orally (PO) for 21–28 days, bortezomib 1.3 mg/m^2 weekly, and 40 mg of dexamethasone PO weekly. His lambda free light chains reached a nadir of 57 mg/dL but rose to 78 mg/dL on this regimen, and subcutaneous (SC) daratumumab 1800 mg weekly was added, which resulted in a marked decrease in his lambda FLC level to 5 mg/dL. He was referred to radiation oncology for treatment of the plasmacytoma and underwent external beam radiation therapy (EBRT) with 52.2 Gy delivered in 29 fractions. Following radiation, his lambda FLC completely normalized. His therapy was de-escalated to dexamethasone 40 mg PO monthly and daratumumab 1800 mg SC monthly. He has remained stable on this regimen with no biochemical evidence of recurrence at the time of this report. A repeat PET/CT showed a further decrease in the size of the mass, measuring approximately 8.8 cm $\times$ 6.7 cm without significant SUV uptake, consistent with treatment response.

3. Discussion

In this report, we describe a patient who presented to our institution with new-onset renal failure due to biopsy-proven light-chain cast nephropathy from multiple myeloma secondary to a very large plasmacytoma. It is not clear whether this plasmacytoma was extramedullary or whether it initially arose from the patient's right 11th rib lytic lesion and invaded the lung. The rib lesion was not hypermetabolic on PET/CT, which has high sensitivity and specificity in this setting [14], and it is possible that the rib lesion was caused by compression from the adjacent tumor and was not a focus of myeloma at all. However, as the patient received systemic treatment prior to PET/CT, it is also possible that the rib may have lost the PET avidity that was originally present. Ultimately, without a biopsy of the rib lesion at the time of diagnosis, the plasmacytoma's origin cannot be definitively determined.

Regardless of the plasmacytoma's origin, this appears to be the first case reported of a large plasmacytoma without marrow involvement, fulfilling the International Myeloma

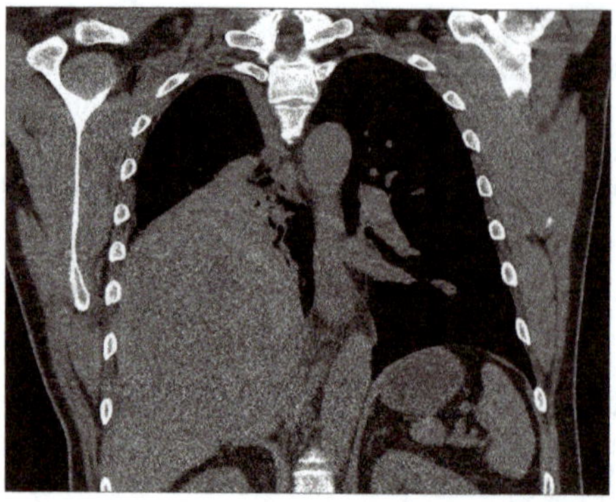

Figure 1: CT scan of the chest on presentation to hospital revealing very large ($14 \times 14 \times 12$ cm) lung mass.

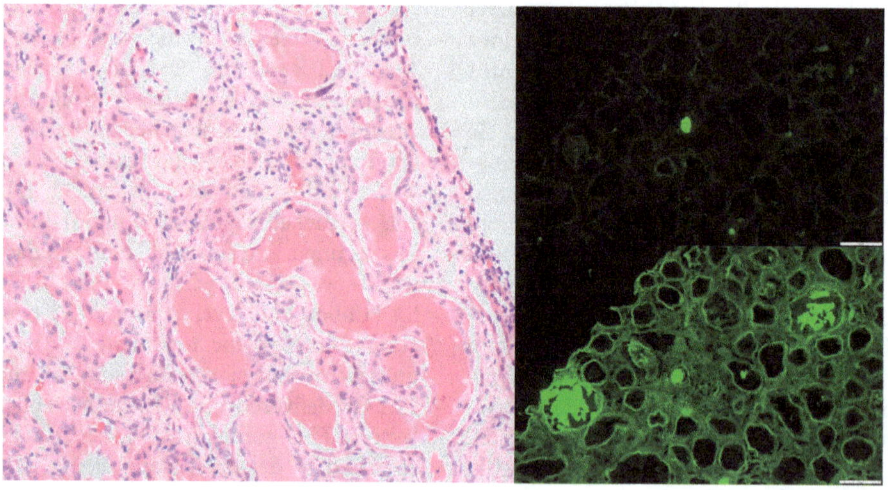

Figure 2: H&E stain of renal biopsy revealing atypical glassy eosinophilic casts associated with cellular reaction in acutely injured tubules (a). Immunofluorescence on renal biopsy is negative for kappa free light chains (b) but shows 2–3+ staining in the atypical casts for lambda free light chains (c).

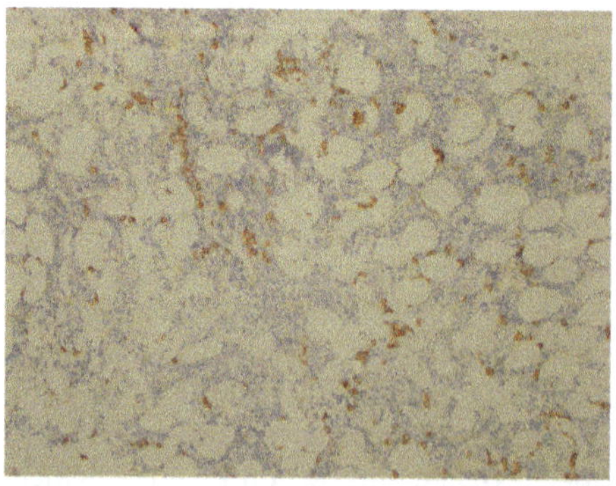

Figure 3: CD138 immunohistochemical stain (Giemsa background) of bone marrow biopsy showing scattered plasma cells in a physiologic distribution with no evidence of neoplasm.

Working Group definition of multiple myeloma [1] by the criteria of renal insufficiency secondary to biopsy-proven cast nephropathy. Although one prior case report described a patient with soft tissue plasmacytoma and myeloma cast nephropathy on renal biopsy, serum free light chains were not quantified in that case and a bone marrow biopsy was not performed prior to systemic therapy [15]. This presentation was similar to but also distinct from the rare phenomenon of macrofocal myeloma, in which multiple bone plasmacytomas are seen in the absence of bone marrow involvement. At this time, the standard of care for macrofocal multiple myeloma is systemic bortezomib-based therapy as a bridge to autologous stem cell transplant [16, 17]. These patients typically respond well to treatment and have a significantly increased overall median survival compared to standard myeloma patients [17].

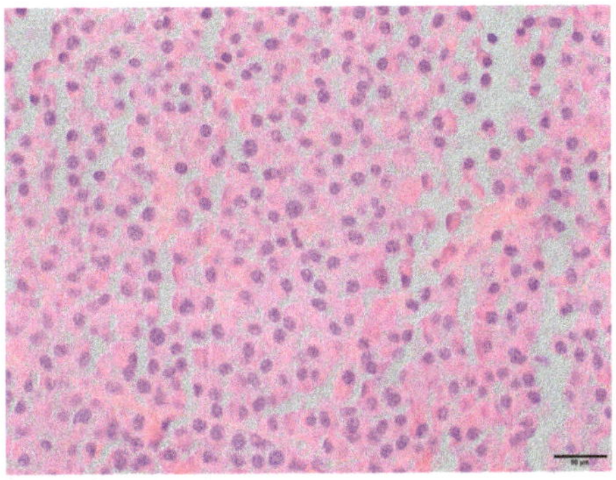

FIGURE 4: H&E stain of lung biopsy consistent with plasmacytoma.

Solitary plasmacytomas with little or no bone marrow involvement do not normally result in light-chain cast nephropathy. While many patients with solitary plasmacytoma have a detectable serum monoclonal protein, the median M spike was 0 g/dL and 0.5 g/dL in two case series [13, 18]. Approximately half of the patients had an abnormal sFLC ratio, but the median involved-to-uninvolved ratio was low at 2.3 [13, 18]. In this case, the large size of our patient's plasmacytoma likely represented a high burden of disease. Previous studies have shown that increased plasmacytoma size is correlated with a higher risk of progression to multiple myeloma [18–20] as well as relapse after radiotherapy [21]. This plasmacytoma was also associated with a significant serum paraprotein, which is independently a poor prognostic factor in extramedullary plasmacytoma [18]. Further investigation into a possible correlation between the size of a solitary plasmacytoma and existence of serum paraprotein could lead to a better understanding of this pathology and lead to a better ability to predict patient outcomes.

Typically, solitary plasmacytomas, with or without the presence of bone marrow involvement, can be treated definitively with radiotherapy [22, 23]. This patient was treated with systemic therapy immediately following the results of his kidney biopsy. At that time, his bone marrow biopsy had not yet resulted, and based on his serum studies with new anemia and renal failure requiring dialysis, it was presumed that he had moderate to high marrow involvement. After his bone marrow biopsy resulted, the decision was made to continue systemic therapy due to his clinically relevant reduction in lambda FLC and improving renal failure. Our patient also received plasmapheresis. The utility of plasmapheresis in patients with myeloma associated with acute renal failure remains unresolved by randomized clinical trials and has been called into question in the era of highly active proteasome inhibitor-based regimens [24, 25]. However, our patient had rapidly progressive renal failure requiring dialysis with a high serum free light-chain level. Thus, plasmapheresis was incorporated into his therapeutic plan to provide the highest likelihood of rapid serum free light reduction and renal recovery pending a more durable response from chemotherapy.

It is possible that the patient's disease could have been controlled with radiotherapy alone. However, recent studies have found a significant benefit to systemic therapy for solitary plasmacytoma, with significantly lower rates of progression to multiple myeloma [26, 27]. Furthermore, in this case, due to the extreme size of the mass, initiating treatment with systemic therapy resulted in the shrinking of the tumor and thus reduction in the area requiring radiation. Further research is needed to determine optimal treatment strategies in patients with very large plasmacytomas that lack significant bone marrow involvement by clonal plasma cells but meet criteria for multiple myeloma based on laboratory findings.

Disclosure

This case was submitted as an abstract for the 2021 URMC Internal Medicine Residency Poster Day.

References

[1] S. V. Rajkumar, M. A. Dimopoulos, A. Palumbo et al., "International Myeloma Working Group updated criteria for the diagnosis of multiple myeloma," *The Lancet Oncology*, vol. 15, no. 12, pp. e538–e548, 2014.

[2] L. Rosiñol, M. Beksac, E. Zamagni et al., "Expert review on soft-tissue plasmacytomas in multiple myeloma: definition, disease assessment and treatment considerations," *British Journal of Haematology*, vol. 194, no. 3, pp. 496–507, 2021, Online ahead of print.

[3] B. LeNoir, E. T. Bruner, C. E. Denlinger, and B. C. Gibney, "Extramedullary plasmacytoma of the right main bronchus," *The Annals of Thoracic Surgery*, vol. 108, no. 2, pp. e119–e120, 2019.

[4] J. I. Park, Y. Y. Lee, S. S. Lee, and J. H. Ahn, "A rare case of primary solitary endobronchial plasmacytoma," *Thoracic Cancer*, vol. 12, no. 6, pp. 958–961, 2021.

[5] A. Codorniz, R. Cunha, F. Fernandes, M. J Pais, T Neves, and C Quintana, "Uterine extramedullary plasmacytoma as a primary manifestation of multiple myeloma," *Revista Brasileira de Ginecologia e Obstetrícia : revista da Federacao Brasileira das Sociedades de Ginecologia e Obstetricia*, vol. 39, no. 9, pp. 516–520, 2017.

[6] Y. J. Gan, A. Chopra, and J. Kanagalingam, "Subglottic extramedullary plasmacytoma with light chain multiple myeloma masquerading as adult-onset asthma," *Journal of Voice : Official Journal of the Voice Foundation*, vol. 28, no. 3, p. 394, 2014.

[7] K. K. Sahu, P. D. Kumar, U. Yanamandra, and P. Malhotra, "Macrofocal multiple myeloma with frontal plasmacytoma," *Case Reports*, vol. 20, no. 1, Article ID bcr2015210759, 2015.

[8] A. Ozkok, O. C. Elcioglu, A. Bakan et al., "An unusual case of renal failure due to solitary plasmacytoma: parenchymal invasion of the kidney," *Renal Failure*, vol. 34, no. 5, pp. 640–642, 2012.

[9] J. Caers, B. Paiva, E. Zamagni et al., "Diagnosis, treatment, and response assessment in solitary plasmacytoma: updated recommendations from a European Expert Panel," *Journal of Hematology & Oncology*, vol. 11, no. 1, 2018.

[10] A. Pham and A. Mahindra, "Solitary plasmacytoma: a review of diagnosis and management," *Current Hematologic Malignancy Reports*, vol. 14, no. 2, pp. 63–69, 2019.

[11] D. Fotiou, M. A. Dimopoulos, and E. Kastritis, "How we manage patients with plasmacytomas," *Current Hematologic Malignancy Reports*, vol. 13, no. 3, pp. 227–235, 2018.

[12] T. D. Ellington, S. J. Henley, R. J. Wilson, M. Wu, and L. C. Richardson, "Trends in solitary plasmacytoma, extramedullary plasmacytoma, and plasma cell myeloma incidence and myeloma mortality by racial-ethnic group, United States 2003-2016," *Cancer Medicine*, vol. 10, no. 1, pp. 386–395, 2020.

[13] D. Dingli, R. A. Kyle, S. V. Rajkumar et al., "Immunoglobulin free light chains and solitary plasmacytoma of bone," *Blood*, vol. 108, no. 6, pp. 1979–1983, 2006.

[14] M. Cavo, E. Terpos, C. Nanni et al., "Role of 18F-FDG PET/CT in the diagnosis and management of multiple myeloma and other plasma cell disorders: a consensus statement by the International Myeloma Working Group," *The Lancet Oncology*, vol. 18, no. 4, pp. e206–e217, 2017.

[15] P. Binnani, M. M. Bahadur, N. Kedia, and P. Sharbidre, "Disease recurrence in a transplant kidney in a patient with extramedullary plasmacytoma," *Indian Journal of Medical and Paediatric Oncology : Official Journal of Indian Society of Medical & Paediatric Oncology*, vol. 31, no. 3, pp. 91–93, 2010.

[16] V. Goranova-Marinova, M. Yaneva, and T. Deneva, "Multiple myeloma with advanced bone disease and low tumor burden - different clinical presentation but similar outcome after bortezomib-based therapy and radiotherapy," *Acta Clinica Croatica*, vol. 56, no. 2, pp. 262–268, 2017.

[17] E. Katodritou, E. Kastritis, M. Gatt et al., "Real-world data on incidence, clinical characteristics and outcome of patients with macrofocal multiple myeloma (MFMM) in the era of novel therapies: a study of the Greco-Israeli collaborative myeloma working group," *American Journal of Hematology*, vol. 95, no. 5, pp. 465–471, 2020.

[18] E. E. Manasanch, C. Kunacheewa, C. M. Claussen et al., "Serum paraprotein persistence and size determine outcome in a cohort of patients with a modern definition of plasmacytoma with up to 19 years of follow up," *Blood Cancer Journal*, vol. 11, no. 2, p. 17, 2021.

[19] P. Finsinger, S. Grammatico, M. Chisini, A. Piciocchi, R. Foà, and M. T. Petrucci, "Clinical features and prognostic factors in solitary plasmacytoma," *British Journal of Haematology*, vol. 172, no. 4, pp. 554–560, 2016.

[20] B. Venkatesulu, S. Mallick, P. Giridhar, A. D. Upadhyay, and G. K. Rath, "Pattern of care and impact of prognostic factors on the outcome of head and neck extramedullary plasmacytoma: a systematic review and individual patient data analysis of 315 cases," *European Archives of Oto-Rhino-Laryngology*, vol. 275, no. 2, pp. 595–606, 2018.

[21] D. A. Barzenje, A. Kolstad, W. Ghanima, and H. Holte, "Long-term outcome of patients with solitary plasmacytoma treated with radiotherapy: a population-based, single-center study with median follow-up of 13.7 years," *Hematological Oncology*, vol. 36, no. 1, pp. 217–223, 2018.

[22] R. W. Tsang, B. A. Campbell, J. S. Goda et al., "Radiation therapy for solitary plasmacytoma and multiple myeloma: guidelines from the international lymphoma radiation oncology group," *International Journal of Radiation Oncology, Biology, Physics*, vol. 101, no. 4, pp. 794–808, 2018.

[23] G. Wen, W. Wang, W. Wang et al., "Management of extramedullary plasmacytoma: role of radiotherapy and prognostic factor analysis in 55 patients," *Chinese Journal of Cancer Research*, vol. 29, no. 5, pp. 438–446, 2017.

[24] W. F. Clark, A. K. Stewart, G. A. Rock et al., "Plasma exchange when myeloma presents as acute renal failure," *Annals of Internal Medicine*, vol. 143, no. 11, pp. 777–784, 2005.

[25] L. J. Costa, J. Abbas, K. L. Ortiz-Cruz, Y. Kang, and R. K. Stuart, "Outcomes of patients with multiple myeloma and renal impairment treated with bortezomib, cyclophosphamide, and dexamethasone without plasma exchange," *European Journal of Haematology*, vol. 89, no. 5, pp. 432–434, 2012.

[26] K. Elsayad, M. Oertel, L. König et al., "Maximizing the clinical benefit of radiotherapy in solitary plasmacytoma: an international multicenter analysis," *Cancers*, vol. 12, no. 3, p. 676, 2020.

[27] F. Mignot, A. Schernberg, A. Arsène-Henry, M. Vignon, D. Bouscary, and Y. Kirova, "Solitary plasmacytoma treated by lenalidomide-dexamethasone in combination with radiation therapy: clinical outcomes," *International Journal of Radiation Oncology, Biology, Physics*, vol. 106, no. 3, pp. 589–596, 2020.

49

Systemic Mastocytosis in a Patient with BCR-ABL1-Positive Chronic Myeloid Leukemia in the Remission Phase

Christos Fokoloros,[1] Periklis Foukas,[2] Nikolaos Georgakopoulos,[3] Zoi Tsakiraki,[2] Anthi Bouchla,[4] Vasilliki Pappa,[4] Alexandros Katoulis,[1] Michael Makris,[1] and Sotirios Papageorgiou[3]

[1]*Allergy Unit "D. Kalogeromitros", 2nd Department of Dermatology and Venereology, Medical School, National and Kapodistrian University of Athens, Attikon University Hospital, Athens, Greece*
[2]*2nd Department of Pathology, Medical School, National and Kapodistrian University of Athens, Attikon University Hospital, Athens, Greece*
[3]*Department of Cytogenetics and Molecular Pathology, Locus Medicus S.A., Athens, Greece*
[4]*Hematology Unit, 2nd Department of Internal Medicine, Propaedeutic, Medical School, National and Kapodistrian University of Athens, Attikon University Hospital, Athens, Greece*

Correspondence should be addressed to Christos Fokoloros; fokomd@gmail.com

Academic Editor: Massimo Breccia

Systemic mastocytosis (SM) comprises a group of rare disorders resulting from tissue infiltration by pathological mast cells. In a percentage ranging from 5 to 40% in various patient series, SM appears to be associated with an accompanying hematologic neoplasm (SM-AHN). The coexistence of SM with chronic myelogenous leukemia (CML) is extremely rare with only 3 cases in the literature. The natural course of CML has changed dramatically over the past 2 decades with the use of tyrosine kinase inhibitors (TKIs). We report a case of diagnosing SM in a patient in complete molecular remission of CML after stopping TKI treatment.

1. Introduction

Systemic mastocytosis (SM) is a rare myeloid neoplasm. According to current guidelines [1], SM is classified into subgroups mainly based on clinical and laboratory findings. Among them, SM with an associated hematologic (non-MC) neoplasm (SM-AHN) was the second most common SM subgroup in data of the European Competence Network on Mastocytosis (ECNM) registry [2].

Chronic myeloid leukemia is a pluripotent stem cell disease characterized by the presence of the Philadelphia chromosome that fuses the BCR gene on chromosome 22 with the ABL1 gene on chromosome 9. The treatment of CML has changed dramatically in the last two decades. According to current guidelines, treatment-free remission is achieved when a patient who has discontinued TKI therapy maintains a deep molecular response (DMR) and does not need to restart treatment [3]. We describe for the first time a case of SM in a patient with CML in the TFR phase.

2. Case Report

A 45-year-old man with a personal history of three episodes of near-fatal anaphylaxis after Hymenoptera stings during the last decade was referred to mastocytosis outpatient clinic due to elevated serum tryptase (27.5 ng/mL). The allergological workup detected IgE sensitization to multiple species of Hymenoptera venoms; *Apis mellifera*, *Vespa crabro*, and *Polistes dominula*. The bone marrow (BM) biopsy revealed multifocal aggregates of spindled CD117+, CD2+, CD25+, and CD30+ mast cells, with more than 15 cells per aggregate. Additional studies on the BM samples showed a normal karyotype (46, XY), while allele-specific polymerase chain reaction for KITD816V detection was positive. Therefore,

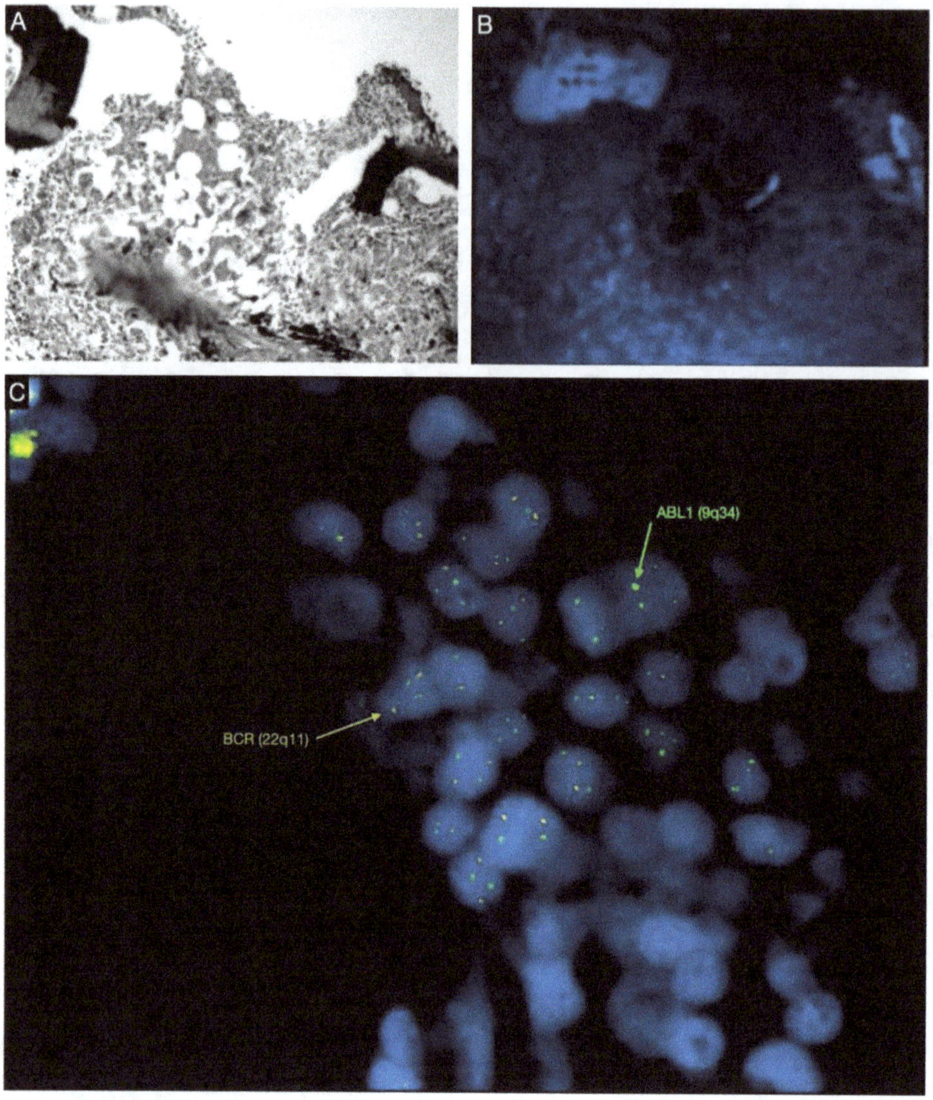

Figure 1: (a): IHC (×10), (b): FISH (×10), and (c): FISH (×100); a fluorescence in situ hybridization (FISH) technique for the detection of the *t* (9; 22) (*q*34; *q*11) reciprocal translocation was performed in samples with mast cell infiltration and was negative.

the diagnosis of SM was documented, according to the recent WHO criteria [1].

The patient reported a diagnosis of chronic myeloid leukemia (CML) BCR-ABL-positive (Ph+), 8 years ago. He was treated with dasatinib (100 mg per day), a second-generation TKI, for almost 7 years with full remission (MR 4.5) after 4 to 5 years of therapy and with no complications during treatment. In the last 16 months, the patient has discontinued TKI therapy and maintains a deep molecular response (treatment-free remission/TFR). According to his history, an additional BM study with a fluorescence in situ hybridization (FISH) technique for the detection of the *t* (9; 22) (*q*34; *q*11) reciprocal translocation was performed in samples with mast cell infiltration and was negative (Figure 1). Bone marrow samples from the initial diagnosis of CML were not available to investigate the presence of mast cell infiltration.

The patient's CML remains in a deep molecular response (MR 4.5) and venom immunotherapy has been initiated in a combination of omalizumab (300 mcg per month) due to anaphylactic episodes during immunotherapy. No other cytoreduction therapy for SM was initiated as the patient does not present any c-finding.

3. Discussion

Up to now, only three cases of SM with associated Ph+ CML have been reported in the literature [4–6]. In our case, the first episode of anaphylaxis occurred before the diagnosis of CML, so we could assume that SM was preexisting. In the other two reported cases of SM-CML, the concomitant SM was present from the initial time point of CML diagnosis [4, 5].

Hymenoptera venom allergy is a typical IgE-mediated disease, in which clinical manifestations are the result of mast cells' (MCs) degranulation. The prevalence of venom allergy in SM patients is higher than in the general population and venom sting represents the most common trigger of anaphylaxis in adult mastocytosis patients. Also, non-IgE degranulation of MCs may occur in patients with SM [7]. A clinical history of multiple near-fatal anaphylactic episodes is strong evidence for additional investigation, especially in a patient with already known myeloid neoplasm.

In conclusion, in this case, the coexistence of two rare genetic aberrations drives the development of two distinct neoplastic diseases, for which the targeted treatment of CML had no effect on the natural history of the SM.

Consent

Informed consent was obtained from all individual participants included in the study.

References

[1] P. Valent, C. Akin, and D. D. Metcalfe, "Mastocytosis: 2016 updated WHO classification and novel emerging treatment concepts," *Blood*, vol. 129, no. 11, pp. 1420–1427, 2017.

[2] P. Valent, J. N. G. Oude Elberink, A. Gorska et al., "The data registry of the European competence network on mastocytosis (ECNM): set up, projects, and perspectives," *Journal of Allergy and Clinical Immunology: In Practice*, vol. 7, no. 1, pp. 81–87, 2019.

[3] Chronic Myeloid Leukemia, "National comprehensive cancer network: NCCN guidelines version 2022," 2022, https://www.nccn.org/professionals/physician_gls/pdf/cml.pdf.

[4] K. Hussein, H. P. Horny, G. Büsche et al., "Systemic mastocytosis (SM) with associated BCR-ABL-positive myelogenous leukaemia (SM-AHNMD): evidence that mast cells do not belong to the leukaemic clone," *Leukemia*, vol. 25, no. 6, pp. 1050–1053, 2011.

[5] H. Agis, K. Sotlar, P. Valent, and H. P. Horny, "Ph-chromosome-positive chronic myeloid leukemia with associated bone marrow mastocytosis," *Leukemia Research*, vol. 29, no. 10, pp. 1227–1232, 2005.

[6] H. P. Horny, K. Sotlar, F. Stellmacher et al., "The tryptase positive compact round cell infiltrate of the bone marrow (TROCI-BM): a novel histopathological finding requiring the application of lineage specific markers," *Journal of Clinical Pathology*, vol. 59, no. 3, pp. 298–302, 2006.

[7] F. Ruëff, B. Przybilla, M. B. Biló et al., "Predictors of severe systemic anaphylactic reactions in patients with hymenoptera venom allergy: importance of baseline serum tryptase—a study of the European academy of allergology and clinical immunology interest group on insect venom hypersensitivity," *The Journal of Allergy and Clinical Immunology*, vol. 124, no. 5, pp. 1047–1054, 2009.

50

An Atypical Presentation of Hemophagocytic Lymphohistiocytosis (HLH) Secondary to Occult Hodgkin Lymphoma

Justin Komisarof,[1] Kevin McGann,[1] Alissa Huston,[1] Hani Katerji,[2] and Mary Anne Morgan[1]

[1]*Department of Medicine, University of Rochester Medical Center, 601 Elmwood Avenue Box MED, Rochester, NY 14642, USA*
[2]*Department of Pathology and Laboratory Medicine, University of Rochester Medical Center, 601 Elmwood Avenue Box 626, Rochester, NY 14642, USA*

Correspondence should be addressed to Justin Komisarof; justin_komisarof@urmc.rochester.edu

Academic Editor: Kiyotaka Kawauchi

Hemophagocytic lymphohistiocytosis (HLH) is a rare and life-threatening syndrome of immune system dysregulation characterized by the phagocytosis of various cells by histiocytes in the bone marrow. HLH can present in one of the two ways: primary HLH, which is caused by mutations in genes essential to T and NK-cell function, and secondary HLH, typically caused by Epstein–Barr virus (EBV) infection or malignancy. Because of the rapid progression and high mortality of this disease, prompt diagnosis is essential to good outcomes. Here, we report the 2-month clinical course of a patient who presented with altered mental status and recurrent fever of unknown origin. Initially, he did not meet diagnostic criteria for HLH and had a negative bone marrow biopsy; however, he eventually progressed to full-blown HLH secondary to occult Hodgkin lymphoma. This case is unusual for the slow and smoldering course of the patient's disease and highlights the importance of aggressively searching for potential malignancies to ensure the initiation of definitive therapy as soon as possible.

1. Introduction

Hemophagocytic lymphohistiocytosis (HLH) is a rare life-threatening syndrome of immune system dysregulation characterized by hypersecretion of inflammatory cytokines due to persistent overactivation of cytotoxic T cells and NK cells, ultimately leading to phagocytosis of hematopoietic cells by histiocytes throughout the reticuloendothelial system [1–3]. While HLH was initially described as a genetic disorder of childhood and much of what is known regarding its pathophysiology, presentation, and management has originated from the pediatric literature, our understanding of secondary HLH in adults continues to grow [4]. While the potential etiologic underpinnings of secondary HLH are exceedingly broad [5–10], principal among them are EBV infection and lymphoma [1, 11–14]. The presentation of HLH is variable and nonspecific, overlapping with many conditions such as sepsis, thereby posing significant challenges for early diagnosis and treatment in what is often a rapidly progressive and fatal picture [15–21].

Diagnostic criteria developed from pediatric patients with familial HLH were first proposed in 1991 [22] and later revised in 2004 [23] to include eight criteria of which a patient must meet at least five: fever (≥38.5°C for ≥7 days), cytopenias (≥2 cell lines affected), splenomegaly (>3 cm below costal margin), hypertriglyceridemia (≥2 mmol/L) and/or hypofibrinogenemia (≤150 mg/dL), hemophagocytosis in the bone marrow, spleen, or lymph nodes, elevated ferritin (≥500 μg/l), elevated soluble IL-2 receptor levels (≥2400 U/mol), and low/absent NK-cell activity. More recently, novel diagnostic criteria known as the HScore have also been developed and validated in a small population of adult patients [24]. These diagnostic criteria align with the most common presenting symptoms of HLH and include fever, splenomegaly, and cytopenias. However, an array of other presenting findings, including skin rash [3, 25, 26], pulmonary symptoms such as dyspnea and cough [27], and neurologic features including encephalopathy, seizure, ataxia, and cranial nerve abnormalities have been reported [28–31]. Treatment of secondary HLH must be initiated early and aims to address the underlying precipitating disorder, with the most commonly used HLH protocol relying on etoposide, dexamethasone, and hematopoietic stem cell transplantation as mainstays of therapy [32]. For HLH secondary to Hodgkin lymphoma, brentuximab therapy has been reported to be successful [33, 34].

2. Case Presentation

A 63-year-old man with a history of remote Hodgkin lymphoma at age 19 years, coronary artery disease (CAD), and recent urothelial carcinoma presented to Highland Hospital with 2-3 months of intermittent fevers and confusion. His initial laboratory values were notable for anemia (hemoglobin 9.0 g/dL) and thrombocytopenia (63,000 platelets/μL) with a normal white blood cell count (5700 WBC/μL). He was hyponatremic with a sodium of 125 mmol/L and had an elevated alkaline phosphatase (300 U/L). He underwent an extensive infectious workup which was notable only for positive Epstein–Barr virus (EBV) viral PCR (7800 copies/mL) but negative EBV IgM. Hematology was consulted out of concern for a hemolytic anemia, but hemolysis labs were unremarkable with normal serum haptoglobin (93 mg/dL) and total bilirubin (0.9 mg/dL). Reticulocyte count was not elevated (2.3%), and schistocytes were not seen on a peripheral smear. The possibility of hemophagocytic lymphohistiocytosis (HLH) was raised at this time due to the patient's cytopenias and recurrent fever. At this time, his ferritin was elevated at 1089 ng/mL and triglycerides were elevated at 153 mg/dL but below the diagnostic cutoff for HLH. However, fibrinogen was normal, and the patient was not observed to have splenomegaly. A bone marrow biopsy was performed and did not show phagocytic histiocytes or evidence of malignancy (Figure 1). NK functional assay was sent but cancelled due to insufficient lymphocyte count. Soluble IL-2 receptor assay was ordered. The patient was treated with a 5-day course of antibiotics, and his fever curve gradually downtrended. His encephalopathy improved with the resolution of his fevers. The patient was afebrile for 72 hours and was able to be discharged from the hospital.

One month later, the patient was admitted to Strong Memorial Hospital with ongoing intermittent fevers and confusion. In the interim, he underwent a positron emission tomography (PET) scan which revealed a hypermetabolic focus in the left palatine tonsil (Figure 2). On admission, triglycerides were slightly higher at 173 mg/dL and ferritin was also slightly higher at 1407 ng/mL. He had a positive blood culture for *Staphylococcus epidermidis* which was believed to be a contaminant. Tonsillar biopsy demonstrated an atypical clonal lymphoid population but no morphologically abnormal lymphoid cells and no Hodgkin Reed–Sternberg (HRS) cells or other evidence for lymphoma. Soluble IL-2 receptor assay from the earlier hospitalization had still not resulted at this time. Ferritin continued to rise climbing steadily to 9573 ng/mL two weeks after admission. The patient became hypotensive and was transferred to the ICU for vasopressor support. He developed acute hypoxic respiratory failure requiring intubation thought to be due to pleural effusions and atelectasis. Soluble IL-2 receptor came back extremely elevated at 17,375 U/mL. Repeat EBV viral PCR was now 40,400 copies/mL. The patient underwent repeat bone marrow biopsy which showed Hodgkin lymphoma with hemophagocytic lymphohistiocytosis (Figure 3), confirming the diagnosis of HLH. Karyotype analysis was 46XY with no apparent clonal chromosomal aberrations, and EBER-ISH was positive. The patient was started on high-dose dexamethasone (20 mg) daily as well as etoposide (100 mg/mL) twice weekly. At this point, ferritin was now 12,130 ng/mL. Dexamethasone was increased shortly after to 40 mg daily, and the patient received a single dose of brentuximab (1.8 mg/kg). After receiving brentuximab, the patient developed progressive renal failure with creatinine increasing from 1.4 to 3.0 mg/dL over the course of a week as well as a lactic acidosis. After discussion with the family, the patient was terminally extubated and passed away.

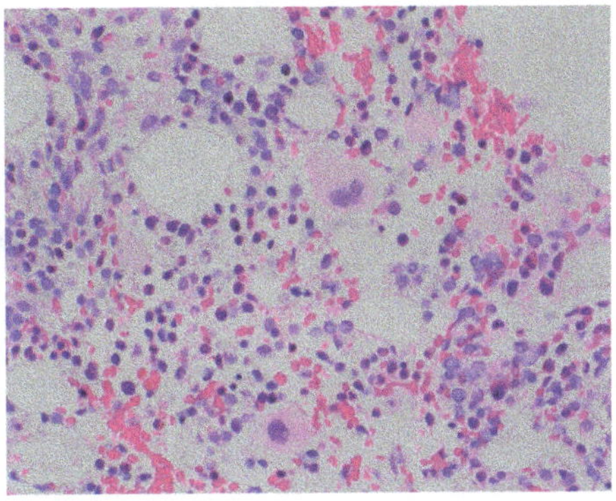

Figure 1: Hematoxylin and eosin (H&E) section of the hypocellular bone marrow with no definitive infiltration by lymphoma.

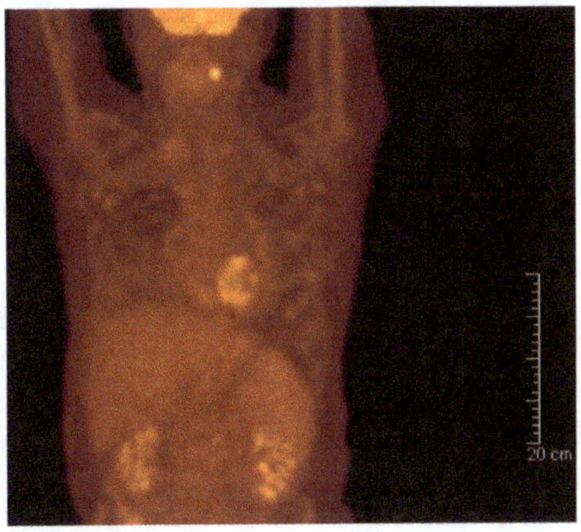

Figure 2: PET scan revealing the hypermetabolic focus localized to the left palatine tonsil.

3. Discussion

Hemophagocytic lymphohistiocytosis (HLH) is a rare life-threatening syndrome of immune system dysregulation typically seen secondary to EBV infection or blood

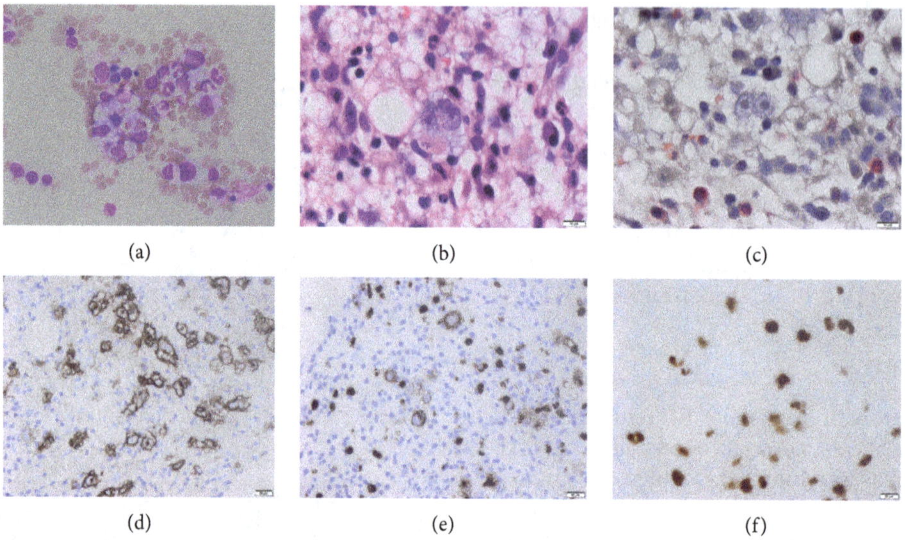

Figure 3: H&E section of the bone marrow revealing hemophagocytosis (a). High-powered H&E section (b) and chloracetate esterase section (c) demonstrating binucleated Reed–Sternberg (RS) cells. Immunohistochemistry showed positivity for CD30 (d) and CD15 (e) in RS cells. Epstein–Barr encoding region in situ hybridization (EBER-ISH) (f).

malignancy. Herein, we describe the detailed 2-month course of a 63-year-old male who presented with altered mental status, recurrent fevers, and fatigue and who was ultimately found to have HLH secondary to occult Hodgkin lymphoma.

This case is unusual for its slow and smoldering presentation. Typically, patients with active HLH present acutely ill, often in multiple organ system failure and requiring ICU level of care. This patient's symptoms fluctuated to an extent that he met criteria for hospital discharge, only to be readmitted four weeks later with ongoing subacute and intermittent symptoms. Although the diagnosis of HLH secondary to new lymphoma was entertained during the patient's first hospital stay, the bone marrow biopsy was unrevealing. During his second hospital stay, despite multidisciplinary subspecialty consultation and interdepartmental review, the diagnosis was clinched only when the bone marrow aspirate was repeated. As no malignant cells were found outside the bone marrow, it is possible that this represented primary bone marrow Hodgkin lymphoma. While this is quite rare and typically associated with HIV infection, for which our patient tested negative, several previous cases have been described of HIV-negative primary bone marrow Hodgkin lymphoma [35, 36]. Alternatively, it is possible that the tonsillar biopsy was a false negative and that this represented stage 4 Hodgkin lymphoma.

The most notable feature of this case that delayed diagnosis was the first bone marrow biopsy which did not show any evidence of phagocytic histiocytes or underlying malignancy. While HLH is characterized by hemophagocytosis, it is important to note that the sensitivity of bone marrow biopsy for HLH is relatively low at 83% and that hemophagocytosis can be seen in the bone marrow of patients without HLH [37]. Similarly, it is becoming clear that bone marrow biopsy false negatives are fairly common in Hodgkin lymphoma and that patients should undergo PET/CT as part of their initial workup [38]. HLH is treated primarily with a regimen of dexamethasone and etoposide, and HLH secondary to malignancy must be treated by addressing the underlying cancer [39]. In all cases where HLH is suspected, an aggressive approach must be taken both to work up all HLH diagnostic criteria as well as to identify any underlying malignancy present and initiate definitive treatment as quickly as possible.

Acknowledgments

The authors would like to thank Dr. Andrew Evans for assistance with pathology figures.

References

[1] H. Al-Samkari and N. Berliner, "Hemophagocytic lymphohistiocytosis," *Annual Review of Pathology: Mechanisms of Disease*, vol. 13, no. 1, pp. 27–49, 2018.

[2] N. S. Bhatt, B. Oshrine, and J. An Talano, "Hemophagocytic lymphohistiocytosis in adults," *Leukemia & Lymphoma*, vol. 60, no. 1, pp. 19–28, 2019.

[3] M. V. Maus, M. B. Leick, K. M. Cornejo, and V. Nardi, "Case 35-2019: a 66-year-old man with pancytopenia and rash," *New England Journal of Medicine*, vol. 381, no. 20, pp. 1951–1960, 2019.

[4] M. Campo and N. Berliner, "Hemophagocytic lymphohistiocytosis in adults," *Hematology/Oncology Clinics of North America*, vol. 29, no. 5, pp. 915–925, 2015.

[5] C. Bailey, C. Dearden, and K. Ardeshna, "Haemophagocytic lymphohistiocytosis as a consequence of untreated B-cell chronic lymphocytic leukaemia," *Case Reports*, vol. 2017, 2017.

[6] J. Chen, X. Wang, P. He et al., "Viral etiology, clinical and laboratory features of adult hemophagocytic lymphohistio-

cytosis," *Journal of Medical Virology*, vol. 88, no. 3, pp. 541–549, 2016.

[7] R. Assi, P. Boddu, T. M. Kadia, Z. E. Estrov, G. Garcia-Manero, A. Abou Zahr et al., "Characteristics and outcomes of patients (pts) with malignancy-associated hemophagocytic lymphohistiocytosis (M-HLH) in adults: a single-center, prospective analysis of 36 pts," *Blood*, vol. 132, no. 1, p. 3689, 2018.

[8] C. Y. Dumancas, H. A. G. Reyes, J. Cosico, A. Savadkar, and S. Lah, "Streptococcus pneumoniae-related hemophagocytic lymphohistiocytosis treated with IVIG and steroids," *American Journal of Case Reports*, vol. 19, pp. 25–28, 2018.

[9] F. E. Elzein, N. Al Sherbini, M. M. Alotaibi, and W. M. Al-Hassan, "Brucellosis accompanied by haemophagocytic lymphohistiocytosis and multiple splenic abscesses in a patient with depression," *Case Reports*, vol. 2018, 2018.

[10] C. Kennedy-Snodgrass, M. Obayomi, R. Muddasani, L. B. Slonim, and M. Braunstein, "Hemophagocytic lymphohistiocytosis secondary to babesia in an immunocompetent adult," *American Journal of Hematology*, vol. 94, no. 3, pp. 379–383, 2019.

[11] W. Lai, Y. Wang, J. Wang, L. Wu, Z. Jin, and Z. Wang, "Epstein-Barr virus-associated hemophagocytic lymphohistiocytosis in adults and adolescents-a life-threatening disease: analysis of 133 cases from a single center," *Hematology*, vol. 23, no. 10, pp. 810–816, 2018.

[12] C. Bigenwald, L. Fardet, P. Coppo et al., "A comprehensive analysis of Lymphoma-associated haemophagocytic syndrome in a large french multicentre cohort detects some clues to improve prognosis," *British Journal of Haematology*, vol. 183, no. 1, pp. 68–75, 2018.

[13] A. Iardino, Z. Amar, and Y. Ahmed, "Epstein-barr-positive classical hodgkin lymphoma-associated haemophagocytic lymphohistocytiosis: a rare case," *Case Reports*, vol. 2018, 2018.

[14] Z. Jin, Y. Wang, N. Wei, and Z. Wang, "Hodgkin lymphoma-associated hemophagocytic lymphohistiocytosis-a dangerous disease," *Annals of Hematology*, vol. 99, no. 7, pp. 1575–1581, 2020.

[15] F. G. N. Rosado and A. S. Kim, "Hemophagocytic lymphohistiocytosis," *American Journal of Clinical Pathology*, vol. 139, no. 6, pp. 713–727, 2013.

[16] Z. K. Otrock and C. S. Eby, "Clinical characteristics, prognostic factors, and outcomes of adult patients with hemophagocytic lymphohistiocytosis," *American Journal of Hematology*, vol. 90, no. 3, pp. 220–224, 2015.

[17] Z. K. Otrock, N. Daver, H. M. Kantarjian, and C. S. Eby, "Diagnostic challenges of hemophagocytic lymphohistiocytosis," *Clinical Lymphoma Myeloma and Leukemia*, vol. 17, pp. S105–S110, 2017.

[18] S. Birndt, T. Schenk, B. Heinevetter et al., "Hemophagocytic lymphohistiocytosis in adults: collaborative analysis of 137 cases of a nationwide German registry," *Journal of Cancer Research and Clinical Oncology*, vol. 146, no. 4, pp. 1065–1077, 2020.

[19] M. Zhou, L. Li, Q. Zhang et al., "Clinical features and outcomes in secondary adult hemophagocytic lymphohistiocytosis," *QJM: An International Journal of Medicine*, vol. 111, no. 1, pp. 23–31, 2018.

[20] J. A. Carcillo, B. Podd, and D. W. Simon, "From febrile pancytopenia to hemophagocytic lymphohistiocytosis-associated organ dysfunction," *Intensive Care Medicine*, vol. 43, no. 12, pp. 1853–1855, 2017.

[21] B. C. Prokesch, S. Nagalla, F. Ezzati et al., "What's in a name? the heterogeneous clinical spectrum and prognostic factors in a cohort of adults with hemophagocytic lymphohistiocytosis," *Transfusion and Apheresis Science*, vol. 57, no. 6, pp. 779–784, 2018.

[22] J. I. Henter, G Elinder, and A Ost, "Diagnostic guidelines for hemophagocytic lymphohistiocytosis. The FHL study group of the histiocyte society," *Seminars in Oncology*, vol. 18, pp. 29–33, 1991.

[23] J.-I. Henter, A. Horne, M. Aricó et al., "HLH-2004: diagnostic and therapeutic guidelines for hemophagocytic lymphohistiocytosis," *Pediatric Blood & Cancer*, vol. 48, no. 2, pp. 124–131, 2007.

[24] L. Fardet, L. Galicier, O. Lambotte et al., "Development and validation of the HScore, a score for the diagnosis of reactive hemophagocytic syndrome," *Arthritis & Rheumatology*, vol. 66, no. 9, pp. 2613–2620, 2014.

[25] M. Khairoun, F. Meynen, W. Vercoutere, and H. L. Leavis, "Case series of three adult patients with exceptional clinical presentations of haemophagocytic lymphohistiocytosis," *The Netherlands Journal of Medicine*, vol. 78, no. 3, pp. 136–141, 2020.

[26] A. M. Schram, P. Comstock, M. Campo et al., "Haemophagocytic lymphohistiocytosis in adults: a multicentre case series over 7 years," *British Journal of Haematology*, vol. 172, no. 3, pp. 412–419, 2016.

[27] A. Seguin, L. Galicier, D. Boutboul, V. Lemiale, and E. Azoulay, "Pulmonary involvement in patients with hemophagocytic lymphohistiocytosis," *Chest*, vol. 149, no. 5, pp. 1294–1301, 2016.

[28] G. Cai, Y. Wang, X. Liu, Y. Han, and Z. Wang, "Central nervous system involvement in adults with haemophagocytic lymphohistiocytosis: a single-center study," *Annals of Hematology*, vol. 96, no. 8, pp. 1279–1285, 2017.

[29] D. M. Pastula, M. Burish, G. F. Reis et al., "Adult-onset central nervous system hemophagocytic lymphohistiocytosis: a case report," *BMC Neurology*, vol. 15, no. 1, p. 203, 2015.

[30] S. Magaki, N. Ostrzega, E. Ho, C. Yim, P. Wu, and H. V. Vinters, "Hemophagocytic lymphohistiocytosis associated with epstein-barr virus in the central nervous system," *Human Pathology*, vol. 59, pp. 108–112, 2017.

[31] Y. Song, R.-J. Pei, Y.-N. Wang, J. Zhang, and Z. Wang, "Central nervous system involvement in hemophagocytic lymphohistiocytosis in adults," *Chinese Medical Journal*, vol. 131, no. 7, pp. 776–783, 2018.

[32] A. M. Schram and N. Berliner, "How i treat hemophagocytic lymphohistiocytosis in the adult patient," *Blood*, vol. 125, no. 19, pp. 2908–2914, 2015.

[33] K. Nagaharu, M. Masuya, Y. Kageyama et al., "Successful treatment of primary bone marrow hodgkin lymphoma with brentuximab vedotin: a case report and review of the literature," *Journal of Medical Case Reports*, vol. 12, no. 1, p. 151, 2018.

[34] B. Knox, D. Singh, H. Mai, and K. Mirza, "Hodgkin's lymphoma with HLH and complete remission with brentuximab-based therapy," *BMJ Case Reports*, vol. 12, no. 12, Article ID e231629, 2019.

[35] Y. Morita, M. Emoto, K. Serizawa et al., "HIV-negative primary bone marrow hodgkin lymphoma manifesting with a high fever associated with hemophagocytosis as the initial symptom: a case report and review of the previous literature," *Internal Medicine*, vol. 54, no. 11, pp. 1393–1396, 2015.

[36] C. Laurent, D. A. Arber, P. Johnston, F. Fend, A. Zamo, and A. D. Attygalle, "Diagnosis of classic hodgkin lymphoma on bone marrow biopsy," *Histopathology*, vol. 76, no. 7, pp. 934–941, 2020.

[37] S. Goel, J. M. Polski, and H. Imran, "Sensitivity and specificity of bone marrow hemophagocytosis in hemophagocytic lymphohistiocytosis," *Annals of Clinical and Laboratory Science*, vol. 42, no. 1, pp. 21–25, 2012.

[38] C.-A. Voltin, H. Goergen, C. Baues et al., "Value of bone marrow biopsy in hodgkin lymphoma patients staged by FDG PET: results from the german hodgkin study group trials HD16, HD17, and HD18," *Annals of Oncology*, vol. 29, no. 9, pp. 1926–1931, 2018.

[39] S. Ehl, I. Astigarraga, T. von Bahr Greenwood et al., "Recommendations for the use of etoposide-based therapy and bone marrow transplantation for the treatment of HLH: consensus statements by the HLH steering committee of the histiocyte society," *The Journal of Allergy and Clinical Immunology: In Practice*, vol. 6, no. 5, pp. 1508–1517, 2018.

Permissions

All chapters in this book were first published by Hindawi Publishing Corporation; hereby published with permission under the Creative Commons Attribution License or equivalent. Every chapter published in this book has been scrutinized by our experts. Their significance has been extensively debated. The topics covered herein carry significant findings which will fuel the growth of the discipline. They may even be implemented as practical applications or may be referred to as a beginning point for another development.

The contributors of this book come from diverse backgrounds, making this book a truly international effort. This book will bring forth new frontiers with its revolutionizing research information and detailed analysis of the nascent developments around the world.

We would like to thank all the contributing authors for lending their expertise to make the book truly unique. They have played a crucial role in the development of this book. Without their invaluable contributions this book wouldn't have been possible. They have made vital efforts to compile up to date information on the varied aspects of this subject to make this book a valuable addition to the collection of many professionals and students.

This book was conceptualized with the vision of imparting up-to-date information and advanced data in this field. To ensure the same, a matchless editorial board was set up. Every individual on the board went through rigorous rounds of assessment to prove their worth. After which they invested a large part of their time researching and compiling the most relevant data for our readers.

The editorial board has been involved in producing this book since its inception. They have spent rigorous hours researching and exploring the diverse topics which have resulted in the successful publishing of this book. They have passed on their knowledge of decades through this book. To expedite this challenging task, the publisher supported the team at every step. A small team of assistant editors was also appointed to further simplify the editing procedure and attain best results for the readers.

Apart from the editorial board, the designing team has also invested a significant amount of their time in understanding the subject and creating the most relevant covers. They scrutinized every image to scout for the most suitable representation of the subject and create an appropriate cover for the book.

The publishing team has been an ardent support to the editorial, designing and production team. Their endless efforts to recruit the best for this project, has resulted in the accomplishment of this book. They are a veteran in the field of academics and their pool of knowledge is as vast as their experience in printing. Their expertise and guidance has proved useful at every step. Their uncompromising quality standards have made this book an exceptional effort. Their encouragement from time to time has been an inspiration for everyone.

The publisher and the editorial board hope that this book will prove to be a valuable piece of knowledge for researchers, students, practitioners and scholars across the globe.

List of Contributors

Julian Verran and Vidya Mathavan
Department of Haematology, Waikato Hospital, 183 Pembroke Street, Hamilton 3204, New Zealand

M. S. Cruz, J. Santillan, J. Lesser, J. Ortiz, L. Forzani and P. Plaza
Fundación de la Hemofilia de Salta, Salta, Argentina

Marcela Osovská and Andrea Janíková
Department of Hematology and Oncology, University Hospital Brno, Faculty of Medicine, Masaryk University Brno, Brno, Czech Republic

Leoš Křen
Department of Pathology, University Hospital Brno, Faculty of Medicine, Masaryk University Brno, Brno, Czech Republic

Andrea Marečková
Department of Molecular Biology and Genetics, University Hospital Brno, Faculty of Medicine, Masaryk University Brno, Brno, Czech Republic

Madiha Iqbal, Prachi Jani, Salman Ahmed and Taimur Sher
Department of Hematology and Oncology, Mayo Clinic, Jacksonville, FL, USA

Yoshiki Uemura
Department of Hematology, Chikamori Hospital, 1-1-16, Okawasuzi, Kochi-shi, Kochi- ken 780-8522, Japan

Marina Komoto
Department of Cardiology, Chikamori Hospital, 1-1-16, Okawasuzi, Kochi-shi, Kochi- ken 780-8522, Japan

Mitsuo Okada
Department of Gastroenterology, Chikamori Hospital, 1-1-16, Okawasuzi, Kochi-shi, Kochi-ken 780-8522, Japan

Kunio Hayashi
Division of Hematology, Meiwa General Hospital, 4-31 Agenaruocho, Nishinomiya, Hyogo 663-8186, Japan

Kazuhiro Ikegame
Division of Hematology, Hyogo College of Medicine, Mukogawacho, Nishinomiya, Hyogo 663-8501, Japan

Naoto Takahashi
Department of Hematology Nephrology and Rheumatology, Akita University, 1-1 Hondo 1-Chome, Akita 010-8543, Japan

Yuki Kageyama
Department of Hematology, Yokkaichi Municipal Hospital, 2-2-37 Shibata, Yokkaichi 510-8567, Japan
Department of Hematology and Oncology, Mie University Graduate School of Medicine, 2-174 Edobashi, Tsu 514-8507, Japan

Kenshiro Tsuda
Department of Dermatology, Yokkaichi Municipal Hospital, 2-2-37 Shibata, Yokkaichi 510-8567, Japan

Yuma Nato
Department of Hematology, Yokkaichi Municipal Hospital, 2-2-37 Shibata, Yokkaichi 510-8567, Japan

Keiki Nagaharu
Department of Hematology and Oncology, Mie University Graduate School of Medicine, 2-174 Edobashi, Tsu 514-8507, Japan

Nicholas B. Burley, Paul S. Dy, Suraj Hande, Shreyas Kalantri and Chirayu Mohindroo
Department of Internal Medicine, Sinai Hospital of Baltimore, Baltimore, MD, USA

Kenneth Miller
Department of Hematology/Oncology, Sinai Hospital of Baltimore, Baltimore, MD, USA

S. Kartthik
Department of Haematology–Oncology, GKNM Hospital, Coimbatore, Tamilnadu, India

Prakas K. Mandal
Department of Haematology, NRS Medical College and Hospital, Kolkata, West Bengal, India

Saleh Mohammed Abdullah
Department of Medical Laboratory, Faculty of Applied Medical Sciences, Jazan University, Jazan, Saudi Arabia

Mert Erciyestepe
Istanbul University, Istanbul Medical Faculty, Department of Internal Medicine, Istanbul, Turkey

Tarık Onur Tiryaki, Meliha Nalçacı and İpek Yönal Hindilerden
Istanbul University, Istanbul Medical Faculty, Department of Internal Medicine, Division of Hematology, Istanbul, Turkey

Gülçin Yeğen
Istanbul University, Istanbul Medical Faculty, Department of Pathology, Istanbul, Turkey

John S. Wang, Omar Elghawy, Brett R. Kurpiel and Michael G. Douvas
School of Medicine, University of Virginia, Charlottesville, Virginia, USA

Heather Katz
Department of Hematology/Oncology, Donald and Barbara Zucker School of Medicine at Hofstra/Northwell, 500 Hofstra Blvd, Hempstead, NY 11549, USA

Mina Shenouda
Department of Hematology/Oncology, Joan C. Edwards School of Medicine, Marshall University, 1600 Medical Center Dr., Huntington, WV 25701, USA

Deena Dahshan
Joan C. Edwards School of Medicine, Marshall University, 1600 Medical Center Dr., Huntington, WV 25701, USA

George Sonnier
Department of Dermatology, University of Louisville School of Medicine, Louisville, KY 40203, USA

Yehuda Lebowicz
Department of Hematology/Oncology, UPMC Hillman Cancer Center, 1030 Beaver Hollow Rd., Beaver, PA 15009, USA

Matilda Ongóndi
Department of Internal Medicine; Hemato-oncology Unit, Kenyatta National Hospital, Nairobi, Kenya

Elizabeth Kagotho
Department of Pathology and Laboratory Medicine, Aga Khan University hospital, Nairobi, Kenya

Jiankun Tong and Sana Jadallah
Department of Pathology, New York–Presbyterian Queens, 56-45 Main Street, Flushing, NY 11355, USA

William H. Rodgers
Department of Pathology, New York–Presbyterian Queens, 56-45 Main Street, Flushing, NY 11355, USA
Weill Cornell Medical College, 525 East 68th Street, Box 130, New York, NY 10065, USA

Gabriel Jung, Malvina Fulman and Abhisek Swaika
Hematology & Medical Oncology, Queens Medical Associates, 176-60 Union Tpke # 360, Fresh Meadows, NY 11366, USA

Laura M. Stanko
Internal Medicine Program, University of Alabama at Birmingham, Birmingham, AL, USA

Vishnu Reddy
Division of Anatomic Pathology and Neuropathology, University of Alabama at Birmingham, Birmingham, AL, USA

Fady M. Mikhail
Department of Genetics, University of Alabama at Birmingham, Birmingham, AL, USA

Nikolaos Papadantonakis
Division of Hematology/Oncology, University of Alabama at Birmingham, Birmingham, AL, USA

Adelaide Moutinho, Rita Gamboa Cunha, Sheila Koch Jamal, Marta Meleiro Lisboa and Sandra Tavares
Department of Internal Medicine, Hospital de Chaves—Centro Hospitalar de Trás-os-Montes e Alto Douro, Vila Real, Portugal

Sarah Premji
Department of Medicine, Baylor College of Medicine, Houston 77030, TX, USA

Andreia Barbieri and Christine Roth
Department of Pathology and Immunology, Baylor College of Medicine, Baylor St. Luke's Medical Center, Houston 77030, TX, USA

Eric M. Rohren
Department of Radiology, Baylor College of Medicine, Houston 77030, TX, USA

Gustavo Rivero and Sravanti P Teegavarapu
Department of Medicine, Section of Hematology-Oncology, Baylor College of Medicine, Houston 77030, TX, USA
Dan L Duncan Comprehensive Cancer Center, Baylor College of Medicine, Houston, TX 77030, USA

J. J. Lipof, E. J. Huselton and C. S. Zent
Division of Hematology/Oncology, University of Rochester Medical Center, James P. Wilmot Cancer Institute, Rochester, NY, USA

A. Evans, B. Zhang and P. G. Rothberg
Department of Pathology and Laboratory Medicine, University of Rochester Medical Center, Rochester, NY, USA

J. M. Bennett
Division of Hematology/Oncology, University of Rochester Medical Center, James P. Wilmot Cancer Institute, Rochester, NY, USA
Department of Pathology and Laboratory Medicine, University of Rochester Medical Center, Rochester, NY, USA

Laura Alder
Department of Medicine, VCU Health, 1201 E Marshall St, Richmond, VA 23298, USA

Scott Graupner and Victor Yazbeck
Department of Hematology Oncology, Massey Cancer Center, VCU Health, 401 College St, Richmond, VA 23298, USA

Guanhua Lai
Department of Pathology, VCU Health, 1201 E Marshall St, Richmond, VA 23298, USA

Prarthna V. Bhardwaj
Resident, Department of Internal Medicine, Baystate Medical Center, Springfield, MA, USA

Shrinkhala Khanna
Assistant Professor, Department of Hematology/Oncology, UMass Medical Center, Worcester, MA, USA

Majd D. Jawad
Resident, Department of Pathology, Baystate Medical Center, Springfield, MA, USA

Syed S. Ali
Assistant Professor, Department of Hematology Oncology, Baystate Medical Center, Springfield, MA, USA

Ashish Bains
Department of Pathology and Laboratory Medicine, Lewis Katz School of Medicine at Temple University, Philadelphia, PA, USA

Pedro Covas
Department of Internal Medicine, George Washington University, Washington, DC, USA

Olga Timofeeva
Department of Pathology, Georgetown University Hospital, Washington, DC, USA

Michael Bromberg
Department of Internal Medicine, Section of Hematology, Lewis Katz School of Medicine at Temple University, Philadelphia, PA, USA

Bicky Thapa, Gulrayz Ahmed, Meera Mohan and Parameswaran Hari
Division of Hematology and Oncology, Department of Medicine, Medical College of Wisconsin, Milwaukee, WI, USA

Volodymyr Shponka
Division of Pathology and Laboratory Medicine, Department of Medicine, Medical College of Wisconsin, Milwaukee, WI, USA

Deborah Osafehinti and Kaveh Zivari
Department of Internal Medicine, Maimonides Medical Center, Brooklyn, NY, USA

Maris Bartkevics and Alexander Kadner
Center for Congenital Heart Disease, Department of Cardiovascular Surgery, Inselspital University Hospital, Bern University, Bern, Switzerland

Bert Hennig and Roland Ammann
Department of Pediatrics, University Children's Hospital, Bern University, Bern, Switzerland

Tayfun Gungor
Department of Stem Cell Transplantation, University Children's Hospital Zurich, University Zurich, Zürich, Switzerland

Anindita Ghosh and Joshua Baalwa
Departments of Pathology, Laboratory Medicine, McGovern Medical School, University of Texas Health Sciences Center at Houston, Houston, Texas, USA

Rodrick Chitaurirwa Zvavanjanja
Diagnostic and Interventional Imaging, McGovern Medical School, University of Texas Health Sciences Center at Houston, Houston, Texas, USA

Motoharu Shibusawa
IMS Group, Shinmatsudo Central General Hospital, Department of Hematology, Chiba, Japan

Kazuya Sato, Nodoka Tsukada and Junki Inamura
Department of Hematology/Oncology, Asahikawa Kosei General Hospital, 1-24, Asahikawa 078-8211, Japan

Shigetsuna Komatsu
Department of Dermatology, Asahikawa Kosei General Hospital, 1-24, Asahikawa 078-8211, Japan

Keisuke Sato
Department of Clinical Laboratory, Asahikawa Kosei General Hospital, 1-24, Asahikawa 078-8211, Japan

Masayo Yamamoto, Motohiro Shindo, Kentaro Moriichi, Yusuke Mizukami, Mikihiro Fujiya, Yoshihiro Torimoto and Toshikatsu Okumura
Division of Gastroenterology and Hematology/Oncology, Department of Medicine, Asahikawa Medical University, Asahikawa, Hokkaido, Japan

Michela Staderini, Valentina Carrai, Alberto Bosi, Elisabetta Antonioli and Benedetta Puccini
Haematology Unit, Careggi University Hospital, Florence, Italy

Lara Mannelli
Medical Genetics, University of Siena, Siena, Italy

Valentina Berti
Nuclear Medicine Unit, Department of Biomedical, Experimental and Clinical Sciences, Careggi University Hospital, Florence, Italy

Francesco Mungai
Diagnostic Radiology Unit, Careggi University Hospital, Florence, Italy

Federica Vergoni
Pathological Anatomy Unit, Careggi University Hospital, Florence, Italy

Luigi Rigacci
Haematology Unit, Careggi University Hospital, Florence, Italy
Hematology and Stem Cell Transplant Unit, San Camillo Forlanini Hospital, Rome, Italy

Di Wu, Wenlan Chen, Zhichao Chen and Qiubai Li
Institute of Hematology, Union Hospital, Tongji Medical College, Huazhong University of Science and Technology, Wuhan 430022, Hubei, China

Zoe L. Lyski and David Xthona Lee
Department of Molecular Microbiology & Immunology, Oregon Health & Science University (OHSU), Portland, OR 97239, USA

David Sampson, Vikram Raghunathan, Debbie Ryan, Stephen E. Spurgeon and Myung Sun Kim
Knight Cancer Institute, Oregon Health & Science University (OHSU), Portland, OR 97239, USA

Hans-Peter Raué and Mark K. Slifka
Division of Neuroscience, Oregon National Primate Research Center, Oregon Health & Science University, Beaverton, OR 97239, USA

Amanda E. Brunton
OHSU-PSU School of Public Health, Portland, OR 97239, USA

William B. Messer
Department of Molecular Microbiology & Immunology, Oregon Health & Science University (OHSU), Portland, OR 97239, USA
Division of Neuroscience, Oregon National Primate Research Center, Oregon Health & Science University, Beaverton, OR 97239, USA
Department of Medicine, Division of Infectious Diseases, Oregon Health & Science University (OHSU), Portland, OR 97239, USA

Johanne Marie Holst and Marie Beck Enemark
Department of Hematology, Aarhus University Hospital, Palle Juul-Jensens Boulevard 35, Aarhus N 8200, Denmark
Department of Clinical Medicine, Aarhus University, Palle Juul-Jensens Boulevard 82, Aarhus N 8200, Denmark

Trine Lindhardt Plesner
Department of Pathology, Copenhagen University Hospital, Blegdamsvej 3B, København N 2200, Denmark

Martin Bjerregaard Pedersen
Department of Hematology, Aarhus University Hospital, Palle Juul-Jensens Boulevard 35, Aarhus N 8200, Denmark

Maja Ludvigsen and Francesco d'Amore
Department of Hematology, Aarhus University Hospital, Palle Juul-Jensens Boulevard 35, Aarhus N 8200, Denmark
Department of Clinical Medicine, Aarhus University, Palle Juul-Jensens Boulevard 82, Aarhus N 8200, Denmark

Lucas Oliveira Cantadori, Rafael Dezen Gaiolla and Ligia Niero-Melo
São Paulo State University (UNESP), Medical School of Botucatu, Department of Internal Medicine, Botucatu, SP, Brazil

Cristiano Claudino Oliveira
São Paulo State University (UNESP), Medical School of Botucatu, Department of Pathology, Botucatu, SP, Brazil
São Luiz/D'or Hospital, Department of Pathology, São Paulo, SP, Brazil

Adam Khorasanchi, Zachary Benson, Patrick Willard and John McKay
Department of Internal Medicine, Virginia Commonwealth University, Richmond, VA, USA

Misty Hall
Department of Pathology, Virginia Commonwealth University, Richmond, VA, USA

Nelya Ebadirad and Mohammad H. Gharavi
Department of Radiology, Virginia Commonwealth University, Richmond, VA, USA

Miranda Chimzar
School of Medicine, Virginia Commonwealth University, Richmond, VA, USA

Gary Simmons and Victor Yazbeck
Massey Cancer Center, Virginia Commonwealth University, Richmond, VA, USA

Osama N. Dukmak, Hamzeh M. I. Abugharbieh, Salem M. Tos and Iman Khamayseh
Al-Quds University, Faculty of Medicine, Jerusalem, State of Palestine

Mohammad Farid Emar and Rafiq Salhab
Al-Ahli Hospital, Hebron, State of Palestine

Abdul Moiz Khan and Ibrahim Azar
Department of Internal Medicine, Albany Medical College, Albany, NY, USA

Saleh Najjar
Department of Pathology, Albany Medical College, Albany, NY, USA

Travis Bevington
Department of Radiology, Albany Medical College, Albany, NY, USA

Syed Mehdi
Section of Hematology/Oncology, Stratton VA Medical Center, Albany, NY, USA

Christopher G. Burkeen, David Pottinger, Chaitanya Iragavarapu, Reshma Ramlal and Gerhard Hildebrandt
University of Kentucky Markey Cancer Center, 800 Rose Street, Lexington, KY 40536, USA

Rehman Faryal and Amjad Hayat
Haematology Department, University Hospital Galway, Galway, Ireland

Karen Nalbandyan, Daniel Benharroch and Benzion Samueli
Department of Pathology, Soroka University Medical Center, Faculty of Health Sciences, Ben-Gurion University of the Negev, Beer-Sheva, Israel

Michael Kafka
Division of Hematology, Hematology Laboratory, Soroka University Medical Center, Faculty of Health Sciences, Ben Gurion University of the Negev, Beer-Sheva, Israel

Anna Gourevitch
Division of Hematology, Soroka University Medical Center, Faculty of Health Sciences, Ben-Gurion University of the Negev, Beer-Sheva, Israel

Abdul Moiz Khan, Zainub Ajmal and Fatima Tuz Zahra
Department of Internal Medicine, Albany Medical Center, Albany, NY, USA

Ananthakrishnan Ramani
Department of Infectious Diseases, Albany Medical Center, Albany, NY, USA

Ira Zackon
New York Oncology Hematology, Albany Medical Center, Albany, NY, USA

Mbarek Yaka
Department of Surgery, Military University Hospital Med V, University Hassan II of Casablanca, Casablanca, Morocco

Farid Chehab
Department of Surgery, Ibn Rochd University Hospital, University Hassan II of Casablanca, Casablanca, Morocco

Mohmed Allaoui
Department of Pathology, Military University Hospital Med V, Rabat, Morocco

Abdelmonaim Ait Ali and Aziz Zentar
Department of Surgery, Military University Hospital Med V, Rabat, Morocco

Ulkuhan I. Koksal, Janeiro Valle Goffin, Brian Lewis, Oliver A. Sartor, Elizaveta Belyaeva, Francisco Socola and Pedro C. Barata
Tulane Cancer Center, School of Medicine, Tulane University, New Orleans, LA, USA

Maria Eduarda Couto, Nelson Domingues, Isabel Oliveira and Mário Mariz
Onco-hematology Department, Instituto Portugu^es de Oncologia Do Porto F.G. E.P.E., Porto, Portugal

Susana Bizarro
Genetics Department, Instituto Português de Oncologia Do Porto F.G. E.P.E., Porto, Portugal

Domingos Sousa
Internal Medicine Department, Centro Hospitalar e Universitário Do Algarve E.P.E., Porto, Portugal

Gabriela Martins
Immunology Department, Instituto Português de Oncologia Do Porto F.G. E.P.E., Porto, Portugal

Manuel R. Teixeira
Genetics Department, Instituto Portugu^es de Oncologia Do Porto F.G. E.P.E., Porto, Portugal
Biomedical Sciences Institute, University of Porto, Porto, Portugal

Carolina Afonso, Adriana Roque, Cátia Almeida, Catarina Geraldes and Marília Gomes
Hematology Unit, Hospitais da Universidade de Coimbra, Centro Hospitalar e Universit´ario de Coimbra, Coimbra, Portugal

Maria Beatriz Pimentão and Maria José Julião
Pathology Unit, Hospitais da Universidade de Coimbra, Centro Hospitalar e Universit´ario de Coimbra, Coimbra, Portugal

Rodolfo Silva
Nuclear Medicine Unit, Hospitais da Universidade de Coimbra, Centro Hospitalar e Universit´ario de Coimbra, Coimbra, Portugal

Oluomachi Charity Nnachi, Innocent Paul Ezenwenyi, Augustine Ejike Okoye, Chinedu Obasi Akpa and Gabriel Chima Ugwu
Department of Haematology, Alex Ekwueme Federal University Teaching Hospital, Abakaliki, Ebonyi, Nigeria

Chukwuma Joseph Uzoigwe
Department of Histopathology, Alex Ekwueme Federal University Teaching Hospital, Abakaliki, Ebonyi, Nigeria

Chimezie Mbachi, Estefania Flores and Benjamin Mba
Internal Medicine, John H. Stroger Jr. Hospital of Cook County, Chicago, IL 60612, USA

Rita Igwilo and Ezekiel Chukwujindu
Internal Medicine, University of Nigeria Teaching Hospital, Ituku-Ozalla, Enugu, Nigeria

Oluwadunni E. Emiloju
Department of Medicine, Einstein Medical Center, Philadelphia, PA 19141, USA

Sorab Gupta and Claudia Dourado
Department of Hematology and Medical Oncology, Einstein Medical Center, Philadelphia, PA 19141, USA

Vivian Arguello-Guerra
Department of Pathology and Laboratory Medicine, Einstein Medical Center, Philadelphia, PA 19141, USA

Justin Komisarof and Joseph DiTursi
Department of Medicine, University of Rochester Medical Center, 601 Elmwood Avenue, Rochester, NY 14642, USA

Jodi Lipof and Frank Passero
Department of Hematology and Oncology, Wilmot Cancer Institute, 601 Elmwood Avenue, Rochester, NY 14642, USA

Amit Chowdhry and Louis Constine
Department of Radiation Oncology, Wilmot Cancer Institute, 601 Elmwood Avenue, Rochester, NY 14642, USA

Hae Yoon Grace Choung and W. Richard Burack
Department of Pathology and Laboratory Medicine, University of Rochester Medical Center, 601 Elmwood Avenue, Rochester, NY 14642, USA

Christos Fokoloros, Alexandros Katoulis and Michael Makris
Allergy Unit "D. Kalogeromitros", 2nd Department of Dermatology and Venereology, Medical School, National and Kapodistrian University of Athens, Attikon University Hospital, Athens, Greece

Periklis Foukas and Zoi Tsakiraki
2nd Department of Pathology, Medical School, National and Kapodistrian University of Athens, Attikon University Hospital, Athens, Greece

Nikolaos Georgakopoulos and Sotirios Papageorgiou
Department of Cytogenetics and Molecular Pathology, Locus Medicus S.A., Athens, Greece

Anthi Bouchla and Vasilliki Pappa
Hematology Unit, 2nd Department of Internal Medicine, Propaedeutic, Medical School, National and Kapodistrian University of Athens, Attikon University Hospital, Athens, Greece

Justin Komisarof, Kevin McGann and Alissa Huston
Department of Medicine, University of Rochester Medical Center, 601 Elmwood Avenue Box MED, Rochester, NY 14642, USA

Hani Katerji and Mary Anne Morgan
Department of Pathology and Laboratory Medicine, University of Rochester Medical Center, 601 Elmwood Avenue Box 626, Rochester, NY 14642, USA

Index

www.ingramcontent.com/pod-product-compliance
Lightning Source LLC
LaVergne TN
LVHW082123200926
848484LV00008B/2001